Congratulations for winning
the 2018 Top Gun
Competition. at UF Urology!

Atlas of Robotic Urologic Surgery

Li-Ming Su

Editor

Atlas of Robotic
Urologic Surgery

Second Edition

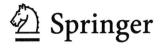

Editor
Li-Ming Su, M.D.
Department of Urology
University of Florida College of Medicine
Gainesville, FL, USA

Videos can also be accessed at http://link.springer.com/book/10.1007/978-3-319-45060-5

ISBN 978-3-319-45058-2   ISBN 978-3-319-45060-5   (eBook)
DOI 10.1007/978-3-319-45060-5

Library of Congress Control Number: 2017932443

Printed on acid-free paper

This Springer imprint is published by Springer Nature
The registered company is Springer International Publishing AG
The registered company address is: Gewerbestrasse 11, 6330 Cham, Switzerland

I would like to dedicate this book to my parents, Stanley and Phek Su, whose continued love, support, and sage advice have endured throughout my life and career. I also want to thank my immediate family, Maria and Sean as well as Cooper and Reilly for making me laugh and smile on a daily basis.

Li-Ming Su, M.D.

Preface

The introduction of robotic surgery to the field of urology has had a dramatic impact on practice patterns worldwide. Few events have had as significant an impact on the field of urology even greater than the introduction of shock wave lithotripsy, lasers, percutaneous surgery, and laparoscopy. Despite the widespread adoption of robotics into urologic practice, robotic urologic procedures remain technically complex and the skill sets required to perform robotic surgery differ significantly from that of traditional open surgery. Unlike open surgery where tactile feedback is frequently used as an intraoperative tool to provide the surgeon with critical information, during robotic surgery, the surgeon is immersed in an environment absent of haptic feedback where operative decisions are made based instead on subtleties and nuances provided primarily by visual cues. Visual cues such as vascularity, organ movement, tissue distortion, and adherence offer different and unique insights into the nature and behavior of organs and their interaction with surrounding structures such as blood vessels, fat, nerves, and muscles. As a result, surgeons are required to think and interpret surgical dissection in a way that is unique and different from their training in open surgery.

Since the introduction of robotic prostatectomy, there has been continued enthusiasm and expansion of robotic surgery in other areas of urologic surgery. The largest growth has been in the area of oncologic procedures with rapid adoption of robotic partial nephrectomy and radical cystectomy. In addition, robotic reconstructive and pediatric procedures continue to expand. As a result, the second edition of the Atlas of Robotic Urologic Surgery was compiled to address the continued expansion of robotics in the field of urologic surgery. As with the first edition of the Atlas, a detailed, step-by-step description of all currently performed robotic urologic procedures is provided by internationally recognized experts in the field. Each chapter is highly illustrated by the same artist to provide uniformity and standardization. Each procedural chapter is complemented by figures and intraoperative photographs, detailing the nuances of each technique. Emphasis is placed on operative setup, instrument and equipment needs, and surgical techniques for both the primary surgeon and the operative assistant. As such, this comprehensive surgical atlas provides educational value to both novice and advanced robotic surgeons as well as the operative assistant. My hope is that this atlas will provide unique insights into robotic urologic surgery and reduce the challenging learning curve of accomplishing these increasingly popular procedures.

Gainesville, FL, USA   Li-Ming Su, M.D.

Contents

Contributors

Editor

Li-Ming Su, M.D. Department of Urology, University of Florida College of Medicine, Gainesville, FL, USA

Authors

Ronney Abaza, M.D., F.A.C.S. Department of Robotic Surgery, Ohio Health Dublin Methodist Hospital, Dublin, OH, USA

Haidar M. Abdul-Muhsin, M.B., Ch.B. Department of Urology, Mayo Clinic Hospital, Phoenix, AZ, USA

Monish Aron, M.D. Catherine & Joseph Aresty Department of Urology, USC Institute of Urology, Keck School of Medicine, University of Southern California, Los Angeles, CA, USA

Kenan Ashouri, M.S. Department of Urology, Bethesda Hospital, Boynton Beach, FL, USA

Ravi Barod, M.B.B.S., Ph.D., F.R.C.S. (Urol) Vattikuti Urology Institute, Henry Ford Hospital, Detroit, MI, USA

Sam B. Bhayani, M.D., M.S. Department of Surgery and Urology, St. Louis, MO, USA

Alfredo Maria Bove, M.D. Catherine & Joseph Aresty Department of Urology, Keck School of Medicine, University of Southern California, Los Angeles, CA, USA

Jamin V. Brahmbhatt, M.D. Department of Urology, The PUR Clinic, South Lake Hospital, Orlando Health, Clermont, FL, USA

Peter Y. Cai, M.D. Department of Urology, University of Florida College of Medicine, Gainesville, FL, USA

Erik P. Castle, M.D., F.A.C.S. Department of Urology, Mayo Clinic Hospital, Phoenix, AZ, USA

Sameer Chopra, M.S., M.D. Catherine & Joseph Aresty Department of Urology, Keck School of Medicine, University of Southern California, Los Angeles, CA, USA

George K. Chow, M.D. Department of Urology, Mayo Clinic, Rochester, MN, USA

Justin Dersch, M.D. Department of Urology, University of Florida College of Medicine, Gainesville, FL, USA

Daniel S. Elliott, M.D. Department of Urology, Mayo Clinic, Rochester, MN, USA

Matthew T. Gettman, M.D. Department of Urology, Mayo Clinic, Rochester, MN, USA

Inderbir S. Gill, M.D., M.Ch. Catherine & Joseph Aresty Department of Urology, Keck School of Medicine, University of Southern California, Los Angeles, CA, USA

Christopher Giordano, M.D. Department of Anesthesiology, University of Florida College of Medicine, Gainesville, FL, USA

David M. Golombos, M.D. Department of Urology, New York Presbyterian Hospital—Weill Cornell Medical College, New York, NY, USA

Nikolaus Gravenstein, M.D. Department of Anesthesiology, University of Florida College of Medicine, Gainesville, FL, USA

Hariharan Palayapalayam Ganapathi, M.D. Global Robotic Institute, Florida Hospital, Celebration, FL, USA

Ashok K. Hemal, M.D. Department of Urology, Wake Forest Baptist Health, Winston-Salem, NC, USA

S. Duke Herrell, M.D. Department of Urologic Surgery, Vanderbilt University Medical Center, Nashville, TN, USA

David Horovitz, M.D., F.R.C.S.C. Department of Urology, Strong Memorial Hospital, University of Rochester Medical Center, Rochester, MN, USA

Micah Jacobs, M.D., M.P.H. Department of Urology, Children's Medical Center, University of Texas Southwestern, Dallas, TX, USA

Isuru S. Jayaratnam, M.D. Department of Urology, UT MD Anderson Cancer Center, Houston, TX, USA

Jason Joseph, M.D. Department of Urology, University of Florida College of Medicine, Gainesville, FL, USA

Jean V. Joseph, M.D. Department of Urology, Strong Memorial Hospital, University of Rochester Medical Center, Rochester, NY, USA

Christopher J. Kane, M.D. Department of Urology, University of California San Diego Health System, San Diego, CA, USA

Jihad H. Kaouk, M.D. Glickman Institute of Urology and Nephrology, Cleveland Clinic, Cleveland, OH, USA

Steven V. Kheyfets, M.D. Department of Urology, Indiana University School of Medicine, Indianapolis, IN, USA

Tony Kim, M.D. Baylor St. Luke's Medical Center, Houston, TX, USA

John J. Knoedler, M.D. Department of Urology, Mayo Clinic, Rochester, MD, USA

Jennifer Kuo, M.D. Department of Urology, University of Florida College of Medicine, Gainesville, FL, USA

Weil R. Lai, M.D. Department of Urology, Tulane University School of Medicine, New Orleans, LA, USA

Jessica N. Lange, M.D. Department of Urology, Wake Forest Baptist Health, Winston-Salem, NC, USA

Huong Thi Thu Le, M.D. Department of Anesthesiology, University of Florida College of Medicine, Gainesville, FL, USA

Davi I. Lee, M.D. Department of Surgery/Urology, University of Pennsylvania, Philadelphia, PA, USA

J. Joy Lee, M.D. Department of Urology, Swedish Medical Center, Seattle, WA, USA

Raymond J. Leveillee, M.D., F.R.C.S.-G. Department of Urology, Florida Atlantic University, Bethesda Hospital, Boynton Beach, FL, USA

Richard E. Link, M.D., Ph.D. Division of Endourology and Minimally Invasive Surgery, Scott Department of Urology, Baylor College of Medicine, Houston, TX, USA

Matthew Lux, M.D. Department of Urology, Kaiser Permanente Medical Center, San Diego, CA, USA

James Mason, M.D. Department of Urology, University of Florida College of Medicine, Gainesville, FL, USA

Surena F. Matin, M.D., F.A.C.S. Department of Urology, UT MD Anderson Cancer Center, Houston, TX, USA

Mani Menon, M.D. Department of Urology, Vattikuti Urology Institute, Henry Ford Health System, Detroit, MI, USA

Pascal Mouracade Glickman Institute of Urology and Nephrology, Cleveland Clinic, Cleveland, OH, USA

Vladimir Mouraviev, M.D., Ph.D. Global Robotic Institute, Florida Hospital, Celebration, FL, USA

Gabriel Ogaya-Pinies, M.D. Global Robotic Institute, Florida Hospital, Celebration, FL, USA

Padraic O'Malley, M.D. Department of Urology, New York Presbyterian Hospital—Weill Cornell Medical College, New York, NY, USA

Brandon J. Otto, M.D. Department of Urology, University of Florida College of Medicine, Gainesville, FL, USA

Sijo J. Parekattil, M.D. Department of Urology, The PUR Clinic, South Lake Hospital, Orlando Health, Clermont, FL, USA

Nishant D. Patel, M.D. Department of Urology, Cleveland Clinic Foundation, Cleveland, OH, USA

Vipul R. Patel, M.D., F.A.C.S. Global Robotic Institute, Florida Hospital, Celebration, FL, USA

Craig A. Peters, M.D. Pediatric Urology, Children's Medical Center, University of Texas Southwestern, Dallas, TX, USA

Curtis A. Pettaway, M.D. Department of Urology, UT MD Anderson Cancer Center, Houston, TX, USA

Steven P. Petrou, MD Department of Urology, Mayo Clinic, Jacksonville, FL, USA

James R. Porter, M.D. Department of Urology, Swedish Medical Center, Seattle, WA, USA

Daniel Ramirez, M.D. Glickman Institute of Urology and Nephrology, Cleveland Clinic, Cleveland, OH, USA

Randee Regan, B.S.N., R.N., C.N.O.R. Surgical Services Administration, Houston Methodist Hospital, Houston, TX, USA

Craig G. Rogers, M.D. Vattikuti Urology Institute, Henry Ford Hospital, Detroit, MI, USA

Douglas S. Scherr, M.D. Department of Urology, New York Presbyterian Hospital—Weill Cornell Medical College, New York, NY, USA

Carlos Eduardo Schio Fay, M.D. Catherine & Joseph Aresty Department of Urology, USC Institute of Urology, Keck School of Medicine, University of Southern California, Los Angeles, CA, USA

Bruce J. Schlomer, M.D. Pediatric Urology, Children's Medical Center, University of Texas Southwestern, Dallas, TX, USA

Eric A. Schommer, M.D. Department of Urology, Mayo Clinic Florida, Jacksonville, FL, USA

John M. Shields Department of Urology, University of Florida College of Medicine, Gainesville, FL, USA

Mark S. Shimko, M.D. Department of Urology, Mayo Clinic, Rochester, MN, USA

Michael Stifelman, M.D. Department of Urology, Hackensack University Medical Center, Hackensack, NJ, USA

Chandru P. Sundaram, M.D. Department of Urology, Indiana University School of Medicine, Indianapolis, IN, USA

David D. Thiel, M.D. Department of Urology, Mayo Clinic Florida, Jacksonville, FL, USA

Raju Thomas, M.D., F.A.C.S., M.H.A. Department of Urology, Tulane University School of Medicine, New Orleans, LA, USA

Friedrich-Carl von Rundstedt, M.D. Department of Urology, Friedrich-Schiller University, Jen, Germany

Gerald J. Wang, M.D. Department of Urology, New York Presbyterian Queens, Flushing, NY, USA

Mary E. Westerman, M.D. Department of Urology, Mayo Clinic, Rochester, MN, USA

Yuka Yamaguchi, M.D. Department of Urology, Highland Hospital, Oakland, CA, USA

Lawrence L. Yeung, M.D. Department of Urology, University of Florida College of Medicine, Gainesville, FL, USA

Lee C. Zhao, M.D., M.S. Department of Urology, NYU Langone Medical Center, NYU Urology Associates, New York, NY, USA

Matthew J. Ziegelmann, M.D. Department of Urology, Mayo Clinic, Rochester, MN, USA

Part I

Getting Started in Robotic Surgery

Establishing a Robotics Team and Practice

Friedrich-Carl von Rundstedt, Randee Regan,
Tony Kim, and Richard E. Link

The successful formation of a highly functional team depends on three core principles: (a) clearly define the goals to be accomplished, (b) select capable individuals invested in accomplishing these goals, and (c) assign clear responsibilities to each member of the team. Modern team building does not require a rigid hierarchical structure but rather strives to implement a high degree of autonomy for each operating element. Here, we outline a framework for establishing a robotic surgical practice that may streamline this process and allow new practitioners to avoid pitfalls that may inhibit progress.

F.-C. von Rundstedt, M.D.
Department of Urology, Friedrich-Schiller University,
Jen, Germany

R. Regan, B.S.N., R.N., C.N.O.R.
Surgical Services Administration, Houston Methodist
Hospital, Houston, TX, USA

T. Kim, M.D.
Baylor St. Luke's Medical Center,
Houston, TX, USA

R.E. Link, M.D., Ph.D. (✉)
Division of Endourology and Minimally Invasive
Surgery, Scott Department of Urology, Baylor
College of Medicine, 7200 Cambridge St.,
Houston, TX 77030, USA
e-mail: link@bcm.edu

Market Analysis

Before committing to development of a robotic program, it is imperative to understand the regional environment within which this program will function. Robotic surgery entails very substantial capital and consumable costs that will impact feasibility and put financial pressure on program success. A market analysis focusing on the healthcare competition and available patient population should be completed prior to moving forward with purchasing robotic hardware [1]. If the surrounding competition is fierce and the patient referral base is questionable, then a large expenditure to build a robotics program may be hard to justify. At the very least, these challenges should be clearly outlined and the timeline transparent to all parties with a stake in program success (including hospital administrators who approve millions of dollars in expenditures for robotic hardware). In some cases, a robotics program may yield benefits to the institution that far outweigh financial concerns including establishing a local reputation for innovation and advancing a training mission [2].

The Surgeon(s)

There is significant potential benefit to building a robotics program around one or more experienced robotic surgeons rather than solely around individuals who have just completed training and are still mastering these procedures. A wealth of literature supports improvement in outcomes and efficiency as surgeons ascend the robotics learning curve [3–5], factors that are particularly critical during the early days of a new program. Moreover, operative time (along with case volume) is a major factor determining the cost-effectiveness of robotic surgery [6, 7].

Robot Coordinator

When first starting out, it is advantageous for the institution to identify a Robotic Coordinator who serves as the coordinating liaison between Intuitive Surgical Inc. (Sunnyvale, CA), the manufacturer of the da Vinci® Surgical System, and the hospital robotics team. Intuitive Surgical offers a 1-week course for liaison staff that comprehensively addresses all aspects of coordinating a robotic surgical program. The robotic coordinator should ideally be recruited from within the operating room (OR) staff and be familiar with daily operations within the OR. In our experience, there is great value in selecting an OR technician or nurse from the Urology Service for the position of coordinator, if the bulk of the early caseload will be urologic cases. These specific individuals already have a detailed understanding of the specific challenges involved in urological procedures and may be able to anticipate potential problems as these cases are transitioned to robotic-assisted laparoscopic approaches.

The primary responsibility of the coordinator is to ensure the operational status of the da Vinci® robotic hardware and to proactively recognize problems with the unit that may require repair. This includes generalized maintenance planning as well as coordinating any necessary robot service. The Readiness Guide by Intuitive Surgical is a comprehensive user manual that may be valuable during the initial phase of setting up a team. The robotic coordinator also has a primary role in assuring that the necessary consumables (such as drapes and robotic instruments) are available prior to cases and that a functional system is in place to assure appropriate restocking.

The Robotic Coordinator is the go-to person responsible for assuring that all elements of the program interact together productively. It is important to have an easily identifiable individual who is ultimately responsible for the day-to-day activities of the robotic program. This individual takes a lead role in addressing concerns from all team members and eliminating roadblocks that threaten efficiency and patient safety.

Staffing

No matter the anticipated surgical volume, it is highly advantageous to organize a dedicated OR team to staff all robotic cases. Ideally, these are volunteers who have expressed a specific interest in robotic surgery and wish to establish specialized expertise in this area within the OR. As the caseload increases, the robotic team should expand to allow coverage of robotic cases by team members under all circumstances. Nurses and OR technicians who were early team members can play a critical role in training new personnel to expand the team.

Basic training offered by Intuitive Surgical includes a da Vinci® system component and room setup overview, system connection orientation, and an introduction to the patient cart and control console. The training also incorporates important practical aspects of arm draping, lens calibration, and sterilization procedures. The goal of this process is to familiarize the participant with all relevant technical details of the da Vinci® robotic unit.

As a general rule, we have found value in the OR team being acquainted with the subspecialty of surgery and understanding the critical aspects of each type of procedure. In setting up a team for urologic robotic surgery, it is advantageous to pick personnel with previous urologic experience. Robotic procedures in resident training are usually broken down into step-by-step modules. It is critical that the entire team is made familiar with these steps and how the addition of robotics may alter them. In more complex cases, it may be helpful to provide written flow sheets to allow preparation before the procedure.

Following the standard time out prior to incision, the surgeon should verbally rehearse the sequence of steps and identify specific events that may be unfamiliar to new scrub technicians and circulators without extensive robotic experience. The surgical team should ideally predetermine standardized instrument setup, lens settings, robotic arm selection, and consumables such as sutures, staplers, or sealing devices. Taking time before the case to review the instruments available will help to avoid delays during the procedure. Robotics adds a level of instrumentation complexity on top of an already intricate procedure. The more the surgeon can anticipate procedure trouble spots in advance and communicate these to the team, the more chaos and frustration can be avoided.

Finally, it is important to have a discussion with the operating room staff concerning an action plan in the event of conversion to standard laparoscopic or open surgery in response to an urgent problem. What other equipment (self-retaining retractors, open surgical instruments, standard laparoscopic towers, a handport, etc.) might be needed to convert to open or standard laparoscopic surgery and is this equipment easily accessible? What sequences of events are required for rapid undocking of the robot and stowing of the equipment out of the way efficiently? In the case of poorly controlled hemorrhage, a one-ton robot attached to the patient can be a formidable barrier to safe open conversion unless all team members have anticipated that eventuality in advance and know their roles. Some of these factors will also be influenced greatly by the available space in the room assigned for robotic cases.

Anesthesia

Robotic surgery is essentially robotic-assisted laparoscopic surgery, and the same anesthetic considerations apply [8]. When putting together a primary anesthesia team, it would certainly be advantageous to select an anesthesiologist and a nurse anesthetist with previous laparoscopic experience. This may simply result in a higher comfort level when dealing with the physiologic challenges associated with positioning and abdominal insufflation. In robotic surgery, special attention is placed on patient positioning since repositioning is particularly difficult after the docking of the robotic unit. It is also critical for the anesthesia team to help monitor patient position throughout the case. Shifting of the patient after robotic docking may not be evident to the surgeon at the console or even to the bedside assistant due to extensive draping and heavy equipment cantilevered over the operating table. Patient positioning concerns include padding of all pressure points, securing the patient from sliding on the operating room table, preventing accidental injury from the movement of robotic arms, and optimizing positioning of IV lines and monitoring cables. In particular, obese and morbidly obese patient may present additional challenges for positioning. This patient population warrants additional time in properly positioning and safeguarding the patient from perioperative injury. Urologic robotic surgery often requires patients to be placed into extreme Trendelenburg or lateral flank positions and patients may shift during the procedure if not adequately fixed in place. The anesthesia team has a unique perspective of the patient under the drapes and should be on the lookout for shifting in position that might result in patient injury. During urologic robotic procedures, the anesthesia team is often located at the head of the patient but may not have ready access to the patient due to equipment and space constraints. All intravenous lines as well as monitors such as the blood pressure cuff and pulse-oximeter should be double checked as functional before the patient is surgically draped.

While performing robotic procedures, the surgeon at the console has excellent visibility of the instruments within the field of view. However, due to the very limited tactile feedback provided by the current da Vinci® robotic systems, the surgeon may not have a good sense of the location of the robotic arms outside the patient. It is critically important to assure that these arms do not have the potential to injure the patient during normal motion or inadvertently dislodge the endotracheal tube or vascular lines. While the surgeon and bedside assistant may be distracted, the anesthesia team can play a very important role in monitoring the positions of these external arms and their relation to the patient and anesthesia equipment. An atmosphere of easy and frequent communication between the surgical and anesthesia teams during robotic surgery about any concerns should be encouraged.

In all of these situations, the whole operative team (including the anesthesia team) should be cognizant of the need to abort the robotic procedure, especially in the case of an emergency. Clear and proactive communication between the surgeon, the OR staff, and the anesthesia team is even more important in robotic cases during which bulky equipment may block line of sight between team members. The team should be familiar with the emergent undocking procedure and strive to avoid any obstacles behind the robot cart that could impede rapid undocking of the robot if required. It is imperative that the team assigns a role to everyone present in the room as to what to do in such an emergency situation including how to quickly access a laparotomy set with vascular instruments. While no special setup is required for the anesthesia bay, consideration for the ability of the anesthesia team to access the patient should be considered. For example, a large volume of equipment may need to be repositioned rapidly should chest compressions be required in an emergency.

Performance Improvement

After the initial groundwork is laid to start a robotic surgical program, a process should be implemented to optimize workflow and improve outcomes. We have had an excellent experience with instituting a regular cadence of meetings in which all personnel including nurses, techs, surgeons, anesthesiologists, nurse anesthetists, and preoperative screening staff have been able to contribute their thoughts and perspectives. A monthly meeting can address any current challenges such as the introduction of new equipment or logistical problems with supplies. Any quality initiative that is launched for the robotics program should be discussed within this context.

Important examples are the identification of high-risk patients, patient optimization, standardized preoperative procedures as well as postoperative pathways, family preparation, and family communication during cases.

Stationary vs. Mobile Setup

The storage location of the robot may be an underappreciated issue in planning a smooth operative experience during initial program development. If the hospital has distinct operating suites and the robot needs to be divided up amongst different surgical disciplines, it may be necessary to move the robot between facilities. With only one da Vinci® robotic unit utilized by different services, the workflow can be improved by creating a mobile rather than a stationary setup. The robot coordinator is generally in charge of moving the robot and confirming the setup required for each procedure. This includes details such as the parking location of the robot and the appropriate placement of the console so no major changes have to be made once the patient enters the room. The goal is to have the robot operate in the setting where all equipment potentially needed for the case are within reach and all personnel are appropriately trained and experienced to assist effectively.

Storage Management

Robotic surgery requires an intelligent storage management and restocking plan for surgical instruments and accessory material. Robotic consumables are expensive and can be fragile if mishandled by inexperienced personnel. To keep costs down, we tend to limit the number of robotic instruments stocked and utilize an onsite sterilization unit that allows fast sterilization within 30 min. This prevents the need to stockpile multiple costly instrument replacements. This will not be feasible for every institution but as a general consideration all instruments need to be available at least in duplicate sets. Every OR tech and circulating nurse involved should know all items of equipment and their exact location in the storage room. There are circumstances during robotic surgery when an instrument fails and a replacement must be rapidly introduced into the case during critical portions of the surgery. Precise labeling and consistency in organizing the storage room keeps the procedure moving forward and protects patient safety.

OR Room Setup

The single most important consideration when planning the OR setup is the actual size of the room. Does the room have enough space to store all the equipment potentially needed in a given case? The list of equipment may be long (including video tower, video recording device, robot cart, surgeon console, insufflation device, and ultrasound cart) so a larger room should be designated for robotic cases if feasible. A primary goal is to minimize the need for equipment shuffling around the patient within a constrained space during surgery.

Hospital Support: Troubleshooting

For any problems with the system connection or vision system dedicated flow charts should be used at first to troubleshoot the da Vinci® unit. During every case, Intuitive Surgical can monitor the robot through live data transfer and provide real-time feedback if problems occur. The room should have an available wired Ethernet connection to allow Internet access for the equipment. Especially in a setting with only one available robot, when equipment failure may necessitate conversion to standard laparoscopic or open surgery, a plan for addressing system faults and a streamlined communication path to technical support staff should be in place before starting a case.

Establishing a Robotic Practice: Important Considerations

Successfully establishing a robotic practice depends on surgical volume and securing referrals of appropriate patients. For the surgeon setting out

to establish a new robotic practice, it is important to understand the local referral patterns. Are other practitioners already established in providing robotic surgical options or is the new practitioner the first to do so? Will a robotic-capable surgeon be viewed as a resource or a threat by other surgeons in the community? While many physicians are averse to advertise for themselves, it is very important to promote a specialized skill set to potential referring physicians both within and outside your specialty in the community. Personal interactions tend to be the most valuable to get the word out about your capabilities, particularly if referrals for robotic surgery are not currently being done within your practice community. Giving lectures about robotic surgery at local meetings with nurses, referring doctors or even patients will allow you to outline the focus of your practice. Serving as a proctor at robotic courses is also an excellent opportunity to pass on your knowledge and meet other accomplished robotic surgeons in your field. Through teaching, you can establish your position as an expert and potentially enhance referrals from colleagues for more complex surgical problems.

On an administrative level, it is wise to be engaged with the robotic surgery steering committee at your institution. Management decisions involving the infrastructure for robotic procedures should not be made without surgeon input as the operational experience allows him or her to specify problems or deficits that need to be resolved.

Communication with referring physicians is the centerpiece of building a strong referral base to support your practice. This generally involves written or verbal communication concerning the assessment of the patient and the role (and potential advantages) of a robotic approach after the initial consultation. We also recommend a follow-up communication after surgery, which may stress to the referring physician the rapid patient recovery and good outcomes associated with the robotic approach. It is also important for potential referring physicians to know your level of training and any special expertise you may have in robotic surgery.

Within a group practice, it is advantageous to nurture a rapport with non-robotic-trained colleagues. It has been our philosophy to be available for others if help is needed and to be a resource rather than a competitor. While the indications for robotic surgery continue to expand, collaboration with open and traditional laparoscopic surgeons should be the foundation of your practice and is of mutual benefit to both surgeons and their patients.

References

1. Luthringer T, Aleksic I, Caire A, Albala DM. Developing a successful robotics program. Curr Opin Urol. 2012;22(1):40–6.
2. Steers WD, LeBeau S, Cardella J, Fulmer B. Establishing a robotics program. Urol Clin North Am. 2004;31(4):773–80.
3. Davis JW, Kreaden US, Gabbert J, Thomas R. Learning curve assessment of robot-assisted radical prostatectomy compared with open-surgery controls from the premier perspective database. J Endourol. 2014;28(5):560–6.
4. Hanzly M, Frederick A, Creighton T, Atwood K, Mehedint D, Kauffman EC, et al. Learning curves for robot-assisted and laparoscopic partial nephrectomy. J Endourol. 2015;29(3):297–303.
5. Porpiglia F, Bertolo R, Amparore D, Fiori C. Margins, ischaemia and complications rate after laparoscopic partial nephrectomy: impact of learning curve and tumour anatomical characteristics. BJU Int. 2013;112(8):1125–32.
6. Scales Jr CD, Jones PJ, Eisenstein EL, Preminger GM, Albala DM. Local cost structures and the economics of robot assisted radical prostatectomy. J Urol. 2005;174(6):2323–9.
7. Yu HY, Hevelone ND, Lipsitz SR, Kowalczyk KJ, Hu JC. Use, costs and comparative effectiveness of robotic assisted, laparoscopic and open urological surgery. J Urol. 2012;187(4):1392–8.
8. Cockcroft JO, Berry CB, McGrath JS, Daugherty MO. Anesthesia for major urologic surgery. Anesthesiol Clin. 2015;33(1):165–72.

Steven V. Kheyfets and Chandru P. Sundaram

Introduction

Minimally invasive surgery (MIS) originated in the 1970s in Germany where Kurt Semm, a gynecologist and engineer at the University of Kiel, headed a team that constructed laparoscopic instrumentation to successfully perform various laparoscopic gynecological procedures, as well as the first "endoscopic appendectomy" in 1982. The general surgery community adopted this early laparoscopic technology and successfully performed the first laparoscopic cholecystectomy in 1985. Ultimately, with the advent of video recording and widespread transmission, general surgeons were able to create significant headway in the global adoption and advancement of laparoscopic surgery [1].

Compared to an open approach, advantages to MIS are well established and include reduced postoperative wound infections, blood loss, length of hospital course, postoperative analgesic requirement, and improved wound aesthetics. Disadvantages to MIS include the fulcrum effect, which requires the inversion of hand-instrument movements. In addition, there is restricted hepatic feedback, loss of depth perception, and at times, challenging ergonomics, all of which create a significant learning curve to overcome [2, 3]. With its approval in 2000 by the United States Food and Drug Administration (FDA), the da Vinci surgical system was implemented in an attempt to overcome many of the MIS limitations; its innovative design incorporated high definition three-dimensional (3D) vision, optimal visualization with 10 times magnification, elimination of the fulcrum effect, reduction of hand tremor, and vastly improved surgeon ergonomics [4]. The system is currently in its fourth generation (da Vinci Xi) and includes the following components: a surgeon console that allows the surgeon to view the operative area and manipulate the robotic instruments, a patient side cart that maintains the camera and endowrist instruments with seven degrees of freedom via articulated arms, and a 3D visualization cart [5, 6].

Rise of Robotic Surgery

The robotic surgery boom has experienced far-reaching success across the globe. Since its inception in 2000, over 1.5 million procedures have been performed using the da Vinci surgical system across many surgical specialties, including gynecology, urology, general surgery, cardiothoracic surgery, and otolaryngology. Specifically in urology, the robotic platform has rapidly overtaken open surgery as the standard way of performing a prostatectomy; in fact, 83% of

S.V. Kheyfets, M.D. • C.P. Sundaram, M.D. (✉)
Department of Urology, Indiana University
School of Medicine, 535 Barnhill Drive, Suite 150,
Indianapolis, IN 46202, USA
e-mail: sundaram@iupui.edu

© Springer International Publishing Switzerland 2017
L.-M. Su (ed.), *Atlas of Robotic Urologic Surgery*, DOI 10.1007/978-3-319-45060-5_2

prostatectomies are performed with robotic assistance [7]. According to the most recent 2015 statistics, 3317 da Vinci surgical systems exist worldwide with 2254 within the United States (68%), 556 in Europe (17%), 194 in Japan (6%), and 313 (9%) in the remainder of the world [8]. That represents a 43% rise seen just in the United States, alone, since 2010 [4].

With the exponential rise and adoption of robotic technology and the equally rapidly evolving landscape of the health care system, the question of how to most effectively train current and future surgeons comes into the forefront. Patient safety and its litigious ramifications are a prime concern in today's health care climate. In 1999, the Institute of Medicine published its "To Err is Human" report, revealing that as many as 98,000 preventable deaths occur in hospitals each year resulting from medical errors [9]. More recent 2013 estimates report that between 210,000 and 440,000 preventable patient deaths occur per year [10]. Astoundingly, this would place medical errors as the third leading cause of death in the United States, trailing only heart disease and cancer [11]. This issue is further compounded by mandatory reductions in duty hours allotted for resident training. Thus, the all-important question becomes how do surgical residencies incorporate robotic training into their programs while simultaneously considering patient safety, resident work hour restrictions, and procedure outcomes?

Surgical Training and Credentialing

The conventional Halstedian surgical training model was designed to be a long-term apprenticeship between a junior surgeon and his upper level residents and house staff. This method of training provided young surgeons a graduated responsibility until they were able to perform surgical procedures independently. This model has sustained great longevity; however, its inherent lack of organization can lead to variable outcomes in training [4, 12]. Consequently, in this current modern era of rapidly changing all-pervasive technological advancements in medicine, a more structured surgical training curriculum is necessary to promote effective learning as well as patient outcomes. In 2009, the American Board of Surgery (ABS) required that all general surgeons applying for board certification must have successfully completed the Fundamentals of Laparoscopic Surgery (FLS), a course designed to teach and assess basic laparoscopic skills [13]. Similarly, although not mandated by any formal organizations at this time, the Fundamentals of Robotic Surgery Skills and Training (FRS) is a basic skills proficiency curriculum composed of four modules: introduction to surgical robotic systems, didactic instructions for robotic surgery systems, psychomotor skills curriculum, and team training and communication skills. This program is funded by the Department of Defense as well as by Intuitive Surgical and is currently undergoing a validation study across 15 well-established robotic surgical centers across the world. When the validation study is complete, surgical specialties utilizing the robotic platform will be encouraged to incorporate the FRS concepts into an individualized, specialty-specific core curriculum [14].

Other available training resources include the American Urological Association Education and Research (AUAER) online urologic robotic surgery course; this course is composed of nine modules designed to address the general fundamental aspects of performing robotic surgery as well as focus on key surgical steps, possible complications as well as their management, and troubleshooting during performance of basic (e.g., transperitoneal prostatectomy) and more advanced (e.g., radical cystectomy) robotic procedures. The modules contain specific aims, videos, and posttest evaluations. Additionally, the trainee is required to successfully complete the da Vinci Surgery online fundamental training module prior to starting the AUAER course [15].

Additional online video resources include the da Vinci Surgery Online Community which offers full-length narrated procedures, narrated video clips, and various procedure guides that include patient positioning, port placement, robot docking, and step-by-step surgical instructions [16]. Videourology is an online peer-reviewed videojournal and publishes novel robotic and laparoscopic surgical techniques that are easily accessible [17]. The American Urological Association surgical video library presents an additional (paid) resource for accessing video content [18].

Currently, no streamlined robotic surgery credentialing process exists [3]. Standard Operating Practices (SOPs) for urologic robotic surgery state that robotic surgery credentialing is the sole responsibility of an individual institution. SOPs suggested basic requirements include successful completion of an Accreditation Council for Graduate Medical Education (ACGME) urology residency as well as proof of the graduate's robotic surgical competence from the residency's program director. SOPs recommend that existing practitioners without prior robotic surgical experience should complete a training course, which includes basic online training modules, observation of procedures performed by an expert, and active participation using the robotic surgical system with an instructor to perform basic system functions, troubleshooting, and inanimate/animate skills exercises [19]. Such MIS training courses are available as week-long mini-fellowships at the University of California and through the da Vinci Training Pathway [20, 21]. After completion of a structured course, it is recommended that the physician undergoes proctoring by an experienced robotic surgeon until competency is deemed adequate to perform robotic surgical procedures independently [19]. As the current robotic surgery credentialing process is rather vague, the FRS will likely have ramifications for more specific institutional certification and credentialing.

Learning Curve

It is clear that a paradigm shift to performing robotic MIS has quickly occurred since the launch of the robotic surgical platform. Adaptation to robotic surgery once thought to represent a straightforward transition for experienced open surgeons, however, has proven to require a significant adjustment period. Sood et al. [3] convey this point in a robotic kidney transplantation study where the learning curves of three groups of surgeons with different levels of robotic and open experience are evaluated based on performance of the critical steps of the operation, including venous, arterial, and ureterovesical anastomoses, as well as the period of ischemia. The results clearly revealed that the group with the least amount of prior robotic experience required a significantly longer learning curve to achieve proficiency for each critical step of the procedure [14].

The notion of a "learning curve" was first applied to the airplane manufacturer industry in 1936 by Wright [22] where he hypothesized that the cost of labor in production of an airplane decreases over time with quantity produced. This concept has since been applied to various fields, including surgery, where it highlights the number of required cases a surgeon must perform to attain competence in a specific procedure. The learning curve applies to both beginner surgeons training under a supervised environment and to experienced surgeons incorporating novel techniques into their armamentarium. Along the same vein, in robotic surgery, a learning curve also pertains to the bedside surgeon as well as the entire surgical team [3].

Surgical Simulation

Surgical simulation is a field that has risen out of necessity to help shorten the learning curve and help surgeons safely adapt to the rise in widespread adoption of minimally invasive surgery. In fact, in 2008, the American Council on Graduate Medical Education (ACGME) set a requirement that all general surgery residency programs must provide simulation and skill laboratories for its trainees [23]. Surgical simulation is not a novel idea and follows suit after the success of flight simulation in the aircraft industry, where it has proven benefits [24]. Surgical simulation has evolved over the past 20 years, first with the introduction of laparoscopic surgery and subsequent development of the robotic platform. [25] Simulation involves various types of simulator training models with the goals of reproducing an accurate depiction of the surgical field and developing a specific set of skills in the trainee that can be used effectively during an actual surgical procedure [26]. Surgical simulators can be divided into low fidelity, high fidelity, and virtual reality (VR) simulators [25, 27]. Examples of low fidelity simulators are pelvic laparoscopic trainers, which do not represent a high level of operating room realism nor do they simulate an operative procedure; however, they are cost-effective, and have been shown to improve basic laparoscopic skills. High fidelity simulators use live or cadaveric animal models with the main advantage of simulating a realistic operating room environment. Disadvantages include their substantial cost of use, difficulty with accessibility, poor tissue compliance and deficient bleeding in cadaveric models, and adjunctive requirement of veterinary support for live animal models [27]. Virtual reality simulation offers computer-generated digital reproduction of a real-world operating room experience [25].

The benefits of virtual reality surgical simulation are multiple: It fosters a safe, realistic, trainee-centered environment with the ability to make mistakes while acting out various clinical scenarios, including portions of and/or entire surgical procedures, and performing varying degree of difficulty technical skill tasks without compromising patient safety, all while tracking the surgeon's progression [24]. VR simulation has been validated for use in surgical training; the technology has been tested for face validity (realism), content validity (appropriateness), construct validity (capacity to discern between inexperienced and experienced users), concurrent validity (performance on simulator versus a gold standard), and predictive validity (capacity to predict future performance) [28, 29].

Robotic Simulators

Although numerous models are described in the literature, the following mainstream simulators will comprise the focus of discussion for VR robotic simulation training: Mimic DV-trainer, Xperience team trainer, Maestro™ AR, da Vinci skills simulator, RoSS, and SEP robot.

Mimic Technologies, Inc. (Seattle, WA) introduced the first robotic simulator, the Mimic dV-Trainer®, and installed its early version in 2007 at Indiana University's urology department. It is a portable, desktop-sized trainer and, unique in its class, in that it has the ability to simulate all three *da Vinci*® models (S™, Si™, and Xi™) via its MSim™ simulation technology that is able to generate a wide array of updatable 3D, surgical skill training exercises and requires a desktop computer to power the software. Over 60 surgical training exercises validated for face, content, and construct are included with concentration on the trainee's ability to attain competence in various robotic skill sets, including *EndoWrist*® manipulation, knot tying, camera use, needle control and driving, clutching, vessel dissection, basic and advanced (i.e., tube closure and anastomosis) suturing, energy control and robotic arms' movements [30, 31]. The MScore™ proficiency scoring allows the user to immediately receive objective performance metrics and compare them to experienced users' results, which may assist as a tool in the credentialing and certification process. Custom curricula can be tailored for individual users, and MShare™ enables online users to share their effective skills curricula with each other [32]. The system costs between $85,000 and $105,000 with a service contract [26].

In 2014, Mimic introduced the Xperience™ Team Trainer as well as the Maestro AR™ (Augmented Reality). The Xperience™ Team Trainer is an optional hardware add-on for the dV-Trainer; it includes an interface complete with two laparoscopic instrument ports and a built-in video monitor. This simulator enables the coordinated training to both the console surgeon and bedside surgeon through 13 skill exercises emphasizing effective object transfers, assistance with retraction, and clip application. It provides the opportunity for both surgeons to develop psychomotor tasks as well as communication skills and rehearse them in a safe setting outside of the operating room. The MScore™ performance evaluation system allows for objective skills measure of the overall team and each individual surgeon [32, 33]. Validation studies are pending for the Xperience™ Team Trainer.

The MSim™ simulation platform enabled the production of the Maestro AR™. This advanced simulation has the ability to overlay interactive 3D virtual instruments onto actual footage of a previously performed procedure. This allows the user to obtain procedure-specific skills, including identification of critical anatomical landmarks, plane dissection, and tissue retraction in this 3D "augmented reality." The partial nephrectomy and hysterectomy procedures are currently available for use on the Maestro AR™, and low anterior resection and prostatectomy modules are scheduled for future release. Validation studies are pending for this new technology [34].

The *da Vinci Skills Simulator* (dVSS) was produced by Intuitive surgical in collaboration with Mimic Technologies in 2011. The simulator serves as a hardware backpack that attaches and fully integrates with the *da Vinci® Si™, Si-e™,* and *Xi™* robotic platforms. The surgical skill exercises are partially based on Mimic's dV-Trainer software and have been previously discussed. Learners have the ability to receive immediate feedback and track their progress over time [35]. Face, content, and construct validity has been proven for the dVSS [36, 37]. The simulator costs roughly $90,000 [26].

The Robotic Surgical Simulator (RoSS™) is manufactured by Simulated Surgicals and represents a stand-alone robotic platform capable of simulating the da Vinci® robotic system. It includes 16 training modules that develop the trainee's orientation, cognitive, motor, basic and more advanced surgical skills via various training tasks. The RoSS™ incorporates the Fundamental Skills of Robotic Surgery (FSRS) and uses a standardized scoring performance system [38]. Additionally, RoSS™ boasts its HoST (Hands-on Surgical Training) system, which enables the trainee's hands to be guided through a previously performed real procedure; this provides an interactive environment for the user to perform the critical steps of a procedure in a virtual environment. Thus far, radical prostatectomy, radical hysterectomy, radical cystectomy, and lymph node dissection modules are available for the

HoST system [39]. The RoSS II™ is an updated, redesigned, more compact version of the platform that possesses improved graphics and visualization. It also incorporates the RSA (Robotic Skills Assessment) Score, which provides users real-time feedback based on a timed assessment as part of the RoSS™ training curriculum measuring the trainee's safety, critical error, economy of motions, dexterity, time, and metrics [38]. Face and content, however, not construct, validity has been proven for the RoSS™ simulator [25].

The SimSurgery Educational Platform (SEP) Robot is a modified version of its laparoscopic VR platform; the laparoscopic arms of the basic VR trainer are replaced for robotic arms on the SEP robot. It offers multilevel skill training, and only includes 6 tissue manipulation, 7 basic suturing, and 8 advanced suturing exercises [40–42]. Its limitations are its lack of 3D visualization, fourth-arm manipulation, objective feedback, and procedure-specific modules [27]. However, compared to its competitors, it does represent a cost-conscious VR system ($45,000) and has proven face, content, and construct validity [25–27].

Efficacy data directly comparing various VR simulators is sparse in the literature; Table 2.1 summarizes the validity data for aforementioned VR simulators and their associated costs. Figure 2.1 displays their images.

Surgical Skills Training

The merits of VR simulation in surgical training have been established. Its use has been shown to help novice surgical trainees quickly acquire and improve a basic laparoscopic skill set. Grantcharov et al. [43] studied three groups of surgeons with varying levels of laparoscopic expertise (advanced, intermediate, and novices) using the Minimally Invasive Surgical Trainer-Virtual Reality (MIST VR), which entails six different and increasingly difficulty skill exercises, including grasping, transference, use of energy, and combinations of these tasks. Subjects in each group completed ten sessions of all tasks over a 1-month block of time. Their performance metrics were measured via

Table 2.1 Summary of the validity data for VR simulators and their associated costs

Virtual reality simulators						
	Face validity	Content validity	Construct validity	Concurrent validity	Predictive validity	Price
Mimic dV-T	+	+	+	–	–	$85–100,000
Xperience Team Trainer	n/a	n/a	n/a	n/a	n/a	
Maestro AR	n/a	n/a	n/a	n/a	n/a	
dVSS	+	+	+	–	–	$85–90,000
RoSS	+	+	n/a	–	–	$100–125,000
SEP	+	+	+	–	–	$40–45,000

dV-T dV-Trainer, *AR* augmented reality, *dVSS* da Vinci skills simulator, *RoSS* robotic surgical simulator, *SEP* SimSurgery educational platform, – no, + yes, *n/a* not available

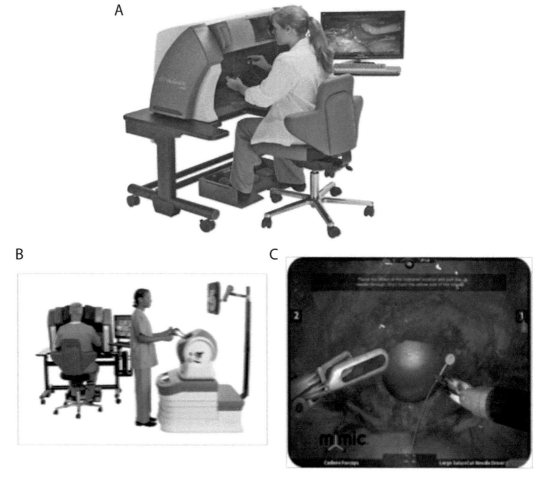

Fig. 2.1 VR Simulators: (**a**) Mimic Dv-T (courtesy of Mimic Technologies, Inc.); (**b**) Xperience Team Trainer (courtesy of Mimic Technologies, Inc.); (**c**) Maestro AR (courtesy of Mimic Technologies, Inc.); (**d**) dVSS [35]; (**e**) RoSS [38]; (**f**) SEP [42]

time to completion of tasks, errors committed, and economy of motion utilized. Although performance scores for the beginner group were significantly lower compared to the intermediate and advanced cohorts after the first trial run, the results were not significantly different after the final session, revealing that basic laparoscopic skill attainment is possible in a relatively short period of time. In fact, the beginner group's learning curves reached a steady stage just after seven, six, and five sessions for time, economy of motion, and error scores, respectively.

Furthermore, in a randomized, double-blinded study, Seymour et al. [44] showed that the surgical resident group who underwent basic task training using the MIST VR platform proved to perform subsequent laparoscopic cholecystectomy procedures faster and with a reduced error rate compared to the control group. This study pioneered the concept that transference of a surgical skill set from a simulation platform to an operative venue is, indeed, possible. Calatayud et al. [45] furthered this idea from a different training angle: the operative warm-up setting. In this randomized crossover study, surgical residents functioned as their own controls, and each group performed a total of two laparoscopic cholecystectomy procedures 2 weeks apart. The first group was randomized to perform the procedure without VR warm-up, followed 2 weeks later by undergoing VR warm-up exercises and subsequently performing the procedure. The second group first completed a VR surgical warm-up and performed the procedure; 2 weeks later, this group performed an additional laparoscopic cholecystectomy without the benefit of VR warm-up exercises. VR warm-up training constituted executing three exercises (object manipulation, clip application, and dissection) for 15 min using the Lapsim VR simulator just prior to the start time of the operative procedure. The results of the study revealed significantly higher operative surgical performance scores in the groups who performed laparoscopic cholecystectomy cases with prior surgical warm-up as measured by a validated objective structure of technical skills (OSATS) global rating scale. Lee et al. [46] helped to cement that surgical warm-up is a beneficial practice; this randomized crossover study included three junior urology residents, two senior urology residents, and three urology fellows. Each subject performed a total of four laparoscopic renal procedures in two sets divided by more than 1 week apart. During each session consisting of two procedures, each subject had the opportunity to either first perform warm-up exercises or directly proceed with the operative procedure; the actual order of events (i.e., warm-up vs. surgical procedure) was randomized. Surgical warm-up was composed of performing a 5 min electrocautery exercise on the LAP Mentor VR simulator as well as a 15 min laparoscopic suturing/knot tying task 1 h prior to the operative procedure. Psychomotor and cognitive data was obtained using electroencephalography (EEG), eye tracking technology, and video recording of the operative procedures. Mean psychomotor performance scores, as measured by hand movement smoothness, tool movement smoothness, and postural stability, proved to be significantly higher in the surgical warm-up group. The warm-up group also showed improved cognition during performance of renal surgery, as measured by mean attention, distraction, and mental workload scores. Furthermore, the surgical rehearsal cohort achieved significantly higher technical performance scores when evaluating its ability to mobilize the colon during an early portion of a renal procedure. However, during a later step of the procedure (retroperitonealizing the colon), surgical warm-up was not found to improve surgical task scores, thus, lending theory that warm-up may be applicable for a short period of time. Lendvay et al. [47] performed a trial designed to test whether VR surgical warm-up proved beneficial in a robotic dry lab situation. The group consisted of a total of 51 subjects across various fields (urology, gynecology, and general surgery) and training levels (residents and attendings). All subjects underwent robotic proficiency training and were subsequently randomized to either the surgical warm-up group or the control group. All subjects completed four trial runs: the initial three involved completion of the da Vinci VR rocking pegboard task while the final one comprised a robotic intracorporeal suturing exercise.

In all trials, the surgical warm-up group completed a brief (3–5 min) VR pegboard warm-up task while the control group read a book for 10 min prior to the required exercise. In the first three repetitions that tested similar VR exercises, the VR warm-up group proved to show significantly improved performance metrics (task times and tool path lengths) compared to the control group. The fourth trial sitting evaluated a different and more complex VR task (robotic intracorporeal suturing) designed to test generalizability of the warm-up task; results revealed the warm-up group had a significantly decreased error rate when performing this exercise compared to the control group. The next step in robotic VR warm-up training is to assess whether it transfers dry lab skills to the operating room and impacts patient safety.

Patient-specific simulation is a technological concept/advancement that is intricately related to surgical warm-up. It allows for two-dimensional data from CT scans and MRIs to be uploaded onto a VR simulator and rendered into an interactive 3D image on the stereoscopic field. In this fashion, surgeons are given the opportunity to rehearse the planned procedure using a patient's unique anatomical data in a VR environment, a concept similar to augmented reality. Currently, Simbionix holds the only commercially available patient-specific VR simulator (AngioMentor) designed for carotid endovascular stent placement.

It has proven face, construct, and content validity and enables the user to track objective measures over time [48].

In addition to VR simulation, the robotic platform can also be effectively utilized to develop a basic robotic skill set using inanimate exercises. Jarc and Curet [49] proved the construct validity of nine ex-vivo tasks designed to test camera control, clutching, instrument manipulation, needle positioning, and suturing. In this study, advanced robotic surgeons significantly outperformed novice surgeons, as evident by quicker task completion times and performance scores. Furthermore, Raza et al. [50] used a commercially available inanimate vesicourethral anastomosis kit (Fig. 2.2) (3-Dmed) to prove content, construct, and concurrent validity in performing a vesicourethral anastomosis using the da Vinci robotic platform.

Novel Avenues of Surgical Grading

In this ever-expansive online technological age, novel avenues of surgical grading have been explored and developed. Crowdsourcing is one such method and involves seeking out responses from a large, heterogeneous cohort of people from an online community to assist in finding a solution to a problem, in this case, evaluating surgical performance; this has been termed crowd-sourced

Fig. 2.2 Inanimate vesicourethral anastomosis model (courtesy of 3-DMED)

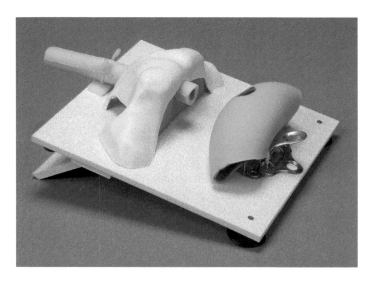

assessment of technical skills (C-SATS). Studies involving C-SATS have recently revealed that the surgically inexperienced online community is equally effective as experienced surgeons in evaluating performance during dry lab robotic videos as well as brief animate videos performed by surgeons of varying experience levels. Surgical performance was graded using a validated surgical grading tool, the Global Evaluative Assessment of Robotic Skills (GEARS), which evaluates the following five domains: depth perception, bimanual dexterity, efficiency, force sensitivity, and robotic control [51, 52]. While C-SATS will certainly not serve to replace a surgical trainee's invaluable feedback from his experienced mentor, it may have a supplementary role for receiving further feedback in a timely fashion [51].

Along a similar train of thought, video-based peer evaluation via social networking is another innovative surgical evaluation grading tool. In a recent randomized control trial, a total of 41 urology and gynecology residents performed a running anastomosis exercise (Tubes simulator task) in three different sessions over 6 weeks. The 20 subjects in the intervention group received peer feedback after each session after their videos were de-identified and uploaded to a social networking site while the control group did not receive video-based peer feedback. Feedback was provided using GEARS as well as summative remarks. While mean scores for both subject groups were similar for the first session, the intervention residents scored significantly higher and completed the tasks substantially faster than the control group after the second and third sessions [53]. Consequently, this method has shown to improve simulation training performance metrics and holds promise for the evaluation and improvement of real-world robotic operative procedures.

Conclusion

It is clear that the booming use of robotic technology has brought an overwhelming sense of enthusiasm to the field of minimally invasive surgery. In turn, with the pervasive acceptance of this technology, efficiently training the new wave of surgeons as well as existing ones comes into the forefront, as this is essential to patient safety, medicolegal aspects, and health care expenditure. VR robotic simulation has clearly shown to be beneficial in helping trainees rapidly acquire a basic surgical armamentarium that can be transferred to the operative theatre. Furthermore, VR simulation is currently being used to create training curriculums and potentially play a role in credentialing and licensing. While the benefits of VR simulation are clear, however, one also has to take into account its substantial cost, and the fact that it has not yet been studied or shown to ultimately impact patient outcomes, the overarching driving force in the medical landscape. Thus, while new technology continues to become incorporated into mainstream medicine, we must find a way to utilize it in a safe, smart, and effective manner.

References

1. Blum CA, Adams DB. Who did the first laparoscopic cholecystectomy? J Minim Access Surg. 2011;7(3):165–8.
2. Passerotti CC, Franco F, Bissoli JC, Tiseo B, Oliveira CM, Buchalla CA, et al. Comparison of the learning curves and frustration level in performing laparoscopic and robotic training skills by experts and novices. Int Urol Nephrol. 2015;47(7):1075–84.
3. Sood A, Jeong W, Ahlawat R, Campbell L, Aggarwal S, Menon M, et al. Robotic surgical skill acquisition: what one needs to know? J Minim Access Surg. 2015;11(1):10–5.
4. Jenison EL, Gil KM, Lendvay TS, Guy MS. Robotic surgical skills: acquisition, maintenance, and degradation. JSLS. 2012;16(2):218–28.
5. Liu M, Curet M. A review of training research and virtual reality simulators for the da Vinci surgical system. Teach Learn Med. 2015;27(1):12–26.
6. The da Vinci® Surgical System [Internet]. 2015 [updated 2015; cited 15 June 2015]. http://intuitive-surgical.com/products/davinci_surgical_system/.
7. da Vinci® Procedures [Internet]. 2015 [updated 2015; cited 15 June 2015]. http://www.davincisurgery.com/da-vinci-surgery/da-vinci-procedures/.
8. Investor FAQ [Internet]. 2015 [updated 2015; cited 15 May 2015]. http://phx.corporate-ir.net/phoenix.zhtml?c=122359&p=irol-faq.
9. Institute of Medicine Committee on Quality of Health Care in America. To err is human: building a safer health system. In: Kohn LT, Corrigan JM, Donaldson MS, editors. To err is human: building a safer health

system. Washington: National Academies Press; Copyright 2000 by the National Academy of Sciences. All rights reserved; 2000.

10. James JT. A new, evidence-based estimate of patient harms associated with hospital care. J Patient Saf. 2013;9(3):122–8.

11. Leading Causes of Death [Internet]. [updated 2015; cited 20 June 2015]. http://www.cdc.gov/nchs/fastats/leading-causes-of-death.htm.

12. Rankin JS. William Stewart Halsted: a lecture by Dr Peter D. Olch. Ann Surg. 2006;243(3):418–25.

13. ABS to Require ACLS, ATLS and FLS for General Surgery Certification [Internet]. 2015 [cited 20 June 2015]. https://www.absurgery.org/default.jsp?news_newreqs.

14. Fifteen Institutions Selected to Participate in the Validation Study for Fundamentals of Robotic Surgery [Internet]. 2015 [cited 21 June 2015]. http://frsurgery.org/news/.

15. Urologic Robotic Surgery Course. 2015 [cited 15 July 2015].https://www.auanet.org/education/modules/robotic-surgery/.

16. da Vinci Surgery Online Community [Internet]. 2015 [cited 15 July 2015]. https://www.davincisurgery-community.com/home-auth?tab1=HO.

17. Videourology [Internet]. 2015 [15 July 2015]. http://www.liebertpub.com/videourology.

18. Videos and Webcasts [Internet]. 2015. http://www.auanet.org/education/videos-and-webcasts.cfm.

19. Standard Operating Practices (SOPs) for Urologic Robotic Surgery [Internet]. 2013 [updated April 2013; cited 11 Aug 2015]. http://www.auanet.org/common/pdf/about/SOP-Urologic-Robotic-Surgery.pdf.

20. Mini-Fellowship in Minimally Invasive Urologic Surgery [Internet]. 2015 [updated 2015; cited 11 Aug 2015]. http://www.urology.uci.edu/education_fellowship_mini.shtml.

21. da Vinci Training [Internet]. 2015 [updated 15 July 2015; cited 15 July 2015]. http://www.intuitivesurgical.com/training/.

22. Wright TP. Factors affecting the cost of airplanes. J Aeronaut Sci. 1936;3(4):122–8.

23. ACGME Program Requirements for Graduate Medical Education in General Surgery [Internet]. 2014 [updated 1 July 2014; cited 28 June 2015]. http://www.acgme.org/acgmeweb/portals/0/pfassets/programrequirements/440_general_surgery_07012014.pdf.

24. Yiannakopoulou E, Nikiteas N, Perrea D, Tsigris C. Virtual reality simulators and training in laparoscopic surgery. Int J Surg. 2015;13:60–4.

25. Abboudi H, Khan MS, Aboumarzouk O, Guru KA, Challacombe B, Dasgupta P, et al. Current status of validation for robotic surgery simulators—a systematic review. BJU Int. 2013;111(2):194–205.

26. Lallas CD, Davis JW. Robotic surgery training with commercially available simulation systems in 2011: a current review and practice pattern survey from the society of urologic robotic surgeons. J Endourol. 2012;26(3):283–93.

27. Kumar A, Smith R, Patel VR. Current status of robotic simulators in acquisition of robotic surgical skills. Curr Opin Urol. 2015;25(2):168–74.

28. McDougall EM. Validation of surgical simulators. J Endourol. 2007;21(3):244–7.

29. Hung AJ, Shah SH, Dalag L, Shin D, Gill IS. Development and validation of a novel robotic procedure specific simulation platform: partial nephrectomy. J Urol. 2015;194(2):520–6.

30. Lendvay T, Casale P, Sweet R, Peters C. Initial validation of a virtual-reality robotic simulator. J Robotic Surg. 2008;2(3):145–9.

31. Sethi AS, Peine WJ, Mohammadi Y, Sundaram CP. Validation of a novel virtual reality robotic simulator. J Endourol. 2009;23(3):503–8.

32. Are you prepared to deliver exceptional care in robotic surgery? [Internet]. 2014 [updated August 2014; cited 25 June 2015]. http://pages.mimicsimulation.com/rs/mimictechnologies/images/Mimic_dV-Trainer_.pdf.

33. Empower teamwork for the robotic surgeon and first assistant [Internet]. 2014 [updated August 2014; cited 25 June 2015]. http://pages.mimicsimulation.com/rs/mimictechnologies/images/Mimic_XTT_bro_update_14-07_FNL.pdf.

34. Maestro AR [Internet]. 2015 [updated 2015; cited 25 June 2015]. http://www.mimicsimulation.com/products/maestro-ar/.

35. da Vinci Skills Simulator [Internet]. 2015 [updated 2015; cited 25 June 2015]. http://www.intuitivesurgical.com/products/skills_simulator/.

36. Schreuder HW, Persson JE, Wolswijk RG, Ihse I, Schijven MP, Verheijen RH. Validation of a novel virtual reality simulator for robotic surgery. ScientificWorldJournal. 2014;2014:507076.

37. Alzahrani T, Haddad R, Alkhayal A, Delisle J, Drudi L, Gotlieb W, et al. Validation of the da Vinci Surgical Skill Simulator across three surgical disciplines: a pilot study. Can Urol Assoc J. 2013;7(7-8):E520–9.

38. Robotic Surgery Simulator [Internet]. 2015 [cited 25 June 2015]. http://www.simulatedsurgicals.com/ross2.html.

39. Hands-On Surgical Training [Internet]. 2015 [cited 25 June 2015]. http://www.simulatedsurgicals.com/host.html.

40. SEP Robot [Internet]. 2015 [cited 25 June 2015]. http://www.simsurgery.com/robot.html.

41. Xperience Team Trainer Picture [Image on the Internet]. 2015 [updated 2015; cited 25 June 2015]. https://pydio.mimicsimulation.com/public/7bbae4.

42. SimSurgery Picture [Image on the internet]. 2015 [cited 25 June 2015]. https://www.google.com/search?q=SimSurgery+Educational+Platform&biw=1491&bih=852&source=lnms&tbm=isch&sa=X&ved=0CAkQ_AUoBGoVChMIj8rhpIPPxwIVzwOSCh0jjAVZ&dpr=1.5#imgrc=opMI_gRPghgtOM%3A.

43. Grantcharov TP, Bardram L, Funch-Jensen P, Rosenberg J. Learning curves and impact of previous operative experience on performance on a virtual reality simulator to test laparoscopic surgical skills. Am J Surg. 2003;185(2):146–9.

44. Seymour NE, Gallagher AG, Roman SA, O'Brien MK, Bansal VK, Andersen DK, et al. Virtual reality training improves operating room performance: results of a randomized, double-blinded study. Ann Surg. 2002;236(4):458–63; discussion 63–4.

45. Calatayud D, Arora S, Aggarwal R, Kruglikova I, Schulze S, Funch-Jensen P, et al. Warm-up in a virtual reality environment improves performance in the operating room. Ann Surg. 2010;251(6):1181–5.

46. Lee JY, Mucksavage P, Kerbl DC, Osann KE, Winfield HN, Kahol K, et al. Laparoscopic warm-up exercises improve performance of senior-level trainees during laparoscopic renal surgery. J Endourol. 2012;26(5):545–50.

47. Lendvay TS, Brand TC, White L, Kowalewski T, Jonnadula S, Mercer LD, et al. Virtual reality robotic surgery warm-up improves task performance in a dry laboratory environment: a prospective randomized controlled study. J Am Coll Surg. 2013;216(6): 1181–92.

48. Willaert WI, Aggarwal R, Van Herzeele I, Cheshire NJ, Vermassen FE. Recent advancements in medical simulation: patient-specific virtual reality simulation. World J Surg. 2012;36(7):1703–12.

49. Jarc AM, Curet M. Construct validity of nine new inanimate exercises for robotic surgeon training using a standardized setup. Surg Endosc. 2014;28(2): 648–56.

50. Raza SJ, Field E, Jay C, Eun D, Fumo M, Hu JC, et al. Surgical competency for urethrovesical anastomosis during robot-assisted radical prostatectomy: development and validation of the robotic anastomosis competency evaluation. Urology. 2015;85(1): 27–32.

51. Holst D, Kowalewski TM, White LW, Brand TC, Harper JD, Sorensen MD, et al. Crowd-Sourced Assessment of Technical Skills (C-SATS): differentiating animate surgical skill through the wisdom of crowds. J Endourol. 2015;29:1183–8.

52. Chen C, White L, Kowalewski T, Aggarwal R, Lintott C, Comstock B, et al. Crowd-Sourced Assessment of Technical Skills: a novel method to evaluate surgical performance. J Surg Res. 2014;187(1):65–71.

53. Carter SC, Chiang A, Shah G, Kwan L, Montgomery JS, Karam A, et al. Video-based peer feedback through social networking for robotic surgery simulation: a multicenter randomized controlled trial. Ann Surg. 2015;261(5):870–5.

Robotic Instrumentation, Personnel, and Operating Room Setup

Matthew J. Ziegelmann, Matthew T. Gettman, and John J. Knoedler

Introduction

Over the past decade and a half, the field of robotic-assisted surgery has evolved from endoscope positioning to "master-slave systems," where the surgeon's hand movements are translated to robotic instrument arms positioned inside the patient several feet away [1, 2]. The da Vinci® (Intuitive Surgical; Sunnyvale, CA) is currently the most commonly utilized "master-slave system" system. Since the first robotic-assisted prostatectomy was performed in 2000 and subsequent Federal Drug Administration approval, the da Vinci® system has become a cornerstone of urologic surgery, and it is increasingly utilized in upper and lower urinary tract procedures. Its use is also expanding rapidly in the field of pediatric urology, along with other surgical specialities outside the realm of urology [3]. Over the years, five different da Vinci® models have been introduced—standard, streamlined (S), S-high definition (HD), S-integrated (1) systems, and most recently the new Xi system. This chapter will review the da Vinci® robotic operating system, equipment, necessary personnel, and operating room setup for standard urologic surgical procedures. We will also briefly touch on the new features associated with the Xi platform. Please note that this chapter does not replace the required video and hands-on training sessions provided by Intuitive Surgical. Instead, this chapter is meant to serve as a reference for members of the robotic surgical team.

Surgical Team

The surgical team consists of the surgeon, circulating nurse, surgical technician, and surgical assistant(s). To maximize efficiency, it is essential that each team member is knowledgeable in robotic-assisted surgery. Communication between each of these individuals is vital for successful outcomes [4, 5]. Intuitive surgical offers training courses for the surgical team, and each member should complete the course modules prior to starting with the surgical team. Separate courses are available based on the specific da Vinci® model, as there are important differences between each model's interface and components. It is also important for the surgical team to remain consistent, and it is generally recommend to have a dedicated team to work through the learning curve and, if possible, all robotic cases [4].

The surgeon will lead the team and should not only master driving the robot, but also possess expertise with the setup, basic operation, and troubleshooting the system. The circulating nurse and surgical technician are critical for operating

M.J. Ziegelmann, M.D. • M.T. Gettman, M.D.
J.J. Knoedler, M.D. (✉)
Department of Urology, Mayo Clinic,
200 1st St SW, Rochester, MD 55901, USA
E-Mail: knoedler.john@mayo.edu

the robot and should become experts on system startup, draping, docking, instruments, troubleshooting, exchanging instruments, and turnover. The surgical assistant should have similar knowledge, but will also need to understand the basics of laparoscopic surgery and be comfortable assisting with trocar placement, clipping, suction, irrigation, retraction, and cutting [1, 4].

Operating Room Setup

The operating room should be able to accommodate all of the robotic components such that there is a clear view of the patient from the surgeon console, tension-free cable connections between the equipment, and clear pathways for operating room personnel to move freely around the room in a safe and expeditious manner (Fig. 3.1). In addition, the room should be able to facilitate

docking of the robot from several different angles depending on the type of surgery being performed.

If the team utilizes a standard operating room (Fig. 3.2a) that is converted to a robotics room on operative days, there may need to be additional laparoscopic towers to hold the insufflator, insufflation tank, electrosurgical units, video system, and extra monitors. In this situation, some of the equipment may also be placed on the vision cart. Ideally, the operating room will be in a dedicated room designed for laparoscopic surgery with an integration system to allow DVD recording and telemedicine (Fig. 3.2b). In addition, flat panel monitors are mounted from the ceiling, CO_2 gas is piped directly into the room for insufflation, and ceiling mounted equipment booms can house insufflators, electrosurgical units, laparoscopic camera equipment, and light sources.

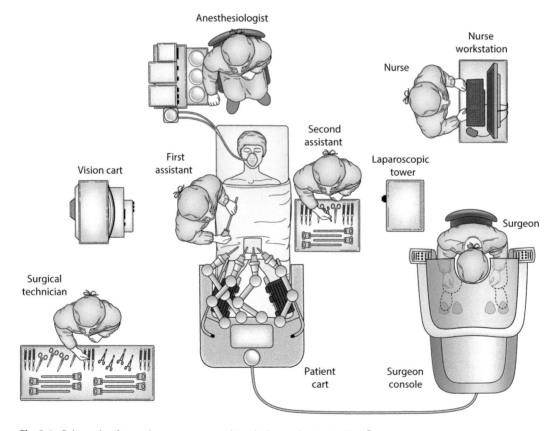

Fig. 3.1 Schematic of operating room setup and surgical team for the da Vinci®

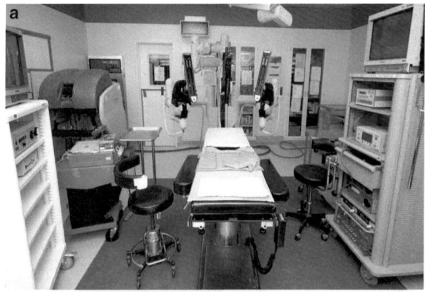

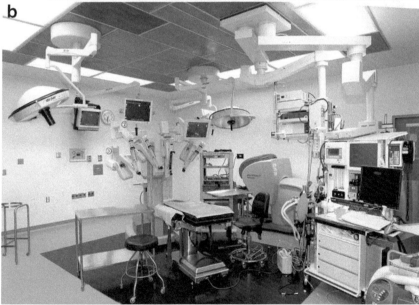

Fig. 3.2 Photograph of operating room for the da Vinci® standard (**a**) and S (**b**) systems. Standard system operating room (**a**) with an additional laparoscopic tower and seating for a second surgical assistant. S system operating room (**b**) where several telemonitors are mounted from the ceiling and a laparoscopic tower is mounted on a ceiling boom with the electrosurgical unit, insufflator, and light source. The room is also equipped with an integration system for DVD recording and telemedicine

Patient Positioning

For surgery of the pelvis and anterior transabdominal surgery, patients are moved directly onto an operating room table with a gel pad (Fig. 3.2) [5, 6]. The gel pad increases friction and prevents patients from sliding during the procedure. The patient is positioned in a modified lithotomy position using yellow fin stirrups (Fig. 3.3a, b) with thromboembolic stockings and

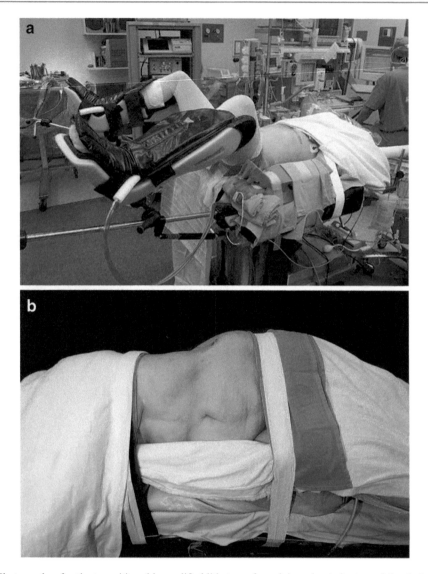

Fig. 3.3 Photographs of patients positioned in modified lithotomy for pelvic and anterior transabdominal surgery (**a**) and flank position for upper urinary tract surgery (**b**)

sequential compression devices. Both arms are padded and positioned along side of the patient on arm boards. A safety strap or tape can be used to secure the patient to the table, and it is recommended that it not be placed across the shoulder to prevent postoperative neuropathy. An upper body Bair Hugger® (Arizant Inc., Eden Prairie, MN) is then placed above the xiphoid and insulated with a blanket. Once the patient is positioned, we secure a face shield plate (Fig. 3.4) to protect the patient's face and endotracheal tube

from inadvertent damage or dislodgement during movement of the robotic endoscope. The patient is then prepped from the xiphoid to perineum to midaxillary lines and draped.

For surgery of the kidney or ureters, the patient is moved onto the surgical table with a beanbag immobilizer and positioned in a 45° modified flank position for transperitoneal access or a full flank position for transperitoneal or retroperitoneal access with the surgical side up (Fig. 3.3b) [7]. The patient is positioned with the

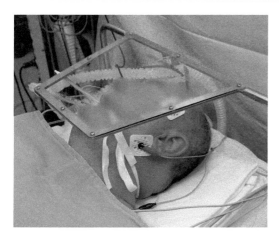

Fig. 3.4 Photograph of patient with a protective face shield plate secured to the operating room table

space between the costal margin and anterior superior iliac spine over the kidney rest. However, the kidney rest is not typically used for these cases. Thromboembolic stockings and sequential compression devices are placed and a urethral catheter is inserted. The surgical side leg is bent slightly and padded with pillows or towels. An axillary roll is placed to prevent postoperative neuropathy, and the arm is padded and secured. The upper arm is padded and secured to an arm board and the table can then be flexed. When flexing the table, the anesthesiologist should be alerted to support the head and place several pillows or towels to avoid hyperextension of the cervical spine. Safety straps or tape can be used over the hip, lower extremity, and thorax to secure the patient to the bed. An upper body Bair Hugger® is placed and insulated with a blanket. The patient is prepped from the nipples to anterior superior iliac spine and midline to erector spinae.

Abdominal Access

Robotic-assisted surgery begins with abdominal access and trocar placement. Pneumoperitoneum may be established using a Veress needle or with open trocar placement by the Hasson technique [5]. The initial trocar can be placed via a direct vision bladed or non-bladed trocar, or a step sys-

tem without direct vision can be used. For the standard and S systems, we typically gain abdominal access by making a small incision and carrying the dissection down to the level of the fascia. The fascia is then elevated with tracheal hooks and the Veress needle is inserted [8]. Placement is verified with the hanging drop test and the abdomen is insufflated to 15 mmHg. A 12 mm trocar is then placed with a Visiport™ device (Covidien, Inc., Dublin, Ireland). This will serve as the trocar for the da Vinci® endoscope, and the robotic camera arm is compatible with most 12 mm laparoscopic trocars. The camera trocar should be placed 15–18 cm from the target anatomy to allow optimal visualization of the surgical field. For obese patients, the camera trocar may need to be placed closer to target anatomy to adjust for abdominal girth. This is especially important when using the da Vinci® standard system [6].

After visual access is obtained, secondary trocars can be placed under laparoscopic vision. The robotic instrument arms are compatible with specific da Vinci® 5 or 8 mm metal trocars that can be placed using blunt or sharp obturators (Fig. 3.5). The da Vinci® system utilizes "remote center technology" to maximize efficiency and minimize trauma to the patient tissues surrounding the robotic trocars. Trocars have three black lines to assist with correct trocar placement. The thick black line located between two thin lines is known as the "cannula remote center." Correct trocar placement can be verified by directly visualizing the trocar during placement. Only the first thin black line should be seen within the abdominal cavity. This allows the thick black line, or remote center, to sit at the level of the abdominal fascia within the boundaries of the abdominal wall, thus minimizing pressure exerted on surrounding tissues. It is recommended that the robotic trocars be placed at least 8–10 cm away from the camera to avoid instrument arm collision and facilitate intracorporeal suturing. In addition, the angle created by the robotic and camera trocars should be greater than 90° to increase instrument arm maneuverability [1, 4]. Other laparoscopic instruments may need to be available for lysis of adhesions prior to

Fig. 3.5 Photograph of 8 mm trocar for the da Vinci® standard (**a**), S (**b**), and Xi systems(**c**). The trocars for the S system also have a trocar that can be connected to the insufflator. Also shown are the sharp and blunt obturators used for trocar placement. Of note, metal trocars are not available for the Xi system

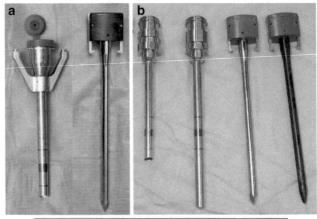

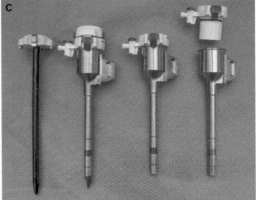

robot docking and for the first assistant to use during the procedure (Table 3.1).

In contrast, with the da Vinci® Xi system, we typically establish pneumoperitoneum using a closed technique with the Veress needled placed through a stab incision at the base of the umbilicus. After pneumoperitoneum is established, an 8-mm trocar for the endoscope is placed using a blind technique. Subsequent trocars are then placed under direct visualization.

The da Vinci® Surgical System

The da Vinci® is available in four generations with five different models—standard, streamlined (S), S-high definition (HD), S-integrated (i)-HD, and most recently, the da Vinci® Xi. Each system has three components: surgeon console, patient cart, and vision cart [2, 8]. There are several sterile accessories and EndoWrist® (Intuitive Surgical, Inc., Sunnyvale, CA) instruments available for each system (Table 3.1). The standard system was released in 1999 and was originally offered with one camera arm and two instrument arms. A third instrument arm was introduced on newer systems or as an upgrade. In 2006, the da Vinci® S system was introduced. This system has a similar platform to the standard system, but added numerous improvements including a motorized patient cart, color coded fiber-optic connections, easier instrument exchanges, quick click trocar attachments, increased range of motion and reach of instrument arms, and interactive video touchscreen display. In 2007, the S system became available with an HD camera and video system, and in 2009 the Si-HD system was released with enhanced HD vision at 1080i, an upgraded surgeon console, and dual console capability. The

Table 3.1 Instruments for robotic-assisted surgery

Laparoscopic instruments
Veress needle
Visiport™ (Ethicon Endo-Surgery, Cincinnati, OH)
12 mm Optiview™ (Ethicon Endo-Surgery, Cincinnati, OH)
12 mm Xcel™ (Ethicon Endo-Surgery, Cincinnati, OH)
6 mm TERNAMIAN EndoTIP™ (Karl Storz Endoscopy America, Inc., Culver City, CA)
Fascial closure device
10 mm ENDO CATCH® entrapment sac (Covidien, Mansfield, MA)
Curved endo Metzenbaum scissors
Maryland dissector
Hook cautery
Needle driver
Endoscopic clip applier
Suction irrigator
0° and 30° laparoscope lens
Camera and fiber optic cords
5 mm and 10 mm Hem-o-lok® clips (Teleflex Medical, Research Triangle Park, NC)
Hot water bath for endoscopes
Robotic instruments
da Vinci® (Intuitive Surgical, Inc., Sunnyvale, CA)
8 mm or 5 mm robotic trocars (2–3 depending on the number of instrument arms)
EndoWrist® instruments (Intuitive Surgical, Inc., Sunnyvale, CA)
Sterile drapes for camera and instrument arms, camera and telemonitor
Sterile camera mount and camera trocar mount (depending on the type of system)
Sterile trocar mount (depending on the type of system)
Sterile instrument adapter (comes attached to the drape for the S)
Sterile camera adapter

dual console feature connects two surgeon consoles to the same patient cart. This allows two surgeons to coordinate a surgical procedure by exchanging control over instruments arms and the endoscope. The dual console feature and HD visions could also be added to existing S systems as an upgrade by the manufacturer.

In 2014, the FDA approved the release of the da Vinci® Xi system. This robot incorporates a different optic system and is designed to enhance four-quadrant surgery. A laser targeting feature is available for docking. The arms are smaller and lighter. The endoscope has been reconfigured to allow placement in any of the four arms. In the next several sections, we describe each of three components that make up the da Vinci® system in detail, and we will highlight new features present with the Xi model. Of note, da Vinci® robots have an optional fluorescence imaging feature that utilizes near infrared light from the endoscope along with administration of intravenous indocyanine green, an agent that binds to plasma proteins and allows identification of vascular structures. Further discussion regarding the exact uses of this new technology is beyond the scope of this chapter.

Surgeon Console

The surgeon console (Figs. 3.6 and 3.7) is the driver's seat for robotic surgery. From here the surgeon views a three-dimensional image of the surgical field through the stereoviewer, adjusts the system with the pod controls, and controls the instruments arms using the master controllers and foot pedals [2, 9]. The standard and S systems have similar surgeon consoles with minor differences (Fig. 3.6), while the Si and Xi surgeon consoles were remodeled, integrating the right and left pod controls into a central touchpad (Fig. 3.7a, b).

The stereoviewer displays the real-time high-resolution three-dimensional image of the surgical field along with system status icons and messages [2]. The system status icons and messages are displayed in specific locations within the stereoviewer and alert the surgeon to any changes or errors with the system. Through the viewer, the surgeon can identify instrument names and the corresponding arms controlling each instrument. The type of energy applied through each instrument can also be seen. Directly adjacent to the stereoviewer are infrared sensors that activate the surgeon console and instruments when the surgeon's head is placed between them. This feature prevents unintentional movement of robotic instruments inside of the patient's body as the robotic instruments are

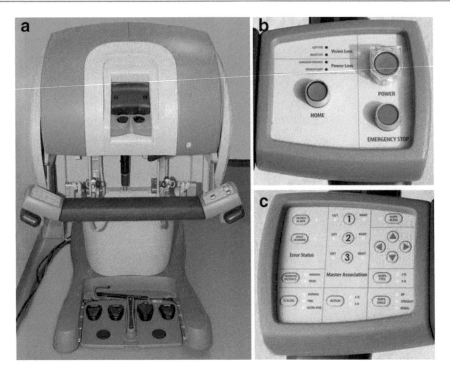

Fig. 3.6 Photograph of da Vinci® S surgeon console (**a**), *right* (**b**), and *left-side* (**c**) pod controls

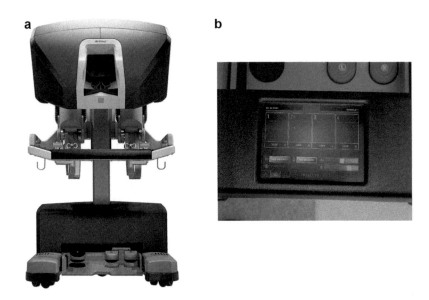

Fig. 3.7 Photograph of da Vinci® Xi surgeon console (**a**) and center touchpad (**b**) (Reproduced with permission from Intuitive Surgical, Inc © 2015)

immediately deactivated when the surgeon looks away from the stereoviewer and removes his head from between the infrared sensors. Below the stereoviewer are knobs to adjust the intraocular distance, intercom volume, brightness, and contrast. Some of these controls may not be equipped on every model. There is a microphone at the bottom of the viewer to allow easy communication between the surgeon and the operating room personnel. The Xi model also contains speakers to allow audio feedback and amplification of OR communication during the procedure.

The da Vinci® standard and S-models (Fig. 3.6) have right- and left-sided pod controls on the end of the arm rest. The right-side pod control allows for communication of major system errors and turns the system on and off, while the left-side pod controls are used to set the system configuration and troubleshoot system faults. On the outside edge of the left-sided pod controls, there are adjustment buttons for raising and lowering the height of the surgeon console. The Si-HD and Xi models have a central touchpad on the arm rest (Fig. 3.7b), along with separate pods located on the right and left sides of the armrest. The left-sided pod allows for adjustment in four different directions in order to facilitate better ergonomics, while the right-sided pod contains the emergency stop and power buttons used to power the system on and off. The middle touchpad has multiple functions. It allows the surgeon to create a profile and store ergonomic settings for future use. It also displays specific information for each robotic arm as well as the endoscope. For instance, there is a lock function for each arm to prevent inadvertent switching between arms. The touchpad also allows access to multiple system settings including motion scaling, haptic zoom, and activation of the Firefly™ system.

For all of the da Vinci® systems, the master controllers (Fig. 3.8) are the manual manipulators used by the surgeon to control the instrument arms and endoscope (Fig. 3.9). For the standard and S-models, the controllers are grasped with the thumb and index or middle finger and movements are translated by a computer that scales, filters, and relays them to the instruments. For the SI and Xi-models, the controllers are grasped by the thumb and middle finger to facilitate finger clutching of the robot. There is no measurable delay between surgeon and robotic instrument movement, and there is a filtering mechanism that eliminates physiologic tremor [9]. Total working area for the master controllers in the da Vinci® standard and S systems is 1 ft³, while the Si-HD has 1.5 times the working space. Surgeons should adjust their working space between the master

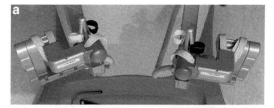
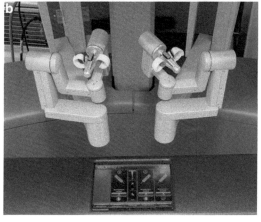

Fig. 3.8 Photograph of master controllers from the da Vinci® S (**a**) and Xi (**b**) systems

controllers to a comfortable working distance using the master clutch (see below) to avoid collision between the master controllers as well as against the walls of the working space. This helps to prevent reaching or stretching with eventual arm and wrist fatigue. The Si-HD and Xi models have an added finger clutch on each of the master controllers that can also be used to adjust the working space of each individual master controller independently. To activate the instrument arms during surgery, the surgeon must "match grips" by grasping the masters to match the position and grip of the EndoWrist® instrument tips as seen within the body. This feature prevents accidental activation of the instrument arms and inadvertent tissue damage. When toggling between two instruments and taking control of an instrument that is retracting tissue, keep the master closed to prevent dropping the tissue.

The footswitch panel (Fig. 3.10) is used in conjunction with the master controllers to drive the surgery. The clutch pedal allows the surgeon to shift to the third arm or adjust the working distance between the master controllers. By quickly tapping the clutch pedal once, the designated

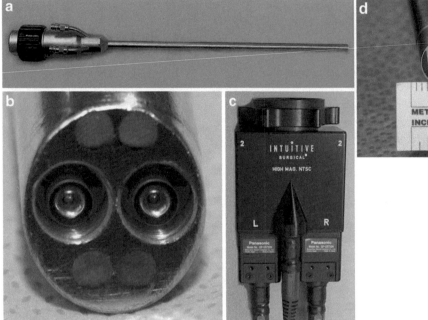

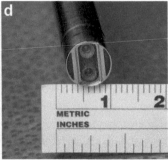

Fig. 3.9 Photograph of da Vinci® stereo endoscope (**a**) showing the two individual 5 mm endoscopes (**b**) and camera (**c**) with right and left optical channels, as well as the new Xi-endoscope (**d**) (Reproduced with permission from Intuitive Surgical, Inc © 2015)

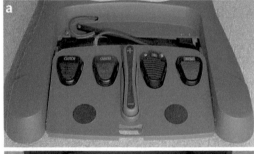

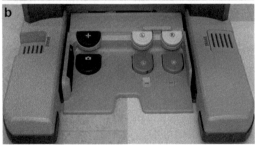

Fig. 3.10 Photograph of foot switch panels from the da Vinci® S (**a**) and Xi (**b**) systems with pedals for clutch, camera, focus control, accessory/bipolar, and monopolar electrocautery

master controller toggles between control of the current arm to the third robotic arm. Tapping the

clutch pedal once again will toggle back to the default settings and control of the original robotic arm. This feature allows the surgeon to toggle control of two different robotic arms using the same master controller. Completely depressing the clutch pedal disengages the master controls from the instrument arms, and the surgeon can readjust their arms to a more comfortable position in the working space. The Xi model has separate pedals for foot clutching and toggling of the robotic arms. Adjusting the working space is similar to moving a computer mouse when the limits of the mouse pad are reached. We generally recommend adjusting the working space when your elbows start to lift off of the armrest, your hands are in an awkward position, or if the master controllers are colliding with the sidewalls or with one another.

Completely depressing the camera pedal disengages the master controls from the instrument arms and instead engages the endoscope. The endoscope may then be moved or rotated to the appropriate area of interest within the body by manipulating the master controllers in a coordinated manner. Tapping the camera pedal on the S system activates the auxiliary visual channels in the lower third of the stereoviewer which can be connected to intraoperative monitors or ultrasound allowing for picture-in-picture view (called TilePro™, Intuitive Surgical Inc., Sunnyvale, CA). There is a focus control pedal on the standard and S systems for the endoscope labeled "+/−" in the center of the footswitch panel. The standard system has an auxiliary pedal, while the S system has a bipolar pedal that can be connected to bipolar energy. The electrocautery pedal is connected to a compatible electrosurgical unit. For instance, the da Vinci® Xi system utilizes the ERBE VIO dV (ERBE USA, Inc, Marietta, GA) electrosurgical unit to provide monopolar and bipolar energy. This system is located on the vision cart and provides the non-sterile OR staff with opportunities to adjust the settings for cut, as well as monopolar and bipolar electrocautery.

With the dual energy capabilities, one instrument arm can be connected to bipolar energy while the other one is connected to monopolar energy. The Si-HD and Xi systems have a completely remodeled foot panel with two tiers of pedals as well as pedals on the side of the panel (Fig. 3.10). The clutch and camera pedals remain on the left side of the panel, while on the right side there is a cut and coagulation pedal for each of the arms currently in use (labeled right and left). The pedals on the side of the panel are used to switch control between the two surgeons in dual console mode. In addition, the footswitch panel on the right can be used to change the coagulation pedal to bipolar mode.

Another interesting feature is present with the newer systems. When the surgeon's foot is held over a set of pedals, prior to depressing the pedal, a green border will be seen around the associated side of the view screen. This function assists with confirming appropriate foot placement prior to initiating electrocautery. This feature prevents inadvertent electrosurgical activation of the wrong instrument arm. On all of the systems, the back of the surgeon console houses the AC power connection, color-coded cable connections, bipolar and monopolar electrocautery inputs, and additional audio and visual connections.

Patient Cart

The patient cart for the standard and S systems houses the camera and instrument arms (Figs. 3.11 and 3.12) [2, 9]. Each arm has several clutch

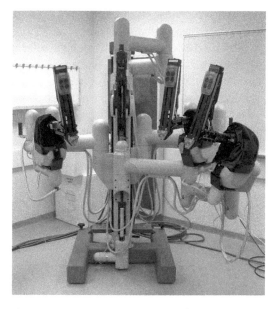

Fig. 3.11 Photograph of the da Vinci® standard patient cart with optional third instrument arm

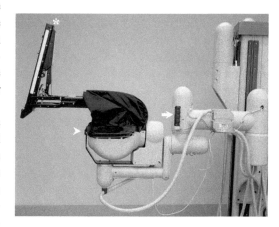

Fig. 3.12 Photograph of the da Vinci® standard instrument arm showing the port clutch joystick button (*arrow*), port clutch button (*arrowhead*), and instrument clutch button (*asterisks*) used to position the arm for draping, docking, and storage

buttons that assist with the gross movements of the arm and to insert or withdraw instruments. To activate the clutch, the buttons are depressed and the arm is moved. Otherwise, there will be resistance encountered and the arm will return to the original position. Each arm has two port clutch buttons used for gross movements of the instrument arm, and there is a specific camera or instrument clutch button located at the top of each arm to adjust the final trajectory of the arm during docking and to insert or withdraw endoscope/instruments. Each arm requires several sterile accessories that are placed during the draping procedure (Fig. 3.13).

The standard system was originally offered with a camera arm and two instrument arms. Later, an optional third instrument arm became available for new standard systems or could be added as an upgrade to existing systems. The third instrument arm is mounted on the same axis as the camera arm (Figs. 3.14 and 3.15). Therefore, care must be taken when positioning the third arm so that it does not collide with the other arms or operating room table. Each arm on the standard system is color coded with the camera arm (blue) and the instrument arms (yellow, green, and red). When moving the instrument arms using the trocar clutch, you should use your free hand to brace the instrument arm for better control. With the standard system, you can only use one clutch at a time to move the instrument arm. With the S, Si, and Xi systems you can use the trocar clutch and camera/instrument clutch simultaneously to maneuver the arm into position in a more dynamic manner.

Similar to the standard system, the S and Si systems have a camera arm and two instrument arms and are available with an optional third instrument arm. Each instrument arm is numbered. These models also added an LED light below the camera/instrument clutch and a touchscreen monitor. The LED light communicates the status of the arm to the surgical team using a preset color scheme. The touchscreen monitor is synchronized with the surgeon's view and displays all of the system status icons and messages. It can be used for endoscope alignment, telestration, or to toggle between video inputs. The telestration feature can be used to draw real-time images on the screen that are relayed to the ste-

reoviewer. This feature is especially useful for training residents or fellows. The touchscreen monitor can also be mounted on the vision cart. The patient side cart of the S, Si, and Xi systems also feature a motor drive (Fig. 3.16a, b), which assists in docking the patient cart to the operating table and trocars. All cable connections are located at the back of the cart.

The Xi system patient cart is equipped with several other new features. The boom height can be adjusted by both the sterile or non-sterile personnel during the procedure, allowing real-time adjustments to be made during cart positioning. To help with this, there is a horizontal laser mounted to the superior most aspect of the patient care. A green horizontal line is projected outwards to help guide cart movement and prevent inadvertent collisions with other operating room equipment. There is a patient cart touchpad located on the back of the patient cart (Fig. 3.16b). The touchpad allows the non-sterile staff to select target anatomy as well as place the patient cart in stow mode. Just below the touchpad there is a boom control joystick that can be activated by pressing the "Enable Joystick" button located in the upper right of the touchpad. This allows non-sterile OR personnel to manually control the boom position. On the downside of the boom, there is another targeting laser that projects downward. The patient cart should be positioned such that the target laser projects onto the area of target anatomy, allowing optimal positioning of the endoscope and robotic arms. Finally, there are a total of four separate arms. An important feature unique to the Xi model is the ability to interchange the endoscope between all arms, allowing more versatility for approaching different procedures. For the Xi system, the arms are still denoted by numbers. However, the number sequence is reversed on the Xi when compared to the S and SI-systems.

Vision Cart

The vision cart (Fig. 3.17) contains the light source, video processing equipment, camera focus control, and camera storage bin [2, 9]. There are also several empty storage areas that

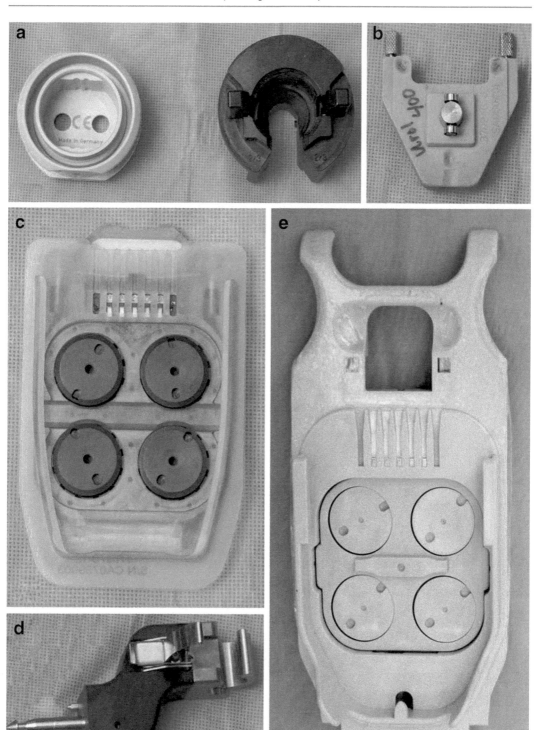

Fig. 3.13 Photographs of sterile accessories placed during the draping procedure. (**a**) Camera sterile adapter (*left*) and camera arm sterile adapter (*right*). Da Vinci® standard trocar mount (**b**), instrument arm sterile adapter (**c**), and camera trocar mount (**d**). The instrument arm sterile adapter may be reused 50 times (**e**). Da Vinci® S instrument arm sterile adapter can only be used one time before being discarded

can be used for insufflators, electrosurgical units, or a DVD recording device. A telemonitor may be placed on the top of the tower. In the newer models, this telemonitor is equipped with a touchscreen. As was mentioned previously, this allows non-sterile OR team members to assist with adjustment of endoscope alignment, make changes in the video input, and utilize the telestration feature.

The system's light source is a xenon fiber optic system with a lamp life of approximately 500 h. On the standard and S systems, the light source is connected to the endoscope by a sterile bifurcated cable to illuminate the right and left channels, while the Si has a single cable. On some of the standard systems, two light sources and two cables were required. The lamp on the S and S-HD systems can be changed by a member from the surgical team, while the standard systems require a service visit.

The endoscope is available as a 0° and 30° lens. We typically use the 30° downward lens for most robotic procedures in the pelvis, while a variety of endoscopes (i.e., 0°, 30° upward, 30° downward) are used for interventions of the upper urinary tract depending on the particular procedure and approach as well as surgeon preference. With the standard and S systems, the endoscope is connected to either a high-magnification (×15 magnification with 45° view) or wide-angle (×10 magnification with 60° view) camera head with right and left optical channels. The HD systems only come with one camera (see below). The right and left optical channels are connected to two 3-chip camera control units

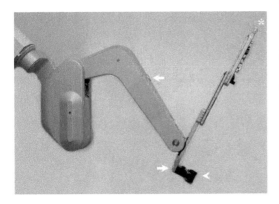

Fig. 3.14 Photograph of the da Vinci® S and HD instrument arm showing the port clutch buttons (*arrows*) and instrument clutch button with LED indicator (*asterisks*). Also seen is the trocar mount (*arrowhead*)

a   b

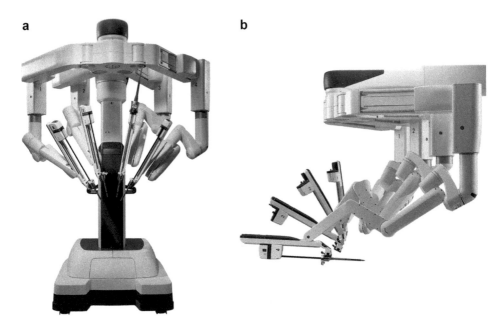

Fig. 3.15 Photograph of the da Vinci® Xi patient cart (**a**) and surgical arms (**b**) (Reproduced with permission from Intuitive Surgical, Inc © 2015)

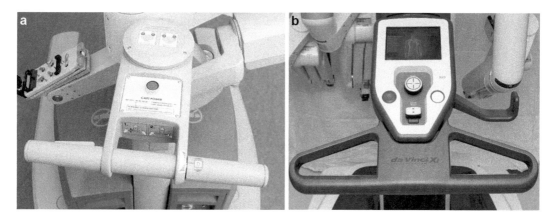

Fig. 3.16 Photograph of the back of the da Vinci® S (**a**) and Xi (**b**) patient cart showing the power switch and motor drive controls

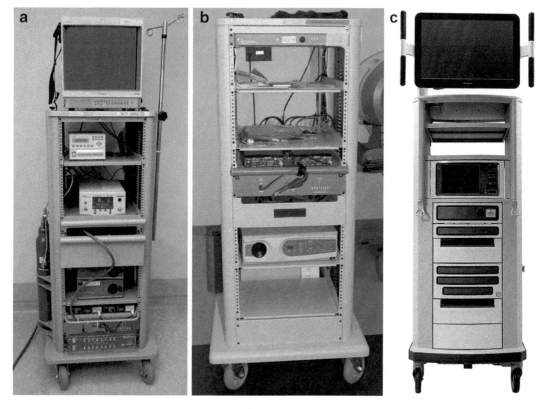

Fig. 3.17 Photographs of vision cart for the da Vinci® standard (**a**), S (**b**), and Xi (**c**) systems (Reproduced with permission from Intuitive Surgical, Inc © 2015)

(CCU). The input from these CCUs is integrated in the surgeon console to produce the three-dimensional image. The camera head is also connected to an automatic focus control that is linked to the surgeon console. The S-HD system adds a high definition camera and CCUs to increase resolution and aspect ratio. The first generation HD system had a resolution of 720p (1280×720) which is significantly increased from standard NTSC 720×480. The aspect ratio also increases to 16:9, which improves the viewing area by 20%. The system also has a digital zoom that allows the surgeon to magnify the tissue without moving the endoscope. This is done by pressing the left and right arrow keys on the left-side pod controls or depressing the camera pedal and moving the masters together or apart. The Si-HD system is equipped with increased resolution to 1080i (1920×1080). The patient cart for the Si-HD was remodeled to integrate the light source and camera control unit into single connections. In addition, the camera adjustments and white balance are performed using the central touchpad or telemonitor.

The Xi model contains a new vision system. In comparison to prior models, control selection of the endoscope (30° up/down, 0°) can be made at the surgeon's console. At the time of this writing, software enhancements continue to be made to the optic system to make the images as realistic as possible compared with traditional open surgery. For instance, at times, the source of intraperitoneal bleeding can appear "white" with the current vision system. The smaller (8-mm) optic has also been associated with an increased need for optic cleaning secondary to splatter from the surgical field and steam production clouding the vision of the optic field.

EndoWrist® Instruments

The EndoWrist® instruments (Fig. 3.18) carry out motions originating from the master controllers. The instruments have seven degrees of freedom with 180° of articulation and 540° of rotation simulating a surgeon's hand and wrist movements (Fig. 3.19). The instruments are designed to actually reduce surgeon tremor.

Each instrument has a fixed number of uses before becoming deactivated. The system automatically tracks the number of uses remaining on each instrument and communicates this in the stereoviewer. An instrument arm will not function if an outdated instrument is loaded [9]. We have found that some EndoWrist® instruments, particularly the monopolar scissors, tend to degrade and become ineffective before all lives are exhausted. We recommend, from a standpoint of patient safety, that only fully functional instruments be used for robotic procedures.

EndoWrist® instruments are composed of an instrument housing with energy cable attachments and release levers, instrument shaft, wrist, and a variety of instrument tips (Fig. 3.18). The housing also has a manual instrument release socket available in the event that the surgeon is unable to release the grip via control at the surgeon console. The da Vinci® standard instruments are 52 cm with grey housing compared to the S systems arm length of 57 cm with blue housing. The working length for the da Vinci® Xi instruments ranges from approximately 30 to 34 cm. The instruments are not interchangeable between the systems. Currently, there are more than 40 EndoWrist® instruments available in 8 mm or 5 mm shaft diameters and several have been designed specifically for urologic surgery. The 8 mm instruments operate on an "angled joint" compared to the 5 mm on a "snake joint" (Fig. 3.20). The angled joint allows the tip to rotate using a shorter radius compared to the snake joint. We have consistently used the 8 mm ProGrasp™ forceps (Intuitive Surgical, Inc., Sunnyvale, CA), monopolar curved shears, large needle driver, and Maryland bipolar forceps for our robotics practice.

Fig. 3.18 Photograph of an EndoWrist® instrument for the standard (**a**) and S (**b**) systems

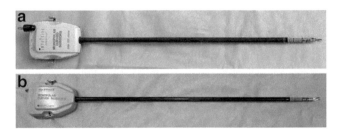

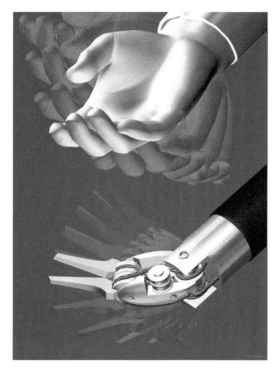

Fig. 3.19 Illustration comparing surgeon hand movements to EndoWrist® instrument

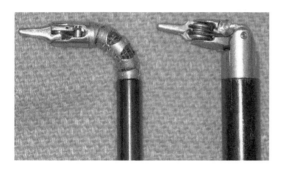

Fig. 3.20 Photograph of EndoWrist® needle drivers. On the left is a 5 mm needle driver with the "snake joint" compared to the 8 mm needle driver with an "angled joint"

Preparing the da Vinci® for Surgery

Preparing the operating room for robotic-assisted procedures begins well before the patient enters the room. Once the equipment is positioned, the surgical team can prepare the system [8].

1. Connect system cables, optical channels, focus control, and power cables, and turn the system on. The system will then perform a self-test. During this time, do not attempt to manipulate the system or a fault may be triggered.

2. Position the instrument and camera arms so they have adequate room to move.

3. Initiate homing sequence.

4. Drape the patient cart arms. This takes a coordinated team effort between surgical technician and circulating nurse and uses system-specific sterile drapes and accessories. Make sure the drapes are not too tight as this may decrease the range of motion of the robotic arms.

   (a) The instrument arms are draped to completely cover the arm and the sterile instrument adapter is locked into the instrument arm carriage. For the standard system, the sterile trocar mount is also locked into position, while the S system has the trocar mount permanently attached and the drape is placed over the mount.

   (b) The camera arm is draped in a similar fashion. For the standard system, a sterile endoscope trocar mount and camera arm sterile adapter are also placed at this time. The S system also requires a camera arm sterile adapter. Depending on when the S system was purchased, some use a sterile endoscope trocar mount, while others have the mount permanently attached. There are different robotic camera arm trocar mounts for each trocar manufacturer.

   (c) The touchscreen monitor is draped for the S systems.

5. Drape the endoscope by connecting the camera sterile adapter to the endoscope and then taping the drape to the sterile adapter. The camera head is connected, and the drape is inverted over the camera head and optical cables.

6. Connect the light source to the endoscope with the sterile light cable. Perform a black and white balance.

7. Align the endoscope and set endoscope settings (three dimensional vs. two dimensional, 0° vs. 30° up or down).

8. Set the "sweet spot" of the camera arm by aligning the trocar mount with the center of

the patient cart column and extending the camera arm so there is approximately 20″ between the back of the camera arm and patient cart. The S systems have a guide on the camera arm to assist with setting the sweet spot. This allows maximal range of motion of the camera and instrument arms and prevents collisions. The Xi system features a targeting laser to help with trocar alignment at the time of patient cart docking.

Patient Cart Docking

After abdominal access is obtained, and trocars are placed, the patient cart is maneuvered into position to align the patient cart tower, camera arm, and target anatomy. One member of the surgical team drives the patient cart while another member guides the driver. To avoid any confusion during docking, it is recommended that the navigator use anatomic or room references versus directional cues. The surgical table should be placed in the desired position (Trendelenburg, etc.) prior to docking the patient cart.

The standard system is pushed into position and the brakes at the base of the cart are hand-tightened. The S, Si, and Xi systems have a motor drive to assist with docking. However, use of the motor drive is not mandatory for the docking process (Fig. 3.16). To operate the motor drive, unlock the brakes and turn the shift switches on the base of the cart to the drive position. Engage the motor drive by holding the throttle-enable switch on the left and turning the throttle forward or backward with the right hand. To move the cart without the motor drive assist, turn the shift switches to neutral. With the newer systems, there is no mechanical brake, and once an instrument arm is connected to a trocar, the motor drive brakes automatically to keep the cart from moving.

The endoscope arm should be the first one connected to the patient by locking the endoscope trocar mount to the endoscope trocar. It is important to use the camera setup joint buttons to move the camera arm into position and the camera clutch to adjust the final trajectory of the arm.

Exclusively using the camera clutch to move the camera arm may limit the range of motion of the camera during surgery. The instrument arms are then attached to the robotic trocars and screwed into place using a twist-lock device when using a standard system. When using the S or Si system, snap mounted devices are used to engage the robotic trocars. When using the Xi system, a "click-in" type engagement system is used. Again, use the port clutch for gross movements of the instrument arms and the instrument clutch for the final trajectory. When using the standard system with the third instrument arm for surgery of the pelvis, the arm comes from below the table and wraps around the patients leg. Care must be taken when docking to avoid collision, contact, or pinching the patient's arm, body, or leg.

Once all of the robotic arms are connected, the surgical team should check each of the arms for proper working distance and make sure the arms are not compressing the patient. The endoscope is inserted by placing the lens into the trocar and locking it into the camera trocar mount. The endoscope can then be advanced into the surgical field using the camera clutch button. EndoWrist® instruments are inserted by straightening the instrument wrist, placing the closed instrument tip into the trocar, and sliding the instrument housing into the adapter, ensuring that it is seated well and locked into place. The instrument is then advanced into the surgical field using the instrument clutch button. Each instrument should be placed into the patient under direct laparoscopic vision. With the Xi system, there is a longer processing delay that occurs before the instrument can be used in comparison to prior versions.

To remove an instrument, the surgeon should straighten the instrument wrist and the assistant squeezes the release levers and pulls the instrument out. Maintaining close communication between the surgeon and assistant, especially during instrument exchanges, is important so as to avoid inadvertent adjustment, movement, and complete removal of an instrument that is in active use. As a safety measure, the S and Xi systems feature a "guided tool change" where a new instrument can be inserted and placed to a depth

1–3 mm short of the previous instrument position. On the Xi system, when the guided tool change feature is activated, a blinking green light will be seen on the robotic arm. This feature is disabled when the instrument clutch is engaged or when there is a system error. If disabled, the arms should be exchanged under direct laparoscopic visualization.

For surgery of the pelvis, the surgical team can take their positions for the procedure (Figs. 3.1 and 3.2). The surgeon sits at the console, circulating nurse at their workstation, surgical technician on the patient's left, and the surgical assistant on patient's right side. When using a system with two instrument arms, a second surgical assistant or the surgical technician can assist with the procedure from the patient's left side. In this instance, the second assistant uses a separately prepared Mayo stand with the instruments they need to complete the case. Using a third instrument arm can often eliminate the need for a second surgical assistant during the procedure. The cost and benefits of the third instrument arm must be weighed against the cost of a second assistant.

The patient cart docking process is longer and more detailed with the new da Vinci® Xi system. Once abdominal access has been obtained, a non-sterile OR staff member should select the appropriate anatomy and cart location options on the touchpad that is located on the back of the patient cart. Next, the "Deploy for Docking" button should be pressed and held, resulting in movement of the boom as it positions itself for docking. A beeping noise will be heard throughout this step. When this step is complete, a "double chime" can be heard. At this point, the cart can be maneuvered into position. Appropriate patient cart positioning is verified by aligning the cross hairs of the targeting laser to the location of the initial endoscope trocar. The endoscope arm should be locked into position with the endoscope trocar. The patient cart stabilization feet can then be deployed to lock the carts position during the procedure. The endoscope is then locked and the clutch button deployed to move the endoscope into the abdomen, pointing at the target anatomy. The endoscope targeting function is then deployed by pressing the targeting button on the endoscope

itself. The remaining three arms are then attached to their respective trocars. If only three arms are required for a procedure, the remaining arm can be stowed. However, this arm should be draped as it will inevitably come into contact with the operative field. As was previously discussed, the Xi system allows the surgeon to utilize any of the four arms for the endoscope, and the camera location can be switched intraoperatively.

System Shutdown

Once robotic-assisted surgery is completed, all of the instruments are removed first, followed by the endoscope. The arms are disconnected from the trocars, and the patient cart is undocked from the patient. For the S and Si systems, the motor drive system cannot be activated until all the instruments are removed, and the camera and instrument arms are disconnected. The specimen is delivered within a specimen retrieval bag by extending one of the incisions. This incision and any 12 mm trocars made with a cutting trocar require fascial closure to prevent incisional hernias. The 8 and 5 mm trocars generally do not require fascial closure [4, 5]. Once the surgery is completed, the sterile accessories and drapes are removed and the system is cleaned. It is not necessary to power the system off between surgical procedures. With the new Xi-system, the "Stow" button, located on the patient cart touchpad, should be pressed and held. Information regarding instruments used during the procedure will be seen on the screen. Although not necessary, the system can then be powered down by pressing the "Power" button that is located on the patient cart, vision cart, or surgeon console. The power down process takes approximately 10 s to complete.

Conclusions

Robotic-assisted urologic surgery has increased significantly over the past decade. Successful implementation of a robotics program hinges on proper operating room setup and a complete understanding of instrumentation required. Selection of the robotic system is also an important consideration. To date, the benefit from the Xi robot seems greatest when performing multi-quadrant robotic procedures. For procedures involving work in one predominant anatomic area, any robotic model will typically suffice. In addition, a knowledgeable, well-trained and collegial surgical team is crucial for operating room dynamics and likely contributes to positive patient outcomes.

References

1. Gettman MT, Cadeddu JA. Robotics in urologic surgery. In: Graham SD, Keane TE, Glenn JF, editors. Glenn's urologic surgery. Philadelphia: Lippincott Williams & Wilkins; 2004. p. 1027–33.
2. Narula VK, Melvin SM. Robotic surgical systems. In: Patel VR, editor. Robotic urologic surgery. London: Springer; 2007. p. 5–14.
3. Mahida JB, et al. Utilization and costs associated with robotic surgery in children. J Surg Res. 2015;199(1): 169–76.
4. Gettman MT, et al. Current status of robotics in urologic laparoscopy. Eur Urol. 2003;43(2):106–12.
5. Su LM, Smith Jr JA. Laparoscopic and robotic assisted laparoscopic radical prostatectomy and pelvic lymphadenectomy. In: Wein AJ, Kavoussi LR, Novick AC, Partin AW, Peters CA, editors. Campbell-Walsh urology. Philadelphia: Saunders Elsevier; 2007. p. 2985–3005.
6. Gettman MT, et al. Laparoscopic radical prostatectomy: description of the extraperitoneal approach using the da Vinci robotic system. J Urol. 2003;170(2 Pt 1):416–9.
7. Gettman MT, et al. Robotic-assisted laparoscopic partial nephrectomy: technique and initial clinical experience with DaVinci robotic system. Urology. 2004;64(5):914–8.
8. Joyce AD, Beerlage H, Janetscheck G. Urological laparoscopy for beginners. Eur Urol. 2000;38(3):365–73.
9. Bhandari A, Hemal A, Menon M. Instrumentation, sterilization, and preparation of robot. Indian J Urol. 2005;21(2):83–5.

Anesthetic Considerations with Robotic Surgery

4

Christopher Giordano, Nikolaus Gravenstein, and Huong Thi Thu Le

Introduction

The popularity of minimally invasive surgery has increased exponentially over the past two decades, and urologic robotic surgery has been at the forefront. This rapid growth has been accompanied by many lessons on how to best manage the complex set of physiologic perturbations that patients experience during these procedures. In particular, the typical urologic surgery combines requirements of lithotomy, steep Trendelenburg, and pneumoperitoneum, which create unique challenges for the patient and anesthesiologist. Also challenging are the limited access to the patient, the generally longer duration of surgery, and the complexities of having a docked robot. This chapter will cover the pearls and pitfalls of considerations for robotic urologic surgery from an anesthetic perspective.

C. Giordano, M.D. (✉) • N. Gravenstein, M.D.
H.T.T. Le, M.D.
Department of Anesthesiology, University of Florida College of Medicine, 1600 SW Archer Road, PO Box 100254, Gainesville, FL 32608, USA
e-mail: cgiordano@anest.ufl.edu

Pneumoperitoneum

To best visualize internal structures, the pelvis and abdominal cavities are insufflated with carbon dioxide (CO_2) to create a pneumoperitoneum. Because CO_2 is inert (i.e., does not support combustion) and is most easily accommodated by the physiologic systems if it becomes intravascular or subcutaneous, it is the exclusive gas of choice for pneumoperitoneum insufflation and maintenance. The first major effect of a CO_2 pneumoperitoneum is an abrupt increase in intra-abdominal pressures, which is often accompanied by a vagal response. The vagal response follows peritoneal distension and manifests as a decrease in heart rate—especially with rapid insufflation (>2 L/min). The rate of insufflation is controlled by the access device (needle < port) and the insufflating gas flow rate. If a vagal response does occur, it is treated by desufflation and administration of an anticholinergic such as atropine or glycopyrrolate. Table 4.1 summarizes the impact of the pneumoperitoneum on normal physiology. Increased intra-abdominal pressures compress the inferior vena cava and decrease venous return. In addition, there are the accumulating effects of absorbed CO_2 on the homeostasis of different organ systems. Patients generally tolerate hypercapnia, and human physiology is well adapted to compensate for mild acidosis. However, if the pH falls below 7.1 as a consequence of arterial CO_2 ($PaCO_2$) rising to 80 mmHg, normal hemostatic functions such as drug metabolism and coagulation, as well

© Springer International Publishing Switzerland 2017
L.-M. Su (ed.), *Atlas of Robotic Urologic Surgery*, DOI 10.1007/978-3-319-45060-5_4

Table 4.1 Impact of pneumoperitoneum and steep Trendelenburg position on physiology

Source	Pneumoperitoneum (PP)	Steep Trendelenburg (ST)	PP + ST
CVP	↑	↑	↑
CO	↔	↑	↑
SVR	↑	↑	↔
MAP	↑	↑	↑
Airway compliance	↓	↓	↓
Airway pressure	↑	↑	↑
FRC	↓	↓	↓
ICP	↑	↑	↑
CBF	↑ *	↔	↑ *
VBF	↓	↓	↓
Ocular pressure	↑	↑	↑
CPP	↓	↔	↔

PP + ST = partially additive effects
= changes due to intra-abdominal compression of aorta
* = if hypercarbic

as the cardiopulmonary system, become compromised. Additionally, the increased $PaCO_2$ from intraoperative CO_2 deposition can be troublesome if the elevated $PaCO_2$ is coupled with narcotic administration, obesity, or a pulmonary disease state such as chronic obstructive pulmonary disease, which limits ventilation. For these reasons, vigilant postoperative anesthesia care unit monitoring is needed.

Reflexively correcting an acidosis from hypercarbia with sodium bicarbonate actually intensifies the CO_2 burden (>1 L of CO_2 released per 50 meq ampule of sodium bicarbonate) and will also increase intravascular volume from the hypertonicity of the sodium bicarbonate. This increased fluid volume may exacerbate the development of orbital, corneal, pulmonary, and laryngeal edema.

Insufflation Techniques

The first consideration for pneumoperitoneum is the choice of entry into the abdominal cavity. The most widely used technique is the Veress needle (VN) despite it having a slower insufflation rate and potentially life-threatening complications. The VN may accidentally and undetectably puncture a vessel and lead to occult bleeding into the retroperitoneum or blood pooled away from surgical view due to positioning. A more immediate and catastrophic injury is introduction of the VN into a major blood vessel, resulting in brisker bleeding or a CO_2 embolus. If the rate and volume of intravascular CO_2 is large enough, right heart and pulmonary circulation will be obstructed, which leads to cardiovascular collapse. Similarly, if the insufflation tubing is not first bled of air, which is 78% nitrogen, with CO_2 gas, intravascular penetration could create a lethal nitrogen venous air embolism. A nitrogen venous air embolism is more likely to cause cardiac arrest then a CO_2 embolus because of nitrogen's much lower solubility in blood. A symptomatic air or CO_2 embolism is treated by placing the patient in the head down left lateral decubitus position (Durant maneuver), administering fluid and inotropic support, and performing chest compressions during low or no cardiac output.

An alternative technique to insufflation with a VN is direct trocar insertion. This technique decreases the opportunities of insufflating areas other than the peritoneal cavity because it is done under direct visualization, but it affords a greater likelihood of extensive subcutaneous emphysema that extends along contiguous fascial planes up to and including the face. Once properly positioned, the trocar can deliver higher a CO_2 insufflation flow rate. A faster insufflation rate has two drawbacks: it increases the likelihood of cardiac bradyarrhythmias and it contributes to the referred pain from pneumoperitoneum. The surgeon should be prepared to quickly desufflate the abdomen in the cases of severe bradycardia or asystole, and the anesthesiologist should consider administering anticholinergic drugs to attenuate the bradycardia and hypotension. In severe cases, low doses of epinephrine are given.

A third approach is the open entry technique, which is typically only used with patients who have undergone previous abdominal operations and who are thus at risk for multiple adhesions. This entry approach includes many of the same insufflation and hemodynamic concerns as the direct trocar insertion approach.

Insufflation Pressures

Following the entry of the insufflating device, the surgeon may commence to the target insufflation pressure or briefly exceed the goal in order to place trocars into a maximally dilated cavity.

The goal pressure for creating a pneumoperitoneum has been much debated. The consensus appears to be 12–15 mmHg of pressure. Insufflation pressures of 12–15 mmHg will increase CO_2 absorption progressively throughout the case and require ventilator adjustments to increase the patient's minute ventilation. Increasing the insufflation pressure to 20 mmHg slightly improves surgical visualization and reduces blood loss by tamponading venous oozing, but these elevated pressures incrementally add risk and increase CO_2 absorption in the patient. Some of these risks include cardiac arrhythmias, lung barotrauma, renal and hepatic hypoperfusion, respiratory acidosis, increased postoperative pain, and postoperative nausea and vomiting. Thus, from a physiologic standpoint and in the Trendelenburg position, pressures above 15 mmHg may be tolerated but should be used conservatively.

Complications of the Pneumoperitoneum

Subcutaneous Emphysema
Subcutaneous emphysema is found on the x-ray films of approximately 34–77% patients after laparoscopic operations [1]. Subcutaneous emphysema (Fig. 4.1) occurs when insufflated CO_2 extravasates from the peritoneal space into the subcutaneous tissues. The palpable crepitus of subcutaneous emphysema can extend from the

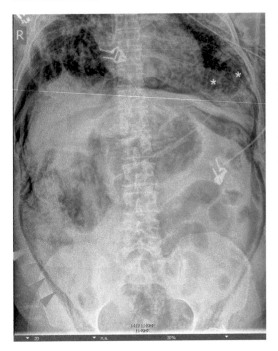

Fig. 4.1 Subcutaneous emphysema occurs when insufflated CO_2 extravasates from the peritoneal space into the subcutaneous tissues

abdomen to the genitalia to the eyes. Patient risk increases for such a situation as age increases and body mass index drops below 25. Additional risk factors include duration of surgery, insufflation pressures, number of ports, direct trocar insertion, and extraperitoneal and retroperitoneal approaches. Although subcutaneous emphysema is generally thought of as a benign postinsufflation finding, it can be misdiagnosed as necrotizing fasciitis. The crepitus will usually resolve within hours to several days after the discontinuation of insufflation. However, severe subcutaneous emphysema may lead to postoperative hypercarbia as CO_2 reenters the bloodstream from tissue deposition.

Capnothorax, Capnomediastinum, and Capnopericardium

Capnothorax is not an infrequent complication following CO_2 pneumoperitoneum. The first indication of a developing capnothorax is progressive hypercapnia despite appropriate escalation in minute ventilation. It should concern the

anesthesiologist that the CO_2 pneumoperitoneum is dissecting through pleuro-peritoneal connections and is increasing the normal rate of CO_2 absorption. Alternatively, the anesthesiologist may observe that pulmonary compliance becomes progressively lower. This phenomenon is more common in patients who have incompetent diaphragms or hiatal hernias. In such patients, the abdominal pneumoperitoneum dissects into the thoracic cavity, compresses lung parenchyma, decreases V/Q matching, and creates a shunt physiology from atelectasis. Transthoracic ultrasound is a useful and readily accessible tool for detecting capnothorax in the operating room because the normal visceral pleural movement is absent with gas outside the lung and in the thorax.

Interventions for capnothorax include desufflation or at least lowering the insufflation pressure to 10 mmHg or less in the presence of hemodynamic compromise, increasing positive end-expiratory pressure, increasing the inspiratory-to-expiratory ratio to lengthen inspiratory pressure time, and switching to pressure-controlled ventilation. If there is a decrease in blood pressure, elevated jugular venous distension, and hypoxemia, the capnothorax may be under tension and immediate desufflation is required. Most commonly, capnothoraces reabsorb on their own and do not require chest tube drainage, as there is no visceral pleural injury.

Capnomediastinum can develop from progressive CO_2 dissection from a capnothorax into the mediastinum. The mediastinum, which contains the heart and major vessels, esophagus, and trachea, can become so compressed from CO_2 that there is obstruction of venous return to the heart. Capnopericardium has been reported as a predominantly incidental finding but can result in cardiac tamponade in patients who have been mechanically ventilated. Due to the high solubility of CO_2, conservative management of capnopericardium and capnomediastinum is advised in clinically stable patients. A more aggressive approach may be recommended for symptomatic or unstable patients. The first step is always to desufflate. If reinsufflation is needed, a lower insufflation pressure is recommended. As a frame of reference, most patients do not tolerate intra-thoracic pressures (capnothorax) >10 mmHg, while most laparoscopic abdominal and pelvic procedures are done at >10 mmHg insufflation pressures.

Postoperative Pneumoperitoneum

Postoperative pneumoperitoneum is the presence of free air in the abdomen after surgery. In lapa-roscopy, the free air usually occurs because of CO_2 insufflation, and the expected amount of intraperitoneal air is less than that seen after a laparotomy. This is possibly due to the rapid absorption of CO_2 and the small ports used in robotic or laparoscopic surgery. Postoperative pneumoperitoneum is considered to be a self-limiting process. Forty percent of patients will have more than 2 cm of free air below the dia-phragm on upright radiographs obtained 24 h after laparoscopy with minimal effects on post-operative pain by 48 h after surgery [2].

Choice of Anesthesia

General Anesthesia

General anesthesia with an endotracheal tube and controlled mechanical ventilation is the most common choice for laparoscopic and robotic urologic surgery. This technique neces-sitates a secured airway, controlled ventilation, and muscle relaxation. Not only is general anes-thesia the most comfortable option for most patients, but endotracheal intubation is also rec-ommended to protect the patient's airway from aspiration. This is especially important for patients with frank gastroesophageal reflux. Suggestions for pre-, intra-, and postoperative management of these patients is highlighted in Fig. 4.2a–c, which is modified from the "verti-cals and threads" describing the University of Florida perioperative approach [3].

Complete muscle paralysis is highly recom-mended to prevent any patient movement while the robot is docked, as any patient movement can easily injure the patient. Using dense neuromus-cular blockade with paralytic drugs has been

shown to provide minor improvements in peritoneal cavity size with 12 mmHg of insufflation pressure. Along with facilitating the creation of pneumoperitoneum and the introduction and exchange of robotic instruments, muscle relax-ation improves mechanical ventilation by relax-ing the intra-abdominal and intrathoracic musculature, which increases thoracic compli-ance and helps reduce the airway pressures nec-essary to ventilate the patient in the presence of a pneumoperitoneum and steep Trendelenburg.

Controlled mechanical ventilation also allows the intraoperative team to optimize $PaCO_2$ levels. $PaCO_2$ is usually reflected by end-tidal CO_2 (Et-CO_2) on the capnograph. Using volume-controlled ventilation keeps minute ventilation constant in the presence of fluctuating intra-abdominal pressure.

Although not reported for robotic surgery, laparoscopic urologic surgery can be performed under general anesthesia using a laryngeal-mask airway (LMA). Compared to general anesthesia with an endotracheal tube, using an LMA makes it much more difficult to control $PaCO_2$ and achieve necessary airway pressures, and may place the patient at elevated risk for aspiration.

General anesthesia can be maintained with exclusively inhalational agents, a total intrave-nous anesthetic technique, or a combination of the two. These are choices of style rather than substance. Inhalational anesthetics include des-flurane, isoflurane, sevoflurane, and nitrous oxide. When administered over several hours, nitrous oxide will diffuse into the bowel, obstruct-ing the surgical field as well as introducing the risk of fire in the case of a bowel perforation due to its combustibility. Nitrous oxide has also been purported to increase the incidence of postopera-tive nausea and vomiting (PONV). Subsequently, the authors do not recommend its use in these cases or at least limiting its use to the end of the procedure.

Intravenous anesthetics include propofol, midazolam, narcotics, and ketamine. The decision to choose one specific drug or drug combination to accomplish general anesthesia depends on the patient's coexisting diseases and PONV risk. The total intravenous anesthetic technique has been

a

Decisions for Up to Day of Surgery	Minimal Complexity	Moderate Complexity	Maximum Complexity
Labs	none except for co-morbidities	CBC, BMP,ABO screening	CBC, BMP,eGFR, ABO screening
Anesthesia PreOp Visit status	Phone PreOp Eligible	Clinic Preop	Clinic Preop
Nutrition	Usual NPO startegies	Complex CHO loading	Complex CHO loading
Age > 80	none except for co-morbidities	ECG, GUGT	ECG, GUGT,prealbumin,MMCT
CHF, compensated	Echo in past 2 yrs if no change in functional capacity for EF % 30	Echo in past 2 yrs if no change in functional capacity for EF % 30	Cardiology assessemnt with UF Health clearance form
CHF, decompensated	Obtain dry weight, Echo, optimize	Obtain dry weight, Echo, optimize, risk stratification review	Obtain dry weight, Echo, optimize, risk stratification review
CAD > 4 METS	Continue Beta Blocker and ASA	ECG, continue Beta Blocker	ECG, continue Beta Blocker
CAD < 4 METS	ECG, continue Beta Blocker and ASA	ECG, continue Beta Blocker, cardiology consult is patient optimal,Risk stratification review	ECG, continue Beta Blocker, cardiology consult is patient optimal, Risk Stratification review
Unstable angina	Evaluation by cardiology	Evaluation by cardiology	Evaluation by cardiology
ESRD	K+ post last dialysis CBC BMP	K+ post last dialysis CBC BMP, detailed cardiac assessment	K+ post last dialysis CBC BMP, Risk Stratification review
Chronic Kidney Disease	eGFR, UA, BMP	eGFR, UA, BMP	eGFR, UA, BMP
Chronic pain > 30 mg MSO per day	Continue home pain medications on day of surgery	1. Prescribing pain physician contact information for follow up appointment post operatively; 2. Continue home pain medications on day of surgery; 3. Acute Pain Service Consult on admission; 4. Start preemptive pain protocol	1. Prescribing pain physician contact information for follow up appointment post operatively; 2. Continue home pain medications on day of surgery; 3. Acute Pain Service Consult on admission; 4. Start preemptive pain protocol
Diabetes, no history of DKA	Hgb A-1-C in past 6 months, optimize prior to surgery > 11	Hgb A-1-c in past 3 months, >9% acute care diabetes appt	Hgb A-1-c in past 3 months, > 9 acute care diabetes appt
Diabetes with history of DKA	Hgb A-1-C in past 3 months, optimize prior to surgery >11	Internal medicine	Internal Medicine consult
PONV risk	Multimodal antiemetics	Multimodal antiemetics	Multimodal antiemetics
Anticipate ICU stay	No	No except CHF	Yes

Fig. 4.2 (a) Considerations for preoperative management of patients up to the day of surgery are based on complexity of the disease and medical history. *eGFR* estimated glomerular filtration rate, *UA* urinanalysis, *BMP* basic metabolic panel, *Hgb A-1-c* hemoglobin A1C, *ECG* electrocardiogram, *MMCT* mini-mental cognitive test, *CHO* carbohydrate, *CBC* comprehensive blood count, *GUGT* Hopkins Frailty Exam; (b) Considerations for management of patients on the day of surgery are based on complexity of the disease and medical history. *BMP* basic metabolic panel, *Hgb A-1-c* hemoglobin A1C, *ECG* electrocardiogram, *CBC* comprehensive blood count; (c) Considerations for management of patients during their hospitalization are based on complexity of the disease and medical history. *MMCT* mini-mental cognitive test, *APS* acute pain service

b

Decisions for Day of Surgery	Minimal Complexity	Moderate Complexity	Maximum Complexity
Labs	none except for co-morbidities	Hct, BMP, ABO screening	CBC, T&S
Age > 80	Consider reduce induction meds	Consider reduce induction meds	Consider reduce induction meds
CAD	ECG filter set	ECG filter set	ECG filter set
IVF management	Consider 10cc/kg ideal 20cc/kg max	Consider 10cc/kg ideal 20cc/kg max replace UOP, EBL	Consider 10cc/kg ideal 20cc/kg max replace UOP, EBL
BMI > 35	Prepare CPAP for PACU	Consider extubation to BiPAP	Consider extubate to BiPAP
Chronic pain > 30 mg MSO per day	Instruct to continue meds	Pain management plan established preop	Pain management plan established preop
ESRD	Minimize fluids	Minimize fluids	Minimize fluids
Diabetes	Hgb A-1-c in past 6 months, >11 Acute Care Diabetes appointment	Hgb A-1-c in past 6 months, >10 acute care diabetes appt	Hgb A-1-c in past 6 months, > 9 acute care diabetes appt

c

Decisions for Hospitalization	Minimal Complexity	Moderate Complexity	Maximum Complexity
Age > 80		MMCT POD #1	MMCT POD #1
CHF	Daily weights. Obtain weight at POD#2	Daily weights. Obtain weight at POD#2	Daily weights. Obtain weight at POD#2
BMI > 35	Require OOB for meals and TID, SCD's in bed	Require OOB for meals and TID consider PT evalution, SCD's in bed	PT evaluation, SCD's in bed
Chronic pain > 30 mg MSO per day	Continue usual meds. Appt with usual pain provider prn.	Multi modal analgesia with APS consult, establish follow up plan. Appt with usual pain provider within 7 days of discharge	Multi modal analgesia with APS consult, establish follow up plan. Appt with usual pain provider within 7 days of discharge
ESRD	Continue usual dialysis schedule	Continue usual dialysis schedule	Renal consult
Hospitalist Comanagement		if 2> comorbidities	yes
Diabetes	restart home meds	postop glucose >250 insulin infusion	postop gluose > 250 insulin infusion

Fig. 4.2 (continued)

shown to improve PONV when compared to inhalational anesthetics. The choice of which intraoperative narcotic to use is based on cost, onset, side effect profile, and duration of action. A typical approach combines short-duration, fast-onset drugs such as fentanyl, remifentanil, or sufentanil for the maintenance portion of the case, followed by titration of a longer-acting narcotic such as hydromorphone or morphine at the end for postoperative analgesia.

Regional Anesthesia

Given the benefits of general anesthesia, regional anesthesia is rarely used as the primary anesthetic modality for laparoscopy because of surgical positioning requirements, the discomfort of a pneumoperitoneum, duration of the case, and the mentioned benefits of muscular relaxation. The risk of performing robotic surgery without muscular relaxation is of significant concern because of the potential injury from the patient moving while the robot is docked. However, regional anesthesia has been successfully used in laparoscopic urologic cases. In these cases, establishing a thoracic-to-lumbar epidural level between T3 and L4 is necessary to provide acceptable patient comfort. Other major concerns of a solely regional approach include CO_2 absorption, patient ventilation in the presence of a pneumoperitoneum-induced restrictive ventilatory defect, and pulmonary or abdominal pain during the operation. Therefore, regional anesthesia has only been used for short laparoscopic cases with low insufflation pressures (8-0 mmHg) in which general anesthesia is not a viable option. The placement of transversus abdominis plane local anesthetic blocks may reduce intraoperative and postoperative opioid use following laparoscopic cases.

IV Fluid Management

Intraoperative fluid management for robotic cases focuses on optimizing the surgical field as well as maintaining appropriate intravascular volume and cardiac output. Robotic urologic pelvic surgery places the patient in lithotomy and/or steep Trendelenburg. These positions significantly augment preload and coronary perfusion pressure. This autotransfusion from the lower extremities limits the need for additional fluid administration and helps offset the caval compression effect of the pneumoperitoneum on venous return. However, over time, the steep Trendelenburg position will increase upper body hydrostatic pressure in the vasculature and cause fluid to leak out of intravascular vessels and into interstitial and extracellular spaces, resulting in facial, orbital, pulmonary, and laryngeal edema. In cases such as prostatectomies and cystectomies, urinary fluid leaking into the abdomen and then suctioned into the suction bucket may lead to an overestimation of blood loss. Absent unusual bleeding, a typical fluid resuscitation during a robotic prostatectomy or cystectomy should range from 1.5 to 2 L of crystalloid solution, with the majority administered after the urinary anastomosis is completed. Additional fluids should be consistent with surgical blood loss and fluid loss due to bowel prep.

Monitoring

The American Society of Anesthesiology (ASA) has specific recommendations for monitoring patients based on the depth of anesthesia provided (Table 4.2). The components of basic monitoring include a noninvasive blood pressure cuff, pulse-oximetry, capnography, temperature monitoring, and electrocardiogram [4].

CO_2/EtCO_2

EtCO_2 monitoring guides ventilator management to offset the additional CO_2 absorption from the pneumoperitoneum. EtCO_2 is a surrogate for $PaCO_2$. In healthy adults, EtCO_2 levels are approximately 5–10 mmHg lower than arterial levels. Because of this relationship, preventing physiologic derangements from elevated $PaCO_2$ levels occurs by using a target EtCO_2, which is achieved by adjusting the ventilator settings as well as decreasing insufflation pressures, and altering patient positioning. This typically requires increasing the minute ventilation 20–50% over baseline during robotic and laparoscopic cases based on the length of time.

The predictable relationship between EtCO_2 and $PaCO_2$ can be inaccurate if ventilation-to-perfusion (V/Q) matching is unequal. In scenarios of V:Q mismatching, incomplete emptying of CO_2 may be evident on the capnogram by an inclination of the plateau phase during exhalation. In the presence of an inclination of the plateau phase, attempts to counteract hypercapnia

Table 4.2 Standards for basic anesthesia monitoring

Standard	Method
Oxygenation	A quantitative method of assessing oxygenation such as pulse oximetry shall be employed
Ventilation	Every patient receiving general anesthesia shall have the adequacy of ventilation continually evaluated
Circulation	Every patient receiving anesthesia shall have the electrocardiogram continuously displayed from the beginning of anesthesia until preparing to leave the anesthetizing location
	Every patient receiving anesthesia shall have arterial blood pressure and heart rate determined and evaluated at least every 5 min
Body temperature	Every patient receiving anesthesia shall have temperature monitored when clinically significant changes in body temperature are intended, anticipated, or suspected

Adapted from the American Society of Anesthesiology Guidelines [4]

by increasing the respiratory rate may actually result in EtCO$_2$ levels that are lower than actual PaCO$_2$ (Fig. 4.3). Uncoupling the predictable EtCO$_2$ and PaCO$_2$ relationship may result in mismanagement [5]. In cases where CO$_2$ management is critical (e.g., pulmonary hypertension or significant metabolic or respiratory acidosis), prolonging exhalation time will allow EtCO$_2$ to better represent PaCO$_2$. Alternatively, blood gas analysis can be used to correlate with capnography. Independent risk factors for the development of hypercarbia (EtCO$_2$ of 50 mmHg or greater) are operative time greater than 200 min and patient age over 65 years. If the minute ventilation requirement more than doubles from baseline, consideration needs to be given that CO$_2$ has tracked into another cavity (e.g., thorax and mediastinum) or subcutaneously via an access port track or hernia defect.

Temperature

Ideally, all patients should be kept normothermic as hypothermia is associated with an increased risk of surgical site infection and altered enzymatic function (i.e., altered drug metabolism,

coagulation, catecholamine function, electrical conductivity, and renal excretion). Normothermia can be maintained by warming the supporting gel pads prior to use, placing fluid warming blankets beneath the patient, using IV fluid warmers, or covering exposed patient areas with forced air-warming blankets. If these measures fail, increasing the room temperature will attenuate heat transfer from the patient.

For robotic cases, the most accurate way to monitor temperature is with a nasal or esophageal temperature probe. The target temperature should be >36 °C. Proper placement of the temperature probe avoids influence by the cooler airway gas temperatures. Nasal probes should not be advanced deeper than the distance from the nare to the external auditory meatus. An esophageal temperature probe should be advanced into the distal third of the esophagus so that it is retrocardiac rather than retro-tracheal. Alternatively, a heat and moisture exchange filter can be inserted between the endotracheal tube and the breathing circuit to passively increase airway gas temperature and thereby give a better representation of the patient's core temperature.

Invasive Monitoring

Invasive monitoring is rarely necessary for robotic urologic surgery, except in the case pheochromocytoma patients. The decision to place an arterial catheter is based on the patient's preexisting medical diseases, anticipated blood loss, need for repeated arterial blood gas monitoring, inability to use a noninvasive blood pressure cuff, or need for beat-to-beat blood pressure monitoring. Many early robot-assisted procedures used arterial catheters, but it is now commonplace to use only a noninvasive blood pressure cuff cycled every 3–5 min for interval blood pressure monitoring. Central venous access is useful for medications needing direct and reliable deposition into the central venous system. Otherwise, peripheral access usually provides greater flow capabilities for resuscitation. Central venous pressure (CVP) has been shown to be a generally inaccurate surrogate of intravascular volume status, and is even more unreliable in this population

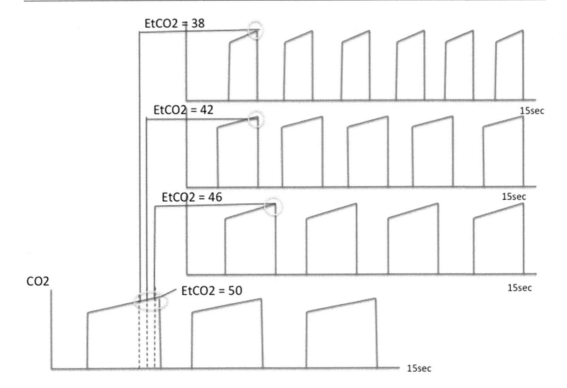

Fig. 4.3 This capnography illustrates the truncation of the expiratory time by increasing the respiratory rate in attempt to lower the $EtCO_2$. There is often a gradient between end-tidal CO_2 ($EtCO_2$) and arterial CO_2 ($PaCO_2$). The $EtCO_2$ value results from the permitted expiratory time, thus increasing the respiratory rate will decrease the expiratory time and consequentially lower the $EtCO_2$ value. Unfortunately, simultaneous measurement of $PaCO_2$ would recognize an elevated or unchanged $PaCO_2$ despite a lowered $EtCO_2$

where Trendelenburg and/or lithotomy positioning, in combination with a pneumoperitoneum, confound the value.

Positioning

Practical Concerns Regarding Positioning

Robotic-assisted surgeries create unique positioning challenges for the anesthesiologist because of limited access to the patient, an inability to alter positioning after docking the robot, and the duration of the procedure. The docked robot displaces the operating room table away from the anesthesiologist. This, coupled with the bedside surgeon and surgical technician, allows very limited access for any intraoperative adjustments to the patient, making proper initial positioning a critical part of the procedure. For these reasons, the desired intravascular access, monitoring, and positioning should be meticulously adjusted prior to docking the robot (Table 4.3). Planning and preparation for accidental extubation must also always be a universal concern because access to the airway will be substantially limited once the robot is docked and the patient is positioned. In the event of an unanticipated extubation, mask ventilation or LMA placement may be the best alternative until the robot is undocked and the patient can be repositioned appropriately for placement of a secure airway. The optimal manner in which to manage these critical and nonroutine events is through undocking simulation drills that can streamline the process for rare, high-acuity episodes such as major hemorrhage, cardiac arrest, or lost airways.

Awareness of intraoperative monitors should focus on minimizing tissue and nerve compression, kinking, and inadvertent disconnections of tubes and cables and their connection points. For instance, turning around the noninvasive blood pressure cuff with the inflation tubing exiting outside the patient's proximal arm prevents kinking of the tube as well as ulnar nerve compression injury to the patient. The same considerations for peripheral intravenous (PIV) lines should be made regarding the directionality and course traversed by the tubing, the appropriate length of tubing, and any possible compression or injury from stopcocks or flow locks located on PIVs. In those cases where the patient's arms are tucked, two PIV lines should be considered in the event one becomes infiltrated, accidentally removed, or intraoperative changes require additional IV access. Universal patient identification bands on limbs may also become a source of injury either by direct compression on the patient's extremities or creation of a tourniquet effect if IV access becomes infiltrated and there is any swelling near the band.

Sequential compression devices (SCDs) mitigate deep vein thrombosis secondary to the inflammatory stress of the surgery and the low flow states of positioning. However, SCDs must be delicately placed, especially when the patient is in lithotomy positioning because the connective tubing may cause pressure injuries analogous to the noninvasive blood pressure cuff and PIV. As with all of the other monitoring devices and intravascular access points, visibility and impact on the patient is lost after draping.

Table 4.3 Positioning checklist

• Ears
• Ulnar nerves
• Peroneal nerves
• Chin
• Neck
• Breath sound symmetry
• Vitals
• IV function
• Axilla if lateral

Specific Positioning Concerns

The major organ system concerns for patient positioning include the nervous system, musculoskeletal system, eyes, and respiratory system. These systems are impacted differently depending on the particular surgical positioning.

Lithotomy

Patients undergoing prostatectomies in the lithotomy position are at greater risk for neurologic injuries if they have a history of diabetes mellitus, thin body habitus, inadequate padding, or improper placement of the robot's arm. The lithotomy positioning endangers the obturator, saphenous, and lateral femoral cutaneous nerves in the lower limbs; therefore, careful attention must be made with hip flexion and lower limb abduction (Fig. 4.4a, b). The lithotomy position with SCD placement also puts at risk the common peroneal nerve due to compression from the lithotomy boots. Nerve injury associated with robotic-assisted urological surgery was much more likely in cases lasting over 5.5 versus 4 h, and that the incidence of injury increased with higher ASA physical status scores. This increased incidence of position injury in relation to surgical time is consistent with the author's experience related to robotic and laparoscopic surgery.

There have been multiple case reports documenting compartment syndrome during open prostatectomies in lithotomy position. Prolonged lithotomy compromises arterial perfusion pressure (combination of hydrostatic and direct calf pressure effects), resulting in compartment syndrome in the lower extremities. The addition of pneumoperitoneum and steep Trendelenburg positioning for robotic prostatectomies exacerbates this risk and should alert the physician to the possibility of rhabdomyolysis with hypotension in the calves (much higher positioned than the blood pressure cuff in Trendelenburg position) or if a metabolic acidosis is identified. Additionally, Gaylon et al. warn that the combination of pro-

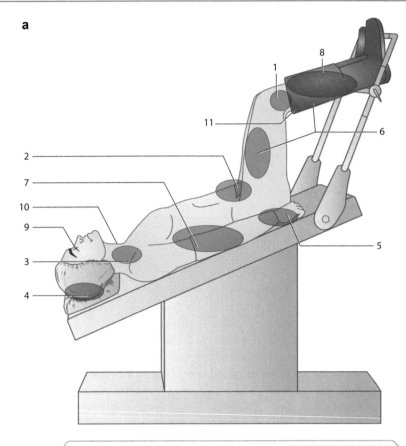

a

1. Peroneal nerve injury (foot drop)
2. Femoral and LFC nerves injury in inguinal crease from prolonged hip flexion
3. Brachial plexus injury (compression between clavicle and first rib vs stretch)
4. Alopecia
5. Injury to hand and fingers that are tucked
6. Compartment syndrome for LE due to prolonged lithotomy position
7. Injury to soft tissue of UE from cables, tubing and connectors (iv, a-line, blood pleasure, pulse oximeter)
8. Injury to soft tissue of LE from tubing and wrinkles of SCDs
9. Eye injury (increased IOP and edema from TDB) corneal abrasion
10. Airway edema from prolonged steep TDB position
11. Soft tissue injury from boots (heel ulcers and muscle necrosis)

Fig. 4.4 (**a**, **b**) This illustration depicts the many opportunities for position injuries that can occur in robotic cases. Some of these injuries are unique to the positioning for the case. The at-risk areas include nerves and nerve plexus, pressure points, foreign body compression, and edematous concerns. The illustration is numbered and color coded to highlight common themes and risks

longed lithotomy positioning, extended SCD usage, hypotension, vasopressor usage, and body mass index > 25 kg/m^2) significantly increase the risk of rhadomyolysis [6].

Steep Trendelenburg

This positioning maneuver allows for optimal exposure of the pelvis and the lower abdomen, but it introduces two particular challenges for the

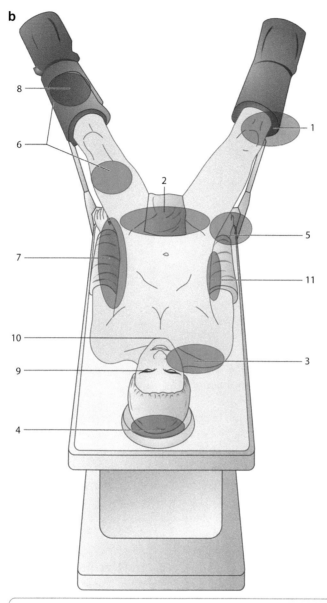

1. Peroneal nerve injury (foot drop) at the boot edge
2. Femoral and LFC nerves injury in inguinal crease from prolonged hip flexion
3. Brachial plexus injury (compression between clavicle and first rib vs stretch) Body weight vs straps to prevent sliding
4. Alopecia
5. Injury to hand and fingers that are tucked
6. Compartment syndrome for LE due to prolonged lithotomy position
7. Injury to soft tissue of UE from cables, tubing and connectors (iv, a-line, blood pleasure, pulse oximeter)
8. Injury to soft tissue of LE from tubing and wrinkles of SCDs
9. Eye injury (increased IOP and edema from TDB) corneal abrasion
10. Airway edema from prolonged steep TDB position
11. Ulnar nerve injury

Fig. 4.4 (continued)

operative team. First, this position places the patient at risk for sliding off the table. This can be averted with different approaches, each with its own concerns of which the operative team should be aware. Shoulder braces placed behind the patient will prevent sliding, but also introduce the real risk of brachial plexus nerve injury. Therefore, if used (we do not), shoulder braces should be applied over the acromio-clavicular joint to avoid compression of the upper trunk of the brachial plexus against the first rib and to avoid pushing by the humerus into the axilla and further stretch the plexus. Other institutions use a body-fitting bean-bag that functions as a torso-securing brace with a gel pad placed between the patient and the bean-bag. This prevents sliding and the injury of the brachial plexus that occurs from traction on the shoulders during positioning slips. Third, the patient may be strapped to the operating room table with chest binding in an "x" like pattern (Fig. 4.5). This binding limits chest excursion and may significantly decrease pulmonary compliance. The anesthesiologist should evaluate the change in pulmonary compliance after chest binding and consider the additional reduction in compliance that will occur after steep Trendelenburg positioning. We have also found it useful to draw lines on the bed sheets by the patient's shoulders as a reference point to identify if a patient has slid toward the head of the bed.

Another concern with steep Trendelenburg positioning is the displacement of the abdominal organs against the diaphragm. This significantly increases intrathoracic pressure. Danic et al. found that chest binding, pneumoperitoneum, and steep Trendelenburg decreased pulmonary compliance by 68% [7]. The combination of chest binding, Trendelenburg, and pneumoperitoneum may severely limit ventilation and increase airway pressures, which increase the risk of barotrauma. This positioning may also compress the lung fields enough to displace the endotracheal tube into a main stem bronchus. Therefore, bilateral breath sounds should be verified after final positioning.

To allow maximum exposure of the patient for a second surgeon, surgical assistant, and docked robot, the patient's arms must be tucked. To

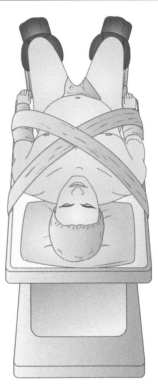

Fig. 4.5 The patient may be strapped to the operating room table with chest binding in an "x" like pattern. This binding limits chest excursion and may significantly decrease pulmonary compliance

prevent ulnar nerve injury, the hands should be mildly supinated, the elbow padded, and not flexed more than 90°. All foreign body objects such as wrist-bands, PIV, monitors, and connections should be reevaluated after padding and tucking.

Lateral Decubitus

For robotic renal and adrenal surgery, the patient is placed into a flexed lateral decubitus position to create maximal exposure. A pillow should be placed between the up, straight leg and the down, flexed leg to elevate the up leg to the level of the pelvis as well as pad the bony prominences to prevent pressure injury. A chest roll should be placed just caudal to the axilla to prevent brachial plexus injury; however, enough room should remain to not directly compress the brachial plexus. A useful strategy is to verify that you can place your hand between the chest roll and the axilla after positioning. Patients with a body mass index greater than 25 kg/m², full table flexion (as opposed to half-table flexion), and the use of a kidney rest are all associated with increases in table–patient interface pressures. This interface creates enough compression to precipitate rhabdomyolysis with kidney rest usage as the greatest risk factor. Attention to cervical neutrality is important and typically requires several folded blankets to reestablish a neutral cervical spine after turning and flexing.

Specific Position-Related Injuries

Ocular Injury

Patients undergoing robotic surgery may experience eye injury such as ischemic optic neuropathy, glaucoma, and corneal abrasion. The most common anesthetic-related injury after robotic surgery is corneal abrasion. It has been reported to occur in up to 3% of cases after robotic surgery [7]. Long-term complications are rare because corneal epithelial cells are able to regenerate; however, scarring may occur. In the short term, the injury is unexpected, painful, anxiety producing, and potentially delays discharge. Patients complain of blurry vision, tearing, redness, photophobia, and a foreign body sensation in the eye. Risk factors for corneal abrasion during urologic surgery include Trendelenburg position, advanced age, general anesthesia, higher estimated blood loss, and increased body mass index. Preventive measures include lubricating and taping the eyes after induction of anesthesia, or placing eye goggles on the patient, and possibly restricting IV fluid. The use of an upper body forced air warming blanket, as is common, provides a high flow of hot, dry air around the face, thus if there is any break in the seal around the eye, the forced air warmer predisposes to corneal desiccation/abrasion. When seen postoperatively, the most common treatment is a combination of antibiotic ointment with artificial tears. Follow-up with an ophthalmologist is only required if symptoms fail to improve within 24 h.

Increased intraocular pressure is inevitable and unavoidable in any head-lowered position. Decrease of cardiac output and increase of venous pressure in the head from steep Trendelenburg leads to an increased intra-ocular pressure. Elevated $PaCO_2$ results in vasodilation in the choroid plexus, which also increases intraocular pressure. In patients with a predisposition to elevated intra-ocular pressure, prolonged placement in the Trendelenburg position may increase the risk for glaucoma. Increased intraocular pressure has also been attributed to complete bilateral visual loss.

Ischemic optic neuropathy results in blindness. It is a rare ischemic event that most likely results from the combination of prolonged steep Trendelenburg position (higher venous and ocular pressures), anemia, and hypotension. Ischemic neuropathy has been reported after robot-assisted laparoscopic prostatectomy.

Laryngeal Edema

Laryngeal edema and postoperative stridor may occur after extubation and result in a tenuous airway with questionable patency requiring emergent reintubation. Risk factors related to this surgery include prolonged surgery, steep Trendelenburg positioning, high endotracheal cuff pressure, large fluid administration, traumatic intubation, and possibly hypoalbuminemia. In the event of significant orbital edema, one should consider placing the patient in reverse Trendelenburg, performing a cuff leak test or video laryngoscopy to evaluate airway patency or edema, and delaying extubation until the edema is reduced if there is no cuff leak or video laryngoscopy reveals significant intraoral/glottic edema.

Position Effects on Physiology

Cardiac

During robotic and laparoscopic surgery, steep Trendelenburg is often necessary for adequate surgical exposure. However, the combination of steep Trendelenburg and pneumoperitoneum creates a number of cardiovascular, neurologic, and pulmonary changes that should be kept within a clinically acceptable range (Table 4.1). These changes can be compared to those in the lateral position and pneumoperitoneum (Table 4.4).

Table 4.4 Impact of pneumoperitoneum and lateral position on physiology

Source	Pneumoperitoneum (PP)	Steep Trendelenburg (ST)	PP + ST
CVP	↓	↑	↑
CO	↑	↓	↓
SVR	↑	↓	↔
MAP	↑	↑	↑
Airway compliance	↓	↓	↓
Airway pressure	↑	↑	↑
FRC	↓	↓	↓
ICP	↑	↑	↑
CBF	↑ *	↔	↑ *
VBF	↓	↓	↓
Ocular pressure	↑	↑ @	↑
CPP	↓	↔	↔

PP + ST = partially additive effects
\# = changes due to intra-abdominal compression of aorta
* = if hypercarbic
@ = particularly in dependent eye

During steep Trendelenburg positioning with pneumoperitoneum, there is a greater than two-fold increase in CVP, mean pulmonary artery pressure, and pulmonary capillary wedge pressure. There is also a 35% increase in left and 65% right ventricular stroke work index [8]. Lateral decubitus can lead to compression of the inferior vena cava in flexed patients when the flex occurs outside of the iliac crest, decreasing venous return and cardiac output.

Pulmonary

In all patients, steep Trendelenburg causes decreases in functional residual capacity, tidal volume, and pulmonary compliance [9], and increases in pulmonary venous pressure and atelectasis with intrapulmonary shunting. A decrease of pulmonary compliance greater than 68% was reported in a review of 1500 robotic-assisted laparoscopic prostatectomies with chest binding, steep Trendelenburg, and pneumoperitoneum [7]. The increased intrapulmonary shunting and decreased delivery of tidal volumes leads to an increased $PaCO_2$, which is exacerbated by CO_2 absorption from insufflation unless corrected by adjusting minute ventilation. This decrease in compliance requires increasing airway pressures to maintain tidal volume, which increases the risk of barotrauma. Both peak and plateau pressures increase by greater than 50% with the cephalad movement of the diaphragm from the Trendelenburg position [10]. Because of the respiratory derangements, the European Association for Endoscopic Surgery recommends avoiding intraabdominal pressures higher than 12 mmHg in the presence of a pneumoperitoneum and steep Trendelenburg [11]. Lateral decubitus can lead to V:Q mismatch with a combination of both increased shunt and dead space, decreased compliance and volume of the dependent lung, and overinflation and barotraumas to the nondependent lung.

Neurologic

The combined effects of steep Trendelenburg and CO_2 pneumoperitoneum is generally well tolerated neurologically. Regional cerebral oxygenation and cerebral perfusion pressures are well preserved [12]. There is evidence that the combination increases intracranial pressure to potentially above 20 mmHg as measured by optic nerve sheath diameter. The elevated $PaCO_2$ levels from the insufflation may contribute to elevating the intracranial pressure as $PaCO_2$ affects cerebral blood flow at 1.8 mL/100 g/min for each 1 mmHg change in $PaCO_2$. However, these findings have not been shown to result in a reduction in cerebral oxygenation or abnormal neurologic signs [13].

Pain Management

Opioid Analgesics

The predominant class of drugs used for postoperative pain after laparoscopic and robotic surgery is opioids. The pure opioid agonists include morphine, hydromorphone, fentanyl, alfentanil,

sufentanil, and remifentanil. Morphine is an agonist at the $\mu 1$ and $\mu 2$ opioid receptors and its actions result in a decrease in the release of substance P. Fentanyl is the most common narcotic used intraoperatively during general anesthesia. Table 4.5 summarizes these drugs.

Opioids have a side effect profile that includes respiratory depression, decreased cough reflex, increased nausea and vomiting, sedation, itching, and urinary retention. Morphine has an active metabolite after liver metabolism that may prolong its action, particularly in patients with renal failure. It is useful to be aware that titration of naloxone can be used to resolve the side effects of opioid narcotics that disappear before the analgesic benefits do. However, naloxone should not be used routinely as its side effects profile includes restlessness, weakness, nausea and vomiting, and tachycardia. To treat non-life-threatening side effects, dosages for naloxone range from 20 to 40 µg boluses alone or followed by an infusion of 40 µg of naloxone per hour (one ampule of 0.4 mg naloxone added to 1 L of maintenance IV fluid running at 100 mL/h). To treat life-threatening side effects, 0.4 mg of naloxone is given.

Nonopioid Analgesics

Limiting narcotic usage has a significant upside for patient care: early ambulation, speed of bowel return, decreased respiratory depression, and the lack of other narcotic side effects. Nonopioid alternative analgesics include salicylates, acetaminophen, ketamine, and nonsteroidal anti-inflammatory drugs (NSAIDs). Selective

Table 4.5 Opioid analgesics

Drug	Onset (min)	Duration (h)	Potency (relative to morphine)
Ketorolac	30	4–6	0.3
Acetaminophen	30	2–4	–
Morphine	15	2–4	1
Codeine	15	3–4	0.1
Hydromorphone	15	2–4	7
Fentanyl	2	0.5–1	100
Sufentanil	2	0.25	500

cyclooxygenase-2 (COX-2) inhibitors (e.g., cele-coxib and rofecoxib) may have a more favorable side effect profile. However, NSAIDs should be used with caution in patients with elevated creati-nine. The FDA has also warned that NSAIDs other than acetylsalicylic acid (aspirin) may increase the risk of heart failure, coronary artery disease, and strokes. All NSAIDs are commonly used in urology patients.

Postoperative Nauseas and Vomiting

PONV affects 25–30% of all surgical patients and up to 70% in certain populations, which includes laparoscopic surgery patients [14]. Minimizing PONV can substantially decrease postoperative anesthesia care unit length of stay, hospital length of stay, and readmission follow-ing same day surgery [15]. Preoperative risk fac-tors for PONV include female gender, history of PONV, nonsmoking history, and postoperative opioid use. Anesthetic-related factors include nitrous oxide, volatile anesthetic use, narcotic use, lack of gastric decompression, and restric-tive IV fluid management. Total intravenous anesthesia with propofol may reduce PONV in the early postoperative period, but there is no strong evidence that a difference exists after 6 h [16]. In patients undergoing surgical procedures lasting greater than 3.5 h, no difference in PONV exists for propofol/remifentanil versus sevoflu-rane/remifentanil [17]. Risk scoring systems exist to assess the likelihood of PONV, with evi-dence suggesting that the prevention of PONV appears to be most cost-effective in patients with a risk of 40% or greater (Table 4.6) [18]. Protocols for managing PONV are institutionally depen-dent because of the number of drug options avail-able to treat each emetogenic pathway. The combination of antiemetics chosen often has to do with the side effect profile of the drug, ease of delivery, cost of the drug, and efficacy. A Cochrane Review from 2006 determined that eight drugs in particular reliably reduced nausea and vomiting after surgery and those are reviewed below [19].

Table 4.6 Apfel risk scoring system for postoperative nausea and vomiting

Risk factors	Points
Postoperative opioids	1
Nonsmoker	1
Female gender	1
History of PONV/motion sickness	1
Risk score = sum	0 … 4

Risk score	Prevalence PONV (%)	Prophylaxis: No. of antiemetics
0	9	0–1
1	20	1
2	39	2
3	60	3
4	78	4

Metoclopramide

Metoclopramide at doses of greater than 20 mg IV are needed for efficacy; it also has a short half-life of approximately 30–45 min. There is an increased incidence of extrapyramidal side effects that include diarrhea and restlessness.

Dexamethasone

The lowest effective dose for dexamethasone is 4 mg. Its mechanism of action for reducing PONV is unclear and its side effects on postop-erative wound healing inhibition, bleeding, and perineal discomfort if given while the patient is awake, and on infection and hyperglycemia in patients with diabetes, are considerations to be kept in mind.

Transdermal Scopolamine

Transdermal scopolamine is a useful medication when used alone or in combination therapy. Scopolamine is particularly useful with patients who have a history of motion sickness. Patients should expect a dry mouth and some experience blurry vision. Patients are instructed to remove the patch if these side effects become unaccept-able. The patch can be applied preoperatively behind the ear or alternatively to the volar forearm where the patient is easily reminded of its presence and it is easier to remove.

Ondansetron

Ondansetron is the most common drug used to prevent and treat PONV and is often considered the "gold standard" when comparing agents for PONV. Ondansetron at 4 mg IV was found have an equivalent effect when compared to ondansetron at 8 mg as an oral disintegrating tablet. This drug is generally given in the last 30 min of surgery so that its effect is established by the time of emergence from anesthesia and the patient experiences the longest awake benefit.

Acupressure

A nonpharmacologic option with various acustimulation devices (e.g., Sea Band®, Relief Band®, and Pressure Right®) work to reduce PONV without drug-related side effects. The devices apply pressure to the Pericardium (P6) or Neiguan pressure point on the inner arm (Fig. 4.6). These devices are more effective when applied to the P6 acupoint during the postoperative period [20]. These disposable devices have been shown to reduce vomiting and retching and may be added

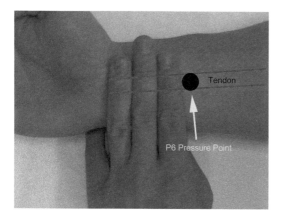

Fig. 4.6 To locate P6, place three middle fingers proximal to the upper wrist crease. The most distal finger will sit just on the wrist crease. The P6 point is located between the two central tendons by the index finger

as part of a multimodal antiemetic routine [21]. It is important to remember that the efficacy of any antiemetic is greater for prevention than it is for rescue and that if PONV occurs despite prophylaxis, using a drug the patient has not already received is more efficacious than repeating a drug that has already been used.

References

1. Wolf JS, Clayman RV, Monk TG, McClennan BL, McDougall EM. Carbon dioxide absorption during laparoscopic operation. J Am Coll Surg. 1995;180:555–60.
2. Stanley IR, Laurence AS, Hill JC. Disappearance of intraperitoneal gas following gynaecological laparoscopy. Anaesthesia. 2002;57(1):57–61.
3. Enneking FK. Verticals and threads™. University of Florida; 2015.
4. ASA House of Delegates. Standards for basic anesthetic monitoring. http://www.asahq.org/~/media/sites/asahq/files/public/resources/standards-guidelines/standards-for-basic-anesthetic-monitoring.pdf. Accessed 14 Oct 2015.
5. Giordano C, Gravenstein N, Rice MJ. Differentiating inspiratory and expiratory valve malfunctions. Anesthesiology. 2013;119(2):489.
6. Gaylon SW, Richards KA, Pettus JA, Bodin SG. Three-limb compartment syndrome and rhabdomyolysis after robotic cystoprostatectomy. J Clin Anest. 2011;23(1):75–8.
7. Danic MJ, Chow M, Alexander G, et al. Anesthesia considerations for robotic-assisted laparoscopic prostatectomy: a review of 1,500 cases. J Robot Surg. 2007;1:119–23.
8. Lestar M, Gunnarsson L, Lagerstrand L, Wiklund P, Odeberg-Wernerman S. Hemodynamic perturbations during robot-assisted laparoscopic radical prostatectomy in 45° Trendelenburg position. Anesth Analg. 2011;113(5):1069–75.
9. Baltayian S. A brief review: anesthesia for robotic prostatectomy. J Robot Surg. 2008;2:59–66.
10. Sharma KC, Brandstetter RD, Brensilver JM, Jung LD. Cardiopulmonary physiology and pathophysiology as a consequence of laparoscopic surgery. Chest. 1996;110:810–5.
11. Neudecker J, Sauerland S, Neugebauer E, Bergamaschi R, Bonjer HJ, Cuschieri A, et al. The European Association for Endoscopic Surgery clinical practice guideline on pneumoperitoneum for laparoscopic surgery. Surg Endosc. 2002;16:1121–43.
12. Kalmar AF, Foubert L, Hendrickx JF, Mottrie A, Absalom A, Mortier EP, Struys MM. Influence of steep Trendelenburg position and CO(2) pneumoperitoneum on cardiovascular, cerebrovascular, and respi-

ratory homeostasis during robotic prostatectomy. Br J Anaesth. 2010;104(4):433–9.

13. Kim MS, Bai SJ, Lee JR, Choi YD, Kim YJ, Choi SH. Increase in intracranial pressure during carbon dioxide pneumoperitoneum with steep Trendelenburg positioning proven by ultrasonographic measurement of optic nerve sheath diameter. J Endourol. 2014;28(7):801–6.

14. Gan TJ, Meyer TA, Apfel CC, Chung F, Davis PJ, Habib AS, et al. Society for Ambulatory Anesthesia guidelines for the management of postoperative nausea and vomiting. Anesth Analg. 2007;105(6): 1615–28.

15. Le TP, Gan TJ. Update on the management of postoperative nausea and vomiting and postdischarge nausea and vomiting in ambulatory surgery. Anesthesiol Clin. 2010;28(2):225–49.

16. Yoo YC, Bai SJ, Lee KY, Shin S, Choi EK, Lee JW. Total intravenous anesthesia with propofol reduces postoperative nausea and vomiting in patients undergoing robot-assisted laparoscopic radical prostatectomy: a prospective randomized trial. Yonsei Med J. 2012;53(6):1197–202.

17. Höcker J, Tonner PH, Böllert P, Paris A, Scholz J, Meier-Paika C, Bein B. Propofol/remifentanil vs sevoflurane/remifentanil for long lasting surgical procedures: a randomised controlled trial. Anaesthesia. 2006;61(8):752–7.

18. Apfel CC, Korttila K, Abdalla M, Kerger H, Turan A, Vedder I, et al. A factorial trial of six interventions for the prevention of postoperative nausea and vomiting. N Engl J Med. 2004;350(24):2441–51.

19. Carlisle J, Stevenson CA. Drugs for preventing postoperative nausea and vomiting. Cochrane Database Syst Rev. 2006;3:CD004125.

20. White PF, Hamza MA, Recart A, Coleman JE, Macaluso AR, Cox L, Jaffer O, Song D, Rohrich R. Optimal timing of acustimulation for antiemetic prophylaxis as an adjunct to ondansetron in patients undergoing plastic surgery. Anesth Analg. 2005; 100(2):367–72.

21. White PF, Zhao M, Tang J, Wender RH, Yumul R, Sloninsky AV, Naruse R, Kariger R, Cunneen S. Use of a disposable acupressure device as part of a multimodal antiemetic strategy for reducing postoperative nausea and vomiting. Anesth Analg. 2012;115(1):31–7.

Part II

Robotic Surgery of the Upper Urinary Tract

Robot-Assisted Total and Partial Adrenalectomy

5

Ravi Barod and Craig G. Rogers

Robot-Assisted Total Adrenalectomy

Patient Selection

Masses of the adrenal gland can be categorized into two main groups, benign and malignant. Benign masses can be further subcategorized into functional and nonfunctional masses. Functional masses are those that secrete hormones, normally produced by the adrenal gland such as aldosterone (Conn's syndrome), cortisol (Cushing's syndrome), virilizing hormones, or sympathetic agents. Hormonally active tumors require extirpative treatment to avoid the long-term consequences caused by the excessive hormone production. Investigation of these tumors is carried out by performing a thorough history and physical, as well as laboratory tests including serum electrolytes, serum or 24 h urinary catecholamines, and urinary-free cortisol [1]. Nonfunctioning adrenal masses tend to be incidental findings during workups for other conditions. Removal of

these masses is generally based on size or for suspicion of malignancy by increasing size on serial imaging [2].

A minimally invasive approach to the treatment of masses of the adrenal gland has been described by several groups [3–28]. These surgeries should be performed by skilled minimally invasive surgeons. Size is considered a relative contraindication to this approach for a malignant mass. Local invasion into adjacent structures is considered a contraindication to a minimally invasive approach.

There are no absolute contraindications to a robotic approach except for uncorrectable bleeding disorders. Any patient who is physically able to undergo general endotracheal anesthesia can have a robotic approach. A relative contraindication to a robotic approach is extensive prior abdominal surgery.

Preoperative Evaluation and Preparation

Patients being considered for robot-assisted adrenalectomy should have preoperative abdominal radiographic imaging with a CT or MRI. All functional masses are evaluated preoperatively and treated appropriately. Patients with pheochromocytoma are placed on several weeks of alpha blockade, followed by beta blockade prior to surgery. Calcium channel blockers can also be used to help control blood pressure and hypertensive episodes.

5

Electronic supplementary material: The online version of this chapter (doi:10.1007/978-3-319-45060-5_5) contains supplementary material, which is available to authorized users.

R. Barod, M.B.B.S., Ph.D., F.R.C.S. (Urol)
C.G. Rogers, M.D. (✉)
Vattikuti Urology Institute, Henry Ford Hospital, 2799 West Gran Blvd, Detroit, MI 48202, USA
e-mail: crogers2@hfhs.org

© Springer International Publishing Switzerland 2017
L.-M. Su (ed.), *Atlas of Robotic Urologic Surgery*, DOI 10.1007/978-3-319-45060-5_5

63

Patients with cortisol-producing masses are given preoperative steroids as the contralateral adrenal is severely suppressed by excessive production of cortisol by the mass. Hormone replacement therapy is continued for a number of weeks postoperatively until the contralateral adrenal has had time to normalize. Patients with aldosterone-secreting tumors receive treatment for any blood pressure issues and any deficiencies in potassium are corrected.

Preoperatively all patients have blood work done including electrolytes, a complete blood count, and coagulation tests. Any patients on anticoagulation therapy are instructed to stop at least 5 days prior to surgery. Patients can be given a bowel preparation, such as one bottle of magnesium citrate, the day before surgery. They are also instructed not to eat or drink anything after midnight the night before surgery. A first-generation cephalosporin is given perioperatively about 30 min prior to skin incision.

Operative Setup

The operative setup, including patient position and trocar placement, is identical for both total and partial adrenalectomy. We use the da Vinci® Surgical System (Intuitive Surgical, Inc., Sunnyvale, CA) to perform robot-assisted adrenalectomies using a three-armed technique. The fourth robotic arm may be used for additional retraction but it is generally unnecessary. The operative setup, including the position of the robot, console surgeon, bedside assistant, scrub technician, and monitors, is illustrated in Fig. 5.1. The robot is docked over the shoulder of the patient at a 45° angle with the long axis of the operating table.

The surgical team includes a minimum of one operating console surgeon, one bedside assistant, an anesthesiologist, a scrub technician, and a circulator. The operating surgeon may scrub initially to assist in patient preparation and trocar placement, and then breaks scrub prior to sitting at the robotic console. The bedside team remains scrubbed throughout the case and assists the console surgeon during the procedure.

Patient Positioning

General endotracheal anesthesia is used for this procedure. A urethral catheter is placed before positioning the patient. The patient is placed in the full flank position with an axillary roll. Moderate table flexion (approximately 15°) is used to increase the space for trocars with the kidney placed at the center of the table break (Fig. 5.2). The arms are padded at the elbows, wrists, and hands, and extended in front of the patient with the upper arm suspended. Alternatively, the upper arm may be tucked behind the patient, rolled in a sheet over foam pads or blankets. The advantage of this position is that the patient's upper arm is less likely to inhibit movement of the cephalad robotic arm. However, care must be taken to prevent over extension of the shoulder, which may precipitate a neuropraxia. The lower leg is flexed, the upper leg is straight, and all lower extremity pressure points are padded. The patient is secured to the table at the chest, iliac crest, and knees with wide cloth tape and Velcro straps to ensure the patient does not move during the procedure. Tape blisters are avoided by placing foam padding or abdominal pads between the skin and the tape. All pressure points including the head, neck, axilla, arms, hip, knees, and ankles are inspected and additional padding is placed if necessary. Security of patient positioning is confirmed prior to draping by "airplaning" the table to expose the patient's abdomen. This is the table position used to close the trocar wounds at the end of the procedure and also to convert to an open procedure in an emergency.

Trocar Configuration

The trocar configuration for left and right robot-assisted adrenalectomy is demonstrated in Fig. 5.3a, b, respectively. Two 12 mm standard trocars and two 8 mm robotic trocars are used for both techniques. An additional 5 mm trocar is used for a right-sided technique for retraction of the liver. Table 5.1 includes an instrumentation list.

Fig. 5.1 (**a, b**) The operative setup. The robot is docked over the shoulder of the patient at a 45° angle with the long axis of the operating table. The bedside assistant and scrub technician are on the opposite side of the patient

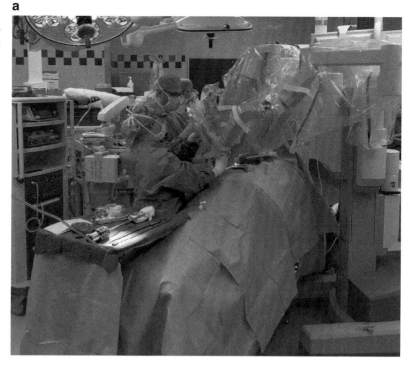

a

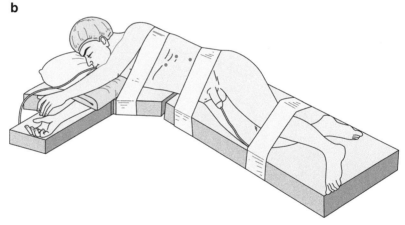

b

Surgical Anatomy

Knowledge of the surgical anatomy of the adrenal gland and the vessels associated with each gland is essential to performing a successful adrenalectomy. Each adrenal is associated with a major vessel and has a unique venous drainage. The adrenal gland receives its arterial blood supply from the branches of the inferior phrenic artery, renal artery,

and aorta. This network of arteries enter the gland along its superior and medial border making the inferolateral, posterior, and anterior surfaces of the gland relatively avascular.

The right adrenal gland is in close relationship with the inferior vena cava (IVC). The right adrenal vein arises from the superomedial surface of the gland and drains into the IVC. The left adrenal vein leaves the adrenal gland via the inferior

a

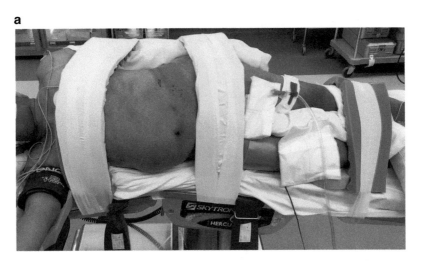

b

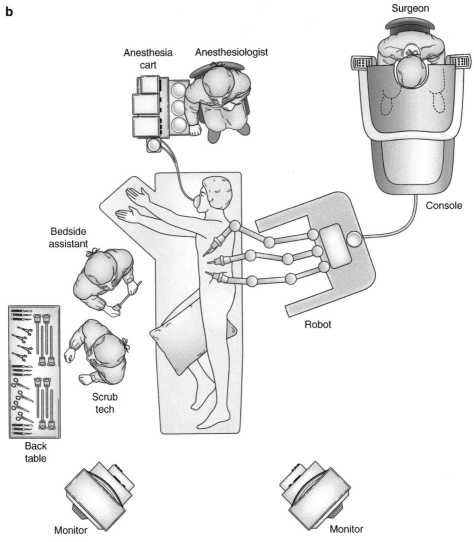

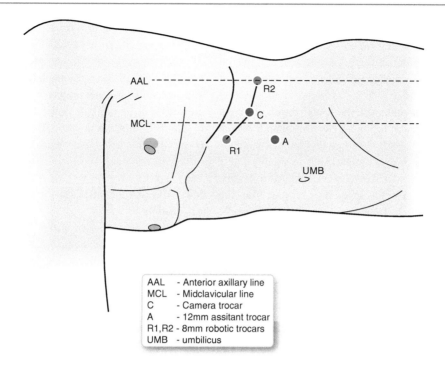

Fig. 5.3 Trocar configuration. The *midline* and lateral border of the ipsilateral rectus abdominis are marked prior to insufflation. The isilateral costal margin and anterior superior iliac spine are marked after insufflation. The tro-cars are placed as shown. *AAL* anterior axillary line, *MCL* midclavicular line, *C* camera trocar, *A* 12 mm assistant trocar, *R1,R2* 8 mm robotic trocars, *UMB* umbilicus

Table 5.1 Instrumentation list

Surgeon instrumentation			Assistant instrumentation
Arm 1—Right	**Arm 2—Left**	**Arm 3 (usually unnecessary)**	• Suction-Irrigator
• Curved monopolar scissors	• Maryland bipolar grasper	Prograsp dissector	• Blunt tip grasper
• Monopolar hook			• Laparoscopic needle driver
• Robotic hem-o-lok applier			• Laparoscopic scissors
			• Hem-o-lok or titanium clip applier
			• 10 mm specimen bag

Fig. 5.2 (**a, b**) Patient positioning. The patient is placed in the full flank position with an axillary roll. The upper arm can be secured behind the hip at the patient's side if it is felt that outward extension might cause collisions with the robotic arms. The lower leg is flexed and the upper leg is straight. The table is flexed approximately 15°. All pressure points are protected. The patient is secured to the table at the chest, hips, and knees with wide cloth tape over foam pads, and Velcro straps

aspect and drains into the left renal vein. It is easiest to identify the left adrenal vein along the superior border of the left renal vein and medial in location as compared to the insertion of the left gonadal vein.

Note that under robotic visualization, the right adrenal vein runs for a few millimeters on the anterior surface of the adrenal gland before entering it. This gives enough room to doubly ligate the vein or place multiple clips. Additionally, there may be collateral veins draining from the adrenal gland. These veins are distinguishable from the adrenal vein in being more tortuous, thin walled, and inferior than the main adrenal vein. The main adrenal vein is high up on the adrenal, has thicker walls, and is shorter.

Step-by-Step Technique (Video 5.1)

Transperitoneal Left Robot-Assisted Adrenalectomy

Step 1: Trocar Placement
Abdominal insufflation is achieved using Veress needle introduced at the level of the umbilicus in the left lateral abdomen, below the costal margin. Insufflation is initiated at 20 mmHg but may be decreased to 15 mmHg during the operation. The midline is marked from the xiphoid to the umbilicus with a marking pen. The lateral border of the ipsilateral rectus abdominis is also marked. A mark for the left robotic trocar is placed on this line, approximately two finger-breadths below the costal margin. A mark for the camera trocar is placed one hands-breadth below and shifted laterally to improve triangulation and focus on the adrenal. The 12 mm camera trocar is placed first and the robotic camera is introduced. Next, the two 8 mm robotic trocars are placed at their previously marked sites, under direct vision. Finally, a 12 mm assistant trocar is placed in the midline, immediately superior to the umbilicus (Fig. 5.3).

Step 2: Mobilization of Colon and Spleen
We use a 0° camera with the Maryland bipolar forceps in the left arm and a monopolar hook or scissors in the right arm (electrocautery settings: 40 W bipolar, 40 W monopolar). The splenic flexure is mobilized along a line between the colon and the line of Toldt. Lienophrenic, lienorenal, and lienocolic ligaments may be taken down to allow the spleen along with the descending colon to fall medially and out of the operating field (Fig. 5.4). This helps to provide optimal exposure of the left adrenal gland.

Step 3: Exposure and Ligation of Left Adrenal Vein
Gerota's fascia is incised at the level of the renal hilum and the left renal vein is identified. The left adrenal vein is identified draining from the inferomedial aspect of the gland into the superior border of the renal vein (Fig. 5.5). The left adrenal vein is isolated circumferentially using robotic instruments (Fig. 5.6). The adrenal vein should be ligated prior to manipulation of the adrenal gland, particularly in cases of pheochromocytoma in which there is potential for release of catecholamines into the systemic circulation during manipulation of the tumor resulting in sudden hypertension. The adrenal vein is ligated using Hem-o-lok® or titanium clips placed by the assistant, or by using robotic Hem-o-lok clips, (Fig. 5.7). The vein should have enough length to be doubly ligated.

Step 4: Dissection of Pancreas Away from Gerota's Fascia
To prevent pancreatic injury, care must be taken during dissection in the plane between the pancreas and Gerota's fascia. Once the plane is identified, it is extended cephalad towards the lienophrenic ligament. The splenic artery and vein are frequently encountered during this dissection and their tortuous course should be noted to avoid injury. Most of the dissection is carried out with the right robotic instrument (hook or scissors), while the shaft of the left robotic instrument (Maryland forceps) is used to retract the pancreas and splenic vessels. The wrist of the Maryland forceps can be angled in such a way that the instrument can still be used for dissection whilst providing atraumatic retraction of the pancreas.

Fig. 5.4 Take down of the lienocolic ligaments (**a**) and lienorenal ligaments (**b**) to free the spleen and expose the left adrenal gland

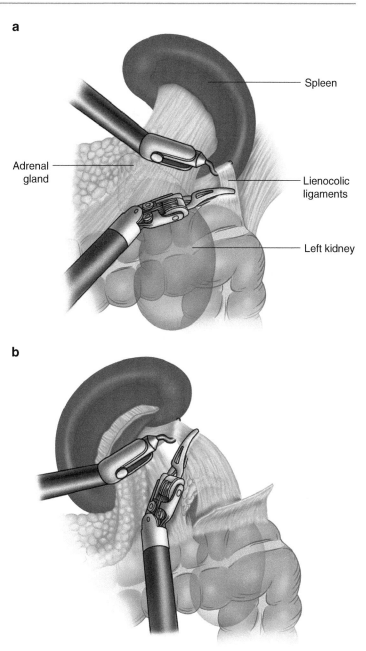

Step 5: Dissection of Upper Pole Renal Attachments

After the adrenal vein is secured and the pancreas has been dissected away from Gerota's fascia, gentle traction on the adrenal gland using the Maryland bipolar forceps and counter traction on the kidney by the assistant aids in the dissection of the gland by opening the space between the adrenal gland and the upper pole of the kidney (Fig. 5.8). Dissection is carried out along the capsule of the upper pole of the kidney as this plane is generally avascular and as well achieves a wide tissue margin around the adrenal tumor. The magnification provided by the robotic camera

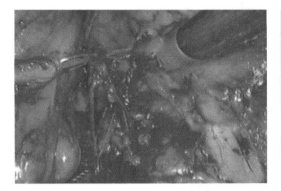

Fig. 5.5 Exposure of left renal vein and adrenal vein

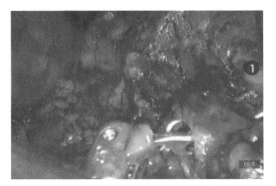

Fig. 5.6 Circumferential robotic dissection of left adrenal vein

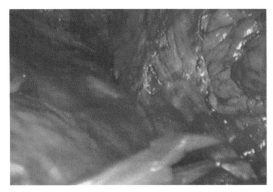

Fig. 5.7 Ligation of left adrenal vein using clips or suture ligation

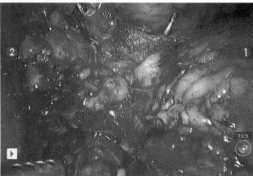

Fig. 5.8 Dissecting the plane between the left adrenal gland (*left*) and the upper pole of the kidney (*right*) following ligation of adrenal vein

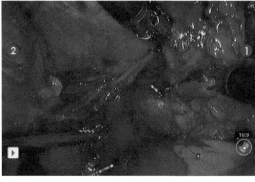

Fig. 5.9 Transecting final superior adrenal attachments to free the left adrenal gland

Step 6: Dissection of Medial, Lateral, and Superior Attachments

Careful, meticulous dissection of the adrenal gland while avoiding grasping the gland directly can help minimize blood loss. Medially, there will be small arterial branches from the aorta, and these can be controlled with clips or electrocautery to help minimize blood loss. The remaining superior and lateral attachments of the gland are dissected free (Fig. 5.9).

Step 7: Entrapment and Extraction of Specimen

The adrenal gland is placed in a 10 mm specimen entrapment bag (Fig. 5.10). Pneumoperitoneum is decreased to 5 mmHg and the adrenal bed is inspected for bleeding. Hemostatic agents such as Floseal or Surgicel may be used to assist

generally allows for identification of small adrenal arteries, which can be clipped or coagulated. Collateral veins may be seen exiting the adrenal gland. These thin walled veins may be either ligated with clips or cauterized.

hemostasis with electrocautery. After adequate hemostasis is confirmed the specimen bag is removed by extending the midline 12 mm assistant trocar.

Transperitoneal Right Robot-Assisted Adrenalectomy

Step 1: Trocar Placement

Trocar placement for a right robot-assisted adrenalectomy is illustrated in Fig. 5.11. A Veress needle is introduced at the level of the umbilicus in the right lateral abdomen, below the costal margin, and pneumoperitoneum is established to 20 mmHg and then dropped to 15 mmHg after placement of

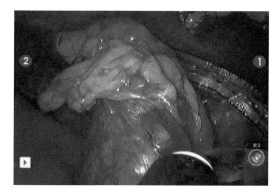

Fig. 5.10 Placement of adrenalectomy specimen into the entrapement bag

all trocars. The midline is marked from the xiphoid to the umbilicus with a marking pen. The lateral border of the ipsilateral rectus abdominis is also marked. A mark for the right robotic trocar is placed on this line, approximately two finger-breadths below the costal margin. A mark for the camera trocar is placed one hands-breadth below this, along the same line. The mark for the left robotic trocar is placed one hands-breadth below this and shifted laterally to improve triangulation and focus on the adrenal. The 12 mm camera trocar is placed first and the robotic camera is introduced. Next, the two 8 mm robotic trocars are placed at their previously marked sites, under direct vision. Finally, a 12 mm assistant trocar is placed in the midline, immediately superior to the umbilicus. For liver retraction, we place a 5 mm subxiphoid trocar and pass a 5 mm locking grasper under the liver and secure it to the abdominal sidewall.

Step 2: Mobilization of Liver, Colon, and Duodenum

We generally use a 0° camera while performing this operation, but a 30 degree lens may also be used per surgeon preference. The console surgeon uses the Maryland bipolar forceps in the left hand and a monopolar hook or monopolar scissors in the right hand. Attachments of the liver are incised allowing for upward traction

Fig. 5.11 Trocar configuration for right robotic adrenalectomy. *AAL* anterior axillary line, *MCL* midclavicular line, *C* camera trocar, *A* 12 mm assistant trocar, *R1,R2* 8 mm robotic trocars, *UMB* umbilicus

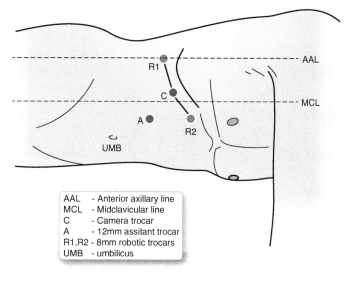

AAL	- Anterior axillary line
MCL	- Midclavicular line
C	- Camera trocar
A	- 12mm assitant trocar
R1,R2	- 8mm robotic trocars
UMB	- umbilicus

applied to the liver by the assistant with a 5 mm blunt tip liver retractor. Mobilization of the hepatic flexure of the colon and kocherization of the duodenum are performed to expose the IVC from the inferior aspect of the liver to the entry of the renal vein.

Step 3: Exposure and Ligation of Right Adrenal Vein

Dissection along the lateral aspect of the IVC is carried out to identify the adrenal vein. During dissection, any collateral adrenal veins which are encountered may be clipped or cauterized. Gentle lateral traction on the adrenal gland and mild medial traction on the IVC helps in dissecting between the IVC and the adrenal gland so as to identify the short right adrenal vein. The adrenal vein generally exits high up from the adrenal gland and runs for a few millimeters on its anterior surface. The adrenal vein is carefully isolated circumferentially and ligated as described for the left-sided procedure (Fig. 5.12).

Step 4: Dissection of Inferior, Posterior, and Superior Attachments

Gerota's fascia is incised and the plane between the upper pole of the kidney and adrenal gland is dissected with the assistance of gentle traction on the kidney by the assistant. A small amount of fat is left on the adrenal to serve as a handle and to minimize direct manipulation of the gland. Small adrenal arteries can be clipped or coagulated as they are identified. Dissection is continued and a

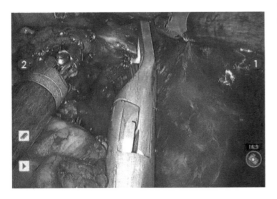

Fig. 5.12 Hem-o-lok® clip being applied to the right adrenal vein at its junction with the inferior vena cava

plane is developed between the posterior surface of the adrenal and the psoas and quadratus lumborum muscles. Finally, the superior attachments are released and the adrenal gland is placed in a 10 mm specimen entrapment bag. The pneumoperitoneum is decreased to 5 mmHg and the adrenal bed is inspected for bleeding. After adequate hemostasis is confirmed, the specimen entrapment bag is removed through the 12 mm assistant trocar.

Robot-Assisted Partial Adrenalectomy

Patient Selection

Indications for partial adrenalectomy include bilateral and hereditary adrenal tumors as well as tumors in a solitary adrenal gland. Hereditary adrenal pheochromocytoma is associated with syndromes such as von Hippel–Lindau disease, multiple endocrine neoplasia type 2, and neurofibromatosis type 1. The goal of partial adrenalectomy is to provide tumor control while preserving adrenocortical function. The safety and feasibility of partial adrenalectomy, particularly by endoscopic techniques, has been shown by several groups [6, 7, 10, 29, 30]. Partial adrenalectomy can provide patients with a greater hormonal reserve, thus decreasing the risk of subsequent adrenal insufficiency and Addisonian crisis as well as the morbidity of lifelong adrenal steroid replacement. The safety and efficacy of robot-assisted adrenalectomy has been described [31]. However, only a few case reports of robot-assisted partial adrenalectomy have been described [32, 33].

Use of Intraoperative Imaging

An important difference in technique while performing partial versus total adrenalectomy is the use of intraoperative ultrasound. Ultrasound allows for more precise demarcation of the limits of the tumor within the adrenal gland during partial adrenalectomy much like the technique used in laparoscopic and robot-assisted partial nephrectomy. The adrenal gland gets its blood supply from multiple blood vessels and thus it may be possible to selectively remove the adrenal tumor while preserving the remaining parenchyma.

Patient Positioning and Operative Setup

Patient positioning, trocar configuration, and operative setup are identical to total adrenalectomy as described previously. Instrumentation and equipment are as described previously with the exception of intraoperative laparoscopic ultrasonography, which is used to detect the size, location, and anatomic boundaries of the tumor within the affected adrenal gland.

Surgical Technique

The same instrumentation and technique is used as in total adrenalectomy to gain access to the adrenal gland. Once the adrenal gland is visualized, a flexible laparoscopic ultrasound probe is inserted through the 12 mm assistant trocar and is used to locate the tumor(s) and to define anatomic margins (Fig. 5.13). Using the TilePro™ (Intuitive Surgical, Inc., Sunnyvale, CA) feature of the da Vinci® S, the console surgeon is able to display the live intraoperative ultrasound images as a picture-in-picture

image on the console screen [34]. The robotic Maryland bipolar forceps and curved monopolar scissors are used to resect the adrenal mass and to free the adrenal tumor from the remaining normal adrenal gland (Fig. 5.14). The adrenal tumor is mobilized and placed in a specimen entrapment bag, which is subsequently removed through the periumbilical trocar incision.

Postoperative Care

A clear liquid diet is started postoperatively and a complete blood count and basic serum chemistries are ordered 12 h postoperatively. Overnight, patients receive intravenous fluids, analgesics as necessary, prophylaxis for deep vein thrombosis with subcutaneous heparin, and antibiotic prophylaxis per hospital protocol. The morning following surgery, the urethral catheter is removed, and patients are encouraged to ambulate. The most important aspect of postoperative care is management of any endocrine dysfunction. Management of these dysfunctions is beyond the scope of this text, and consultation with an endocrinologist may be warranted.

Steps to Avoid Complications

Potential complications associated with this procedure include vascular injury, bowel injury, liver, and splenic injury. The reported rates of vascular injury are about 0.7–5.4% [35–37], but transfusion rates are as high as 10% [38]. While injury to major vessels is often noticed immediately, small vessel

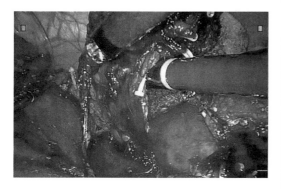

Fig. 5.13 Laparoscopic ultrasound probe is seen underneath a left adrenal tumor defining its anatomic borders prior to transecting the final adrenal attachments to free the tumor

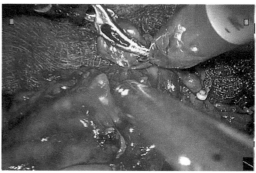

Fig. 5.14 Transecting final adrenal attachments to free an adrenal tumor during a robotic partial adrenalectomy

injury may initially go unrecognized due to the pneumoperitoneum. Manifestations of small vessel injury are not usually seen until the postoperative period when hematomas form or the patient becomes hemodynamically unstable. Bowel injury is also a known complication of minimally invasive adrenalectomy and can be severe if unnoticed. The small bowel is the most commonly injured segment with duodenal injury associated with the most serious sequelae. Thermal injuries are the most common, accounting for up to 50% of bowel injuries [39]. Use of cautery should be minimized when working near the bowel, particularly near the duodenum. Liver and splenic injuries may also occur during adrenalectomy. Capsular tears may be caused by insertion of instruments or aggressive retraction. Adequate lysis of adhesions prior to retracting can help avoid these injuries. All trocars and assistant instruments should enter under direct vision to avoid injuring any viscera.

Conclusion

Robot-assisted adrenalectomy is a feasible and safe procedure. Although adrenalectomy is an extirpative procedure without the need for intracorporeal sutured reconstruction, robotic assistance with wristed instruments and magnified three-dimensional vision can help with precise dissection of large and small vessels. Robotic assistance can facilitate dissection of vessels and adrenal tumors during total adrenalectomy and partial adrenalectomy, potentially allowing more surgeons, even those with limited laparoscopic experience, to offer their patients a minimally invasive approach to adrenalectomy.

References

1. Zeh III HJ, Udelsman R. One hundred laparoscopic adrenalectomies: a single surgeon's experience. Ann Surg Oncol. 2003;10:1012–7.
2. Gill IS. The case for laparoscopic adrenalectomy. J Urol. 2001;166:429–36.
3. Cyriac J, Weizman D, Urbach DR. Laparoscopic adrenalectomy for the management of benign and malignant adrenal tumors. Expert Rev Med Devices. 2006;3:777–86.
4. Liao CH, Chueh SC, Lai MK, et al. Laparoscopic adrenalectomy for potentially malignant adrenal tumors greater than 5 centimeters. J Clin Endocrinol Metab. 2006;91:3080–3.
5. Tsuru N, Ushiyama T, Suzuki K. Laparoscopic adrenalectomy for primary and secondary malignant adrenal tumors. J Endourol. 2005;19:702–8; discussion 708–9.
6. Diner EK, Franks ME, Behari A, et al. Partial adrenalectomy: the National Cancer Institute experience. Urology. 2005;66:19–23.
7. Walther MM, Herring J, Choyke PL, et al. Laparoscopic partial adrenalectomy in patients with hereditary forms of pheochromocytoma. J Urol. 2000;164:14–7.
8. Henry JF, Defechereux T, Gramatica L, et al. Should laparoscopic approach be proposed for large and/or potentially malignant adrenal tumors? Langenbecks Arch Surg. 1999;384:366–9.
9. Liatsikos EN, Papathanassiou Z, Voudoukis T, et al. Case report: laparoscopic adrenalectomy in a patient with primary adrenal malignant melanoma. J Endourol. 2006;20:123–6.
10. Janetschek G, Finkenstedt G, Gasser R, et al. Laparoscopic surgery for pheochromocytoma: adrenalectomy, partial resection, excision of paragangliomas. J Urol. 1998;160:330–4.
11. Gagner M, Lacroix A, Bolte E. Laparoscopic adrenalectomy in Cushing's syndrome and pheochromocytoma. N Engl J Med. 1992;327:1033.
12. Guazzoni G, Cestari A, Montorsi F, et al. Laparoscopic treatment of adrenal diseases: 10 years on. BJU Int. 2004;93:221–7.
13. Hazzan D, Shiloni E, Golijanin D, et al. Laparoscopic vs open adrenalectomy for benign adrenal neoplasm. Surg Endosc. 2001;15:1356–8.
14. Valeri A, Borrelli A, Presenti L, et al. Adrenal masses in neoplastic patients: the role of laparoscopic procedure. Surg Endosc. 2001;15:90–3.
15. Fazeli-Matin S, Gill IS, Hsu TH, et al. Laparoscopic renal and adrenal surgery in obese patients: comparison to open surgery. J Urol. 1999;162:665–9.
16. Hallfeldt KK, Mussack T, Trupka A, et al. Laparoscopic lateral adrenalectomy versus open posterior adrenalectomy for the treatment of benign adrenal tumors. Surg Endosc. 2003;17:264–7.
17. Jacobsen NE, Campbell JB, Hobart MG. Laparoscopic versus open adrenalectomy for surgical adrenal disease. Can J Urol. 2003;10:1995–9.
18. Kirshtein B, Yelle JD, Moloo H, et al. Laparoscopic adrenalectomy for adrenal malignancy: a preliminary report comparing the short-term outcomes with open adrenalectomy. J Laparoendosc Adv Surg Tech A. 2008;18:42–6.
19. Horgan S, Vanuno D. Robots in laparoscopic surgery. J Laparoendosc Adv Surg Tech A. 2001;11:415–9.
20. Brunaud L, Bresler L, Ayav A, et al. Robotic-assisted adrenalectomy: what advantages compared to lateral transperitoneal laparoscopic adrenalectomy? Am J Surg. 2008;195:433–8.
21. Brunaud L, Bresler L, Zarnegar R, et al. Does robotic adrenalectomy improve patient quality of life when

compared to laparoscopic adrenalectomy? World J Surg. 2004;28:1180–5.

22. Desai MM, Gill IS, Kaouk JH, et al. Robotic-assisted laparoscopic adrenalectomy. Urology. 2002;60:1104–7.

23. Gill IS, Sung GT, Hsu TH, et al. Robotic remote laparoscopic nephrectomy and adrenalectomy: the initial experience. J Urol. 2000;164:2082–5.

24. Krane LS, Shrivastava A, Eun D, et al. A four-step technique of robotic right adrenalectomy: initial experience. BJU Int. 2008;101:1289–92.

25. Moinzadeh A, Gill IS. Robotic adrenalectomy. Urol Clin North Am. 2004;31:753–6.

26. Sung GT, Gill IS. Robotic renal and adrenal surgery. Surg Clin North Am. 2003;83:1469–82.

27. Wu JC, Wu HS, Lin MS, et al. Robotic-assisted laparoscopic adrenalectomy. J Formos Med Assoc. 2005;104:748–51.

28. Young JA, Chapman III WH, Kim VB, et al. Robotic-assisted adrenalectomy for adrenal incidentaloma: case and review of the technique. Surg Laparosc Endosc Percutan Tech. 2002;12:126–30.

29. Sasagawa I, Suzuki Y, Itoh K, et al. Posterior retroperitoneoscopic partial adrenalectomy: clinical experience in 47 procedures. Eur Urol. 2003;43:381–5.

30. Walz MK, Peitgen K, Diesing D, et al. Partial versus total adrenalectomy by the posterior retroperitoneoscopic approach: early and long-term results of 325 consecutive procedures in primary adrenal neoplasias. World J Surg. 2004;28:1323–9.

31. Winter JM, Talamini MA, Stanfield CL, et al. Thirty robotic adrenalectomies: a single institution's experience. Surg Endosc. 2006;20:119–24.

32. Rogers CG, Blatt AM, Miles GE, et al. Concurrent robotic partial adrenalectomy and extra-adrenal pheochromocytoma resection in a pediatric patient with von Hippel-Lindau disease. J Endourol. 2008;22:1501–3.

33. Julien JS, Ball D, Schulick R. Robot-assisted cortical-sparing adrenalectomy in a patient with von Hippel-Lindau disease and bilateral pheochromocytomas separated by 9 years. J Laparoendosc Adv Surg Tech A. 2006;16:473–7.

34. Rogers CG, Laungani R, Bhandari A, Krane LS, Eun D, Patel MN, Boris R, Shrivastava A, Menon M. Maximizing console surgeon independence during robotic renal surgery by utilizing the fourth arm and TilePro. J Endourol. 2009;21:115–21.

35. Permpongkosol S, Link RE, Su LM, et al. Complications of 2, 775 urological laparoscopic procedures: 1993 to 2005. J Urol. 2007;177:580–5.

36. Rosevear HM, Montgomery JS, Roberts WW, et al. Characterization and management of postoperative hemorrhage following upper retroperitoneal laparoscopic surgery. J Urol. 2006;176:1458–62.

37. Walz MK, Alesina PF, Wenger FA, et al. Posterior retroperitoneoscopic adrenalectomy—results of 560 procedures in 520 patients. Surgery. 2006;140:943–8; discussion 948–50.

38. Strebel RT, Muntener M, Sulser T. Intraoperative complications of laparoscopic adrenalectomy. World J Urol. 2008;26:555–60.

39. Bishoff JT, Allaf ME, Kirkels W, et al. Laparoscopic bowel injury: incidence and clinical presentation. J Urol. 1999;161:887–90.

Robotic Partial Nephrectomy: Transperitoneal Technique

John M. Shields, Sam B. Bhayani, and Li-Ming Su

Abbreviations

CT   Computerized tomography
MRI   Magnetic resonance imaging

Patient Selection

The American Urological Association includes partial nephrectomy as a standard treatment option for masses <4 cm in size, while select larger masses can be considered on a case-by-case basis [1]. The indications for robotic partial nephrectomy are similar to open surgery, which most notably relates to tumor size, location, and anatomic and clinical conditions. No firm rule for inclusion or exclusion criteria may be universally established as radical nephrectomy is also within the standard of care for suspected renal cell carcinoma. The choice of an open, laparoscopic, or robotic approach is ultimately determined by the surgeon and patient in a concerted discussion of relative experience, risks, and benefits. Robotic partial nephrectomy has become an existing standard for treatment with well-documented and reproducible steps. However, challenges may arise in patients with increased obesity, previous abdominal surgery, dense perinephric fat, or other previous history of infection, inflammation, or biopsy; these features may create challenges with visualization and dissection leading to increased risk of bleeding, injury, and prolonged operative time.

J.M. Shields
Department of Urology, University of Florida College of Medicine, Gainesville, FL, USA

S.B. Bhayani, M.D., M.S. (✉)
Department of Surgery and Urology,
St. Louis, MO, USA
e-mail: bhayanisa@wudosis.wustl.edu

L.-M. Su, M.D.
Department of Urology, University of Florida College of Medicine, 1600 SW Archer Road, 100247, Gainesville, FL 32610-2047, USA
e-mail: sulm@urology.ufl.edu

Preoperative Preparation

Adequate imaging is required not only for diagnosis of the suspected renal mass, but also for a clear understanding of preoperative anatomy including tumor size, location, depth, proximity to deep renal structures (i.e., blood vessels, sinus fat, and collecting system), and especially thorough appreciation of the renal vascular anatomy. Multiphase CT or MRI with axial and coronal views are critical to define tumor and vascular structures. With improved three-dimensional reconstruction of contrasted CT images, improved appreciation of patient's renal vascular anatomy can also be achieved. Preoperative bowel preparation may aid in improved intraoperative visualization through decompression of the bowels and can be used per surgeon preference.

© Springer International Publishing Switzerland 2017
L.-M. Su (ed.), *Atlas of Robotic Urologic Surgery*, DOI 10.1007/978-3-319-45060-5_6

A liquid diet and/or magnesium citrate prior to surgery may also be given to aid in bowel preparation. However, with experience, the authors generally do not perform any specific bowel preparation. Good preoperative practice applies with all medical and surgical comorbidities thoroughly evaluated and cleared by the respective primary teams and specialists, and stopping anticoagulants 7–10 days prior to the procedure, when safely indicated. In the authors' experience, robotic partial nephrectomy can be safely performed in patients who are taking 81 mg of acetylsalicylic acid. Informed consent should include all risks, benefits, and alternatives and patients should be prepared for the possibility of a conversion to either a radical nephrectomy and/or an open procedure, should the need arise. The potential for a urine leak and pseudoaneurysm should also be discussed with the patient as well as need for additional procedures. Parenteral broad-spectrum antibiotics are routinely given upon induction of anesthesia. Subcutaneous heparin is not routinely given upon induction unless there exists a high risk of thromboembolic or cardiovascular disease. Patients should be typed and crossed for blood in the case of unexpected blood loss and need for transfusion.

Operating Room Setup

The operative setup may vary based on surgeon preference and the type of robot used (i.e., daVinci Si vs. Xi); however, it is recommended to keep the operative setup as consistent as possible so that the ancillary members of the team acquire familiarity with one particular routine especially during the learning curve. Figure 6.1 represents the operative setup we routinely use for robotic partial nephrectomy. It is important for the reader to note that this chapter will outline the operative setup and steps when using the daVinci Si robot. When docking the robot, the patient is placed in a lateral decubitus position and the robot is docked from the patient's dorsal side, thereby allowing the surgical assistant and scrub technician to be positioned on the ventral side of the patient. The robot is brought toward

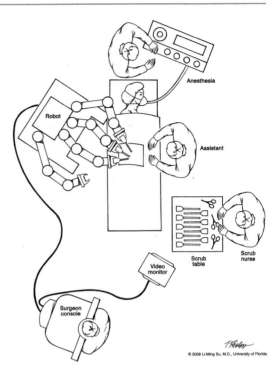

Fig. 6.1 Operating room setup using a three-armed or four-armed robotic technique

the operating table at an approximately 45° oblique angle at the head of the bed. The latest generation daVinci Xi robot allows more flexibility and versatility than the Si robot and can be docked from many different angles with respect to the operating room table due to its unique rotating boom design. Ultrasound and energy sources may come off the table where they are felt least likely to interfere with the moving arms and operating room staff. Video screens are placed throughout the operating room such that the surgical bedside assistant and scrub technician can view the operation and follow the surgeon throughout the procedure.

Patient Preparation and Positioning

The patient is placed under general endotracheal anesthesia and all intravenous lines, arterial lines, and other monitoring equipment are established prior to patient positioning, as access to extremities will be limited once the procedure has commenced. An orogastric tube is inserted and placed on suction to deflate the stomach, thereby minimizing the likelihood of encountering the stomach intraoperatively and sustaining possible injury, particularly during a left-sided procedure. A urethral catheter is also placed with the drainage bag easily accessible by the anesthesia staff. Sequential compression devices are placed on the patient's bilateral lower extremities. The patient is positioned over the table such that the table may be gently flexed at the level just above the anterior superior iliac spine, resulting in increased exposure of the flank for well-spaced trocar placement (Fig. 6.2). The kidney rest on the table is generally not required and may increase the risk of perioperative flank complications. The patient is then placed in the lateral decubitus position; a modified flank position is suitable for anterior renal lesions, whereas a full flank position is preferred for posterior renal lesions. For posterior lesions, where medial rotation of the kidney is expected in order to adequately visualize the renal tumor, the patient should be placed in a full flank (vs. modified) position in efforts to utilize gravity to optimize medial mobilization of the ipsilateral colon and spleen (left) or liver

(right) and allow unimpeded medial rotation of the kidney. An axillary roll is utilized when the patient is placed in a full flank position to prevent brachial plexus injury. To assist with maintaining the flank position, a large gel roll is placed behind the patient, thus supporting the patient's back and pelvis. Pillows are placed between the arms to hold the upper arm in an anatomically neutral position (Fig. 6.3). The pillows are carefully placed such that the endotracheal tube is not compromised. Prior to placing the pillows, the dependent arm is placed on an arm board in a neutral position and is secured with pressure points padded. The pillows are placed over this dependent arm and secured to the arm board. The patient's second arm is placed gently over the pillows, covered with foam padding and secured to the arm board. A shoulder roll is placed such that the shoulder is pulled inferiorly toward the patient's feet to help minimize the risk of brachial plexus injury. The hips are secured to the table with straps and heavy cloth tape placed over foam padding as are the legs with the dependent leg flexed. All pressure points in contact with the table or tape are padded. Pillows are placed between the legs prior to fastening the table strap

Fig. 6.2 The operating table is flexed at the level just above the patient's anterior superior iliac spine, resulting in increased exposure of the flank for well-spaced trocar placement

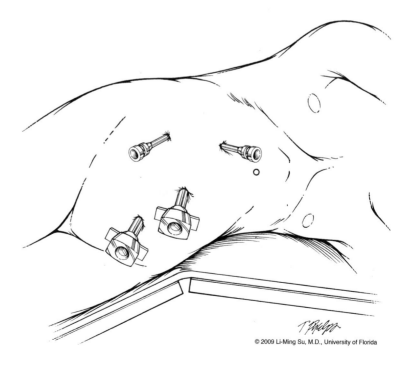

© 2009 Li-Ming Su, M.D., University of Florida

Fig. 6.3 Pillows are placed between the arms to hold the upper arm in an anatomically neutral position

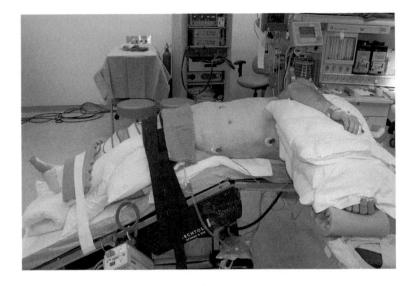

over the superior leg, which is left extended. To confirm that the patient is adequately secured to the operating room table, the table is rotated from one extreme to the other, taking care to ensure the patient's position does not shift.

Instrumentation and Equipment List
- Conventional laparoscope with 0° lens (for entry into the abdominal cavity, trocar placement, specimen extraction, fascial closure)
- EndoWrist® curved monopolar scissors (Intuitive Surgical, Inc., Sunnyvale, CA)
- EndoWrist® curved bipolar Maryland forceps (Intuitive Surgical, Inc., Sunnyvale, CA)
- EndoWrist® ProGrasp™ forceps (Intuitive Surgical, Inc., Sunnyvale, CA) if using a fourth robotic arm
- EndoWrist® large suture cut needle driver (Intuitive Surgical, Inc., Sunnyvale, CA)
- EndoWrist® large needle driver (Intuitive Surgical, Inc., Sunnyvale, CA)
- InSite Vision System with 30° (down) lens (Intuitive Surgical, Inc., Sunnyvale, CA)
- Laparoscopic articulating or robotic drop-in Doppler ultrasound probe; e.g., Aloka (Hitachi Aloka Medical Ltd., Tokyo, Japan) or BK ultrasound probe (BK Ultrasound, Peabody, MA)

Trocars
- 12 mm camera trocar with direct vision obturator
- 12 mm Airseal® System assistant trocar
- 2-3 (depending on whether a three or four-arm technique is performed) × 8 mm robotic standard or extra-long trocars (in case of obese patients)

Instruments Used by the Surgical Assistant
- Suction-irrigator device
- Laparoscopic needle driver
- Laparoscopic blunt tip grasper
- Laparoscopic scissors
- Hem-o-lok® clip applier (Teleflex Medical, Research Triangle Park, NC)
- Large (purple) Hem-o-lok® clips (Teleflex Medical, Research Triangle Park, NC)
- Lapra-Ty® clip applier (Ethicon, Somerville, NJ)
- Lapra-Ty® absorbable suture clips (Ethicon, Somerville, NJ)
- Atraumatic laparoscopic bulldog vascular clamps (six available: three short, three long), or alternatively, robotic bulldog vascular clamps and applicator (Scanlan International, St. Paul, MN)
- Surgicel® hemostatic gauze (Ethicon, Inc., Cincinnati, OH)

- FloSeal® (Baxter Int. Inc., Fremont, CA, USA)
- 10 mm Endocatch® specimen retrieval bag (Covidien, Irvine, CA, USA)
- 8 French Blake round closed suction drain
- Airseal® System and tubing for insufflation (Conmed, Surgiquest Inc., Milford, USA)

Sutures
- 3-0 Polyglactin suture on an SH needle × 5; cut to 7″-secured at distal end with Lapra-Ty® clip and knot (Fig. 6.4a)
- 0 Polyglactin suture on CT-1 needle × 7; cut to 8″-secured at distal end with Hem-o-lok® clip, Lapra-Ty® clip, and knot (Fig. 6.4b)
- 0 Polydiaxanone suture on a CT-1 needle
- 4-0 Monofilament absorbable suture on a PS-2 needle
- 2-0 Monofilament non-absorbable suture on an FS needle

Available and in the Room
- Laparoscopic reticulating Endo GIA™ (Covidien, Irvine, CA, USA) stapling device with a 30 mm cartridge length and vascular load
- Laparoscopic Satinsky vascular clamp

Step-by-Step Technique

Step 1: Insufflation

Prior to placing the Veress needle, with the surgeon facing the patient's abdomen, the operating table is rotated away from the surgeon, placing the patient in a relatively supine and horizontal position. A Veress needle is placed in a standard fashion within the umbilicus, penetrating the skin and abdominal fascia. Once satisfied with Veress placement, a drop test is performed and insufflation is commenced with CO_2 to a maximum pressure of 12–15 mmHg. We routinely use the Airseal® System for insufflation. Once four-quadrant pneumoperitoneum is achieved, we commence placement of the trocars.

Step 2: Trocar Placement

Given the high variability of trocar placement, three- vs. four-arm approach, lateral vs. medial camera port placement, daVinci Si vs. Xi robot, tumor location, and body habitus, a number of trocar configurations can be used. Several literature reports document trocar placement. In general, it is important to place trocars at least 8 cm apart from one another to prevent internal and external instrument collision [2, 3]. With the advent of the daVinci Xi robot, the arms are much smaller in profile and more agile, making collisions minimal when compared to older model robots. As stated before, we will describe our institution's technique using the daVinci Si robot, based upon a three-arm technique. Reference will be made to maneuvers using a four-arm technique when necessary.

We use a total of four trocars; a 12 mm trocar for the robotic camera, two 8 mm metallic robotic trocars, and a fourth 12 mm trocar to be used by the assistant (Fig. 6.5a, b). A fifth 5 mm trocar may also be placed, particularly for right-sided

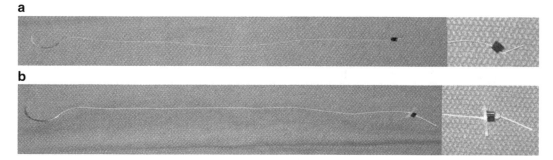

Fig. 6.4 (**a**) 3-0 Polyglactin suture on an SH needle × 5; cut to 7″-secured at distal end with Lapra-Ty® clip and knot. (**b**) 0 Polyglactin suture on CT-1 needle × 7; cut to 8″-secured at distal end with Hem-o-lok® clip, Lapra-Ty® clip, and knot

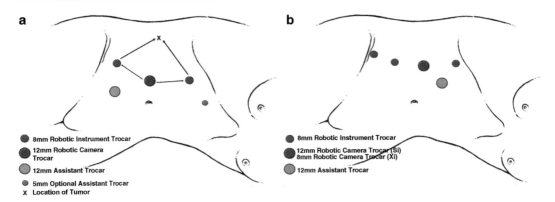

Fig. 6.5 (**a**) Three-arm trocar placement for daVinci Si. (**b**) Four-arm trocar placement for daVinci Si and Xi

procedures to assist with liver retraction. Using a direct vision 12 mm trocar and 0° standard laparoscope, the robotic camera trocar is the first trocar to be placed once insufflation is achieved. Placement of this primary trocar for the endoscope is critical to the success of robotic partial nephrectomy and should be tailored according to the unique location of the renal tumor and not based on standard anatomic landmarks. Using the preoperative imaging films (both axial and coronal imaging) and the location of the renal tumor as a guide, the 12 mm camera trocar is placed so as to achieve a proper view of the tumor once dissected and fully exposed. It is critical not to have the camera trocar directly above or too far away from the tumor, compromising instrument maneuverability or visualization of the tumor base, respectively. Ideally, the camera trocar should be strategically placed to allow a 45° downward view of the renal tumor. For posterior renal lesions where the kidney and tumor will need to be rotated medially into view, the camera trocar should be placed further laterally to be able to peer along the posterior surface of the kidney. Once this primary trocar is placed into the abdomen, the Veress needle is identified and surrounding structures visualized to ensure no injury has been sustained. The Veress needle is then removed. At this point, the anterior abdominal wall can be inspected for adhesions, which if present are carefully lysed.

Prior to secondary trocar placement, the operating room table is rotated to the abdominal side to achieve the final position that the patient will remain in for the duration of the operation. This allows for bowels to fall away from the affected renal unit. The approximate location of the kidney and tumor is estimated based upon visual landmarks such as the contour of the kidney, ipsilateral colon, spleen (on left), and liver (on right). On the outside of the body, with the camera pointing in the direction of the tumor, an "X" is marked on the skin as a rough guide to assist in placement of secondary trocars (Fig. 6.5a). Two 8 mm trocars are then placed under direct vision; these 8 mm trocars are placed in such a fashion that they form a broad-based triangle with the "X" (i.e., tumor) forming the apex of this imaginary triangle. The assistant's 12 mm Airseal® trocar is placed under direct vision in a plane that bisects an imaginary line between the camera trocar and the inferolateral 8 mm robotic trocar. Some surgeons opt to use a fourth robotic arm to assist with retraction that is placed through a trocar located dependent and inferior to the most inferior robotic trocar (Fig. 6.5b). Placement of these trocars may need to follow a different order depending on the nature of any adhesions encountered. With obese patients or patients with anatomy that will predispose to the robotic arms clashing externally, extra-long trocars (vs. standard size) can be used to decrease the likelihood of clashing. Occasionally, a fifth 5 mm trocar will need to be placed for right-sided procedures in order to aid with liver retraction (Fig. 6.5a).

The robot is then docked as described earlier. It is important to note that the robotic camera arm rests within the area of the "sweet spot" (a pre-determined area on the joint of the camera arm demarcated by a blue line), allowing for optimal range of motion. The 30° down robotic camera lens is then placed. The robotic instruments are then passed slowly into the abdomen under direct vision.

Step 3: Mobilization of Ipsilateral Colon (Table 6.1)

Dissection begins with identification and incision of the white line of Toldt, approximately 2 cm lateral to the ipsilateral colon. The colon is reflected medially and mobilized far enough inferiorly and superiorly so as not to create a "hammock" effect, whereby the extreme ends of the colon are still suspended to the lateral abdominal wall, impeding proper visualization and exposure of the renal hilum. For a left-sided dissection, the descending colon is mobilized from (and including) the spleen down to the pelvic inlet. For a right-sided dissection, the ascending colon is mobilized from (and including) the right lobe of the liver down to the pelvic inlet.

Left-Sided Dissection

For left-sided tumors, reflection of the descending colon toward the splenic flexure should continue lateral to the spleen in order to medially reflect the spleen en bloc with the splenic flexure and tail of the pancreas. With the bipolar forceps elevating and reflecting the spleen medially, monopolar scissors are used to bluntly develop the natural plane between the spleen and the tail of the pancreas and Gerota's fascia. At the most cephalad aspect of this dissect, care must be taken to avoid injury to the stomach as it can

Table 6.1 Instrumentation for colon mobilization

Surgeon instrumentation		Assistant instrumentation
Right arm	Left arm	• Suction-irrigator
• Curved monopolar scissors	• Bipolar Maryland forceps	

occasionally be seen superior-medial to the spleen. It is prudent at this point to recheck with the anesthesia team that an orogastric tube is in place and on suction to decompress the stomach. Once colon and spleen are sufficiently medialized, attention is turned toward identifying the gonadal vein, ureter, and psoas muscle. The gonadal vein and left ureter are retracted upward by the assistant to expose the psoas muscle. The gonadal vein is traced cephalad to its junction with the left renal vein. When using a four-arm technique, the fourth robotic arm is useful during this step to elevate the ureter and lower pole of the kidney with a Prograsp™ forceps, allowing for a two-handed dissection of the renal hilum.

Right-Sided Dissection

For right-sided dissection, the robotic instrument selection is the same as for left-sided dissection. The white line of Toldt is incised and the ascending colon is mobilized medially both in a superior and inferior direction. On the right side, the liver is encountered at the hepatic flexure. In cases where visualization of the upper pole of the kidney is required, the coronary ligament of the right lobe of the liver is divided as are attachments between the liver and right hemidiaphragm. Care is taken when dissecting along the diaphragm as inadvertent injury and trauma to the diaphragm can occur due to sudden muscle contraction especially when using monopolar electrocautery. As the hepatic flexure is further dissected, awareness of the anatomy with particular attention paid toward the duodenum and inferior vena cava is critical in order to avoid injury. In the case of a particularly large liver overhanging the kidney and limiting dissection, a second assistant port can be placed (usually inferior to the xiphoid process) in order to pass a second instrument to aid in fixed liver retraction. As the duodenum is encountered, it is kocherized medially in order to expose the inferior vena cava, right renal vein, and right renal hilum. Inferior to the lower pole of the kidney, a plane is identified between the ureter and psoas muscle, taking care to avoid these structures as well as the right gonadal vein.

Fig. 6.6 Illustration depicting surgeon's left instrument providing anterior traction of lower pole to assist with dissection of renal hilum

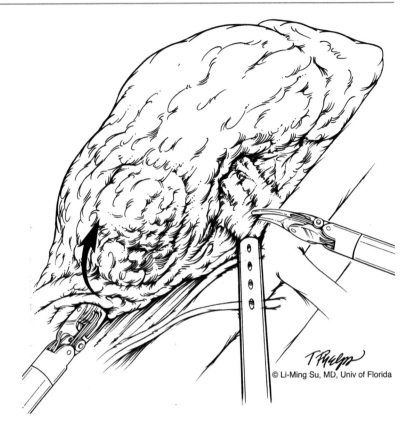

© Li-Ming Su, MD, Univ of Florida

Cephalad dissection is carried out toward the renal hilum. Either the surgeon's left instrument or the assistant can provide anterior traction on the ureter and lower pole perinephric fat to allow dissection of the renal hilum (Fig. 6.6). Again, if a fourth robotic arm has been placed, retraction of the ureter can be accomplished using blunt anterior traction with a Prograsp™ forceps.

Step 4: Renal Hilar Dissection (Table 6.2)

Using preoperative cross-sectional imaging as a guide, all arteries and veins are carefully identified both in the axial and coronal views. This provides the surgeon with a mental "road map" so as to anticipate each vessel during hilar dissection. More specifically, the precise number of renal arteries must be identified as this can lead to unwanted bleeding during tumor excision if an

Table 6.2 Instrumentation for renal hilar dissection

Surgeon instrumentation		Assistant instrumentation
Right arm	Left arm	• Suction-irrigator
• Curved monopolar scissors	• Bipolar Maryland forceps	• Laparoscopic blunt tip grasper
		• Large Hem-o-lok® clip applicator
		• Large Hem-o-lok® clips
		• Red and blue vessel loops

unidentified renal artery is not addressed. All arteries and veins are skeletonized in anticipation of clamping of these vessels. However, in the authors' experience, only the renal arteries are routinely clamped during most tumor excisions. On occasion, with deep endophytic or hilar tumors, significant venous backbleeding is encountered from larger subsegmental veins during tumor excision, resulting in poor visualization warranting clamping of the renal vein(s). It is important to make every attempt to free up all connective tissue around the renal vessels in order to facilitate ease of applying the bulldog clamps and their subsequent ability to adequately occlude the vessels without entrapment of adjacent perivascular fat. Clamping the renal artery along sites of atherosclerosis (often at the renal artery origin off the aorta) should be avoided as this may lead to incomplete occlusion of the artery. Non-contrasted CT views of the renal vessels can help delineate sites of atherosclerosis. Once the hilar vessels are skeletonized, vessel loops are introduced by the assistant and placed around the renal vessels (e.g., red vessel loop for arteries and blue vessel loop for veins), which allow for prompt identification of the vessels during the operation. The tail ends of the vessel loops are then clipped together using a Hem-o-lok® clip.

Step 5: Dissection and Exposure of the Renal Tumor (Table 6.3)

Prior to tumor identification and dissection, 12.5 g of intravenous mannitol are administered. A laparoscopic or robotic drop-in Doppler ultrasound probe can be used to identify the location of the renal tumor within Gerota's fascia. Gerota's fascia is incised and the underlying perinephric fat dissected away to expose the tumor lying beneath. Specific attention should be paid to removing all perinephric fat circumferentially

Table 6.3 Instrumentation for dissection and exposure of the renal tumor

Surgeon instrumentation		Assistant instrumentation
Right arm	Left arm	• Suction-irrigator
• Curved monopolar scissors	• Bipolar Maryland forceps	• Laparoscopic blunt tip grasper
	• ProGrasp™ forceps	• 4″ × 8″ moist gauze (as required)
		• Laparoscopic or Drop-in Doppler ultrasound probe

around the tumor, giving rise to a generous 2–3 cm margin of surrounding normal parenchyma (Fig. 6.7). This affords adequate surgical margin around the tumor specimen and sufficiently exposed parenchyma for eventual renorraphy. A small patch of fat is left overlying the tumor site so as not to violate the tumor capsule.

In the case of more posterior or superior tumors, extensive dissection of the perinephric fat will allow for either medial rotation or even transposition of the kidney upon its long axis, thus relocating the tumor in the anterior position. One or more moist 4″ × 8″ gauzes may be placed, if needed, behind the kidney in order to prop up and support the kidney in the ideal position for tumor excision. Alternatively, a ProGrasp™ forceps placed through a fourth robotic arm may be used for this purpose.

Step 6: Ultrasonic Demarcation of Renal Tumor Margins (Table 6.4)

With the assistance of intraoperative ultrasound, the renal tumor is identified and its margins and depth visualized in comparison to preoperative imaging. This can be done with a drop-in ultrasound probe passed through the assistant port, controlled by the robotic ProGrasp™ forceps. Alternatively, a laparoscopic articulating ultrasound probe can be passed through the assistant port and controlled by the assistant (Fig. 6.7). The ultrasound image can be introduced into the surgeon console view using the TilePro® multi-input display feature. The use of a robotic drop-in probe provides advantages over the laparoscopic probe in that the surgeon can control movement of the ultrasound and clearly demarcate the margin of the tumor along its entire perimeter. This is more challenging when using the laparoscopic hand-held articulating ultrasound probe as its entry point is fixed at the trocar insertion site and not all of the unique angles along the tumor perimeter can be clearly visualized. The amount of margin is dependent on each patient's clinical characteristics. Monopolar scissors are used to mark an adequate margin around the tumor where the subsequent incision will take place (Fig. 6.7).

Fig. 6.7 Illustration depicting identification of tumor with laparoscopic ultrasound probe and demarcation of margin around tumor with monopolar cautery

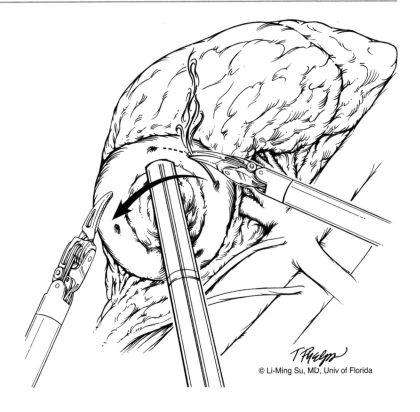

© Li-Ming Su, MD, Univ of Florida

Table 6.4 Instrumentation required for laparoscopic ultrasound assessment and demarcation of renal tumor margins

Surgeon instrumentation		Assistant instrumentation
Right arm	Left arm	• Suction-irrigator
• Curved monopolar scissors	• ProGrasp™ forceps	• Laparoscopic or Drop-in Doppler ultrasound probe

Step 7: Pre-clamp Checklist and Suture Preparation

At this point, prior to proceeding to further incision of the renal capsule and clamping of the renal vessels, we review a pre-clamp checklist of required instruments, sutures, and products as well as responsibilities of each team member.

Personnel
• Scrub technician and anesthesiologist who will remain consistent for the duration of the operation

• Circulating nurse who will manage stopwatch and document warm ischemia clamp time
• Bedside assistant who will apply/remove laparoscopic bulldog clamps, deliver sutures to operating surgeon, retract and expose base of resection site

Instrumentation
• Two functioning (i.e., non-expired) robotic needle drivers
• Sutures for repair of deep base of resection site and renorrhaphy. The number of sutures will depend on the size and complexity of the defect and repair.
• Adequate number of Hem-o-lok® and Lapra-Ty® clips

Prior to proceeding with incision of the renal capsule, the curved monopolar scissor is removed and both needle drivers are tested to ensure they work appropriately and have not expired. We routinely use a suture cutting needle driver in the right arm to obviate the need for the bedside assistant to cut sutures during the remainder of the operation. While testing the needle drivers, we also pre-place two to three 3-0 polyglactin sutures on an SH needle into the abdominal cavity for easy access to the operating surgeon. These are secured out of the way along the lateral abdominal wall. Each suture is placed a reasonable distance apart from each other to avoid tangling.

Step 8: Clamping of Renal Vessels, Tumor Excision, and Renorraphy (Table 6.5)

With a curved monopolar scissor to the right arm, tumor excision is commenced. We start by superficially incising the renal cortex with monopolar electrocautery along the previously demarcated margin to approximately 5 mm depth. This is performed while off clamp as there typically is very

Table 6.5 Instrumentation required for clamping of renal hilar vessels, tumor excision and renorraphy

Surgeon instrumentation		Assistant instrumentation
Right arm	Left arm	• Suction-irrigator
• Curved monopolar scissors	• ProGrasp™ forceps	• Laparoscopic needle driver
		• Bulldog vascular clamps
• Large suture cut needle driver	• Large needle driver	• Laparoscopic bulldog vascular clamp applicator
		• Hem-o-lok® clip applier
		• Lapra-Ty® suture clip applier
		• 3-0 Polyglactin suture on an SH needle; cut to 7″
		• 0 Polyglactin suture on CT1 needle; cut to 8″
		• FloSeal® (Baxter Int. Inc., Fremont, CA, USA)
		• Surgicel® (Ethicon Inc., Somerville, NJ)

little bleeding from the superficial cortex of the kidney. Once this is carried out circumferentially, attention is then turned toward clamping of the renal artery(ies). The artery should be clamped as close to the crotch of the bulldog clamp as possible as the proximal closing strength is much greater than the distal end. In addition, the authors generally place two bulldog clamps on each renal artery (Fig. 6.8). The surgeon will assist with the surgical assistant's placement of the vascular clamps by utilizing the vessel loops to expose the renal artery in a manner best suited for placement of the bulldog clamps. Once the renal artery is clamped, the time is noted by the circulating nurse. As stated previously, a clamp is only placed onto the renal vein in cases of deep or hilar tumor resections. In such cases, large subsegmental veins can become exposed and contribute to significant backbleeding. By clamping the renal vein(s), venous backbleeding is minimized.

It is important that the deeper portions of tumor excision be performed using a cold-cutting technique as the charring effect of electrocautery can make assessment of the surgical margins and accidental tumor violation at the base of the tumor difficult. With the tips of the scissors pointed *away* from the tumor and toward the parenchyma (to prevent violation of the tumor capsule), the parenchyma is incised gradually and in a circumferential manner, taking care not to dig deep into a hole in any one area. As cold-cutting dissection progresses, the assistant provides downward counter-traction on the renal parenchyma as the surgeon lifts upward on the tumor. Occasional spot electrocautery can be used for small exposed vessels. As dissection progresses towards the deepest aspect of the tumor specimen, the scissors are then rotated allowing the tips to point upwards, thereby completing the excision while leaving a concave renal defect (Fig. 6.9). The tumor is placed superiorly toward the diaphragmatic recess of the spleen (left-sided dissection) or liver (right-sided dissection) where it will remain until it can be placed in a laparoscopic entrapment sac toward the end of the procedure.

Fig. 6.8 Illustration
depicting exposure and
clamping of renal artery
with two bulldog clamps

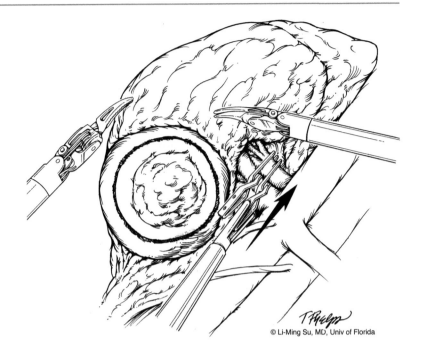

© Li-Ming Su, MD, Univ of Florida

Fig. 6.9 Illustration
depicting retraction,
exposure, and dissection
of renal tumor. Note
assistant's suction-
irrigator providing
counter traction to
surgeon's left instrument

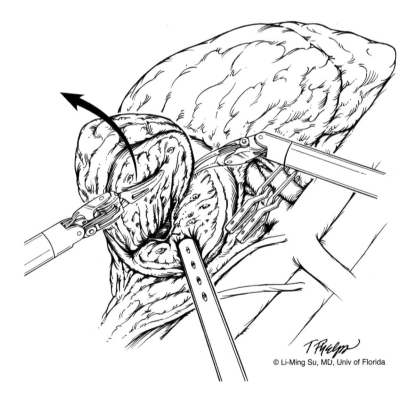

© Li-Ming Su, MD, Univ of Florida

Step 9: Renorrhaphy (Table 6.6)

In order to perform the renorrhaphy, the bedside assistant promptly switches both robotic arms to robotic needle drivers. The renorrhaphy is divided into two layers. The deep layer involves oversewing blood vessels and collecting system in a running continuous manner using two to three 3-0 polyglactin sutures on an SH needle, cut to a length of 7″. A Lapra-Ty® clip is fastened to the end of the suture along with a knot proximal to this (Fig. 6.4a). The second layer involves formal reapproximation of the renal parenchymal edges using multiple 0 polyglactin sutures on a CT-1 needle cut to a length of 7″ with Hem-o-lok® clips placed at the distal end just proximal to a knot (Fig. 6.4b). The 3-0 polyglactin sutures used on the deep base are retrieved from their pre-placed location along the lateral abdominal wall so as to eliminate the time required for the bedside assistant to pass sutures in and out of the abdomen while the artery is clamped. Generally, two running sutures are used for small- to moderate-sized defects; however, for larger defects, three to four running sutures may be required. As each suture run is completed, the needles are cut and securely placed back into the lateral abdominal wall where they will safely remain until they are removed at the end of the procedure. The authors do not generally use hemostatic agents or bolsters within the defect, but have these available if needed. During reapproximation of the parenchymal edges, the 0 polyglactin sutures are driven from the outside edge of the parenchyma with a generous 1–1.5 cm bite, through the renal defect and then to the opposing side. The suture is then secured with a Hem-o-lok® clip through which the suture can be tightened, thereby further closing the gap and compressing the parenchymal edges. Figure 6.10

Illustration depicting renorrhaphy using sliding clip technique. This technique has also been described as the "sliding clip renorrhaphy" [4]. Multiple sutures are placed in a simple interrupted fashion until the entire defect is securely approximated and compressed.

The vascular clamps are then promptly removed noting the end of warm ischemia, and the excision site is observed for signs of bleeding. The parenchymal sutures are then further tightened and reinforced with a second Hem-o-lok® or Lapra-Ty® clip. This maneuver, in addition to simply allowing the kidney to regain perfusion and turgor, results in cessation of most minor bleeding within the defect. On rare occasions, an additional suture may be required if brisk arterial bleeding is noted. The needles are cut and removed with a laparoscopic needle grasper along with the 3-0 polyglactin SH needles.

Step 10: Extraction and Closure (Table 6.7)

Attention is turned toward the renal hilum for reinspection. The renal artery should be inspected for adequate pulsations and the renal vein for adequate filling. The vessel loops are cut by the assistant with laparoscopic scissors and removed with laparoscopic spoons. Any 4″ × 8″ gauze is also removed with the laparoscopic spoons. A specimen entrapment sac is then passed through the assistant port and the specimen and any surrounding perinephric fat is retrieved from the diaphragmatic recess and placed carefully into the bag. The bag is then closed and the tail end of the string fed into the abdominal cavity. The string may then be removed with a laparoscopic blunt tip grasper depending on which trocar site will be used for specimen extraction. The drain may be placed through the inferolateral robotic trocar after removing the robotic arm, allowing the surgeon to place the drain in its desired location within the abdomen. The drain is externally secured to the skin using a 2-0 monofilament suture on an FS needle. Once the drain is secured, the robotic arms may be removed. The camera

Table 6.6 Instrumentation required for renorrhaphy

Surgeon instrumentation		Assistant instrumentation
Right arm	Left arm	
• Suture cut needle driver	• Large needle driver	• Suction-irrigator • Laparoscopic bulldog applicator • Laparoscopic needle driver

Fig. 6.10

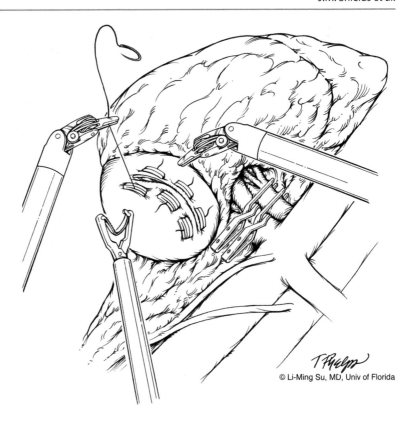

© Li-Ming Su, MD, Univ of Florida

Table 6.7 Instrumentation for specimen extraction and closure of incisions

Surgeon instrumentation		Assistant instrumentation
Right arm	Left arm	• Suction-irrigator • Laparoscopic needle driver • Laparoscopic scissors • Laparoscopic spoons • Laparoscopic specimen entrapment sac • Laparoscopic blunt tip grasper • 8 French suction drain • Carter-Thomason CloseSure System (Cooper Surgical, Trumbull, CT, USA) • 0 Polydiaxanone suture on a CT-1 needle • 2-0 Monofilament suture on an FS needle • 4-0 Monofilament absorbable suture on a PS-2 needle
• Large suture cut needle driver	• Large Needle driver	

can then be removed and the robot undocked from the operating table.

Closure of the fascia depends on the size of the extraction site. For smaller tumors, the laparoscopic bag may be removed under direct vision without extending the fascial opening. When extracting in this manner, care must be taken to avoid iatrogenic fragmentation of the specimen when extracting through a tight extraction site. The trocar site and fascia can subsequently be closed using a Carter-Thomason CloseSure System. For larger tumors, a larger extraction site is required and the fascia closed using 0 polydiaxanone sutures on a CT-1 needle, in an interrupted figure-of-eight fashion. The wound site is then irrigated and the skin is approximated using a 4-0 monofilament absorbable suture on a PS-2 needle, in a subcuticular fashion.

Postoperative Management

Intraoperative initiation of ketorolac and intravenous acetaminophen can be routinely used in appropriate patients who do not have bleeding tendencies or renal insufficiency. Patients are started on a clear liquid diet on the evening of surgery and advanced to a regular diet on postoperative day one. Patients are encouraged to ambulate as soon as possible. Criteria for discharge differ markedly as per the patient and comorbid medical status; however, patients at our institution tend to routinely be discharged home on postoperative day one. In general, both the drain and urethral catheter are removed prior to discharge. However, if considerable output (i.e., over 100 cc per day) is noted from the operative drain, a sample can be sent for creatinine analysis, and if negative, the drain can be removed. If there is confirmation of a urine leak, the drain may be left off suction to allow for the leak to seal, while the urethral catheter remains in place for 5–7 days until the drain output is low. Rarely, a ureteral stent may be required to manage a significant urine leak.

Complications

Complications following robotic partial nephrectomy are rare, but can include bleeding, transfusion, pseudoaneurysm, and urine leak. Pseudoaneurysms and urine leak are minimized by meticulous hemostasis and suture closure of exposed calyces along the deep resection base prior to renorrhaphy. Conversion to an open partial nephrectomy or radical nephrectomy is uncommon with experienced teams. Prolonged surgery can lead to the rare case of rhabdomyolysis of the dependent thigh and hip, especially in patients with high body mass index.

Conclusion

Robotic partial nephrectomy is an excellent procedure for patients desiring a minimally invasive approach to excision of a renal mass. Overall results are similar to the open approach with improved convalescence and cosmesis. Unlike other robotic surgeries, many aspects of this procedure can vary from surgeon to surgeon including basic trocar placement and technique, differences in tumor location, amount of fat around the kidney, body habitus, size of tumor, and other considerations. However, once a routine is adapted with defined roles among team members in the operating room, the learning curve for all involved can be significantly improved.

References

1. Andrew Novick. Guideline for management of the clinical stage 1 renal mass. AUA guidelines. 2009. Cited March 5, 2017. https://www.auanet.org/common/pdf/education/clinical-guidance/Renal-Mass.pdf.
2. Bhayani SB. Da Vinci robotic partial nephrectomy for renal cell carcinoma: an atlas of the four-arm technique. J Robot Surg. 2008;1(4):279–85.
3. Patel MN, Bhandari M, Menon M, Rogers CG. Robotic-assisted partial nephrectomy. BJU Int. 2009;103(9):1296–311.
4. Benway BM, Wang AJ, Cabello JM, Bhayani SB. Robotic partial nephrectomy with sliding-clip renorrhaphy: technique and outcomes. Eur Urol. 2009;55(3):592–9.

Robotic Partial Nephrectomy: Advanced Techniques and Use of Intraoperative Imaging

Sameer Chopra, Alfredo Maria Bove, and Inderbir S. Gill

Abbreviations

CT   Computed tomography
GFR   Glomerular filtration rate
JP   Jackson-Pratt
PN   Partial nephrectomy
RAPN   Robotic-assisted partial nephrectomy

Introduction

Although the role of partial nephrectomy (PN) in the management of small renal masses is still debated for certain indications [1, 2], it is generally agreed that the significant prevalence and morbidity of chronic kidney disease validate the importance of nephron-preserving approaches in patients with small renal masses [3–7]. Laparoscopy and robotics have become increasingly utilized for PN due to the equivalent oncologic and functional outcomes and decreased morbidity when compared to open PN [7].

Post-PN function of the operated kidney depends primarily upon the quantity and quality of preserved, vascularized renal parenchyma, and secondarily upon the duration of warm ischemia [8]. Warm ischemic duration should be preferably restricted to 20–25 min or less [9, 10]. The volume of kidney excised and the duration of ischemia during PN are closely and inextricably inter-linked. Technological refinements of PN surgery are aimed at optimizing surgically modifiable factors, such as sculpted tumor excision, meticulous renorrhaphy and decreased ischemia, maximize the preservation of vascularized, functioning, normal kidney tissue [11]. Surgical attempts at minimizing warm ischemic injury began initially with "early-unclamping" techniques, then evolved to selective arterial clamping to achieve tumor-specific devascularization in an attempt to eliminate global ischemia [12]. In addition to minimizing ischemia duration, techniques involving sculpted tumor excision with pin-point sutured hemostasis further minimize functional parenchymal loss [13].

In this chapter, we focus on advanced PN surgical techniques that are aimed at minimizing global ischemia, preserving as much normal kidney parenchyma as possible and performing meticulous sutured renal reconstruction with minimal blood loss and complications. We also demonstrate imaging modalities that assist in the propagation of these techniques.

Electronic supplementary material: The online version of this chapter (doi:10.1007/978-3-319-45060-5_7) contains supplementary material, which is available to authorized users.

S. Chopra, M.S., M.D. • A.M. Bove, M.D.
I.S. Gill, M.D., M.Ch. (✉)
Catherine & Joseph Aresty Department of Urology, Keck School of Medicine, University of Southern California, Los Angeles, CA 90089, USA
e-mail: inderbir.gill@med.usc.edu

L.-M. Su (ed.), *Atlas of Robotic Urologic Surgery*, DOI 10.1007/978-3-319-45060-5_7

Pre-operative Preparation

Pre-operative Evaluation

Pre-operative evaluation includes history and physical examination, routine laboratory tests such as serum creatinine and estimated glomerular filtration rate, which is calculated using the modification of diet in renal disease formula. A dedicated three-dimensional abdominal computed tomography (CT) or magnetic resonance imaging scan with 0.5–2 mm slice thickness is obtained to delineate details about tumor location, depth, and proximity to the collecting system. The arterial and venous phases of the scan provide a detailed vascular road-map as regards extra-renal hilar arterial and venous anatomy.

Patients are counseled as to all treatment alternatives and surgical options. Risks, benefits, potential complications, and the possibility of conversion to open surgery or radical nephrectomy are discussed during informed consent.

Antiplatelet and anticoagulant medications are discontinued or bridged before surgery, as clinically indicated. Medical and anesthesia clearance are obtained. We do not routinely perform any formal bowel preparation; however, per surgeon preference, a clear liquid diet the evening before surgery augmented by Dulcolax suppository or an oral saline cathartic (e.g., magnesium citrate or Fleet Phospho-Soda) can be administered.

Intravenous antibiotics, such as one gram of cefazolin, are administered pre-operatively. For deep venous thrombosis prevention, pneumatic compressive stockings and 5000 U subcutaneous heparin is administered 2 h prior to procedure and continued every 12 h post-operatively; anticoagulation is continued for 1 month after discharge, per surgeon preference. At commencement of the robotic procedure, 1.5–2 L of crystalloid intravenous fluids are administered to expand the intravascular volume.

Operative Room Set-up

We routinely employ a 4-arm robotic technique. The assistant is positioned facing the patient's abdomen; the scrub technician is positioned behind the assistant. Video monitors are placed at the head and foot end of the patient on the side of the robot for easy viewing by the surgical team. A Mayo stand is placed next to the assistant where frequently used instruments are placed. The da Vinci® Surgical System (Intuitive Surgical, Inc., Sunnyvale, CA) is docked posterior to the patient with the camera arm coming in to the patient at an angle of 15° in line with the camera trocar site (described in detail below) (Fig. 7.1).

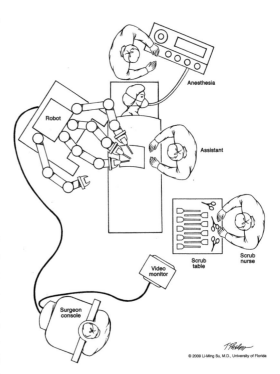

Fig. 7.1 (**a**) Operative room set-up for right partial nephrectomy; (**b**) Operative room set-up for left partial nephrectomy

Patient Positioning

Under general endotracheal anesthesia, the patient is placed in a modified (30°–70°) lateral decubitus position, with the umbilicus over a mild break in the table. An axillary roll is placed, the table is flexed as necessary (usually minimally compared with open flank surgery), and copious padding is used and positioned to support the buttocks and flank. Pillow(s) are placed between the flexed lower and straight upper leg. The upper arm rests on a well-padded arm board (or pillows) without tension on the brachial plexus. Tape is used to secure the patient around the hips, shoulders, and thighs to ensure stability when rolling the table to facilitate bowel retraction (Fig. 7.2). Care is taken to adequately pad all pressure points and place all limbs in neutral position to minimize positioning injuries. The abdominal skin is shaved with clippers and the patient is prepped and draped in standard sterile fashion for a trans-peritoneal robotic surgery. An 18-French urethral catheter is inserted and an orogastric tube is placed. A standard timeout is called prior to incision.

Instrumentation and Equipment List

Equipment
- Da Vinci® Si or Xi Surgical System (Intuitive Surgical, Inc., Sunnyvale, CA)
- 0° and 30° robotic scope (Intuitive Surgical, Inc., Sunnyvale, CA)
- Monopolar Scissors (Intuitive Surgical, Inc., Sunnyvale, CA)
- ProGrasp™ Forceps (Intuitive Surgical, Inc., Sunnyvale, CA)
- Bipolar Grasper™ Forceps (Intuitive Surgical, Inc., Sunnyvale, CA)
- Needle Drivers (Intuitive Surgical, Inc., Sunnyvale, CA)
- Clip Appliers (Intuitive Surgical, Inc., Sunnyvale, CA)

Trocars
- 12-mm visual obturator trocar (Visiport, Medtronic Parkway, Minneapolis, Minnesota)
- 5-mm trocar × 2
- 8-mm trocar × 2
- Bariatric 8-mm trocar × 2

Assistant Instruments
- Suction irrigator device (Bariatric length)
- Laparoscopic spoon forceps
- 5-mm locking atraumatic grasper

Fig. 7.2 Patient positioning

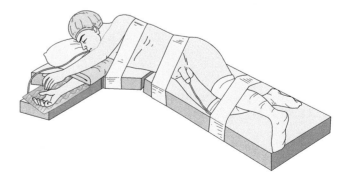

- Hem-o-lok applier (Teleflex Medical, Research Triangle Park, NC)
- Medium (purple) Hem-o-lok clips (Teleflex Medical, Research Triangle Park, NC)
- Small (green) Hem-o-lok clips (Teleflex Medical, Research Triangle Park, NC)
- 10-mm LigaSure Atlas™ Sealer/Divider device (Valleylab, Tyco Healthcare Group LP, Boulder, CO)
- Laparoscopic Needle driver
- Laparoscopic scissor
- 0-mm specimen entrapment bag
- Sponge on a stick
- Laparoscopic Doppler ultrasound probe
- Surgicel® hemostatic gauze (Ethicon, Johnson & Johnson, New Brunswick, NJ, USA)
- Hemovac or Jackson Pratt
- FloSeal hemostatic matrix (Baxter International, Deerfield, IL)
- FloSeal laparoscopic applier with obturator (Bariatric length) (Baxter International, Deerfield, IL)
- Laparoscopic bulldog clamps
- Neurosurgical aneurysm micro bulldog clamps (Bear™ disposable vascular clamp, AROSurgical, Newport Beach, CA)
- Mini-vessel loops (Devon Dev-o-loops, Tyco Healthcare, Mansfield, MA).
- Indocyanine Dye (Akorn, Lake Forest, IL)

Recommended Sutures

- 4-0 Prolene suture or 3-0 Vicryl suture on a SH needle (Ethicon, Johnson & Johnson, New Brunswick, NJ, USA)
- 4-0 Monocryl or V-Loc barbed suture (Ethicon, Johnson & Johnson, New Brunswick, NJ, USA)

Step-by-Step Technique (Videos 7.1, 7.2 and 7.3)

Step 1: Pneumoperitoneum and Trocar Placement (Fig. 7.3)

A transperitoneal approach is typically used for most tumors. Our standard trocar placement configuration allows for treatment of all renal tumors irrespective of location, whether upper pole, lower pole, or hilar. We employ four robotic trocars with 1–2 assistant ports. Veress needle pneumoperitoneum (13–15 mmHg) is established and the first trocar (12-mm for the Si robot; 8-mm for the Xi) is inserted on the same level as the 12th rib just lateral to the para-rectus line. The robotic camera is inserted and the peritoneal cavity inspected to ensure safe entry. Bariatric 8 mm trocar is placed at the costal margin just slightly cephalad and lateral to the pubic bone (just lateral to the medial umbilical ligament). A standard 8 mm trocar is placed two fingerbreadths above the anterior superior iliac spine. Assistant trocars are placed in their traditional locations: one trocar between the camera trocar site and upper-most robotic arm, another between the camera and the lower robotic arm. Both assistant trocars are placed slightly more medial than the other trocars.

To reduce instrument clashing, the trocar configuration should form an equilateral triangle between the camera port, the lower bariatric port, and the lateral traditional robotic port. For a right partial nephrectomy, an additional incision is made at the xiphoid sternum where the liver retractor is inserted. In this trocar configuration, the lower bariatric trocar is the most "active" arm, regardless of laterality. The use of a bariatric, and thus longer, trocar enhances our reach when treating upper pole tumors. Specimen retrieval typically occurs in the more caudal assistant port, though this is patient dependent. The surgical table is tilted, and the da Vinci® is docked posterior to the patient with the camera arm coming in to the patient at an angle of 15° in line with the camera port. Robotic instruments are inserted into the peritoneal cavity under direct vision.

Steps 2-3: Bowel Mobilization and Hilum Dissection

These steps are standard procedural steps for RAPN and have been discussed elsewhere. We present a brief summary of these steps. The

Fig. 7.3 (**a**) Trocar placement for left partial nephrectomy. (**b**) Trocar placement for right partial nephrectomy

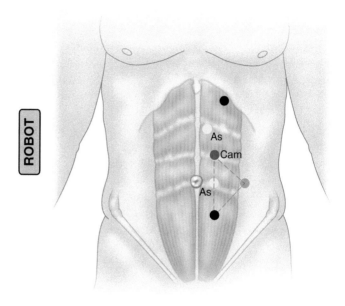

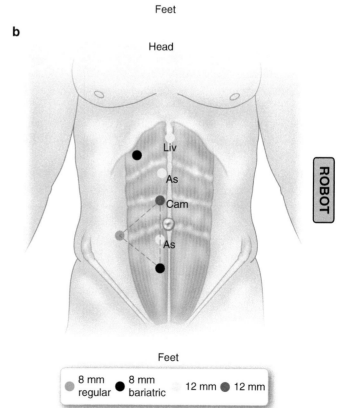

Gerota's fascia-covered kidney and the uretero-gonadal packet are visualized and retracted later-ally. The main renal artery and vein are circumferentially mobilized and each is encircled with mini-vessel loops.

Steps 4–5: Hilar Micro-dissection and Super-Selective Arterial Clamping

Medially Located Tumors and Visible Confirmation of Interrupted Perfusion

The pre-operative CT-reconstructed 3D renal arterial images help guide and orient the surgeon during arterial micro-dissection. The main renal artery and vein remain unclamped during this procedure. Delicate and selective anatomical vascular micro-dissection of tumor feeding arterial branches (tertiary, quaternary or higher order) is performed deep into the renal hilum in a medial-to-lateral direction. Micro-dissection of tertiary renal arterial branches is advanced by dissecting into the renal sinus by developing the peri-pelvic plane of Gil-Vernet. A small radial nephrotomy incision is initiated on the concave, hilar edge of the kidney directly overlying the tumor-feeding arterial branch. Mini-vessel loops can be used to isolate and atraumatically retract higher-order arterial branches as the surgeon advances the micro-dissection toward the tumor; the small radial nephrotomy incision is extended to 2–3 cm to extend the micro-dissection intra-renally, if necessary. If a nephrotomy incision is deemed necessary, it should be made on the hilar edge of the kidney directly overlying the anterior surface of that specific arterial branch. Once the per-ceived terminal, tumor-feeding arterial branch is identified, a neuro-surgical aneurysm micro-bulldog is placed temporarily to confirm selective devascularization of the tumor. Visual (normal color and turgor), color-Doppler and "fire-fly" indigo-cyanine green fluorescence inspection of the surrounding normal kidney is performed to confirm that this super-selective clamping did not interrupt perfusion to the normal kidney. Topical

papavarine can be applied onto the renal hilar vessels to counteract any vasospasm.

Laterally Located and Intra-renal Tumors and Doppler Use

If the tumor is located at a significant trans-parenchymal distance from the renal hilum, or if the tumor is completely intra-renal and endo-phytic (thus not visible on inspection with the robotic camera), real-time intra-operative imag-ing is necessary to facilitate micro-dissection and identify the specific arterial branch or branches that supply blood to the tumor. Laparoscopic color Doppler ultrasound is placed on the kidney parenchyma to locate the tumor and identify inter-lobar arteries. The sus-pected tumor-specific arterial branch is identi-fied and test-occluded transiently with a micro-bulldog clamp; Doppler re-examination of kidney parenchyma simultaneously confirms occlusion of the tumor-specific vessel and devascularization of peri-tumor region (Fig. 7.4). In event this targeted arterial branch does not feed the tumor (i.e., tumor vascularity remains unchanged despite test-clamping), vas-cular dissection continues until the correct feed-ing arterial branch(es) is/are identified.

Steps 6–8: Tumor Scoring, Excision, and Renorrhaphy

Again, these steps are detailed elsewhere in the book. Specific steps for this technique include circumferential scoring of the tumor and tumor excision using a combination of electrocautery and cold scissors. The tumor is separated from its point(s) of contact with the underlying renal vessels, preserving intact the intra-renal and hilar vessels. Hemostasis in the partial nephrec-tomy bed is achieved using a combination of Hem-o-lok clips and point-specific intra-corpo-real suturing. Hem-o-lok clips are applied to the vessels feeding the tumor from the deep resec-tion bed; these are subsequently under-sown to prevent migration into the calyceal system. The

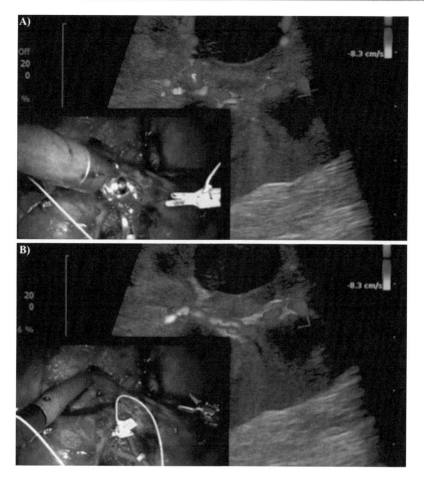

Fig. 7.4 Ultrasound color Doppler-guided super-selective clamping of a renal arterial branch. A segmental artery is identified. (**a**) Doppler ultrasound is placed onto the renal parenchyma to determine blood flow prior to temporary cessation. (**b**) A micro-bulldog is placed onto the segmental artery, and Doppler confirms cessation of blood-flow to the tumor-specific region

collecting system is suture-repaired with a running 3-0 Polyglactin on SH-1 needle. Sutured renorrhaphy of the partial nephrectomy bed is performed deep to the clips, typically without use of a bolster; however, a bolster can certainly be used to maximize parenchymal hemostasis, a critical priority, per surgeon preference. Watertightness of the repair is confirmed by repeat retrograde injection of dilute methylene blue through the indwelling ureteral catheter. A biologic hemostatic agent is layered onto the partial nephrectomy bed.

Step 9: Completely-Unclamped ("Zero-Ischemia"), Minimal-Margin Partial Nephrectomy

This technique is a more recent advance upon our prior, super-selective segmental arterial clamping technique, described above. Herein, all vascular clamping is completely eliminated; thus, neither vascular micro-dissection nor use of micro-bulldog is necessary. Furthermore, herein, tumor excision maintains only a minimal-margin (1–2 mm) adjacent to the capsular edge. This technique is based on the following anatomic facts: (a) intrarenal architecture, both parenchymal and vascular, is radially oriented; (b) there is a distinct intra-renal pseudo-capsule on the vast majority of small clinical T1 renal tumors; (c) the tumor-parenchyma inter-face is histologically altered with sclerotic changes; and (d) the intra-renal arteries at this junctional interface immediately adjacent to the tumor edge are typically smaller in diameter and fewer in number. These anatomic facts inform the basis for performing a sculpted enucleo-resection in the plane immediately adjacent to the tumor capsule—the "minimal-margin" plane. The technical goal herein is to maintain a uniform, 1-mm sliver of parenchymal tissue on the tumor capsular surface, without completely denuding the capsule, which occurs routinely during classic tumor enucleation.

Using ultrasound guidance, the tumor edge is scored with electrocautery approximately 2 mm from the tumor edge. Using the fourth robotic arm, the peri-renal fat directly overlaying the tumor is retracted, thereby elevating the tumor from the kidney. A 2–3 mm deep radial nephrotomy is made along the cephalad and caudal edges of the tumor, along the scored margin, using electrocautery (setting at 100 W). This relatively bloodless incision is further developed bluntly by placing the tip of the robotic bipolar forceps in the left robotic arm into the nephrotomy incision and gently opening its jaws (Fig. 7.5). This starts to open the kidney "like a book" along the naturally existing radial plane adjacent to the tumor by cold dissection, with point coagulation used strategically to guide the enucleation. The capsular incision is circumferentially developed around the tumor and deepened with blunt dissection, and the tumor is retracted away off the partial nephrectomy bed with robotic forceps. During this excision, the renal parenchyma is bluntly separated, not incised. By doing this, the dissection is kept along the natural, relatively avascular intra-renal plane and avoids injuring the interlobar vessels. Any small intra-renal vessel(s) directly entering the tumor is/are defined and controlled with Hem-o-lok clips before transection. Important technical point: this technique requires two suction apparatuses, one strictly for parenchymal compression, and the second for

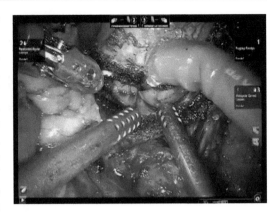

Fig. 7.5 Further development of the incision of a minimal-margin, zero-ischemia partial nephrectomy. The radial nephrotomy incision is relatively bloodless and is further developed bluntly by placing the tip of the robotic bipolar forceps (left robotic arm) into the nephrotomy incision and gently opening its jaws, thus initiating the avascular plane of dissection

suction and irrigation. The bed-side assistant uses the suction cannula to transiently compress any bleeding vessel until point-specific suturing can be performed. Once the tumor is completely excised, hemostasis is achieved with point-specific suturing. Repair of the caliceal system is done by using 3-0 Polyglactin on a SH-1 needle. Use of a bolster depends upon individual surgeon preference.

Step 10: Intraoperative Near Infrared Fluorescence Using Indo-cyanine Green

The use of Doppler ultrasound to assist facilitating super-selective partial nephrectomy has been mentioned previously in the super-selective operative technique. Similarly, intravenous indo-cyanine green dye can be used to confirm tumor devascularization. Additionally, indo-cyanine green dye can also be used to confirm ongoing global perfusion of the normal kidney, thus providing graphic visual confirmation that the clamping of the proposed terminal artery does not devascularize the non-tumor bearing normal kidney (Fig. 7.6).

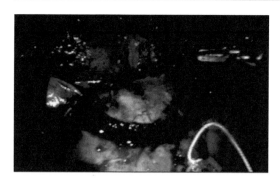

Fig. 7.6 Indo-cyanine green infrared fluorescence, confirming cessation of blood flow to the tumor bed

Post-operative Management

Appropriate pain control is administered, typically with Ketorolac (Toradol) 15 mg every 6 h for the first 3 days. Oral narcotics can also be prescribed if needed. Clear liquid diet is administered and advanced as soon as the patient can tolerate it. On post-operative day 1, parenteral antibiotics are discontinued and the patient is encouraged to ambulate and prepared for discharge the subsequent day. The Jackson-Pratt (JP) drain is removed on post-operative day 2–3, or later once JP-output has decreased to <50 mL per day. If a urinary leak is suspected, a JP drain fluid creatinine is assessed. Out-of-town patients from longer distances are required to stay in a nearby hotel for 3–4 days to ensure smooth recovery before returning home. Post-operative follow-up depends upon individual patient histology.

Special Considerations

Complications associated with PN surgery include positive cancer margins; compromise of renal function; and urological complications (urine leak, bleed). These and other common complications have been described in the book chapter regarding PN.

References

1. Marconi L, Dabestani S, Lam TB, Hofmann F, Stewart F, Norrie J, et al. Systematic review and meta-analysis of diagnostic accuracy of percutaneous renal tumour biopsy. Eur Urol. 2016;69(4):660–73.
2. Bjurlin MA, Walter D, Taksler GB, Huang WC, Wysock JS, Sivarajan G, et al. National trends in the utilization of partial nephrectomy before and after the establishment of AUA guidelines for the management of renal masses. Urology. 2013;82(6):1283–9.
3. Hafez KS, Novick AC, Butler BP. Management of small solitary unilateral renal cell carcinomas: impact of central versus peripheral tumor location. J Urol. 1998;159(4):1156–60.
4. Gratzke C, Seitz M, Bayrle F, Schlenker B, Bastian PJ, Haseke N, et al. Quality of life and perioperative outcomes after retroperitoneoscopic radical nephrectomy (RN), open RN and nephron-sparing surgery in patients with renal cell carcinoma. BJU Int. 2009;104(4):470–5.
5. D'Armiento M, Damiano R, Feleppa B, Perdona S, Oriani G, De Sio M. Elective conservative surgery for renal carcinoma versus radical nephrectomy: a prospective study. Br J Urol. 1997;79(1):15–9.
6. Van Poppel H, Da Pozzo L, Albrecht W, Matveev V, Bono A, Borkowski A, et al. A prospective randomized EORTC intergroup phase 3 study comparing the complications of elective nephron-sparing surgery and radical nephrectomy for low-stage renal cell carcinoma. Eur Urol. 2007;51(6):1606–15.
7. Lane BR, Campbell SC, Gill IS. 10-year oncologic outcomes after laparoscopic and open partial nephrectomy. J Urol. 2013;190(1):44–9.
8. Go AS, Chertow GM, Fan D, McCulloch CE, Hsu CY. Chronic kidney disease and the risks of death, cardiovascular events, and hospitalization. N Engl J Med. 2004;351(13):1296–305.
9. Volpe A, Blute ML, Ficarra V, Gill IS, Kutikov A, Porpiglia F, et al. Renal ischemia and function after partial nephrectomy: a collaborative review of the literature. Eur Urol. 2015;68(1):61–74.
10. Hung AJ, Tsai S, Gill IS. Does eliminating global renal ischemia during partial nephrectomy improve functional outcomes? Curr Opin Urol. 2013;23(2):112–7.
11. Klatte T, Ficarra V, Gratzke C, Kaouk J, Kutikov A, Macchi V, et al. A literature review of renal surgical anatomy and surgical strategies for partial nephrectomy. Eur Urol. 2015;68(6):980–92.
12. Desai MM, de Castro Abreu AL, Leslie S, Cai J, Huang EY, Lewandowski PM, et al. Robotic partial nephrectomy with superselective versus main artery clamping: a retrospective comparison. Eur Urol. 2014;66(4):713–9.
13. Hung AJ, Cai J, Simmons MN, Gill IS. "Trifecta" in partial nephrectomy. J Urol. 2013;189(1):36–42.

Retroperitoneal Robotic Partial Nephrectomy

J. Joy Lee and James R. Porter

Abbreviations

PN   Partial nephrectomy
RP-RPN   Retroperitoneal robotic partial nephrectomy
TP-RPN   Transperitoneal robotic partial nephrectomy

Patient Selection

The retroperitoneal approach for robotic partial nephrectomy is particularly well suited for patients with prior abdominal surgery in whom exposure of the kidney and retroperitoneum may be more difficult due to adhesions or distorted anatomy. The retroperitoneal approach is also ideal for renal masses located posteriorly or laterally, as in the transperitoneal approach access to the tumor would require significantly more mobilization of the kidney. The retroperitoneal approach allows for direct and rapid access to the renal artery [1–3]. The challenge of retroperitoneal surgery however is a smaller working space and the need for the surgeon to become oriented to a new set of anatomic landmarks to avoid potential disorientation and inadvertent injury to surrounding tissues. While the physiologic effects of insufflation are lessened by inflating the retroperitoneum instead of the peritoneal cavity, patient who have tenuous cardiopulmonary or hepatic status are not good candidates for a robotic approach. Likewise, patients with bleeding diatheses or who cannot hold anticoagulation are poor candidates. Prior retroperitoneal or percutaneous renal surgery is not an absolute contraindication to a retroperitoneal approach, but these patients may be better served transperitoneally.

Preoperative Preparation

All patients should undergo a thorough preoperative evaluation. Any blood thinners, including aspirin and ibuprofen, should be discontinued 7 days prior to surgery. As part of the informed consent process, all patients are counseled that there is a possibility of conversion to a radical nephrectomy and/or open surgery if intra-operative complications occur.

Because the retroperitoneal working space is not significantly limited by the bowels, no bowel preparation is required. Knee-high sequential

Electronic supplementary material: The online version of this chapter (doi:10.1007/978-3-319-45060-5_8) contains supplementary material, which is available to authorized users.

J.J. Lee, M.D. • J.R. Porter, M.D. (✉)
Department of Urology, Swedish Medical Center,
1101 Madison Street, Suite 1400, Seattle,
WA 98104, USA
e-mail: porter@swedishurology.com

compression devices are placed. We have not routinely given subcutaneous heparin to patients unless they are at high risk for thromboembolic events. A parenteral antibiotic such as cefazolin is given prior to skin incision. A type and cross is verified prior to incision as well. We do not perform cystoscopy and open-ended ureteral stent placement for retrograde injection of dye, as we feel the magnification and optics of the daVinci® system allow for adequate visualization of entry into the collecting system [4].

Operative Setup

Familiarity of the operating team with the positioning and subsequent operation are paramount in promoting efficiency and helping minimize risks for the patient. To that end, we keep as consistent a setup as possible as shown in Fig. 8.1a. The robot is draped for a three-arm technique, but the fourth arm can also be used according to surgeon preference (the kidney can be elevated by the ProGrasp™, thus freeing both robotic arms) or if the peritoneum is inadvertently entered. For right-sided masses, following intubation and patient positioning, the patient bed is turned 135° counterclockwise so that the patient's head is at approximately 7 o'clock. For left-sided masses, the patient bed is turned 135° clockwise so that the patient's head points toward 5 o'clock. The robot is thus able to be docked directly over the patient's head in line with the patient's spine, while allowing the anesthesiologist to maintain access to the head as well.

The Bovie electrocautery unit and insufflation tower are positioned next to the patient's feet. The assistant is positioned on the anterior side of the patient and scrub technician is on the posterior side of the patient. Monitors are positioned such that the assistant, scrub technician, and anesthesiologist all have a clear direct view (Fig. 8.1b).

Patient Positioning and Preparation

After induction of general endotracheal anesthesia, the anesthesiologist places all necessary lines for monitoring and fluids, particularly as the subsequent lateral decubitus position may limit access to the extremities. No orogastric or nasogastric tube is required for the retroperitoneal approach. An 18 French urethral catheter is inserted. The patient is then placed in full 90° flank position with the side of the renal mass up, taking care to ensure that the hips are in line with the shoulder. Maintaining alignment of the hip and shoulder during patient flexion is essential for maximizing working space in the retroperitoneum. If the hips and shoulders are not in line however, flexion of the table will accentuate any rotation and will result in distortion and compression of the retroperitoneum. Some patients may have a prominent hipbone, in which case we make sure to place the hip below the break in the table.

To help maintain the full flank position, we use two rolled blankets folded in thirds, and rolled under the drawsheet to support the patient's spine. One blanket (likewise folded in thirds) is rolled under the drawsheet in front of the patient so provide a low profile support to the patient's abdomen (Fig. 8.2a). The rolled blankets allow for adequate exposure of both the retroperitoneal space as well as the whole abdomen in the event of a conversion to a transperitoneal approach. Blankets also allow stable patient positioning without the need for a hard surface such as a beanbag. The bottom leg is bent, and the top leg is left straight and resting on pillows. An axillary gel roll is placed. The dependent arm is supported by an arm board, tilted toward the head as much as possible, and secured with tape. Two or three pillows are then placed over the arm, and the ipsilateral arm placed over this pillow tower and secured. We use 2-in. cloth tape over the ipsilateral shoulder and arm, and another piece perpendicular to this to help prevent the arm from falling toward the patient's head. The bed is then fully flexed to maximize the space between the 12th rib and iliac crest, and reverse Trendelenburg used to make sure that the flank is parallel to the floor. Lastly, we use cloth tape to secure the hips and legs. The final position is shown in Fig. 8.2b. An upper-body warming device is placed. Depending on the side of the mass, the bed is then rotated as described above to allow for the robot to be docked directly over the head.

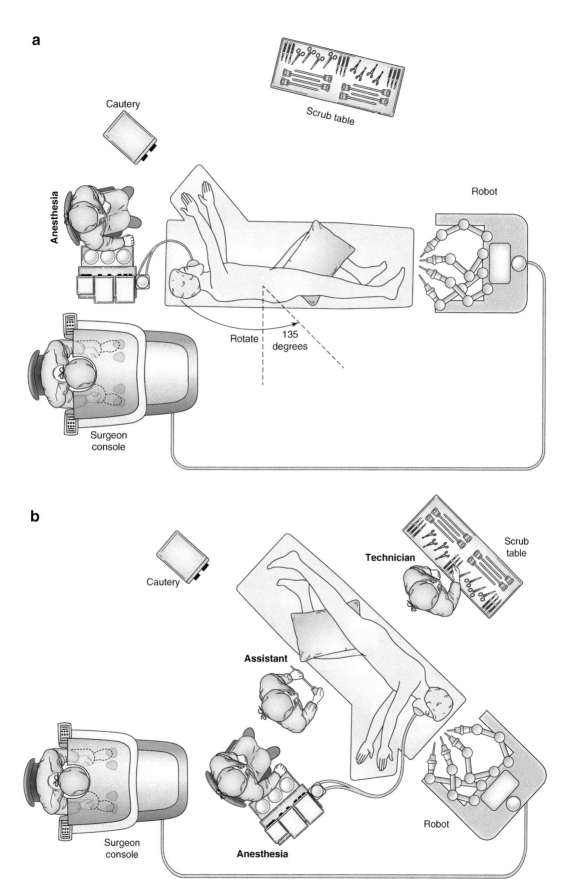

Fig. 8.1 (**a**) Initial operating room setup for a right-sided retroperitoneal robotic partial nephrectomy. (**b**) Final operating room setup once the patient and operating table have been turned 135° to allow for the robot to be docked over the patient's head

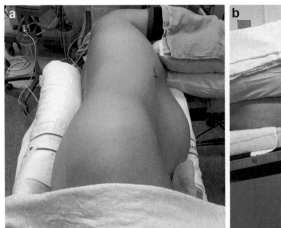
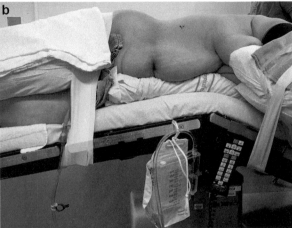

Fig. 8.2 (**a**) The patient is placed in full flank position, with one rolled blanket anteriorly and two rolled blankets posteriorly to help maintain the body perpendicular to the bed. (**b**) The table is fully flexed with slight reverse Trendelenberg

Throughout the case, it is important to maintain clear and effective communication with the anesthesiologist. Once all the positioning has been completed, we verify that they are satisfied with their access to the airway, all IVs and monitoring lines. We request that they run intravenous fluids at a brisk rate as tolerated, and after 2 L of fluids have been given, to administer Furosemide 20 mg IV all prior to any ischemia time.

Trocar Configuration

A total of four trocars are used: a 12-mm camera trocar, two 8-mm robotic trocars for the right and left robotic arms, and a 12-mm assistant trocar. If the surgeon wishes to use the fourth robotic arm, an additional 8-mm robotic trocar is opened. The fourth arm is then draped and positioned such that it is the most medial trocar in relation to the patient's midline (i.e., lateral to the left arm for a left-sided tumor, medial to the right arm for a right-sided tumor).

Trocar configurations for a right retroperitoneal robotic partial nephrectomy using the 3-arm technique is shown in Fig. 8.3.

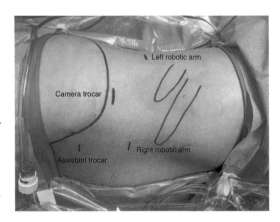

Fig. 8.3 Trocar configuration for a right retroperitoneal robotic partial nephrectomy using a 3-arm technique. If needed, a fourth arm may be placed at the "X"

Instrument and Equipment List

Equipment

- da Vinci® Si Surgical System (4-arm system; Intuitive Surgical, Inc., Sunnyvale, CA)
- EndoWrist® curved monopolar scissors (Intuitive Surgical, Inc., Sunnyvale, CA)
- EndoWrist® fenestrated bipolar grasper (Intuitive Surgical, Inc., Sunnyvale, CA)

- EndoWrist® ProGrasp™ forceps (Intuitive Surgical, Inc., Sunnyvale, CA) if using fourth arm
- EndoWrist® large suture cut needle driver (Intuitive Surgical, Inc., Sunnyvale, CA)
- EndoWrist® needle driver (Intuitive Surgical, Inc., Sunnyvale, CA)
- InSite Vision System with 0° lens (Intuitive Surgical, Inc., Sunnyvale, CA)
- Robotic flexible drop-in Doppler ultrasound probe (BK Ultrasound, Peabody, MA)
- Balloon-dilating device (OMSPDBS2, Kidney Distension Balloon, Covidien, Mansfield, MA)
- Laparoscope with 30° lens

Trocars

- 12-mm trocars (2)
  - A 12-mm Hasson blunt-tip trocar with fixation balloon (OMS-T12BT, Covidien, Mansfield, MA) for the camera
  - A 12-mm trocar for the assistant
- 8-mm robotic trocars (2, or 3 if using the fourth arm)

Recommended Sutures (Fig. 8.4)

- Retraction of perinephric fat as needed: 2-0 Polypropylene on a Keith needle, uncut (not shown)
- Oversewing vessels and collecting system: 4-0 Polyglactin (undyed) on a RB-1 needle. Six sutures are cut to 12 cm, and one suture is cut to 15 cm (not shown).
- Deep renorrhaphy layer: 3-0 Monocryl (dyed) on an SH needle, with a Hem-o-lok® clip and LAPRA-TY® clip on the distal end. One has the Hem-o-lok® clip at 15 cm, and a second suture has the Hem-o-lok® clip at 18 cm.
- Cortical renorrhaphy layer: 2-0 Polyglactin on a CT-2 needle, with a Hem-o-lok® clip and LAPRA-TY® clip on the distal end at 8 cm. An additional 2-armed pledgeted suture is

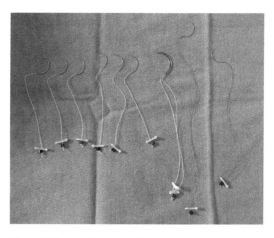

Fig. 8.4 Prepared sutures prior to excision of the renal mass: (from left to right) Six 2-0 Polyglactin CT-2 sutures cut to 8 cm; One 2-armed pledgeted suture made from two 2-0 Polyglactin CT-1 needles clamped together at 12 cm; One 3-0 Monocryl SH cut to 15 cm; One 3-0 Monocryl SH cut to 18 cm

created using two 2-0 Polyglactin CT-1 needles clamped together at 12 cm with a Hem-o-lok® clip and LAPRA-TY® clip and tied together, and a 9.5 × 4.8 mm soft TFE polymer pledget passed through both needles.

Instruments Used by the Surgical Assistant

- Suction irrigator device
- Laparoscopic needle driver
- Laparoscopic blunt tip grasper
- Hem-o-lok® clip applier (Teleflex Medical, Research Triangle Park, NC)
- Large Hem-o-lok® clips (Teleflex Medical, Research Triangle Park, NC)
- LAPRA-TY® suture clip applier (Ethicon, Somerville, NJ)
- LAPRA-TY® absorbable suture clips (Ethicon, Somerville, NJ)
- 10 mm titanium clip applier ML size (Covidien, Mansfield, MA)
- Keith needle with 2-0 Polypropylene suture

- Atraumatic bulldog vascular clamps (six available) (Scanlan International, St. Paul, MN)
- SURGICEL® hemostatic gauze (Ethicon, Inc., Cincinnati, OH)
- 10 mm Endocatch® specimen retrieval bag
- 15 F Blake round closed suction drain
- Available and in the room: Laparoscopic reticulating GIA stapling device with a 30 mm cartridge length and vascular load

Step-by-Step Technique (Videos 8.1, 8.2, 8.3, 8.4, and 8.5)

Step 1: Retroperitoneal Access and Trocar Placement

We begin by gaining access to the retroperitoneal space. To start, the bony landmarks are palpated and marked: the iliac crest, the 12th rib, and the costal margin. A 12 mm transverse incision is made in the midaxillary line, one fingerbreadth above the iliac crest, anterior to the Triangle of Petit [2]. Blunt dissection is carried down to the external oblique fascia. Blunt finger dissection is then used to penetrate the external and internal oblique fascia as well as the transversalis fascia. The finger should then enter the retroperitoneal space, and should be able to palpate the psoas muscle posteriorly, the tip of the 12th rib superiorly, and often the inferior cone of Gerota's anteriorly. The finger is used to gently sweep the peritoneum away. The balloon-dilating device is then placed into this space, taking care to orient the device so that the dimension of maximal expansion is along the cephalo-caudal axis. A 30° laparoscope is inserted into the balloon dissector, and 40 pumps are performed under direct vision. Depending on the dissection of tissues and working space, one can give up to 60 pumps, taking care not to cause undue shearing that may accidentally breach the peritoneum. If the peritoneum is inadvertently entered, we will enlarge the incision and place the robotic fourth arm transperitoneally through this location to help retract the peritoneum and kidney. While pumping the balloon, the landmarks that we identify are the transversus abdominis muscle and anterior layer of

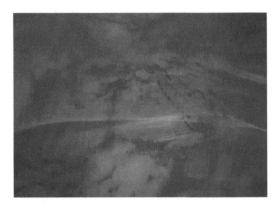

Fig. 8.5 Anatomic landmarks during creation of the retroperitoneal space include the posterior layer of Gerota's fascia on the psoas muscle (shown), as well as the ureter and the peritoneum as it is pushed medially off the tranversus abdominis

peritoneum superiorly, Gerota's fascia as it is pushed off the psoas muscle posteriorly, and the ureter inferiorly (Fig. 8.5). The balloon is then deflated and replaced with the 12 mm Hasson camera trocar.

Once pneumo-retroperitoneum is established to 15 mmHg, the remaining trocars are marked with at least 7 cm (and preferably 8 cm) in between. The lateral robotic trocar site is marked at the apex formed by the erector spinae muscles and 12th rib. The medial robotic trocar site is marked along the anterior axillary line, 7–8 cm away from the camera trocar. The assistant trocar is marked in the anterior axillary line above the anterior superior iliac spine, and 7–8 cm caudal to the medial robotic trocar. If a fourth arm is anticipated to be used, it is placed 7–8 cm medially and ~2 cm inferiorly to the medial trocar. A spinal needle can be inserted under vision to confirm the marked sites. A laparoscopic Kittner can be used through the lateral robotic trocar to sweep away the peritoneum if more space is needed for the medial trocars (Fig. 8.6). All trocars are then placed under direct vision. The robot is then docked over the patient's head, parallel to the spine. The robotic cart is positioned such that the robotic camera arm is in the far end of the "sweet spot" range, which allows for greater range of motion inferiorly in the limited working space. The robotic camera is inserted with a 0° lens, and robotic instruments are advanced into the working field under direct vision. The camera scope is rotated so that the psoas muscle appears horizontal.

Step 2: Management of Paranephric and Perinephric Fat (Table 8.1)

The first step of the retroperitoneal partial nephrectomy is management of the paranephric fat. There is significant variability in the amount of retroperitoneal fat, and the fat is removed if it compromises vision to the kidney. Using monopolar scissors and blunt dissection, the paranephric fat is carefully excised from Gerota's fascia and placed in the lower retroperitoneum (Fig. 8.7). Care must be taken medially and anteriorly so as not to enter the peritoneum. Next, Gerota's fascia is incised 1–2 cm above the psoas muscle, thereby exposing the perinephric fat and kidney (Fig. 8.8). The fenestrated bipolar is used for upward retraction of the kidney while the monopolar scissors methodically dissect toward the hilum in a "hook-and-burn" technique [3]. Not infrequently, we use the blunt shaft of the

robotic monopolar scissors to retract the kidney and use the fenestrated bipolar grasper to gently spread apart tissues, thin them out, and form packets for the monopolar scissors to cauterize. We prefer to control most small vessels with bipolar instead of monopolar electrocautery. The assistant can elevate the perinephric fat with the suction-irrigator, freeing up both robotic arms to establish the plane above the psoas fascia. If there is considerable perinephric fat that keeps dropping into view, a Keith needle can be passed into the retroperitoneum under direct view, passed through the fat, and back out through the skin to

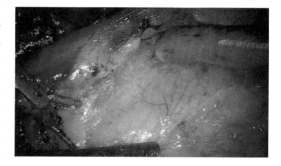

Fig. 8.7 Excision of pararenal fat, exposing Gerota's fascia and the pale yellow perinephric fat beneath

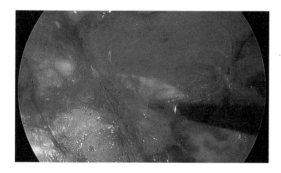

Fig. 8.6 Laparoscopic graspers may be used to sweep away the peritoneal reflection anteriorly from the transversus abdominis muscle

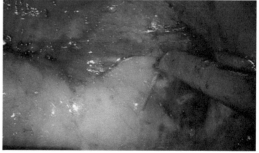

Fig. 8.8 An incision is made in Gerota's fascia 2 cm above the psoas muscle, thereby exposing the perinephric fat

Table 8.1 Management of paranephric and perinephric fat: surgeon and assistant instrumentation

Surgeon instrumentation[a]			Assistant instrumentation
Right arm	Left arm	Fourth arm if used	• Suction-irrigator
• Curved monopolar scissors	• Fenestrated bipolar grasper	• ProGrasp™ forceps	

[a]For simplicity, all instruments used will be in reference to a right-sided robotic retroperitoneal partial nephrectomy

the assistant (Fig. 8.9). The 2-0 Polypropylene suture can then be secured against the skin with gauze and a hemostat to allow for constant retraction of the perinephric fat.

Step 3: Hilar Dissection (Table 8.2)

The renal artery is typically encountered first and closest to the camera in the retroperitoneal approach (Fig. 8.10). The artery is completely skeletonized, and if superselective clamping is planned, the branches are further dissected and exposed. We do not routinely clamp the renal vein except for large tumors or more centrally located tumors. Nonetheless, having the renal vein dissected and exposed can be helpful in the event of bleeding.

Step 4: Tumor Exposure: Defatting the Kidney and Identifying the Renal Mass (Table 8.3)

The robotic flexible drop-in ultrasound probe is placed through the 12 mm assistant trocar and is grasped with the fenestrated bipolar grasper (or, the left arm can by exchanged for a ProGrasp™ grasper). The probe is used to precisely locate the

tumor to guide dissection and avoid entry into the tumor. The upper edge of the previously cut Gerota's fascia serves as a landmark to avoid buttonholing the peritoneum as one begins to defat the kidney (Fig. 8.11). Exposing the posterior surface of the kidney is accomplished by carefully dissecting inside Gerota's fascia to avoid inadvertent entry into the peritoneum. If the peritoneum is entered and the retroperitoneal working space is compromised due to venting into the peritoneal cavity, the entry can be enlarged and a robotic fourth arm docked as described previously. Once the renal parenchyma is adequately defatted around the mass, the ultrasound probe is again used to visualize the extent and depth of

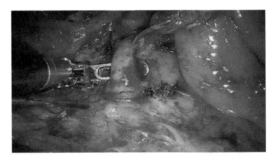

Fig. 8.10 In contrast to a transperitoneal case, in a retroperitoneal approach the renal artery is typically the first structure encountered in the hilum

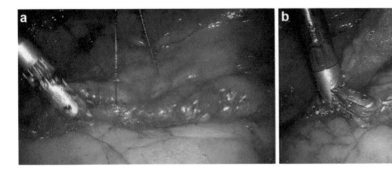

Fig. 8.9 Before (**a**) and after (**b**) use of a Keith needle for retraction of the upper edge of Gerota's

Table 8.2 Hilar dissection: surgeon and assistant instrumentation

Surgeon instrumentation			Assistant instrumentation
Right arm	Left arm	Fourth arm if used	• Suction-irrigator
• Curved monopolar scissors	• Fenestrated bipolar grasper	• ProGrasp™ forceps	

Table 8.3 Tumor exposure: defatting the kidney and identifying the renal mass—surgeon and assistant instrumentation

Surgeon instrumentation			Assistant instrumentation
Right arm	Left arm	Fourth arm if used	• Suction-irrigator
• Curved monopolar scissors	• Fenestrated bipolar grasper	• ProGrasp™ forceps	• Robotic flexible drop-in ultrasound probe

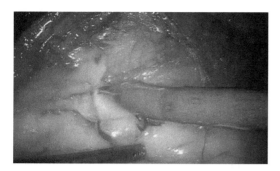

Fig. 8.11 When defatting the kidney it is important to stay within the cut edge of Gerota's fascia so as to avoid inadvertently entering the peritoneum

tumor invasion. The TilePro™ feature is turned on from the surgeon console, allowing a simultaneous view of the endoscopic image and the ultrasound image. The ultrasound probe is used to scan through the tumor in several axes, and monopolar scissors are used to score a 5 mm margin with electrocautery circumferentially. The ultrasound probe is then removed from the field.

Step 5: Tumor Excision and Renorrhaphy (Table 8.4)

At this point, we routinely stop and perform a pre-clamp checklist and safety check so that all members of the team are aware of the surgical plan. We verify with the anesthesiologist that 2 L of intravenous fluids and 20 mg of IV furosemide have been given. We double-check with the scrub tech that all robotic needle drivers have been previously tested and have an adequate number of remaining uses left. We verify that an appropriate number and array of sutures are prepared, based on the anticipated size of the defect. We discuss whether we intend to bag the specimen immediately, or place it to the side to bag after the renorrhaphy is complete. The camera is used to

visualize each trocar sequentially, to make sure that the trocar has not retracted into the abdominal wall, which would inhibit instrument exchange. Lastly, we have the assistant pass an adequate number of bulldog clamps into the field, typically 1–2 clamps per artery, as well as a SURGICEL® cellulose bolster which we use not for the renorrhaphy but as an absorbent tamponading aid if there is bleeding.

We then ask the anesthesiologist to administer 2 mL of indocyanine green intravenously, clamp the main renal artery or one of its branches if superselective clamping is to be used, and verify ischemia to the mass (Fig. 8.12). Cold scissors are used to incise the parenchyma circumferentially along our score mark and then excise the mass. Care is taken to avoid excessive electrocautery which can compromise renal tissue landmarks which are crucial maintaining orientation to the tumor and ensuring a negative margin. If the collecting system is entered or any vascular structures are seen end-on, these are first oversewn with either a figure-of-eight or running 4-0 Polyglactin sutures cut to 12 cm. Next, the base of the defect is brought together using a 3-0 15 or 18 cm Monocryl running suture. Lastly, single 2-0 Polyglactin CT-1 sutures cut to 8 cm are used to reapproximate the cortex using the sliding clip renorrhaphy technique. Because we use the large suture cut needle driver in the right arm, we typically cut each needle once the Hem-o-lok® clip is secured and gives the needle to the assistant for removal when he or she passes in the next suture. Once all the Hem-o-lok® clips are snug, LAPRA-TY® clips are placed behind the Hem-o-lok® clips. The bulldog clamps are then removed and total warm ischemia time recorded.

If there is persistent bleeding from the renorrhaphy, the renorrhapy sutures can be tightened slightly and additional cortical sutures can be placed to help with tamponade. Our preference is

Table 8.4 Tumor excision and renorrhaphy: surgeon and assistant instrumentation

Surgeon instrumentation			Assistant instrumentation
Right arm	Left arm	Fourth arm if used	• Suction-irrigator
• Curved monopolar scissors	• Fenestrated bipolar grasper	• ProGrasp™ forceps	• Laparoscopic needle driver
• Large suture cut needle driver	• Needle driver		• Hem-o-lok® clip applier
			• LAPRA-TY® suture clip applier

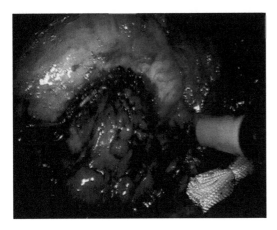

Fig. 8.12 ICG may be used to help identify the region perfused by first and second order branches, or to confirm ischemia to the mass

to use these compression sutures in lieu of hemostatic agents, but acknowledge that many surgeons may choose to use various hemostatic liquids/gels/foams/matrices.

Step 6: Extraction and Closure

The SURGICEL® bolster is removed. All bulldog and suture counts are verified to be correct. If not already entrapped, the specimen is placed in the Endocatch bag. If there was collecting system entry, we generally will leave a 15 French round Blake drain through the anterior-most trocar site. The remaining trocars are removed, and the specimen extracted through the mid-axillary camera trocar. Depending on the size of the extraction incision and visibility, the fascia is closed in 1–2 layers. The external oblique fascia is closed at the camera trocar. Local anesthetic is infiltrated into all the trocar sites, and the skin closed.

Postoperative Management

Patients are started on a clear liquid diet the day of surgery, and advanced to a regular diet on either postoperative day 0 or 1 as tolerated. Patients are given oral acetaminophen around the clock, and are encouraged to try oral narcotic pain medications instead of intravenous narcotics as needed for breakthrough pain. Some studies suggest that the retroperitoneal approach is associated with a decreased [5] or equivalent [6] narcotic requirement compared to transperitoneal cases. Our preference has been to avoid ketorolac given the risk of bleeding and fluctuations in renal function in the acute postoperative setting following a partial nephrectomy. The urethral catheter is removed early on postoperative day 1. If a JP drain was left in place, a JP fluid creatinine is checked after catheter removal to ensure there is no urine leak, and then removed prior to discharge. If there is a urine leak, the drain may be left for a few additional days off suction to allow for the leak to seal. One benefit of retroperitoneal surgery is that any urine leak is contained within the retroperitoneum and would not result in urinary ascites and ileus. The majority of patients are discharged on postoperative day 1.

Special Considerations

With obese patients, substantial abdominal and visceral fat can be avoided by approaching the tumor retroperitoneally. The full flank position allows much abdominal fat to be retracted inferomedially by gravity. Obese patients may still have significant pararenal fat however, and methodical excision of this fat at the beginning of the case is important for adequate exposure of the kidney. As described above, abundant perirenal fat within Gerota's can be managed by passing a Keith needle through Gerota's and creating retraction without the need for an additional trocar.

Large tumors can be particularly challenging in an already limited working space in the retroperitoneum. Use of the robotic fourth arm may be advantageous so that both right and left robotic arms are freed to work on the mass.

Steps to Avoid Complications

As with all operations, the learning curve for robotic retroperitoneal partial nephrectomies can be enhanced with repeated application of this approach in a consistent manner [7]. Familiarity with robotic transperitoneal partial nephrectomy will help greatly. Careful patient selection with small and exophytic tumors (e.g., tumors with a low R.E.N.A.L. nephrometry score) in the initial learning curve can also allow the surgeon to gain familiarity with the retroperitoneal anatomy while minimizing technical challenges with the excision and renorrhaphy portion [8]. As described in the literature, disorientation of the surgeon in retroperitoneal cases can result in major vascular injuries such as vena caval misidentification and transection during laparoscopic nephrectomy [9].

Many details of the operative setup prior to any incision are particularly crucial since there is less working space in the retroperitoneum. Techniques such as maintaining a straight line between the hips and shoulders, docking the robot directly over the patient's head, maximizing space between the trocars, and positioning the camera arm at the outer limit of the "sweet spot" will all help to provide the best exposure possible. In general, bowel injuries are rare with the retroperitoneal approach. Sweeping the peritoneum away and using a spinal needle to test trocar site locations prior to placing the most medial trocars will reduce the risk of transperitoneal trocar placement and inadvertent bowel injury.

Intraoperative bleeding can be a challenging aspect of robotic partial nephrectomies. Close study of preoperative axial imaging and knowledge of the renal vasculature can minimize risk. Early control of the renal hilum is possible with the retroperitoneal approach, as the renal artery is encountered relatively quickly. A skilled bedside assistant is essential not only to keep the field as dry as possible during excision of the mass, but also to help identify and remember open vessels that are subsequently oversewn individually in the first layer. After release of any vessel clamps, we carefully inspect the field for any persistent bleeding. If there is persistent bleeding, additional cortical sutures may be placed to help with tamponade. The pneumoretroperitoneum may also be turned down to 8 mmHg to decrease the tamponade effect of insufflation.

Albeit rare, renal pseudoaneurysms following partial nephrectomy can be a potentially life-threatening complication. Minimally invasive partial nephrectomies appear to have a slightly higher incidence of pseudoaneurysms compared to open surgery, but the cause of this difference remains speculative [10].

Urine leaks are extremely rare in our experience with robotic retroperitoneal partial nephrectomy due to excellent visualization of the collecting system and our practice of separately closing the collecting system with suture. If a urine leak does occur, the drain is taken off suction and the output is closely followed. If the output persists and is confirmed to be urine, a double J stent and urethral catheter are placed to provide maximal antegrade drainage. If the drain output persists despite the stent, the drain can be slowly pulled back 2–3 cm every 2–3 days and re-secured. On occasion the urethral catheter may cause significant bladder spasms such that urine refluxes up the stent; in this case the urethral catheter should be removed. We routinely perform some form of imaging prior to removing the stent. We verify that the drain output does not increase following stent removal, and lastly remove the drain.

References

1. Hollenbeck BK, Taub DA, Miller DC, Dunn RL, Wei JT. National utilization trends of partial nephrectomy for renal cell carcinoma: a case of underutilization? Urology. 2006;67(2):254–9.
2. Ghani KR, Porter J, Menon M, Rogers C. Robotic retroperitoneal partial nephrectomy: a step-by-step guide. BJU Int. 2014;114(2):311–3.
3. Patel M, Porter J. Robotic retroperitoneal partial nephrectomy. World J Urol. 2013;31(6):1377–82.
4. Wright JL, Porter JR. Laparoscopic partial nephrectomy: comparison of transperitoneal and retroperitoneal approaches. J Urol. 2015;174(3):841–5.
5. McDougall EM, Clayman RV. Laparoscopic nephrectomy for benign disease: comparison of the transperitoneal and retroperitoneal approaches. J Endourol. 1996;10(1):45–9.
6. Ng CS, Gill IS, Ramani AP, Steinberg AP, Spaliviero M, Abreu C, Kaouk JH, Desai MM. Transperitoneal versus retroperitoneal laparoscopic partial nephrectomy: patient selection and perioperative outcomes. J Urol. 2005;174(3):846–9.
7. Hu JC, Treat E, Filson CP, McLaren I, Xiong S, Stepanian S, Hafez KS, Weizer AZ, Porter J. Techniques and outcomes of robot-assisted retroperitoneoscopic partial nephrectomy: a multicenter study. Eur Urol. 2014;66(3):542–9.
8. Kutikov A, Uzzo RG. The R.E.N.A.L. nephrometry score: a comprehensive standardized system for quantitating renal tumor size, location and depth. J Urol. 2009;182(3):844–53.
9. McAllister M, Bhayani SB, Ong A, Jaffe W, Malkowicz SB, VanArsdalen K, Chow GK, Jarrett TW. Vena caval transection during retroperitoneoscopic nephrectomy: report of the complication and review of the literature. J Urol. 2004;172(1):183–5.
10. Jain S, Nyirenda T, Yates J, Munver R. Incidence of renal artery pseudoaneurysm following open and minimally invasive partial nephrectomy: a systematic review and comparative analysis. J Urol. 2013;189(5):1643–8.

Robotic Radical Nephrectomy and Nephrectomy with Caval Tumor Thrombus

Ronney Abaza

Patient Selection

The indications for nephrectomy include benign and malignant conditions of the kidney. Benign conditions can include chronic infection (e.g., xanthogranulomatous pyelonephritis) or chronic obstruction causing pain in the setting of minimal remaining renal function. Radical nephrectomy for renal parenchymal tumors is the more common scenario and can be performed in open, laparoscopic, hand-assisted laparoscopic, or robot-assisted laparoscopic fashion.

The use of robotic surgery for nephrectomy is still somewhat controversial for straightforward cases when laparoscopy or hand-assisted laparoscopy is possible [1]. Hand-assisted laparoscopy, while perhaps more available and not dependent on having a robotic surgical system, may not be less expensive or more efficient than robotic nephrectomy as some might believe [2]. Also, for very large tumors upwards of 15–20 cm, robotic nephrectomy is still possible when there would not be room for a hand within the abdomen and ready access to the hilum under the tumor using hand-assisted laparoscopy.

For complex tumors such as those with invasion of contiguous organs or tumor thrombus extending into the renal vein or vena cava, standard laparoscopic instrumentation may be too limited such that the operation might instead be performed open while robotic surgery is increasingly being applied to even such complex surgeries in completely intracorporeal, minimally invasive fashion [3].

Ultimately, the choice of whether to opt for open surgery or minimally invasive surgery as well as the choice of whether to use the surgical robot is up to the surgeon. Various surgeons may have different comfort levels in terms of approaching complex tumors in anything but an open approach while others may philosophically tend to avoid using the robot except when absolutely necessary or at all.

Preoperative Preparation

Patient preparation is similar for robotic nephrectomy as for other intraperitoneal robotic surgery. Avoidance of anticoagulants to the extent possible is preferred although may be less strict than with partial nephrectomy or other procedures with higher bleeding risk. Oral contraceptives taken by fertile females should generally be avoided due to the risk of thrombotic events with general anesthesia and abdominal surgery. Other standard anesthesia and basic surgery-related precautions should be

R. Abaza, M.D., F.A.C.S. (✉)
Department of Robotic Surgery, Ohio Health Dublin
Methodist Hospital, 7450 Hospital Drive, Ste 300,
Dublin, OH 43016, USA
e-mail: ronneyabaza@hotmail.com

© Springer International Publishing Switzerland 2017
L.-M. Su (ed.), *Atlas of Robotic Urologic Surgery*, DOI 10.1007/978-3-319-45060-5_9

taken such as fasting prior to surgery and pre-incision intravenous antibiotics.

A bowel preparation is optional and can be avoided entirely while some surgeons might prefer at least to clear the colon by way of gentle or more rigorous agents to create more intra-abdominal space and ease colon reflection to access the kidney. If preoperative suspicion of bowel invasion is present, a bowel preparation is recommended.

Preoperative patient counseling should include discussion regarding the potential need for open conversion, especially in locally advanced cancers. Imaging studies are essential and should particularly be reviewed carefully to determine vascular anatomy and the potential for tumor invasion into nearby structures. Tumors immediately abutting organs like the colon, duodenum, liver, pancreas, and spleen may be found at the time of surgery to be adherent and inseparable from or invading into these organs. Metastatic evaluation with imaging should also be performed although cytoreductive nephrectomy may still be pursued in proper candidates even in the presence of distant disease.

Operative Setup

As with other upper tract robotic urologic surgery, the robot will approach the patient from the side ipsilateral to the pathologic kidney. The robot can be brought at an angle over the patient's shoulder to ease triangulation of the robotic arms around the kidney and upper abdomen. The daVinci® Xi robot (Intuitive Surgical, Inc., Sunnyvale, CA) has a rotating tower that supports the robotic arms such that the robot can be brought in perpendicular to the patient's side and the tower rotated to the degree necessary to triangulate the arms as desired.

The assistant and scrub nurse will stand on the side of the patient's abdomen across the patient from the robotic patient-side cart. The vision tower of the robot can be positioned at the feet of the bed or elsewhere depending on the preference of the surgical team and size of the operating room.

Another option for positioning of the robot is similar to that used for robotic foregut surgery with the patient in reverse Trendelenburg position with the robot approaching the bed over the patient's head. This approach is less familiar but can be used in select scenarios such as in the setting of bilateral nephrectomy although rare.

Patient Positioning and Preparation

Positioning for robotic nephrectomy is similar to that of laparoscopic nephrectomy with the patient laying on one side with the side of the involved kidney elevated (flank position). Various methods for securing the patient have been described including beanbags, supports attached to the table, and pillows, but regardless of the method used, adequate padding and natural positioning are important to prevent injury.

The operative table can be flexed to extend the space for lateral trocar placement especially in patients with short torsos, but this can also be avoided entirely with the bed remaining flat. The kidney rest is never necessary and does not contribute to the robotic nephrectomy operation such that it should be avoided due to the potential it may increase the risk of injury or rhabdomyolysis particularly in long procedures.

A nasogastric tube on suction should always be placed to decompress the stomach and is particularly helpful in right nephrectomy procedures to keep the duodenum decompressed throughout the surgery. A Foley catheter should be placed in the bladder to monitor urine output. Note can be made just prior to renal artery ligation of urine output before this point so as to be able to monitor urine output from the remaining kidney during the remainder of the procedure. Also, if a port is placed low in the abdomen, decompression of the bladder is important to prevent injury.

The flank positioning of the patient on the bed has been described for laparoscopy as anywhere between 30° and 90° of laterality with some surgeons preferring 45° or 60°. While less than full flank (90°) positioning may ease conversion to open surgery if it becomes necessary, the rarity of need for this and benefit of 90° positioning makes

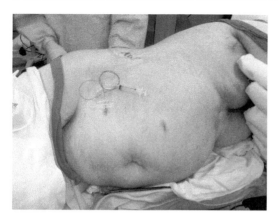

Fig. 9.1 Full flank, 90° patient positioning with beanbag support. Blankets on an arm board are used to support the arm in a neutral position

this our preference (Fig. 9.1). The 90° flank position maximizes gravity retraction of bowels and other intraperitoneal organs (e.g., pancreas on the left) away from the retroperitoneum once the colon is reflected. This then minimizes reliance on a bedside assistant or the robotic fourth arm for retraction throughout the procedure such that most nephrectomies can be performed without an assistant port or bedside assistant trained in laparoscopy.

Trocar Configuration

Basic trocars providing the foundation for robotic nephrectomy include the camera port and at least two other trocars for the robotic left- and right hand instruments. Initially, a surgeon early in his or her experience will add additional trocars for the robotic fourth arm and/or assistant ports. More experience will allow reduction in the number of trocars needed, particularly for more straightforward nephrectomies. The minimum number of trocars with which robotic nephrectomy can be performed is only three (Fig. 9.1). This is particularly beneficial when a bedside assistant skilled in laparoscopy is not available as the procedure can be performed with only a scrub nurse able to change the robotic instruments. Newer surgeons should have a skilled bedside assistant even if this requires having another urol-

ogist when specialized assistants or residents/fellows are not available. This will maximize efficiency and aid in progression of the procedure with an additional level of safety.

For more complex nephrectomy procedures, such as caval thrombectomy, additional trocars allow retraction with the robotic fourth arm and/or one or more assistant ports for suction and retraction as well as introduction of needles, hemostatic agents, bulldog clamps, and the like. Surgeons who prefer to staple hilar vessels will need an assistant trocar large enough to introduce the laparoscopic stapler or can use the robotic stapling device available with the newer generation robots. Surgeons who use Hem-o-lok clips on the renal vessels can simply use the robotic clip appliers or can again place an assistant port of at least 12 mm in diameter for the handheld clip applier used by the bedside assistant.

A dedicated 5 mm trocar can be placed for a liver retractor if desired but is not necessary in straightforward right nephrectomies with experience. If a liver retractor is used, care should be taken to avoid external collisions between the robotic arms and the instrument outside the body being used for liver retraction, which will not be seen by the surgeon at the console. Surgeons avoiding a liver retractor can lift the liver edge and use the shaft of the right robotic arm to keep the liver elevated while they dissect the upper pole of the kidney.

The trocar for the camera has been used by some surgeons at the umbilicus or more laterally for those who prefer. The closer the camera trocar is placed to the midline, the wider the view possible and vice versa. Placing the camera trocar too laterally can cause a view that is too close to the kidney and other relevant anatomy, but a lateral camera port does provide additional room for the bedside assistant. An additional advantage of a periumbilical or midline camera trocar is that this can be extended at the end of the procedure to extract the specimen through the linea alba without any muscle cutting.

After placing the camera trocar at the umbilical level through the midline, the scope can be used to guide optimal positioning of the remaining ports with the goal of triangulating the robotic arms around the affected kidney for ideal access and minimization of external arm clashing. The patient side cart can be docked at an angle over the ipsilateral shoulder to create this angulation or the tower rotated on the da Vinci Xi robot to achieve the same goal. The 30° down lens should be used for midline camera trocar configurations while the 0° lens should be used the more lateral the camera trocar is positioned.

Some surgeons prefer to use ruler measurements and sometimes complex algorithms to decide on trocar positioning, but oftentimes one size does not fit all and an understanding of the individual patient's anatomy is more useful than fixed measurements. Certainly, if measuring and marking the planned trocar sites is done, this is best done after insufflation of the abdomen since pneumoperitoneum will affect the final position and spacing of the trocars.

The working robotic instrument trocars are placed in the lower and upper quadrants ipsilateral to the affected kidney at least 8 in. from the camera trocar and never in line with the camera trocar and patient side cart as this will make docking to the trocars impossible. The exact position of these upper and lower quadrant trocars can be adjusted for better upper pole access when needing to reach high in the abdomen for a predominantly upper pole tumor, for example. In contrast, the trocars can be adjusted for better lower abdominal access, but regardless of minor adjustments in the triangulation of ports, planning must allow adequate access to the hilum for the most critical portion of the procedure.

Assistant ports can be placed before or after the robot is docked, which allows the surgeon to make sure the assistant will have adequate reach to the trocar and to make sure there will be less external collisions with any trocars to be used for static retraction (e.g., liver retractor). On the right side, a 5-mm trocar is adequate for suction or retraction and can be placed in the right upper quadrant for the liver or in the lower quadrant for the colon and/or duodenum.

On the left side, a lower quadrant assistant port is better for retraction of the colon when needed. If the surgeon uses the bedside assistant to clip or staple the renal vessels, a 12 mm port is best placed in the lower quadrant so that the angle of approach to the hilum will be more perpendicular. This way, when clipping or stapling a vessel, visibility will be better, including the back end of the clip or stapler just before deploying to make sure it is all the way across the vessel.

Instrument and Equipment List

Our preference is to use the robotic cautery scissor and fenestrated Maryland bipolar for the entirety of the procedure, using the robotic Hemolock clips for the renal artery, renal vein, and ureter (and gonadal vein when appropriate). Other robotic energy instruments can be substituted, including hook cautery or other robotic bipolar energy instruments. Suction is typically not needed if hemostasis is maintained, but if no assistant port is being used and suction is needed, it can be accomplished through a robotic instrument port by temporarily removing the robotic instrument and applying the included reducer cap on the port valve.

Equipment

- da Vinci® Si HD or Xi Surgical System (three or four-arm system; Intuitive Surgical, Inc., Sunnyvale, CA)
- EndoWrist® Maryland bipolar forceps or PK dissector (Intuitive Surgical, Inc., Sunnyvale, CA)
- EndoWrist® curved monopolar scissors (Intuitive Surgical, Inc., Sunnyvale, CA)
- If using robotic fourth arm, EndoWrist® ProGrasp™ forceps (Intuitive Surgical, Inc., Sunnyvale, CA)
- For caval thrombus cases, two EndoWrist® needle drivers (Intuitive Surgical, Inc., Sunnyvale, CA)
- InSite® Vision System with 30° down lens (Intuitive Surgical, Inc., Sunnyvale, CA)
- EndoWrist® Hem-o-lok clip applier, two for ease of reloading (Intuitive Surgical, Inc., Sunnyvale, CA)
- Large Hem-o-lok® clips (Teleflex Medical, Research Triangle Park, NC)

Trocars

- 12 mm trocars (0 or 1)
- 8 mm robotic trocars (2 or 3)
- 5 mm trocar (0 or 2)

Recommended Sutures

- For caval thrombus cases: 4-0 prolene sutures cut to 6–10 in. for caval reconstruction

Instruments Used by the Surgical Assistant

- Blunt tip grasper (optional for retraction)
- Suction irrigator device (optional)
- Hem-o-lok® clip applier if not using robotic clips or stapler (Teleflex Medical, Research Triangle Park, NC)
- Large Hem-o-lok® clips (Teleflex Medical, Research Triangle Park, NC)
- 10 mm specimen entrapment bag
- SURGICEL® hemostatic gauze (Ethicon, Inc., Cincinnati, OH) or other hemostatic agents (optional)
- Laparoscopic needle driver (for introducing sutures in caval thrombectomy)
- Laparoscopic scissors (for cutting sutures in caval thrombectomy)

Step-by-Step Technique

Right Nephrectomy

Step 1: Colon Reflection

Robotic right and left nephrectomy share many common steps, but the major differences relate to the surrounding anatomy. Colon reflection is easier on the right as the hepatic flexure of the colon is commonly lower in the abdomen than the splenic flexure.

The right colon is reflected by incising the Line of Toldt and gently retracting the colon to develop the natural plane between the colon/mesentery and the Gerota's fascia (Fig. 9.2). The

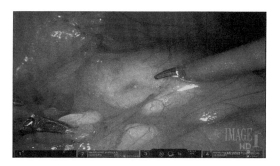

Fig. 9.2 The right colon is mobilized by incising the posterior peritoneal reflection overlying the kidney within Gerota's fascia without violating Gerota's fascia and disrupting the perinephric fat

Line of Toldt should be incised as far down towards the pelvis as possible so that the cecum will not be tethered and keep the colon from falling medially and away from the retroperitoneum.

Step 2: Duodenum and Cava

After mobilizing the colon medially, the duodenum should be identified early to prevent inadvertent injury, which can be catastrophic. The duodenum usually closely overlies the medial aspect of Gerota's fascia and should be carefully dissected away from it and retracted medially until the anterior vena cava is completely cleared. Adequate mobilization of the colon and duodenum will allow gravity to keep them away from the operative field for the rest of the operation. Newer surgeons might inadequately mobilize these structures and consequently will need retraction of them by an assistant or the robotic fourth arm.

Upon visualizing the anterior vena cava, the renal vein will usually be readily identifiable at its junction with the lateral cava, but if it is not, it can be identified after the kidney is lifted off the psoas muscle (Fig. 9.3).

Step 3: Psoas Muscle

The posterior aspect of Gerota's fascia should be identified and elevated from the underlying psoas muscle (Fig. 9.4), but this step can be challenging. One error to be avoided is to mistake the pericaval nodal tissue as being part of the perinephric fat within Gerota's fascia and attempting to lift this with kidney away from the cava and

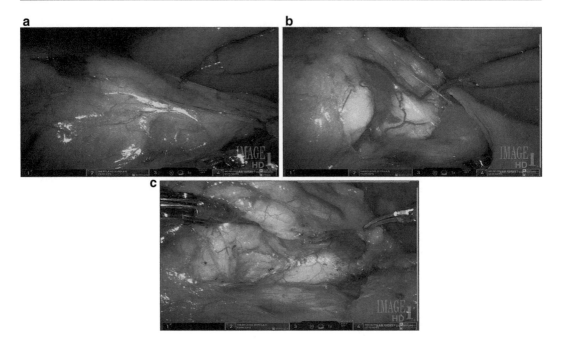

Fig. 9.3 After reflecting the colon, the duodenum will be seen closely adjacent to the medial aspect of Gerota's fascia (*a*) and should be carefully reflected medially (*b*) until completely medialized from the underlying vena cava (*c*)

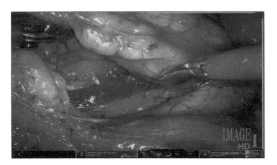

Fig. 9.4 The kidney within Gerota's fascia is lifted off the underlying psoas muscle and allows the kidney to be retracted anteriorly so that the renal hilum is on stretch and ideally positioned for vessel dissection

spine. In almost all patients, there will be fatty tissue comprising the pericaval nodal tissue left behind along the lateral aspect of the cava after lifting the kidney within Gerota's.

Lifting the kidney within Gerota's fascia allows ideal access to the renal hilum and access to the renal artery, which otherwise is difficult to approach behind the renal vein. The safest dissection of the renal artery is when the renal hilum is on stretch with the kidney elevated as this will

minimize inadvertent violation of the artery in attempting to dissect behind the back wall to allow clipping or stapling.

Step 4: Vessel Ligation

With the kidney lifted within Gerota's fascia off of the underlying psoas, the vessels are on stretch for dissection of the artery behind the vein. The artery is usually approached on the caudal aspect of the more anterior renal vein just lateral to the edge of the vena cava. On occasion, the artery will be more cranial and require dissection above the renal vein. The artery can also be approached in the interaortocaval space when difficult to approach behind a very short renal vein or if the artery has already branched into several branches behind the IVC.

The renal artery should be clipped with at least two clips or can be stapled if the surgeon prefers. The renal vein is then dissected and clipped after at least one clip is placed on the renal artery ensuring arterial flow has been interrupted. The renal artery can be completely clipped and divided or simply clipped once until the vein is clipped and divided to provide better access to the artery to complete ligation. The renal vein can be clipped as the renal artery regardless of its width as it is more compressible by clips than an artery. The vein can also be stapled if preferred by the surgeon.

Step 5: Adrenal Plane
The upper pole of the kidney is dissected either to include removal of the adrenal gland when necessary or more commonly to preserve the adrenal when uninvolved by tumor. This is accomplished by dissecting between the lower aspect of the adrenal gland and medial upper pole of the kidney and proceeding directly posterior until seeing the abdominal wall beneath (Fig. 9.5). The upper pole of the kidney can then be lifted off the posterior abdominal wall with the posterior Gerota's fascia intact and the perinephric fat included in the specimen. The upper pole fat can then be followed along the lower edge of the liver all the way until reaching the lateral attachments of the kidney to the abdominal wall (Fig. 9.6).

Step 6: Ureter
The last step before dividing the lateral attachments of the kidney, which should be done last to keep the kidney from falling medially and obscuring the anatomy, is division of the ureter (Fig. 9.7). On the right side, the gonadal vein does not need to be divided and is left medially with the vena cava but can be clipped and divided along with the ureter if needed.

Step 7: Completion
The lower pole is mobilized after clipping the ureter, and the lateral attachments are divided last completing the robotic portion of the procedure. If the kidney is removed without disrupting Gerota's fascia and leaving the perinephric fat intact for ideal margins, the nephrectomy bed will have minimal fat remaining (Fig. 9.8).

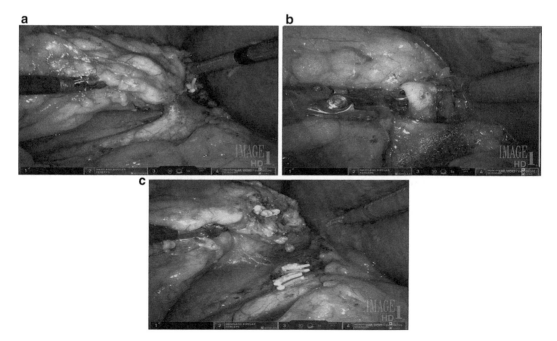

Fig. 9.5 With the kidney lifted to provide stretch on the renal vessels (**a**) and safe access to behind the vessels including circumferential dissection of the renal artery (**b**) whether above or below the renal vein to allow clipping of the artery and then vein (**c**)

a

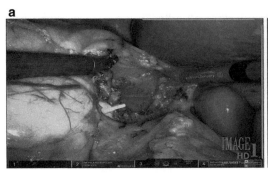

b

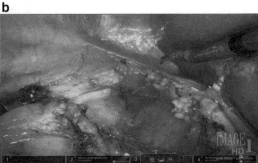

Fig. 9.6 The plane between the adrenal gland and upper pole of the kidney should be identified first (**a**) and then followed posteriorly until the posterior abdominal wall is seen and then used as a landmark for mobilization of the upper pole (**b**)

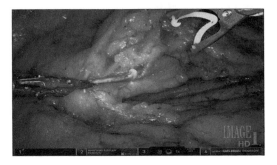

Fig. 9.7 The ureter is clipped and divided

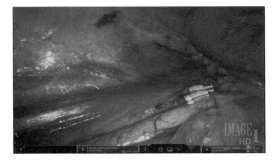

Fig. 9.8 The completed nephrectomy bed after removal of the kidney within Gerota's fascia will have minimal remaining fat and preserved planes

Left Nephrectomy

Step 1: Wide Access to the Retroperitoneum

As with right nephrectomy, the initial step is to reflect the colon away from the underlying retroperitoneum. The splenic flexure of the colon can be reflected partially up to the edge of the level of the spleen allowing access to the renal hilum, but this will leave the colon tethered at this point and require retraction medially by an assistant or the robotic fourth arm for the remainder of the procedure. A better approach is to continue the incision of the line of Toldt more cephalad along the lateral aspect of the spleen all the way to the diaphragm. This will then allow the colon, spleen, and pancreas to reflect medially as one unit such that gravity will keep all of these structures away from the operative field (Fig. 9.9). As on the right side, care should be taken not to violate Gerota's fascia and to respect the natural plane between it and the colon mesentery.

Step 2: Psoas Plane

Similar to the right kidney, the next step is to find the plane between the posterior Gerota's fascia and psoas muscle to allow the kidney to be lifted in approach to the renal hilum. Of course, rather than the vena cava being medial to the kidney, on the left side the aorta is medial. In similar fashion, care should be taken to avoid mistaking the periaortic nodal tissue for perinephric fat as a plane between the two can be identified with proper attention (Fig. 9.10).

Step 3: Vascular Dissection

The renal vein can be found simply by following the plane between the psoas and Gerota's fascia cranially until the vein is encountered or by following the gonadal vein, which will insert into the renal vein on the left. The renal artery is often directly posterior to the vein in most patients as on the right side and can be dissected immediately at its takeoff from the aorta if branching

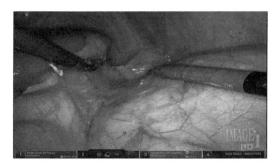

Fig. 9.9 The lateral incision of the line of Toldt is continued beyond the colon all the way to the diaphragm to allow medial retraction of the colon and spleen as one unit by gravity alone

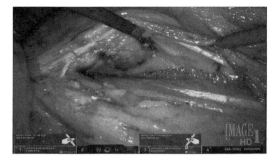

Fig. 9.10 The left kidney within Gerota's fascia is lifted off the underlying psoas muscle while not disturbing the periaortic nodal tissue. Note exposure without any retraction of the colon because of full mobilization of the colon and spleen

early (Fig. 9.11). As on the right side, the artery does not need to be completely controlled and divided prior to addressing the vein. A single clip can be placed on the artery and then further clips and division can be completed after the vein has been clipped and divided to improve visualization and access to the artery (Fig. 9.12). The renal vein is ideally dissected and clipped closer to the kidney than where the adrenal vein enters the renal vein so that the adrenal vein is preserved when possible (Fig. 9.13).

Step 4: Adrenal and Upper Pole

When the adrenal gland is to be spared, Gerota's fascia is entered at the medial upper pole to identify the edge of the adrenal gland and separate it from the upper pole of the kidney (Fig. 9.14). As on the right side, the dissection is carried posteriorly until the posterior abdominal wall is seen,

and then the upper pole of the kidney with its surrounding perinephric fat within Gerota's fascia is lifted intact away with the specimen (Fig. 9.15).

The robotic portion of the procedure is completed by clipping and dividing the ureter and gonadal vein and then lastly dividing the lateral attachments of the kidney. Both in left and right robotic nephrectomy procedures, the kidney is extracted in an extraction bag. Hemostatic agents are typically unnecessary.

If a lymphadenectomy is performed, templates are not well defined for renal cell carcinoma. A thorough dissection can be performed robotically without difficulty [4]. On the right side, caution should be used to avoid injuring lumbar veins entering the vena cava as well as the left renal vein entering the cava medially. On the left side, care should be taken not to injure lumbar arteries or the superior or inferior mesenteric arteries as they leave the aorta (Fig. 9.16).

IVC Tumor Thrombus

Renal cell carcinoma has a tendency to grow by direct extension into contiguous veins and can extend into the renal vein and inferior vena cava (IVC), particularly on the right side where the renal vein is shorter. Robotic nephrectomy can still be performed in the setting of vena caval tumor thrombus with adequate experience and extreme caution given the complexity of the condition and procedure as first described in 2011 [5, 6]. Complete control of the vena cava is necessary to prevent potentially massive bleeding once entered to extract the tumor thrombus. Additionally, care must be taken during circumferential dissection of the IVC not to dislodge the tumor thrombus or any associated bland thrombus as this will lead to potentially fatal pulmonary embolism.

The initial steps of the procedure are similar to any other right nephrectomy except that the renal artery may be more easily and safely accessed in the interaortocaval space when the renal vein is severely distended with tumor and obscuring access to the artery behind (Fig. 9.17). The renal artery can simply be clipped at this point and

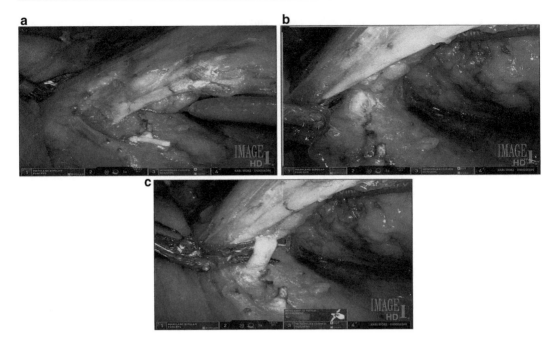

Fig. 9.11 Lifting the kidney to stretch the hilum is essential as this allows access to the renal artery behind the vein as shown. Before lifting the kidney, visualization of the artery is hindered (**a**) while afterwards the artery is identified (**b**) and then dissected circumferentially from the surrounding connective tissues (**c**)

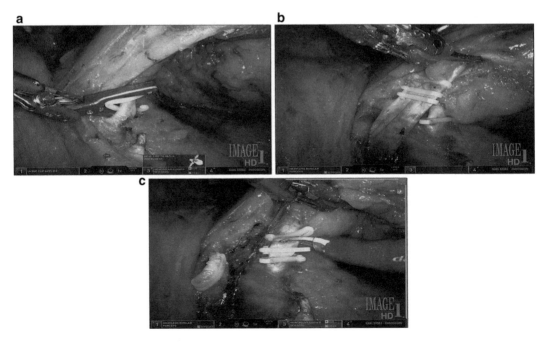

Fig. 9.12 A single clip can be placed on the renal artery to interrupt blood flow to the kidney (**a**), and further clips can be placed after the renal vein is clipped and divided (**b**) since access to the artery will then be easier (**c**)

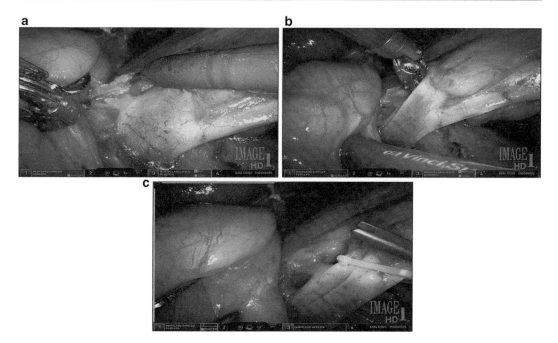

Fig. 9.13 The adrenal vein is found on the cranial aspect of the renal vein (**a**), and the renal vein can be dissected circumferentially closer to the kidney (**b**) to preserve the adrenal vein after the renal vein is clipped and divided (**c**)

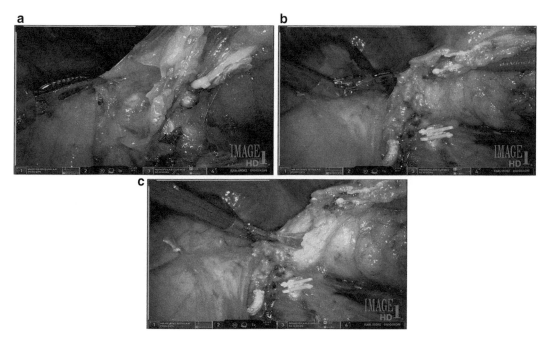

Fig. 9.14 The adrenal is separated from the upper pole of the kidney after completing vascular division by identifying the edge of the adrenal gland within the surrounding fat (**a**) and then following the edge of the adrenal towards the upper pole while lifting the kidney up and laterally (**b**) and then identifying the upper pole (**c**)

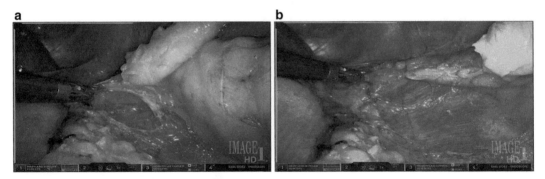

Fig. 9.15 The nephrectomy is completed by continuing division of the attachments around the upper pole (**a**) all the way to the diaphragm above (**b**) until reaching the lateral attachments, which are divided last after the ureter and lower pole are mobilized

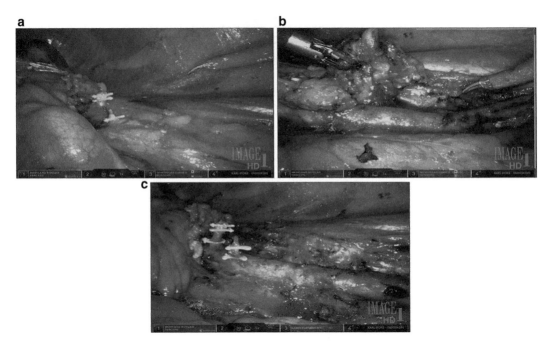

Fig. 9.16 On the *left*, a retroperitoneal lymph node dissection can be performed by removing all of the periaortic and interaortocaval lymphatic tissue seen after completing the nephrectomy (**a**, before node dissection) most easily achieved beginning at the aortic bifurcation and lifting the nodal packet up and away from the aorta (**b**) until the aorta is completely skeletonized of the surrounding tissues (**c**, after node dissection)

does not need to be divided. The IVC must be completely mobilized circumferential along the entire length involved by the tumor thrombus and enough above and below to allow clamping (Fig. 9.18). All lumbar veins entering the cava along this length must be either cauterized or clipped and the left renal vein dissected for clamping so that there is no inflow to the IVC whatsoever before it is opened. Use of laparoscopic ultrasound is critical to identify the upper extent of the thrombus.

Clamping of the IVC can be accomplished with bulldog clamps or more easily with modified Rommel tourniquets by placing vessel loops around the lumen twice. A small cavotomy can be made after tightening the tourniquets around

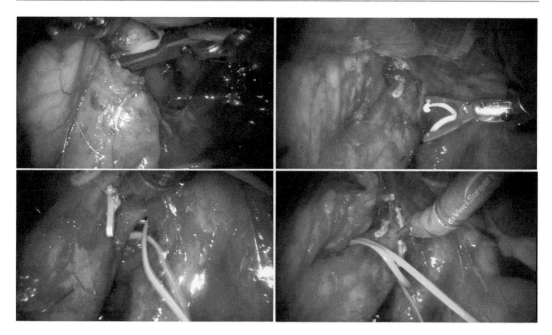

Fig. 9.17 The right renal artery can be accessed in the interaortocaval space and clipped before the IVC is completed dissected (*upper left*), which includes division of the short hepatic veins when needed for high control (*upper right*) and placement of a vessel behind the IVC (*lower left*) twice to create a tourniquet (*lower right*) when later tightened

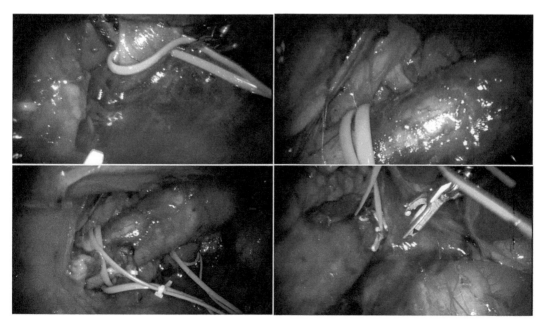

Fig. 9.18 The left renal vein must be dissected for later clamping (*upper left*) and all lumbar vein dissected and ligated (*upper right*) until the IVC has been completely controlled with modified Rommel tourniquets on the left renal vein and above and below the IVC thrombus (*lower left*) before tightening to clamp the cava (*lower right*)

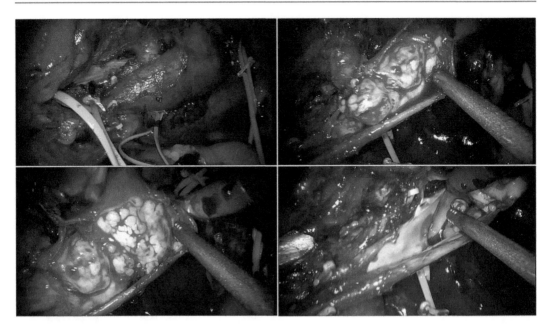

Fig. 9.19 After tightening all three tourniquets, the IVC is opened to extract the tumor thrombus (*upper left*) and should be bloodless as the cavotomy is extended to above the upper extent of the thrombus (*lower left*) to ensure complete removal intact (*lower right*)

the left renal vein and IVC above and below the tumor thrombus to make sure that all inflow has been controlled before widely opening the IVC to extract the tumor. If any continued bleeding is encountered after the IVC is squeezed to empty it, the cavotomy is closed and any missed lumbar veins must be identified and clipped (Fig. 9.19).

Once complete control has been confirmed, the IVC can be further opened until the upper extent of the tumor is identified and extracted intact. The cavotomy is then closed after inspecting the lumen with permanent suture in running, water-tight fashion. The lumen should be flushed with heparinized saline prior to completing the closure to prevent gas embolism upon releasing the tourniquets to reestablish flow (Fig. 9.20).

Postoperative Management

After robotic nephrectomy, patients can be managed based upon surgeon preference in a manner similar to other robotic procedures such as prostatectomy. As with other procedures whether open or robotic, patients managed with a clinical pathway typically have a more expeditious hospi-tal stay [1]. Our preference is to use a subcutaneous catheter for continuous delivery of local anesthetic (ON-Q®, Kimberly-Clark, Lake Forest, CA) at the extraction site with oral acetaminophen for pain, scheduled intravenous ketorolac, oral narcotics for breakthrough pain, and complete avoidance of intravenous narcotics. Oral nutrition can be begun immediately as tolerated after surgery, and ambulation is encouraged beginning on the day of surgery. Most patients can be discharged the day after surgery.

Complications

The potential complicationscomplications following robotic nephrectomy include those of any laparoscopic or robotic procedure as well as those particular to nephrectomy. Access-related complications and injury to nearby organs are included in surgical complications while medical complications include renal insufficiency or failure on rare occasion in those with compromised renal function in the remaining kidney. Although complications are rare, early recognition and appropriate management is key with judicious use of imaging.

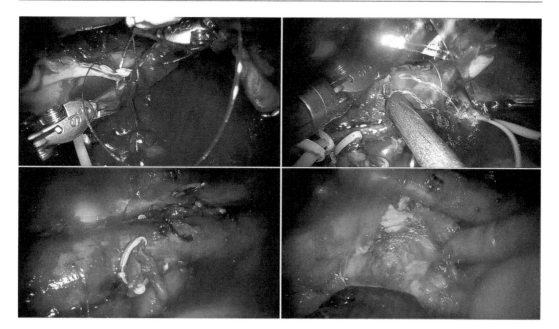

Fig. 9.20 The IVC is closed with running suture (*upper left*) and the lumen flushed with heparinized saline (*upper right*) before completing the closure and removing the tourniquets (*lower left*) after which a node dissection including the retrocaval nodes (*lower right*) can be easily accomplished given previous mobilization of the cava

References

1. Petros FG, Angell JE, Abaza R. Outcomes of robotic nephrectomy including highest-complexity cases: largest series to date and literature review. Urology. 2015;85(6):1352–9.
2. Boger M, Lucas SM, Popp SC, et al. Comparison of robot-assisted nephrectomy with laparoscopic and hand-assisted laparoscopic nephrectomy. J Soc Laparoendosc Surg. 2010;14(3):374–80.
3. Sun Y, Abreu AL, Gill IS. Robotic inferior vena cava thrombus surgery: novel strategies. Curr Opin Urol. 2014;24(2):140–7.
4. Abaza R, Lowe G. Feasibility and adequacy of robotic lymphadenectomy for renal cell carcinoma. J Endourol. 2011;25(7):1155–9.
5. Abaza R. Initial series of robotic radical nephrectomy with vena caval tumor thrombectomy. Eur Urol. 2011;59(4):652–6.
6. Abaza R. Robotic surgery and minimally-invasive management of renal tumors with vena caval extension. Curr Opin Urol. 2011;21(2):104–9.

Robot-Assisted Radical Nephroureterectomy

10

Peter Y. Cai and Li-Ming Su

Patient Selection

Similar to open and laparoscopic approaches, the indications for robot-assisted radical nephroureterectomy (RARNU) include patients with radiographic (by computed tomography or intravenous pyelography) and endoscopic evidence suggestive of upper urinary tract urothelial carcinoma. A positive urine cytology may also provide supportive evidence for the presence of a high-grade urothelial carcinoma. While other therapeutic options, including endoscopic resection or laser ablation, can be applied to select upper tract urothelial tumors, nephroureterectomy remains the "gold standard" therapy. With equivalent oncologic outcomes to open surgery, laparoscopic [1–4] and robotic [5–8] nephroureterectomy may even be applied to high-grade, invasive, and multifocal lesions. RARNU may also be utilized in certain congenital or acquired conditions, such as duplicated renal collecting system and atrophic or nonfunctional renal unit, particularly when associated with recurrent infections, stones, or vesicoureteral reflux.

Absolute contraindications for RARNU include uncorrectable bleeding disorders and inability to undergo general anesthesia due to severe cardiopulmonary compromise or other medical comorbidities. A relative contraindication for RARNU may exist for those patients with locally invasive transitional cell carcinoma with involvement of surrounding structures or lymph nodes. In this setting, an open surgical approach in addition to multimodality therapy (i.e., neoadjuvant chemotherapy) may be prudent, although these patients appear to have poor outcomes regardless of the surgical approach [9]. Prior abdominal and pelvic surgery or morbid obesity make RARNU more challenging but are not absolute contraindications to the procedure depending on the skill and experience of the surgeon.

Preoperative Preparation

Patients are instructed to avoid aspirin, nonsteroidal anti-inflammatories, blood thinners, or vitamin E for 1 week prior to surgery to minimize perioperative bleeding. One bottle of magnesium citrate is taken the day before surgery and the patient's diet is limited to clear liquids 24 h prior to surgery. A single dose of preoperative antibiotics, such as intravenous cefazolin, is administered 30 min prior to skin incision.

Electronic supplementary material: The online version of this chapter (doi:10.1007/978-3-319-45060-5_10) contains supplementary material, which is available to authorized users.

P.Y. Cai, M.D. • L.-M. Su, M.D. (✉)
Department of Urology, University of Florida
College of Medicine, 1600 SW Archer Road, 100247,
Gainesville, FL 32610-2047, USA
e-mail: sulm@urology.ufl.edu

Regarding informed consent, the risks of RARNU are similar to those of laparoscopic and open nephroureterectomy. These include infection, bleeding, blood transfusion, incisional hernia, and the need to convert to open surgery. Adjacent organ injury should be discussed including the possibility for a splenectomy in left-sided lesions and liver or duodenal injury with right-sided lesions. The downstream risk of renal insufficiency and failure should be discussed with patients undergoing nephroureterectomy, especially in those patients with significant comorbid medical conditions such as hypertension, diabetes, long-term nonsteroidal anti-inflammatory use, obesity, smoking and preexisting renal compromise. Finally, the possibility of local and distant tumor recurrence after nephroureterectomy should be discussed with the patient.

Operative Setup

Nephroureterectomy performed by robot assistance creates an operative setup dilemma as a result of the large surgical field extending from the upper pole of the kidney to the deep pelvis where excision of the bladder cuff is performed. Though successful nephroureterectomy using a single docking technique with a hybrid port has been described [8], we favor a two-docking technique to facilitate improved anatomic access and positioning, while avoiding robotic instrument collision [10]. We maintain a single trocar arrangement to minimize time spent on repositioning while preserving access to the deep pelvis. Herein we will describe nephroureterectomy using a two-docking technique with a single trocar arrangement.

At our institution we use the da Vinci® Si-HD system (Intuitive Surgical, Inc., Sunnyvale, CA) with four-arm capabilities, though we generally employ a three-armed technique during RARNU. One surgical assistant is required and is positioned on the contralateral side of the surgical site with a Mayo stand nearby for commonly used instrumentation. A scrub nurse can be positioned on either side depending on operating room space considerations. While setting up for the operation, it is important to consider that in the two-docking RARNU the robot is positioned differently for the nephrectomy and ureterectomy portions of the case. Figure 10.1a shows the operating setup for the nephrectomy portion of the procedure with the surgical robot cart docked posterior to the patient who is in a modified decubitus position. The robot cart is positioned at an approximately 45° angle entering from the head of the table. The robot is then re-docked during the ureterectomy portion of the procedure at a 45° angle entering from the foot of the table at approximately the level of the iliac crest (Fig. 10.1b).

Patient Positioning

The patient is initially placed in the supine position for induction of anesthesia. An orogastric or nasogastric tube and an 18 Fr urethral catheter are placed at the beginning of the case to decompress the stomach and bladder, respectively, to facilitate safe access to the peritoneal cavity for insufflation. The abdomen is then shaved from the xiphoid process to the pubic symphysis. The patient is then positioned in a modified lateral decubitus position at a 45° angle between the patient's back and the surface of the operating room table. This position is maintained with a large gel roll positioned behind the back of the patient for support. Because the patient is not in a full flank position, an axillary roll is generally not required to prevent brachial nerve injury. The bed is flexed to approximately 30° with the break of the bed positioned at the superior margin of the iliac crest to elevate and expand the ipsilateral flank. The dependant leg is flexed to a 90° angle at the knee and is supported at the knee and ankle with gel or foam padding to protect the peroneal nerve and avoid vascular compression. Pillows are placed between the legs to support the nondependant leg which is aligned in a neutral extended position. Sequential compression devices are applied to the lower extremities and activated.

The dependant arm is padded and placed on top of an arm board that is angled slightly cephalad to provide sufficient working space for the robotic arms as well as surgical assistant. The two arms may be separated and padded in a variety of ways in order to maintain a comfortable and neutral position without direct contact with

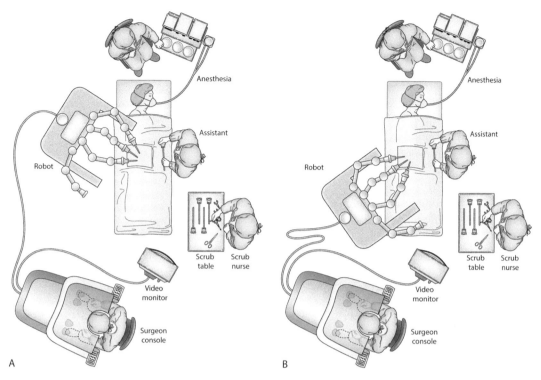

Fig. 10.1 Operating room setup. (**a**) The operating room setup for the nephrectomy portion of the two-docking, right transperitoneal robot-assisted nephroureterectomy including the standard configuration of the personnel and equipment. The robot cart is positioned at a 45° angle entering from the head of the table (Copyright 2009 Li-Ming Su, M.D., University of Florida). (**b**) Operating room setup for the ureterectomy portion of the two-docking, right RARNU. The robotic cart has been repositioned at a 45° angle entering from the foot of the table at the level of the iliac crest (Copyright 2009 Li-Ming Su, M.D., University of Florida)

Fig. 10.2 Patient positioning for a right RARNU. The robot cart is docked posterior to the patient. Note that the 2″ cloth tape used to secure the upper torso and thighs has not yet been placed in this image

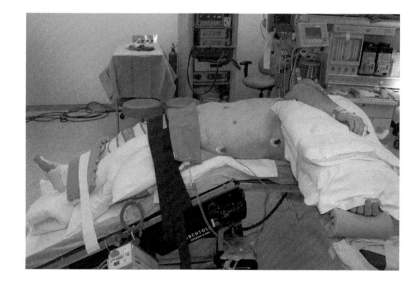

the robotic arms during the operation. We routinely place three to four pillows between the dependant and nondependant arms and then secure the patient to the operative table using 2″ cloth tape at the level of the upper torso and thighs and ankles. Figure 10.2 illustrates proper patient positioning.

Trocar Configuration

Although we utilize a two-docking approach to RARNU, a single trocar configuration allows completion of both the nephrectomy and ureterectomy portions with minimal modifications as shown in Fig. 10.3a, b. Trocar placement begins with a 12 mm paraumbilical trocar for the endoscope. One 8 mm robotic trocar is then placed lateral to the rectus muscle near the anterior axillary line just below the level of the umbilicus. A second 8 mm robotic trocar is placed two to three fingerbreadths below the costal margin lateral to the rectus muscle. These trocars accommodate the left and right robotic arms for the nephrectomy portion of the operation, respectively. For the surgical assistant, a 15 mm metal robotic cannula from the 8/15 mm convertible Hybrid Cannula Trocar (Intuitive Surgical, Inc., Sunnyvale, CA) is placed in the midline midway between the umbilicus and pubic tubercle. This 15 mm trocar has a plastic reducer placed to allow for retraction, suction, and irrigation by the assistant (Fig. 10.4a). While trocar placement is dependent on body habitus, it is important that all trocars are spaced at least 8 cm apart to avoid

external collision. In obese patients with a large abdominal pannus, this trocar configuration may require a slight lateral shift toward the ipsilateral kidney to allow for optimal visualization and to reach the target organ. For right-sided cases, an additional 5 mm laparoscopic trocar can be placed to provide liver retraction at the subcostal margin near the xiphoid process to accommodate a 5 mm grasper for retraction. This should be placed cephalad and more medial with respect to the subcostal 8 mm trocar in efforts to avoid external instrument clashing between the two trocars. For left-sided cases, release of the splenorenal ligament typically leads to adequate visualization of the upper pole of the kidney without the need for an additional trocar for retraction of the spleen.

After the nephrectomy portion of the case, the robot is repositioned as previously described (Fig. 10.1b) and the ureterectomy/bladder cuff excision is performed after making two trocar adjustments. First, the 8 mm cannula of the 8/15 mm Hybrid Cannula Trocar is inserted into the 15 mm assistant trocar for the left robotic arm creating a "hybrid" trocar (Fig. 10.4a, b). Second, the 8 mm subcostal trocar which previously

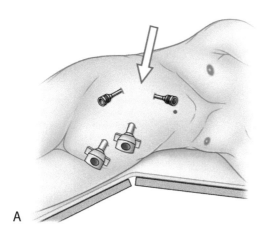
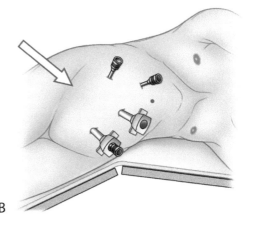
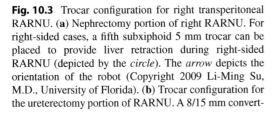

A B

Fig. 10.3 Trocar configuration for right transperitoneal RARNU. (**a**) Nephrectomy portion of right RARNU. For right-sided cases, a fifth subxiphoid 5 mm trocar can be placed to provide liver retraction during right-sided RARNU (depicted by the *circle*). The *arrow* depicts the orientation of the robot (Copyright 2009 Li-Ming Su, M.D., University of Florida). (**b**) Trocar configuration for the ureterectomy portion of RARNU. A 8/15 mm convert-

ible Hybrid Cannula Trocar (Intuitive Surgical, Inc., Sunnyvale, CA) is created by inserting an 8 mm robotic trocar into the assistant 15 mm outer cannula located below the umbilicus. The subcostal trocar becomes the new assistant trocar. The *arrow* depicts the orientation of the robotic cart entering at a 45° angle from the foot of the table (Copyright 2009 Li-Ming Su, M.D., University of Florida)

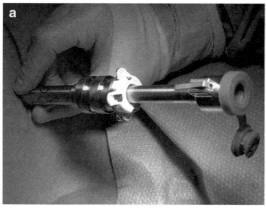 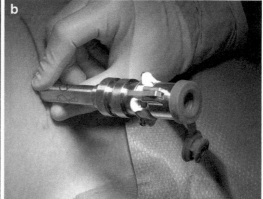

Fig. 10.4 The 8/15 mm Hybrid Cannula Trocar (Intuitive Surgical, Inc., Sunnyvale, CA) is designed to incorporate an 8 mm robotic trocar within a 15 mm outer cannula using a white plastic adapter. To assemble this trocar, (**a**) an 8 mm trocar is inserted into the adapter and (**b**) coupled to the 15 mm outer cannula. This design helps to prevent electrosurgical injury from capacitive coupling (see "Steps to Avoid Complications")

housed the right robotic arm is sealed with the 5 mm trocar valve and becomes the new assistant trocar (Fig. 10.3b). It is important to create the "hybrid" port using the Hybrid Cannula Trocar to prevent capacitive coupling which will be discussed in greater detail later (see "Steps to Avoid Complications").

Instrumentation and Equipment List

Equipment

- da Vinci® Si Surgical System (Intuitive Surgical, Inc., Sunnyvale, CA)
- Endowrist® Maryland bipolar forceps or PK dissector (Intuitive Surgical, Inc., Sunnyvale, CA)
- EndoWrist® curved monopolar scissors (Intuitive Surgical, Inc., Sunnyvale, CA)
- EndoWrist® monopolar hook (Intuitive Surgical, Inc., Sunnyvale, CA)
- EndoWrist® ProGrasp™ (Intuitive Surgical, Inc., Sunnyvale, CA)—optional
- EndoWrist® needle drivers (2) (Intuitive Surgical, Inc., Sunnyvale, CA)
- InSite® Vision System with 0° and 30° lens (Intuitive Surgical, Inc., Sunnyvale, CA)

Trocars

- 12 mm Trocar (1)
- 8 mm Robotic trocars (2)
- 8/15 mm Hybrid Cannula Trocar (Intuitive Surgical, Inc., Sunnyvale, CA)
- 5 mm Trocar (one for right-sided RARNU only)

Recommended Sutures

- 3-0 Polyglactin suture on a SH needle cut to 10 in. for closure of bladder mucosa (1–2 sutures total)
- 2-0 Polyglactin suture on a UR-6 needle cut to 10 in. for closure of the muscularis propria of the bladder (2–3 sutures total)

Instruments Used by the Surgical Assistant

- Laparoscopic needle driver
- Laparoscopic scissors
- Blunt tip grasper
- 5 mm Locking atraumatic grasper (for right-sided technique for liver retraction)
- Suction-irrigator device

- Hem-o-lok® clip applier (Teleflex Medical, Research Triangle Park, NC)
- Small and Medium-Large Hem-o-lok® clips (Teleflex Medical, Research Triangle Park, NC)
- 10 mm LigaSure Atlas™ Sealer/Divider device (Valleylab, Tyco Healthcare Group LP, Boulder, CO)
- Laparoscopic linear stapler with vascular load
- 15 mm Specimen entrapment bag
- Sponge on a stick
- Surgicel® hemostatic gauze (Ethicon, Inc., Cincinnati, OH) (if necessary)
- Hemovac or Jackson Pratt closed suction pelvic drain

Step-by-Step Technique (See Video 10.1)

Step 1: Abdominal Access and Trocar Placement

To begin a transperitoneal RARNU, pneumoperitoneum is established using either a Veress needle inserted at the base of the umbilicus or with an open trocar placement using the Hasson technique. If a Veress needle is used to establish pneumoperitoneum, the 12 mm paraumbilical trocar is placed under direct visualization using a visual obturator and a 0° laparoscope lens. Secondary trocars are then placed as previously described under direct vision and the robot is docked at a 45° angle from the head of the table. Prior to docking the robot to the trocars, the operating table is tilted maximally toward the assistant and opposite to the surgical site and robot to allow for the bowels to fall medially by gravity and provide maximum exposure of the affected kidney, ureter, and bladder.

With intraperitoneal access and establishment of pneumoperitoneum, the 0° stereoscopic camera is inserted through the 12 mm paraumbilical trocar and CO_2 insufflation is maintained at 15 mmHg. For the nephrectomy portion of the operation, a 0° stereoscopic lens is generally used; however, a 30° down lens may be necessary in patients with distended bowels or intraperitoneal fat resulting in poor visualization of the kidney

and renal hilum. Under direct visualization by the console surgeon, the robotic arms are loaded with instruments and are positioned within the operative field. The monopolar scissors are placed in the right robotic arm, while the bipolar forceps are inserted into the left robotic arm. Both monopolar and bipolar electrocautery are set at 30 W throughout the operation.

Step 2: Mobilization of Colon (Table 10.1)

Frequently, adhesions are encountered within the peritoneal cavity, which are released using sharp dissection with curved monopolar scissors in order to gain access to the white line of Toldt. The colon is reflected medially by sharply incising along the relatively avascular white line of Toldt with limited use of electrocautery and gently sweeping the peritoneum and mesocolon medially to reveal Gerota's fascia (Fig. 10.5). The assistant can facilitate this portion of the dis-

Table 10.1 Mobilization of colon: surgeon and assistant instrumentation

Surgeon instrumentation		Assistant instrumentation
Right arm	**Left arm**	• Suction-irrigator
• Curved monopolar scissors	• Maryland bipolar forceps	• Hem-o-lok® clip applier
Endoscope lens: 0°		

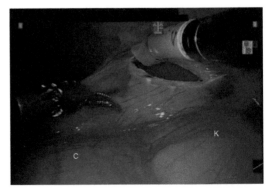

Fig. 10.5 Incision of the white line of Toldt and mobilization of the descending colon. *C* colon, *K* left kidney

section by applying medial traction on the colon and mesocolon using the suction-irrigator device. The colon is dissected as inferiorly as possible into the pelvic inlet to allow for optimal mobilization of the colon and exposure of the kidney and proximal ureter.

During right-sided dissection, the line of Toldt is extended medially between the liver and transverse colon to the space of Morison. The right coronary ligament is incised sharply and the liver retracted anteriorly and superior to expose the kidney. A 5 mm atraumatic locking grasper can be placed through the subxiphoid assistant trocar for this purpose and the liver retracted anteriorly with the tip of the grasper attached to the lateral side wall forming a fixed retractor. Reflection of the hepatic flexure exposes the second portion of the duodenum, which is then kocherized to expose the inferior vena cava. During left-sided dissection, full mobilization of the left colon requires dividing the lienorenal and phrenicocolic ligaments to allow the splenic flexure to retract medially.

Step 3: Dissection and Early Ligation of Ureter

The tail of Gerota's fascia is entered over the lower pole of the kidney and careful dissection is used to expose the ureter and the gonadal vein. A medium-large Hem-o-lok® clip is then placed across the ureter below the index lesion(s) without transection to prevent tumor cells from caudad migration during manipulation of the kidney and ureter. A window to the psoas muscle is created under the ureter using a combination of sharp and blunt dissection. This window is utilized as a traction point to lift the inferior pole of the kidney anteriorly, placing the hilum on slight traction to facilitate dissection of the renal artery and vein. For right-sided dissections, the psoas window is created beneath the ureter and *above* the gonadal vein to minimize its avulsion from the inferior vena cava while lifting the kidney anteriorly. During left-sided cases, the window to the psoas is created under *both* the ureter and gonadal vein, which are simultaneously retracted anteriorly.

Step 4: Dissection of Renal Hilum (Table 10.2)

Fine dissection of perihilar tissue may be aided by use of monopolar hook electrocautery (Fig. 10.6a). Under gentle anterior retraction of the lower pole of the kidney by the assistant using the suction-irrigator device, the renal hilum is carefully and meticulously dissected, bluntly creating small windows within the perivascular tissues parallel to the direction of the renal vessels (Fig. 10.6b). These perihilar tissues are generally avascular and can be divided using hook electrocautery or by the assistant using the LigaSure Atlas™ device. Care must be taken to identify accessory crossing renal arteries or lumbar vessels. The assistant also provides critical medial retraction of the ascending colon, vena cava, and duodenum (for right-sided dissection) and descending colon, pancreas, and spleen (for left-sided dissection) using the suction-irrigator device for exposure to the renal hilum. The hilum can be further exposed by first dissecting the adrenal gland off of the upper pole of the kidney (see "Step 5"). Subsequently, the operating surgeon can lift the kidney anteriorly and laterally with one instrument below the lower pole and the other below the upper pole, applying a gentle stretch to the renal artery and vein (Fig. 10.7a). Proximal dissection of the renal artery should be performed prior to the takeoff of segmental arteries in order to simplify complete arterial ligation. A 2–3 cm proximal segment of renal artery should be dissected free to allow either clipping or stapling of the renal artery based on surgeon preference, although we prefer a vascular laparoscopic linear stapler for this purpose

Table 10.2 Dissection of renal hilum: surgeon and assistant instrumentation

Surgeon instrumentation		Assistant instrumentation
Right arm	**Left arm**	• Suction-irrigator
• Curved monopolar scissors or monopolar hook	• Maryland bipolar forceps	• 10 mm LigaSure Atlas™ device • Laparoscopic linear stapler
Endoscope lens: 0°		

A

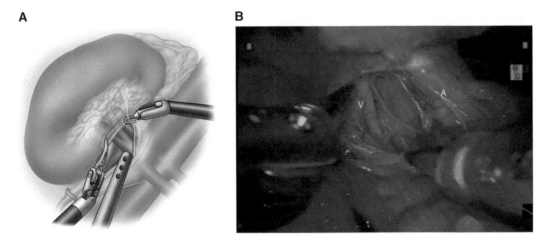

B

Fig. 10.6 Dissection of the renal hilum. (**a**) The renal hilum is carefully dissected by creating small windows within the perihilar tissues parallel to the direction of the renal vessels (right kidney shown). These perihilar tissues can be divided using hook electrocautery (Copyright 2009 Li-Ming Su, M.D., University of Florida). (**b**) Dissection of the left renal hilum. *V* renal vein, *A* renal artery

A

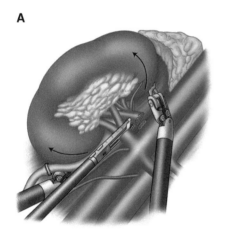

B

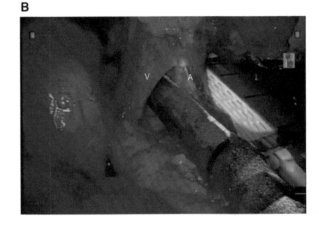

Fig. 10.7 Ligation of the renal hilum. (**a**) The hilum may be further exposed by first dissecting the adrenal gland off of the upper pole of the kidney (right kidney shown). Anterolateral retraction of the kidney applies gentle stretch to the renal artery and vein which facilitates stapling and division of the renal vessels using a laparoscopic linear stapler (Copyright 2009 Li-Ming Su, M.D., University of Florida). (**b**) Ligation of the left renal hilar vessels. *V* renal vein, *A* renal artery

(Fig. 10.7b). It is important to avoid placing the stapler across clips, which can result in misfiring of the stapler and unwanted bleeding. The renal vein is then similarly ligated with the stapler while visualizing the tip of the stapler with respect to the great vessels in order to prevent inadvertent injury to the abdominal aorta or inferior vena cava.

Step 5: Dissection of Adrenal Gland and Posterolateral Renal Attachments

After division of the renal vasculature, the remaining superior attachments of the kidney are divided. Typically, an adrenal sparing approach is utilized unless direct adrenal extension of the tumor is radiographically or visually evident. Care must be employed during dissection of the adrenal gland as its complex arterial blood supply and short adrenal vein, particularly on the right side, may be a source of bleeding. Dissection is carried down to the upper pole parenchyma. This plane of dissection is followed superiorly and posteriorly around the upper pole until the retroperitoneum is reached. Dissection is then carried out between the upper pole of the kidney and perirenal fat which encompasses the adrenal gland. The LigaSure Atlas™ device is a robust hemostatic device and can be used by the assistant to facilitate separation of the adrenal gland from the upper pole of the kidney. Biosealants such as Floseal™ (Baxter, IL) or hemostatic Surgicel™ gauze (Ethicon, NC) are generally not required but may be applied to the adrenal bed if there is any concern for residual minor venous bleeding. The lateral attachments of the kidney are divided and released using the LigaSure Atlas™ in combination with blunt dissection, freeing the kidney and its surrounding perirenal fat completely from their attachments. The renal bed is inspected carefully for bleeding under low insufflation pressure (i.e., <10 mmHg) and meticulous hemostasis is achieved. The kidney specimen is left in the upper abdomen until final extraction of the specimen. Dissection of the ureter is carried out as distally as possible into the true pelvis prior to re-docking the robotic cart to facilitate the subsequent steps of ureteral dissection.

Step 6: Regional Perihilar Lymphadenectomy

Robot-assisted regional perihilar lymphadenectomy can be performed during RARNU especially in patients who present with high-grade disease and/or radiographic evidence of pathologic lymph node enlargement (Fig. 10.8). The lymph node dissection is carried out primarily by blunt dissection with limited electrocautery to minimize the risk of vascular injury. The proximal and distal extents of the lymph node packets are secured with hemoclips to minimize lymphatic leak and postoperative lymphocele.

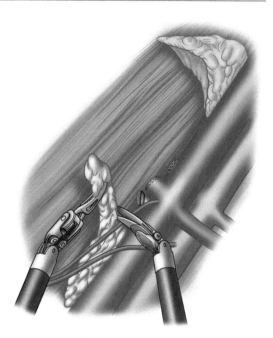

Fig. 10.8 Right regional perihilar lymphadenectomy (Copyright 2009 Li-Ming Su, M.D., University of Florida)

Step 7: Dissection of Distal Ureter and Bladder Cuff (Table 10.3)

The robotic instruments are removed and the arms undocked from the trocars. The robotic cart is then repositioned as previously described for the two-docking RARNU at a 45° angle from the foot of the table. The robot is then re-docked using the revised trocar configuration with an 8 mm trocar placed through the 15 mm outer cannula of the Hybrid Cannula Trocar for the left robotic arm as mentioned previously. Although the 0° lens is generally sufficient to perform the distal ureterectomy and bladder cuff dissection, a 30° down lens may be required in some patients if visualization is limited. The ureter is dissected free from the retroperitoneum and iliac vessels (Fig. 10.9). Access to the distal ureter is enhanced by dividing the vas deferens in the male patient and the suspensory/broad ligaments and round ligament of the uterus in the female patient. The ipsilateral medial umbilical ligament is also divided to allow the bladder to be mobilized medially. If needed, the superior vesical artery may be sacrificed to fully mobilize the lateral portion of the bladder for optimal exposure to the ureterovesical junction. The peritoneal layer covering the bladder and the distal ureter is then incised to reveal the splaying mucosal and muscle fibers of the bladder

Table 10.3 Dissection of distal ureter and bladder cuff: surgeon and assistant instrumentation

Surgeon instrumentation		Assistant instrumentation
Right arm	**Left arm**	• Suction-irrigator
• Curved monopolar scissors	• Maryland bipolar forceps	• 10 mm LigaSure Atlas™ device
• Monopolar hook		
Endoscope lens: 0° or 30° down		

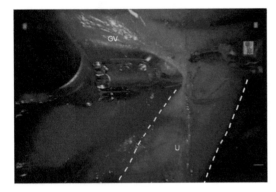

Fig. 10.9 Left ureteral dissection. *GV* gonadal vein, *U* ureter (course of ureter highlighted by *dashed line*)

wall as the ureter enters the bladder at the ureterovesical junction (Fig. 10.10a, b).

Step 8: Excision of Bladder Cuff

The authors have employed the use of intravesical mitomycin C (40 mg in 40 mL saline) instilled for 45–60 min prior to excision of the bladder cuff. This is administered at the beginning of the ureteral dissection. An extravesical approach is used to excise the bladder cuff. Complete evacuation of the bladder of urine and instilled mitomycin C through the urethral catheter is performed with 200–300 mL saline rinse following drainage. Evacuation of all fluid from the bladder is verified prior to opening the bladder at the ureterovesical junction to minimize the risk of urine spillage and potential tumor seeding. The bladder is retracted medially by the assistant using the suction-irrigator device and the monopolar scissors or hook are used to incise the detrusor muscle creating an approximately 2 cm margin around the junction of the ureter and bladder (Fig. 10.11a, b). Once the bladder is entered, the ipsilateral ureteral orifice is visually identified and circumscribed taking care to avoid thermal injury to the contralateral ureteral orifice. Once the bladder cuff is completely freed,

A

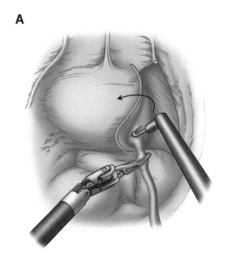

B

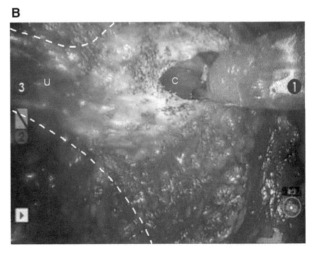

Fig. 10.10 Dissection of the bladder cuff. (**a**) After the bladder is mobilized and retracted medially, the peritoneal layer covering the bladder and the distal ureter (right ureter shown) is incised to reveal the splaying mucosal and muscle fibers of the bladder wall as the ureter enters the bladder at the ureterovesical junction (Copyright 2009 Li-Ming Su, M.D., University of Florida). (**b**) Dissection of bladder cuff during left RARNU. *U* ureter (splaying of the bladder fibers at the ureterovesical junction highlighted by *dashed line*), *C* cystotomy

A

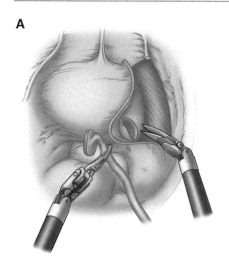

B

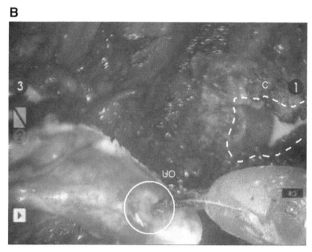

Fig. 10.11 (**a**) Excision of bladder cuff with medial retraction of the bladder, the detrusor muscle is incised creating a 2 cm margin around the junction of the ureter and bladder (right ureter shown). The ipsilateral ureteral orifice is identified and circumscribed with care to avoid thermal injury to the contralateral ureteral orifice (Copyright 2009 Li-Ming Su, M.D., University of Florida). (**b**) After excision of the left ureter and bladder cuff, the ureteral orifice is inspected. *UO* ureteral orifice, *C* cystotomy (highlighted by *dashed line*)

an additional Hem-o-lok® clip may be placed across the distal ureter to prevent tumor spillage. The specimen is then entrapped and stored in the upper quadrants of the abdomen away from the surgical field.

Step 9: Closure of Cystotomy (Table 10.4)

The bladder is then closed in two separate layers using 3-0 polyglactin on a SH needle on the mucosal layer and 2-0 polyglactin suture on an UR-6 needle on the detrusor layer (Fig. 10.12a, b). After closure of the bladder is completed, the integrity of the closure is tested by the circulating nurse by filling the bladder via the urethral catheter with approximately 100–200 mL of saline. The ureterectomy bed is inspected for bleeding under low insufflation pressure (i.e., <10 mmHg).

Step 10: Regional Pelvic Lymphadenectomy (Table 10.5)

Regional pelvic lymphadenectomy, when indicated, can be performed adhering to the standard landmarks used during pelvic lymphadenectomy

Table 10.4 Closure of cystotomy: surgeon and assistant instrumentation

Surgeon instrumentation		Assistant instrumentation
Right arm	**Left arm**	• Suction-irrigator
• Needle driver	• Needle driver	• Laparoscopic scissors
Endoscope lens: 0° or 30° down lens		• Laparoscopic needle driver

for prostate cancer (Fig. 10.13). The proximal and distal extents of the lymph node packets are secured with hemoclips to minimize lymphatic leak and postoperative lymphocele.

Step 11: Entrapment and Delivery of Specimens and Exiting the Abdomen

The 8/15 mm convertible Hybrid Cannula Trocar is removed and closed using a Carter–Thomason fascial closure device. The entrapped lymph node packets and surgical specimen are then delivered via extension of the incision through either a low midline or Pfannenstiel's incision (Fig. 10.14a, b). The 8 mm and 5 mm trocars do not require facial closure but are closed subcutaneously. The 12 mm trocar sites generally do not require fascial closure

A

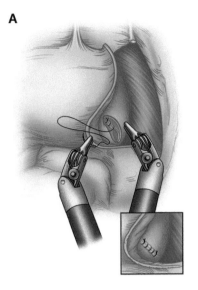

B

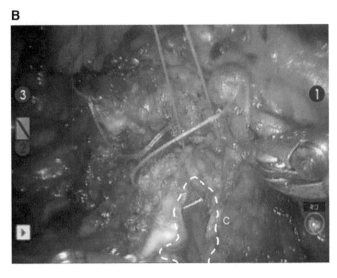

Fig. 10.12 Closure of cystotomy. (**a**) A two-layer repair of a right cystotomy is shown with closure of the mucosal and detrusor (see *inset*) layers (Copyright 2009 Li-Ming Su, M.D., University of Florida). (**b**) Closure of left cystotomy. *C* cystotomy (highlighted by *dashed line*)

Table 10.5 Regional pelvic lymphadenectomy: surgeon and assistant instrumentation

Surgeon instrumentation		Assistant instrumentation
Right arm	**Left arm**	• Suction-irrigator
• Curved monopolar scissors	• Maryland bipolar forceps	• Hem-o-lok® clip applier
Endoscope lens: 0° or 30° lens		

if a non-bladed, self-dilating trocar is used. A closed suction Hemovac or Jackson Pratt pelvic drain is left at the end of the operation exiting through the right robotic arm 8 mm trocar site.

Postoperative Management

Intravenous narcotics are provided for postoperative pain overnight and then switched to oral narcotics on postoperative day 1. Patients are provided clear liquids on postoperative day 1 and advanced to a regular diet as tolerated. Hospital stay is on average 2 days. The pelvic drain is removed prior to discharge if outputs are low (<100 mL/day). The urethral catheter is kept in place for 7–10 days prior to removal at a follow-

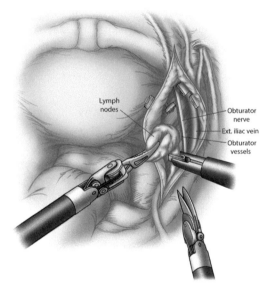

Fig. 10.13 Right ipsilateral, regional pelvic lymphadenectomy (Copyright 2009 Li-Ming Su, M.D., University of Florida)

up clinic appointment with a voiding trial. A cystogram is not generally required but may be performed in patients where a urine leak is suspected based upon intraoperative findings or high postoperative drain output.

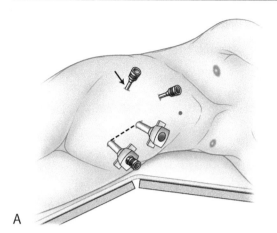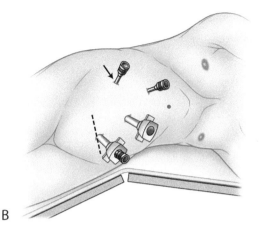

A   B

Fig. 10.14 Specimen extraction. (**a**) Specimen extraction with an infraumbilical incision (Copyright 2009 Li-Ming Su, M.D., University of Florida). (**b**) Specimen extraction with a Pfannenstiel's incision (Copyright 2009 Li-Ming Su, M.D., University of Florida). For both techniques, the *arrow* depicts the port site used to place a pelvic drain at the end of the procedure

Special Considerations

When performing RARNU in a female patient, great care must be taken during dissection of the distal ureter and bladder cuff as these structures are in close proximity to the vagina. A sponge on a stick can be introduced by the assistant into the vagina to delineate its borders during distal ureterectomy and bladder cuff excision to avoid inadvertent entry into the vagina. In order to fully expose the distal ureter in a female patient, the round, infundibulopelvic, and portions of the broad ligament must be divided.

In select patients with a solitary distal ureteral tumor, distal ureterectomy and ureteral reimplantation with or without psoas hitch reconstruction can be considered. These patients should be counseled on the relatively higher risk of ipsilateral tumor recurrence and the need for vigilant endoscopic and radiographic surveillance. Such cases are performed in the lithotomy position similar to a robotic prostatectomy, using a standard trocar configuration as described in the prostatectomy chapters. The affected segment of ureter is isolated between hemoclips and excised including the ipsilateral ureterovesical junction. A biopsy of the proximal ureteral stump margin is sent for frozen section analysis and the ureter is reimplanted into the bladder if adequate length is available. Insufficient ureteral length necessitates a psoas hitch and/or Boari flap. For this, the entire bladder is mobilized by dividing both medial umbilical ligaments and entering into the space of Retzius. The contralateral bladder pedicle is divided allowing the bladder to be pexed to the ipsilateral psoas tendon using two interrupted 2-0 prolene sutures. The ureter is then reimplanted in a refluxing, tension-free manner into the dome of the bladder after spatulation of the ureter using interrupted 4-0 polyglactin sutures. A double pigtail ureteral stent is introduced through the assistant trocar and with the assistance of a guide wire introduced in a retrograde fashion into the proximal ureter and renal pelvis and distally into the bladder prior to completion of the anastomosis. The ureteral stent is kept in place for 4 weeks and the urethral catheter is maintained for 7–10 days postoperatively.

Steps to Avoid Complications

RARNU is a procedure associated with minimal morbidity as long as appropriate anatomic landmarks are identified and precise, careful surgical technique is employed. The use of a laparoscopically trained and skilled bedside assistant is critical to the success of this operation. Judicious use of electrocautery is critically important to prevent a vascular or enteral injury.

It is important to note that the 8/15 mm convertible Hybrid Cannula Trocar used during the ureterectomy portion of the RARNU is specifically designed to minimize the risk of complications arising from capacitive coupling. Capacitive coupling is defined as transfer of current from the source of the active electrode (i.e., monopolar scissors) through intact insulation into adjacent tissues without direct contact and may occur with the use of other hybrid ports that incorporate both metal and plastic components [11]. For example, if a hybrid port is created with a metal trocar placed within an outer plastic conventional trocar, electric current transferred to the metal trocar could not dissipate into the abdominal wall because of the outer plastic sleeve, which acts as an insulator. Instead, capacitive coupling could occur with transfer of current from the metal trocar into adjacent tissues, such as bowel, resulting in unintended injury. The 8/15 mm convertible Hybrid Cannula Trocar has been specifically designed to minimize such complications and its use is strongly advised when performing RARNU.

As previously mentioned, transection of the renal vessels is most easily accomplished using a vascular laparoscopic linear stapler. However, great care must be taken to ensure that the stapler is appropriately placed, avoiding any hemoclips in close proximity that may result in misfiring of the stapler. This can lead to failure of the stapler and partial transection of the renal vessel. The bedside assistant should have a laparoscopic hemoclip immediately available following firing and removal of the laparoscopic linear stapler in case of bleeding at the vessel stump.

At least 11 trocar site metastases have been reported in which either no endobag was used for specimen retrieval, or the bag was torn [12]. While rare, the consequences of this complication are serious and necessitate careful manipulation of the surgical specimen to prevent spillage during handling and extraction. We recommend early entrapment of the specimen during the case. While long-term follow-up is limited, there are no reported cases to date of trocar site recurrences after RARNU. In addition, the authors utilize perioperative intravesical mitomycin C instillation (as described in "Step 8") in efforts to reduce local recurrence of tumor as supported by the bladder cancer literature.

To avoid postoperative lymphocele, during regional lymphadenectomy hemoclips should be used to secure the pedicles to all lymph nodes removed as electrocautery and thermal devices may be inferior to hemoclips in sealing lymphatic vessels.

References

1. Muntener M, Nielsen ME, Romero FR, Schaeffer EM, Allaf ME, Brito FA, Pavlovich CP, Kavoussi LR, Jarrett TW. Long-term oncologic outcome after laparoscopic radical nephroureterectomy for upper tract transitional cell carcinoma. Eur Urol. 2007;51:1639–44.
2. Capitanio U, Shariat SF, Isbarn H, Weizer A, Remzi M, Roscigno M, Kikuchi E, Raman JD, Bolenz C, Bensalah K, Koppie TM, Kassouf W, Fernandez MI, Strobel P, Wheat J, Zigeuner R, Langner C, Waldert M, Oya M, Guo CC, Ng C, Montorsi F, Wood CG, Margulis V, Karakiewicz PI. Comparison of oncologic outcomes for open and laparoscopic nephroureterectomy: a multi-institutional analysis of 1249 cases. Eur Urol. 2009;56(1):1–9.
3. Bariol SV, Stewart GD, McNeill SA, Tolley DA. Oncological control following laparoscopic nephroureterectomy: 7-year outcome. J Urol. 2004;172(5):1805–8.
4. Berger A, Haber GP, Kamoi K, Aron M, Desai MM, Kauok JH, Gill IS. Laparoscopic radical nephroureterectomy for upper tract transitional cell carcinoma: oncological outcomes at 7 years. J Urol. 2008;180(3):849–54.
5. Park SY, Jeong W, Ham WS, Kim WT, Tha KH. Initial experience of robotic nephroureterectomy: a hybrid-port technique. BJU Int. 2009;104(11):1718–21.
6. Park SY, Jeong W, Choi YD, Chung BH, Hong SJ, Rha KH. Yonsei experience in robotic urologic surgery-application in various urological procedures. Yonsei Med J. 2008;49(6):897–900.
7. Eun D, Bhandari A, Boris R, Rogers C, Bhandari M, Menon M. Concurrent upper and lower urinary tract robotic surgery: strategies for success. BJU Int. 2007;100(5):1121–5.
8. Rose K, Khan S, Godbole H, Olsburgh J, Dasgupta P. Robotic assisted retroperitoneoscopic nephroureterectomy—first experience and the hybrid port technique. Int J Clin Pract. 2006;60(1):12–4.
9. Margulis V, Shariat SF, Matin SF, Kamat AM, Zigeuner R, Kikuchi E, Lotan Y, Weizer A, Raman JD, Wood CG. Outcomes of radical nephroureterectomy: a series from the Upper Tract Urothelial Carcinoma Collaboration. Cancer. 2009;115(6):1224–33.
10. Pugh J, Parekattil S, Willis D, Stifelman M, Hemal A, Su LM. Perioperative outcomes of robot-assisted nephroureterectomy for upper urinary tract urothelial carcinoma: a multi-institutional series. BJU Int. 2013;112(4):E295–300.
11. Wu MP, Ou CS, Chen SL, Yen EY, Rowbothom R. Complications and recommended practices for electrosurgery in laparoscopy. Am J Surg. 2000;179:67–73.
12. Zigeuner P, Pummer K. Urothelial carcinoma of the upper urinary tract: surgical approach and prognostic factors. Eur Urol. 2008;53:720–31.

Robot-Assisted Pyeloplasty

Raymond J. Leveillee and Kenan Ashouri

Introduction

Robotic pyeloplasty was first described in 2002 by Gettman et al. using the dismembered Anderson-Hynes technique [1]. Since this initial study, decreased learning curve, decreased suturing time, and improved visualization have been identified as advantages of robotic pyeloplasty over laparoscopic pyeloplasty; however, cost-effectiveness, loss of tactile feedback, limited significant improvement of peri-operative course are important considerations when weighing the two options [2, 3]. Since its origin, robotic pyeloplasty has been proven to be a safe and effective alternative to open pyeloplasty [4, 5].

Patient Selection

Patients typically present with symptomatic hydronephrosis. This may include renal colic exacerbated by fluids, pyelonephritis, or hypertension. Reconstruction is offered after an assessment of the anatomy (intravenous pyelogram, CT, or MR urography) as well as a functional assessment of the split renal function and cortical washout $t_{1/2}$ as noted on diuretic nuclear renal scan (radiolabeled mercaptoacetyl glycine — MAG-3).

In patients with ureteropelvic junction obstruction (UPJO), imaging is essential to evaluate for presence of crossing vessels and to define the extent of hydroureter or hydronephrosis in relation to the renal hilar anatomy (Fig. 11.1a, b). Patients are assessed for their overall renal function, the presence of renal calculi, the level of insertion of the UPJ, the extent of pelvicaliceal dilatation, or the presence of an extrarenal or intrarenal pelvis. Various anatomic presentations may be treated with robotic pyeloplasty, such as high ureteral insertions, redundant renal pelvis, or crossing vessels. The renal scan then provides a practical means for evaluating the relative success of the surgery in the postoperative setting. Any progressive decline in renal function or recurrence of obstruction associated with the ipsilateral renal unit will be noted with sequential follow-up renal scans (Table 11.1).

Preoperative Preparation

We do not routinely utilize a bowel preparation for our patients undergoing pyeloplasty. A clear liquid diet the day prior to surgery is advised. Important consideration for the patient to be aware of is that

Electronic supplementary material: The online version of this chapter (doi:10.1007/978-3-319-45060-5_11) contains supplementary material, which is available to authorized users.

R.J. Leveillee, M.D., F.R.C.S.-G. (✉) • K. Ashouri, M.S.
Department of Urology, Bethesda Hospital,
2800 S. Seacrest Blvd, Ste 140, Boynton Beach,
FL 33435, USA
e-mail: rjleveilleemd@gmail.com

L.-M. Su (ed.), *Atlas of Robotic Urologic Surgery*, DOI 10.1007/978-3-319-45060-5_11

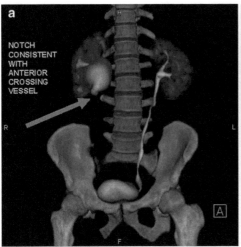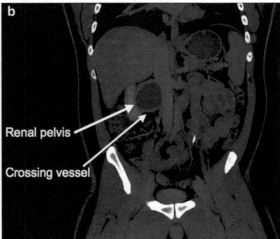

Fig. 11.1 (a) Three-dimensional reconstruction of patient with right UPJO. Note acute termination of proximal ureter with typical "notch," seen when there is pres- ence of anterior crossing vessel. (b) Abdominal CT scan. Note the area of severe hydronephrosis at the renal pelvis and the presence of anterior crossing vessel

the goal of the surgery is to improve the drainage of the affected kidney to preserve/improve renal function as well as avoid renal colic. It may be required in some instances to convert to an open operation. Blood transfusions, devascularization of the lower pole of the kidney, bowel injury, and prolonged urine leaks are extremely rare events. The informed consent should focus primarily on possible stenosis or obstruction after the surgery has been completed but may include comments outlined above.

Operative Setup

At our institution we currently utilize the da Vinci® Xi Surgical System (Intuitive Surgical, Inc., Sunnyvale, CA). The steps described in this chapter were originally developed for the "standard" DaVinci robot, and were modified over the past decade as "DaVinci S' and "Si" models were introduced. Although four robotic arms are available, robotic pyeloplasty is generally and preferably performed using a three-armed technique by the authors. Only one surgical assistant is required in addition to a scrub technician, both of whom stand on the abdominal side of the patient. All accessory instrument exchanges, suction, needle passages are performed by the bedside assistant

utilizing the 8 mm robotic trocar thus eliminating the need for a designated "assistant trocar". Since the point of attack is typically at the lower third of the renal operative field, a "retractor" placed via the assistant trocar is rarely required, even on the right side where the liver can sometimes be overhanging. If, however, the surgeon and patient will benefit from the placement of a fourth and fifth trocar, one should not hesitate to place them in the appropriate locations. The vision cart is positioned so that it is easily seen by both the assistant and scrub technician. The patient-side robotic cart is positioned over the patient's ipsilateral shoulder for the "S" and "Si" models, and directly parallel to the spine when utilizing the "Xi". The final operating room setup is as shown in Fig. 11.2.

Patient Positioning and Preparation

Our technique with robotic pyeloplasty has been previously described and has been modified slightly over the years [6]. After cystoscopy and retrograde pyelography with ureteral stent placement in the lithotomy position (see below) the patient is moved to the operating table. This can be accomplished in the same room with the addition of C-Arm fluoroscopy. Conversely, this can

Table 11.1 Robotic pyeloplasty in literature

Author	Number of patients	Type of repair	Operative time (min)	Anastomosis time (min)	Success (%)	Complication rate (%)	Follow-up (months)	Stay (days)
Mendez et al. [7]	32	Dismembered (31), Fenger (1)	300	n/a	100	3.1	10.3	1.1
Weise et al. [9]	31	Dismembered	271	76	97	6.4	10	n/a
Gettman et al. [1, 10]	9	Dismembered	139	62.4	100	11.1	4.1	4.7
Siddiq et al. [6]	26	Dismembered (23), YV (3)	245	n/a	95	13	6	2
Palese et al. [13]	35	Dismembered	217	63	94	5.6	7.9	2.7
Bentas et al. [14]	11	Dismembered	197	n/a	100	0	21	5.5
Palese et al. [15]	38	Dismembered	226	64.2	94.7	10.5	12.2	2.8
Patel et al. [16]	50	Dismembered	122	20	100	2	11.7	1.1
Mufarrij et al. [17]	140	Dismembered	210	n/a	93	8	26.4	2.5
Schwentner et al. [18]	92	Dismembered	108	24.8	96.7	0	39.1	4.57
Gupta et al. [19]	85	Dismembered (82), YV (3), Fengers (1)	121	47	96.5	9.3	13.6	2.5
Sivaraman et al.	168	Dismembered (161), YV (7)	134.9	n/a	97.6	6.6	n/a	1.48
Moreno-Sierra et al. [20]	11	Dismembered	189.4	n/a	100	9	n/a	4.18
Minnillo et al. [21]	155	Dismembered (153), YV (2)	198.5	54	96.8	11	31.7	1.95
Etafy et al. [22]	57	Dismembered	335	n/a	81	12.2	18	2
Bird et al. [2]	98	Dismembered (88), YV (9)	n/a	48	93.4	5.1	n/a	2.5

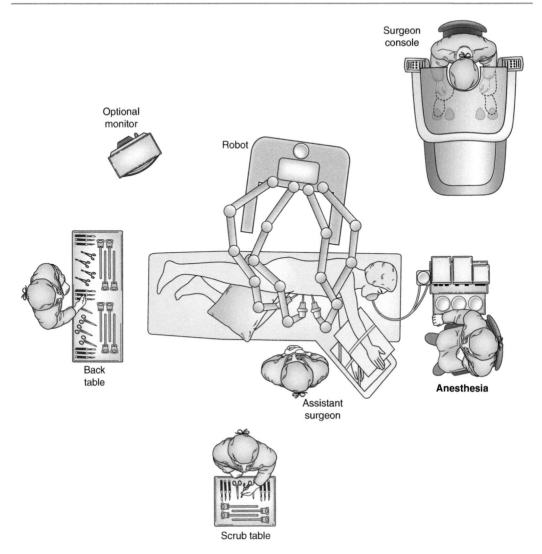

Fig. 11.2 Typical operating room setup for robotic pyeloplasty. The scrub nurse and surgical assistant positions can be interchanged

be done in a standard cystoscopy suite with transfer via gurney to a robotic suite and placed in a supine position on the operating table. Pneumatic compression stockings, urethral catheter, and an orogastric tube are routinely employed. Next, patients are positioned in a modified flank position with a 30° tilt and are held in place with a conformable vacuum "Bean-Bag" (Olympia, Seattle, Washington). It is not generally necessary to "flex the table" to increase space. A sub-axillary roll (gel or 1 L IV bag wrapped in a towel) is employed to prevent brachial plexus injury. The ipsilateral ("up") arm is supported in an Amsco "Krause" arm support that is placed above the chest to allow the arms of the robot sufficient space to maneuver [S; Si]. Alternatively when utilizing the Xi, the ipsilateral arm can be secured along side the patient in a "Marching Soldier" position. The contralateral ("down") arm must lie low and angled slightly cephalad enough to allow for the midline robotic trocar and working element to be positioned without interference (Fig. 11.3a, b). The patient is secured at the arms, chest, hips, and legs with crosstable 3 in. silk tape and Velcro straps (Fig. 11.3b). Finally, the bed is rotated on its

a

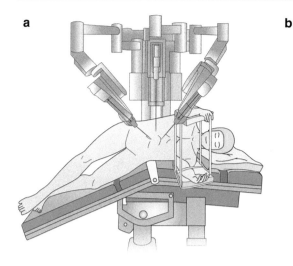

b

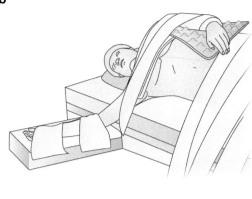

Fig. 11.3 (**a**) Patient positioning for right-sided robotic pyeloplasty, note that flexion of the table is generally not necessary. (**b**) Photo illustrating a patient "Marching Soldier" positioning for left-sided pyeloplasty as used with the Da Vinci Xi system

central axis both clockwise and counterclockwise prior to draping to ensure that the patient is adequately secured to the table.

Trocar Configuration for Da Vinci S and Si Systems

For the majority of patients, a 12 mm camera trocar is placed at the inferior crease of the umbilicus (Fig. 11.4). This allows for wide field of view and is cosmetically appealing. For those with obese or redundant abdominal wall, the initial trocars can be moved laterally at the edge of the rectus muscle. Insertion of the secondary trocars is performed only after careful inspection of the abdomen for the presence of adhesions. One of the 8 mm working arm trocars is placed 8–10 cm superior to the camera trocar in the midline and the second is placed 8–10 cm lateral with a 10° inferior angle from the umbilicus (Fig. 11.5a). A 5 mm assistant trocar can be placed midway and slightly lower than the umbilical and subxyphoid 8 mm robotic trocar. The final trocar configuration for a three armed robotic technique is as shown in Fig. 11.5a. When using the fourth robotic arm, an additional 8 mm robotic trocar is inserted low in the ipsilateral iliac fossa.

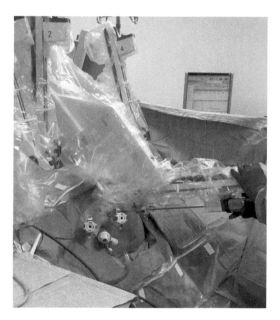

Fig. 11.4 With the Da Vinci S and Si, a 12 mm camera port was required. However, with the Da Vinci Xi any of the 8 mm ports can be used

Trocar Configuration for Da Vinci Xi System

It should be noted that with the Da Vinci Xi system the patient is placed in the "Marching Soldier" position with the ipsilateral arm flexed at the

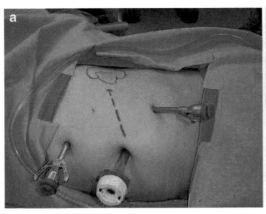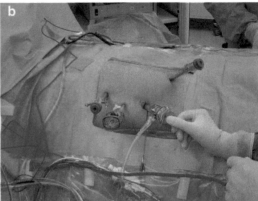

Fig. 11.5 (**a**) Trocar arrangement for left robotic pyeloplasty utilizing three trocars. (**b**) Trocar arrangement for left robotic pyeloplasty with additional 5 mm assistant trocar as utilized with the Da Vinci S or Si

patient's side and the contralateral arm outstretched across an operating table arm board with the operating table flat or slightly flexed as shown in Fig. 11.3b. Trocars can then be placed in a linear fashion as instrumental interference is much less common with the Xi due to improved ergonomics. Conversely, triangulation can be used to try to optimize cosmesis (surgeon preference).

Instrumentation and Equipment List

Equipment

- da Vinci® Xi (four-arm system)
- EndoWrist® Maryland bipolar forceps (Intuitive Surgical, Inc., Sunnyvale, CA)
- EndoWrist® curved monopolar scissors (Intuitive Surgical, Inc., Sunnyvale, CA)
- EndoWrist® Potts scissors (Intuitive Surgical, Inc., Sunnyvale, CA) (optional)
- EndoWrist® ProGrasp™ forceps (optional if using a fourth robotic arm; Intuitive Surgical, Inc., Sunnyvale, CA)
- EndoWrist® needle driver (1) (Intuitive Surgical, Inc., Sunnyvale, CA)
- EndoWrist® suture cut needle driver (1) (Intuitive Surgical, Inc., Sunnyvale, CA)
- InSite® Vision System with 30° lens (Intuitive Surgical, Inc., Sunnyvale, CA)

Trocars for S:Si

- 12-mm Trocar (1)
- 8-mm Robotic trocars (2 alternatively 3 if needing assistant or using a four-armed technique)
- 5-mm Trocar (1) (optional)

Trocars for Xi

- 8-mm Robotic trocars (3 alternatively 4 if using a four-armed technique)
- 5-mm trocar (1) (optional)

Recommended Sutures

- 3-0 Polyglactin suture on RB-1 needle cut to 6–8 in. for the ureteropelvic anastomosis
- 0 Polyglactin suture for closure of the fascia
- 4-0 Monocryl suture for skin closure

Instruments Used by the Surgical Assistant

- Laparoscopic needle driver (5 mm)
- Laparoscopic scissors (5 mm)
- Blunt tip grasper
- Suction irrigator device
- #19 Round, fluted Blake closed suction drain (Ethicon, Somerville, NJ)

Robotic Pyeloplasty: Step-by-Step Technique (see Video 11.1)

Basic Principles

Many of the preoperative steps are common to all robotic ureteral surgery procedures.

1. Preoperative urine culture with culture-specific antibiotics given.
2. Appropriate anatomic definition to determine the treatment options before incision. Judicious use of retrograde pyelography is to be encouraged.
3. Delicate handling of the ureter with minimal use of diathermy.
4. Sufficient mobilization without devascularization of the ureter, any associated vasculature, renal pelvis and the kidney before transection of the UPJ.
5. Clamping of the urethral catheter and forced diuresis can be a useful technique which may aid in hydrodistention (i.e., hydronephrosis) and identification of the Ureteropelvic junction obstruction (UPJO).
6. Spatulation of the ureter and fashioning a wide anastomosis to prevent restenosis.
7. Tension-free anastomosis with use of absorbable material (can be interrupted—our preference—or running) (2).

Step 1: Cystoscopy, Retrograde Pyelogram and Ureteral Stent Placement

A retrograde pyelogram is helpful in evaluating the ureter and delineating the length of obstruction if not seen on other preoperative imaging. Performing both a retrograde pyelogram and preoperative internal double pigtail ureteral stent placement/replacement can be done immediately prior to pyeloplasty to simplify strategic evaluation (Fig. 11.6). At our facility, the preoperative retrograde pyelogram is performed in an adjoining cystoscopy room, but a portable C-arm can be substituted. The ureteral stent placement is performed in the same room as the pyeloplasty. A 6 Fr stent approximately 2 cm

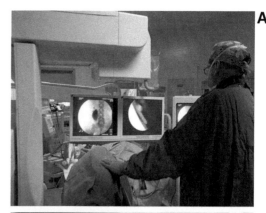

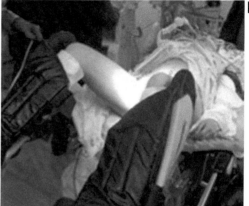

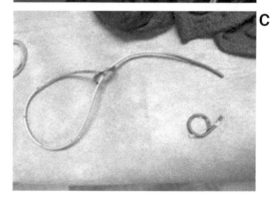

Fig. 11.6 Prior to performance of robotic pyeloplasty, a cystoscopy and retrograde pyelogram with placement of double pig-tail stent is performed. This is usually done on the same day under the same anesthesia. (**a**) Retrograde pyelogram. (**b**) Lithotomy position for retrograde pyelogram. (**c**) It is important to replace old stents that have accumulated biofilm or calcifications

longer than what is usual for the patient's body habitus is chosen to prevent displacement or migration during laparoscopic manipulation of the stent. It should be noted that some authors choose to place the stent in an antegrade fashion after the pyelotomy and ureteral spatulation has been performed.

Step 2: Repositioning and Abdominal Access

Following completion of ureteral stent placement, the patient is repositioned in the modified decubitus position as previously mentioned and reprepped and draped. The abdomen is insufflated to approximately 15 mm using a Veress needle placed at the umbilicus or in the ipsilateral upper quadrant (Fig. 11.7). Alternatively, an open Hasson trocar

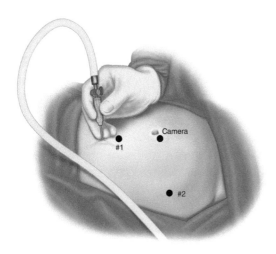

Fig. 11.7 The abdomen is insufflated using a Veress needle or open exposure at the umbilicus or in the ipsilateral upper quadrant. Picture recreates the procedure on the right side

placement can be utilized if the use of a more blunt instrument is preferred. Trocars are then placed as described previously. The operating table is rotated maximally toward the assistant to allow the intestines to migrate medially and provide exposure of the ipsilateral kidney.

Step 3: Docking the Patient-Side Robotic Cart

The patient-side cart is then brought over the patient's ipsilateral shoulder at an approximately 45° angle with the operating room table, entering from the head of the bed (Fig. 11.8a). Following docking of the camera arm to the umbilical trocar, the two robotic arms are docked to their respective trocars, taking great care so as to optimize range of motion while at the same time avoid direct collision with the camera arm as well as the patient's ipsilateral arm and hip (Fig. 11.8b).

Step 4: Mobilization of the Ipsilateral Colon and Small Intestines (Table 11.2)

In general, a 30° down lens is used to perform robotic pyeloplasty; however, in some cases a 0° lens may suffice depending on the patient's body habitus. Monopolar and bipolar electrocautery settings are 30 W. Insufflation pressure is maintained at 15 mmHg throughout the operation.

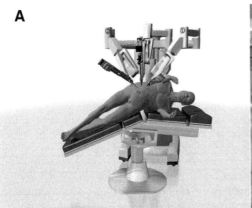

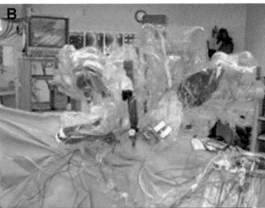

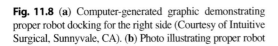

Fig. 11.8 (a) Computer-generated graphic demonstrating proper robot docking for the right side (Courtesy of Intuitive Surgical, Sunnyvale, CA). (b) Photo illustrating proper robot docking for the right kidney using the "standard" Da Vinci system

Table 11.2 Mobilization of the ipsilateral colon and small intestines: surgeon and assistant instrumentation

Surgeon instrumentation			Assistant instrumentation
Right arm	**Left arm**	**Fourth arm**	• Suction-irrigator
• Curved monopolar scissors	• Maryland bipolar grasper	• ProGrasp™ forceps (optional)	• Blunt tip grasper
Endoscope lens: 30° down			

Prior to mobilization of the colon, the renal pelvis is distended via forced diuresis (20 mg of intravenous furosemide and copious intravenous fluids) and clamping of the urethral catheter. Bowel mobilization is performed by incising the line of Toldt and reflecting the ipsilateral colon and small bowel medially. A Kocher maneuver on the right side is rarely needed and if performed is done so without the use of electrocautery. The assistant may use a blunt tip grasper to provide medial traction on the intestines for optimal exposure of the renal hilum (Fig. 11.9).

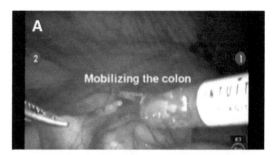

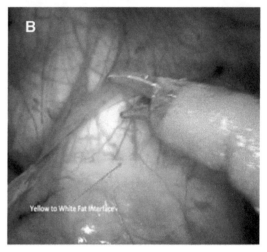

Step 5: Renal Hilar Dissection

Identification of the renal hilar vessels is useful prior to dissection of the ureter. On the right side, this involves skeletonizing the inferior vena cava and localizing the gonadal vein inferiorly and renal vein superiorly. On the left side, this involves identification of the gonadal vein and tracing it cephalad to its origin with the left renal vein. Complete skeletonization of the renal vein and artery may or may not be necessary depending on the location of the ureteropelvic junction. Great care must be taken to look specifically for the presence of a crossing lower pole artery and/or vein. Reference to preoperative cross-sectional imaging is a crucial aspect of assessing the patient's hilar anatomy so as to avoid clipping and transecting a lower pole accessory renal artery.

Fig. 11.9 (**a**) Bowel mobilization is performed, displacing the colon and duodenum medially by dividing the peritoneal attachments. Dissection of the white line of Toldt is primarily executed with cold scissors. Special caution should be used to avoid electrocautery around the duodenum. (**b**) When mobilizing bowel it is useful to identify the change in yellow fat of the bowel mesentery to white fat of the preperitoneum. Incising along the white reduces insult to the mesentery

Step 6: Identification and Dissection of the Ureteropelvic Junction

The ureter is next identified coursing deep and lateral to the ipsilateral gonadal vein (Fig. 11.10). The ureter is carefully dissected avoiding direct manipulation, electrocautery or excessive stripping of periureteral fatty tissues so as to avoid devascularization.

The dilated renal pelvis is skeletonized, and the search for a high insertion of the ureter into the renal pelvis or an anterior crossing vessel is performed (Fig. 11.11). In cases of a crossing vessel or vessels, the vessel(s) and especially the underlying compromised ureteral segment are completely skeletonized. Often adhesions are noted between the two structures. In the absence of a crossing vessel, the entire ureteropelvic junction is skeletonized and inspected for the presence of a kink or stenosis. The

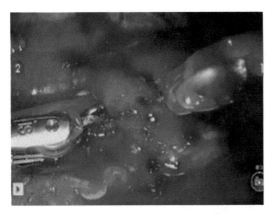

Fig. 11.10 Dissection of the ureteropelvic junction

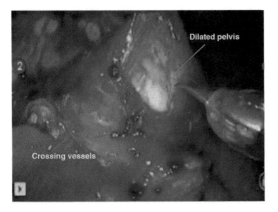

Fig. 11.11 Identification of crossing vessels and exposure of renal pelvis

decision about whether or not to perform an advancement flap (Y-V plasty) or dismembered pyeloplasty is made at this time. For a high inserting ureter, a Y-V plasty may be performed. In cases of an anterior crossing vessel, a dismembered pyeloplasty is preferred.

Step 7: Transecting the Ureteropelvic Junction

The anterior portion of the UPJ is transected horizontally using cold curved monopolar scissors in order to expose the ureteral stent, taking great care not to cut the stent itself. Electrocautery is avoided to reduce the risk of devascularization. Instead, a small amount of bleeding from the ureter and pelvis is tolerated and is typically self-limited or controlled at the time of the anastomosis. The stent is

then pulled out of the renal pelvis and transection of the ureter is completed (Fig. 11.12). The stenotic UPJ segment is excised completely and submitted for pathologic analysis. Crossing vessels are spared (in order to preserve maximal renal perfusion and function) and the ureter and pelvis transposed anterior to the vessels.

Step 8: Reduction of a Redundant Renal Pelvis and Spatulation of the Ureter (Table 11.3)

In cases of a large redundant renal pelvis, the pelvis can be reduced by excising a segment of the medial border (Fig. 11.13). Excessive excision of the renal pelvis should be avoided as this may compromise nearby infundibulum during later closure of the renal pelvis. The ureter is spatulated laterally for at least 2 cm using Potts scissors or curved monopolar scissors (Fig. 11.14). Fresh bleeding may be noted from the ureter, indicating the presence of healthy ureteral tissue. As in all pyeloplasty, it is crucial to minimize excessive handling of ureteral tissue.

Step 9: Anastomosis of the Ureter and Renal Pelvis (Table 11.4)

The anastomosis is carried out in a dependent fashion using interrupted 3-0 polyglactin sutures on RB-1 needle to form a tension-free anastomosis. We perform the suturing in an interrupted manner to allow exact reapproximation of the ureter and renal pelvis without risk of plication. The first stitch is placed outside-in at the fornix of the ureteral spatulation and inside-out at the most dependent portion of the renal pelvis and tied (Fig. 11.15a–c) and is cut 1.5 cm long to use as a retractor. This suture can be passed beneath the anastomosis to better reveal the posterior aspect of the anastomosis. The second suture is placed immediately adjacent and anterior to the first suture. We close the posterior portion of the anastomosis first as visualization of the posterior border is more difficult than the anterior portion (Fig. 11.16). Once the posterior anastomosis is completed, the proximal end of the ureteral stent is replaced into

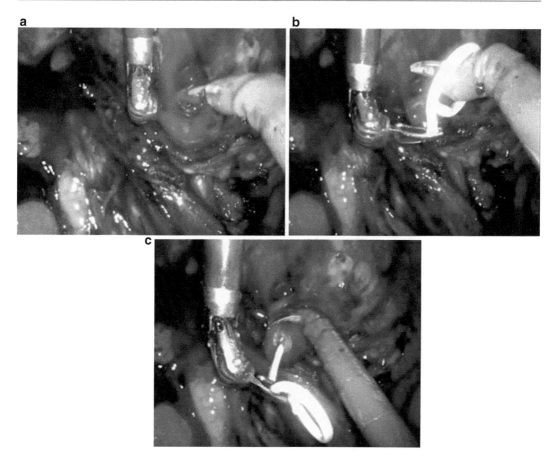

Fig. 11.12 (**a**) Transection of the anterior ureteropelvic junction. Note urine emanating from the incision in the dilated pelvis. (**b**) Exposure of the ureteral stent and removal of proximal portion of ureteral stent. (**c**) Transection of the posterior ureteropelvic junction

Table 11.3 Reduction of a redundant renal pelvis and spatulation of the ureter: surgeon and assistant instrumentation

Surgeon instrumentation			Assistant instrumentation
Right arm	**Left arm**	**Fourth arm**	• Suction-irrigator
• Curved monopolar or Potts scissors	• Maryland bipolar grasper	• ProGrasp™ forceps (optional)	• Blunt tip grasper
Endoscope lens:30° down			

the renal pelvis (Fig. 11.17). Conversely, some authors may choose to perform the ureteral transection without a preplaced stent and place a double J stent antegrade at this point. In this case, a ureteral stent and guide wire are introduced into the abdomen through a trocar and passed down through the ureteropelvic junction and into the bladder. Finally, the anterior portion of the anastomosis is completed (Fig. 11.18). Persisting large defects of the renal pelvis can be closed using a running continuous 3-0 polyglactin suture.

Step 10: Exiting the Abdomen

Prior to the completion of the operation and exiting the abdomen, it is good practice to lower the intra-abdominal pressure to 6–8 mmHg CO_2 pressure to inspect for bleeding and ensure adequate hemostasis. Reapproximation of Gerota's fascia is optional and may help to prevent periureteral fibrosis. At this stage the robot is undocked, a #19 round, fluted Blake® closed suction drain (Ethicon, Somerville, NJ) is placed

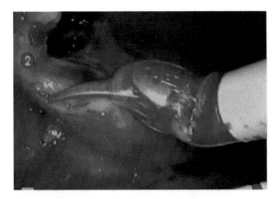

Fig. 11.13 Reduction of the dilated renal pelvis

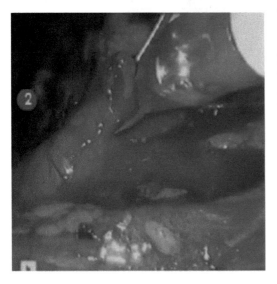

Fig. 11.14 Spatulation of the ureter

exiting the lower 8 mm robotic trocar site and the fascia of the 12 mm umbilical trocar site is closed with interrupted 0 polyglactin sutures. The skin can be reapproximated with 4-0 Monocryl and covered with Dermabond® (Ethicon, Somerville, NJ) or Steristrips®. Final healed postoperative incisions are as shown in Fig. 11.19.

Postoperative Management

Clear liquid diet is resumed the night of surgery with early ambulation. The majority of patients tolerate a regular diet the following day. The urethral catheter is usually removed on postoperative day (POD) 1, and if the drainage from the Blake

drain is <100 cm³ over the next 8 h, the patient is usually discharged home after drain removal. Oral narcotics are typically minimal, but we prescribe oxycodone or codeine for most, with a stool softener. There is no need for a postoperative antibiotic. We see most patients within a week (POD 7) and allow return to non-strenuous activities within 2–3 weeks. The double J stent is removed via office cystoscopy at week 4–6. There is no need for retrograde pyelography. Renal scintigraphy is performed at week 10–12 (approximately 6 weeks after stent removal) and again at 6 months.

Special Considerations

Robot-assisted laparoscopic pyeloplasty poses technical considerations that may differ from a traditional laparoscopic approach. Routine steps (i.e., bowel mobilization) may be more challenging with the robot. This may be due to the robot being designed for precise movements in a small field and not gross extensive movements. Additionally, without haptic feedback the surgeon is forced to rely on visual feedback [7, 8]. Smaller patients (pediatric, BMI < 25) result in the trocars being placed closer together with the potential of more instrument collisions requiring adjustments of the robot arms [1, 9, 10]. Larger patients may need the trocar positions placed more laterally to account for the additional distance that the instruments will traverse to get to the surgical field (e.g., obese pannus). Robotic surgery requires an assistant who is familiar with laparoscopy and the clarity of the surgeon's field of vision is dependent on the assistant's ability to aid with exposure [10, 11]. Secondary Ureteropelvic junction obstruction (UPJOs) (failed endopyelotomy or previous pyeloplasty) may be associated with an increased amount of retroperitoneal fibrosis and poorly vascularized tissues. In our experience, these have involved a previously unidentified anterior crossing vessel. These cases are quite demanding and the surgeon may want to consider reserving these cases until later in their experience [6, 12]. Another special consideration is the treatment of concomitant stones in the kidney during the pyeloplasty. Once a small pyelotomy is made, a flexible cysto-

Table 11.4 Anastomosis of the ureter and renal pelvis: surgeon and assistant instrumentation

Surgeon instrumentation			Assistant instrumentation
Right arm	**Left arm**	**Fourth arm**	• Suction-irrigator
Needle driver	Needle driver	ProGrasp™ forceps	• Laparoscopic scissors
Endoscope Lens: 30° down			• Laparoscopic needle driver

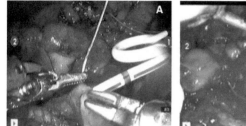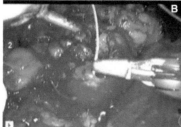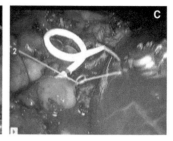

Fig. 11.15 (**a**) Placement of apical suture outside-in on the ureter. (**b**) Placement of proximal suture inside-out on the dependent most portion of the renal pelvis. (**c**) Tying the first knot and reapproximating the ureter and renal pelvis

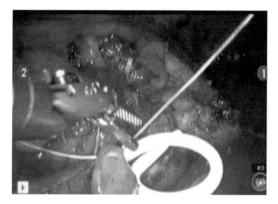

Fig. 11.16 Placement of posterior suture

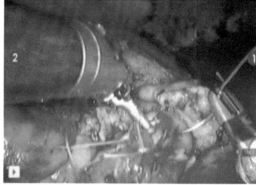

Fig. 11.18 Placement of last anastomotic stitch

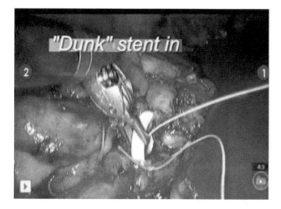

Fig. 11.17 Replacing the proximal end of the ureteral stent into the renal pelvis

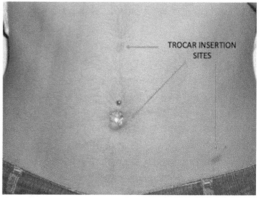

Fig. 11.19 Photo demonstrating healed postoperative incisions (three ports utilized)

scope can be inserted via an accessory trocar and intracorporeal lithotripsy and stone basketing can be performed. If the opening in the renal pelvis is too large, sufficient distention of the renal pelvis cannot occur due to continued loss of irrigant fluid resulting in poor visualization.

Special Considerations Regarding Da Vinci Xi System

At our facility, we use the Da Vinci Xi robot. Considering that many programs use the S or Si system, it is important to note the key differences in the Xi platform. The Xi platform features an overhead arm architecture that facilitates multi-quadrant operation and improved trocar placement (Fig. 11.20), improved endoscopic visualization and definition, improved ergonomics of joints and arms, and longer instrument shafts allowing improved operative reach. Because the 3D camera has been downsized to 8 mm, the angle of view can be altered by placing the camera into ANY of the robotic arms. In addition, switching from 30° up to 30° down can be achieved with the flick of a switch instead of dismount and manual rotation. Due to the fact that there are multiple trocar sizes and configurations, it is our practice utilizing the Xi to not do fascial closure with the 8mm trocar site. When utilizing the S or Si we do recommend fascial closure of the 12mm "camera" trocar site with an absorbable suture.

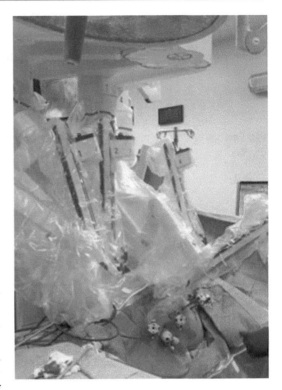

Fig. 11.20 The Da Vinci Xi system has an overhead arm base that allows for improved trocar positioning and multi-quadrant operation

nephrectomy should be considered instead of pyeloplasty if the patient is symptomatic and if clinically warranted. In addition, interrupted suture may have less potential for tying the anastomosis too tight resulting in luminal narrowing.

Steps to Avoid Complications

Proper patient selection and careful positioning are keys to successful outcomes. Sterile urine preoperatively avoids the risk of sepsis and abscess formation. To avoid bowel complications consider open Hasson trocar placement for the initial trocar, especially for patients with a history of prior abdominal surgery and adhesions. Alternatively, a 5 mm insufflating, direct vision trocar with 0° lens may be used instead of Veress needle or Hasson placement (Applied Medical, Rancho Santa Margarita, CA, USA). In patients with poor renal function (i.e., differential renal function <15%), laparoscopic

References

1. Gettman MT, Neururer R, Bartsch G, Peschel R. Anderson–Hynes dismembered pyeloplasty performed using the da Vinci robotic system. Urology. 2002;60(3):509–13.
2. Bird VG, Leveillee RJ, Eldefrawy A, Bracho J, Aziz MS. Comparison of robot-assisted versus conventional laparoscopic transperitoneal pyeloplasty for patients with ureteropelvic junction obstruction: a single-center study. Urology. 2011;77(3):730–4.
3. Riachy E, Cost NG, Defoor WR, Reddy PP, Minevich EA, Noh PH. Pediatric standard and robot-assisted laparoscopic pyeloplasty: a comparative single institution study. J Urol. 2013;189(1):283–7.
4. Autorino R, Eden C, El-Ghoneimi A, Guazzoni G, Buffi N, Peters CA, et al. Robot-assisted and laparoscopic repair of ureteropelvic junction obstruction: a

systematic review and meta-analysis. Eur Urol. 2014;65(2):430–52.

5. Ekin RG, Celik O, Ilbey YO. An up-to-date overview of minimally invasive treatment methods in ureteropelvic junction obstruction. Cent Eur J Urol. 2015;68(2):245–51.

6. Siddiq FM, Leveille RJ, Villicana P, Bird VG. Computer-assisted laparoscopic pyeloplasty: University of Miami experience with the daVinci Surgical System. J Endourol. 2005;19(3):387–92.

7. Mendez-Torres F, Woods M, Thomas R. Technical modifications for robot-assisted laparoscopic pyeloplasty. J Endourol. 2005;19(3):393–6.

8. Leveille RJ, Williams SK. Role of robotics for ureteral pelvic junction obstruction and ureteral pathology. Curr Opin Urol. 2009;19(1):81–8.

9. Weise ES, Winfield HN. Robotic computer-assisted pyeloplasty versus conventional laparoscopic pyeloplasty. J Endourol. 2006;20(10):813–9.

10. Gettman MT, Peschel R, Neururer R, Bartsch G. A comparison of laparoscopic pyeloplasty performed with the daVinci robotic system versus standard laparoscopic techniques: initial clinical results. Eur Urol. 2002;42(5):453–7; discussion 7–8.

11. Yohannes P, Bruno T, Pathan M, Baltaro R. Laparoscopic radical excision of urachal sinus. J Endourol. 2003;17(7):475–9; discussion 9.

12. Yanke BV, Lallas CD, Pagnani C, Bagley DH. Robot-assisted laparoscopic pyeloplasty: technical considerations and outcomes. J Endourol. 2008;22(6):1291–6.

13. Palese MA, Munver R, Phillips CK, Dinlenc C, Stifelman M, DelPizzo JJ. Robot-assisted laparoscopic dismembered pyeloplasty. J Soc Laparoendosc Surg. 2005;9(3):252–7.

14. Bentas W, Wolfram M, Brautigam R, Probst M, Beecken WD, Jonas D, et al. Da Vinci robot assisted Anderson–Hynes dismembered pyeloplasty: technique and 1 year follow-up. World J Urol. 2003;21(3):133–8.

15. Palese MA, Stifelman MD, Munver R, Sosa RE, Philipps CK, Dinlenc C, et al. Robot-assisted laparoscopic dismembered pyeloplasty: a combined experience. J Endourol. 2005;19(3):382–6.

16. Patel V. Robotic-assisted laparoscopic dismembered pyeloplasty. Urology. 2005;66(1):45–9.

17. Mufarrij PW, Woods M, Shah OD, Palese MA, Berger AD, Thomas R, et al. Robotic dismembered pyeloplasty: a 6-year, multi-institutional experience. J Urol. 2008;180(4):1391–6.

18. Schwentner C, Pelzer A, Neururer R, Springer B, Horninger W, Bartsch G, et al. Robotic Anderson–Hynes pyeloplasty: 5-year experience of one centre. BJU Int. 2007;100(4):880–5.

19. Gupta NP, Nayyar R, Hemal AK, Mukherjee S, Kumar R, Dogra PN. Outcome analysis of robotic pyeloplasty: a large single-centre experience. BJU Int. 2010;105(7):980–3.

20. Moreno-Sierra J, Castillon-Vela I, Ortiz-Oshiro E, Galante-Romo I, Fernandez-Perez C, Senovilla-Perez JL, et al. Robotic Anderson–Hynes dismembered pyeloplasty: initial experience. Int J Med Robot. 2013;9(2):127–33.

21. Minnillo BJ, Cruz JA, Sayao RH, Passerotti CC, Houck CS, Meier PM, et al. Long-term experience and outcomes of robotic assisted laparoscopic pyeloplasty in children and young adults. J Urol. 2011;185(4):1455–60.

22. Etafy M, Pick D, Said S, Hsueh T, Kerbl D, Mucksavage P, et al. Robotic pyeloplasty: the University of California-Irvine experience. J Urol. 2011;185(6):2196–200.

Robot-Assisted Laparoscopic Extended Pyelolithotomy and Ureterolithotomy

12

Jessica N. Lange, Mani Menon,
and Ashok K. Hemal

Robotic Pyelolithotomy

Patient Selection

Robot-assisted laparoscopic extended pyelolithotomy (REP) is a relatively new technique with an evolving role in the treatment of nephrolithiasis. This technique is ideally suited for instances when concomitant renal reconstructive procedures such as pyeloplasty and calyceal diverticulectomy are planned; however, it has also been used in the primary treatment of various renal and ureteral stones in patients with normal or complex anatomy. Patients who are appropriate medical candidates for traditional laparoscopy may also be offered robot-assisted surgery. Caution should be used in patients with previous abdominal or renal surgery including shock wave lithotripsy (SWL) as adhesions can make safe dissection problematic. This surgical technique has been used successfully in patients of all ages.

Robot-assisted laparoscopic surgical techniques have been developed for prostate, kidney, and bladder operations over the last two decades [1–5]. Recently, renal stones ranging from 1 to 7 cm in size have been safely treated with REP [6, 7]. However, true staghorn stones with secondary calculi have been associated with increased risk of open conversion, residual stone fragments, and the need for additional procedures to attain stone-free status. Therefore, we feel that REP is best suited for large renal pelvic stones, partial staghorn stones, or complete staghorn stones in hydronephrotic kidneys. The constraints on stone size and location stem from renovascular anatomy as well as lack of tactile sensation and angulation of the robotic approach. Through the use of adjunctive techniques such as intraoperative flexible nephroscopy, none of these constraints are absolute. Robotic dissection may be limited by aberrant renal vessels, and even normal renal vasculature may compromise the superior extent of renal pelvis dissection. Thus, complex upper pole stones which involve calyces at obtuse angles to the renal axis may be problematic. Most authors prefer computed tomography imaging and nuclear medicine renography to precisely define stone anatomy, evaluate renal function, and provide anatomic information prior to surgery. Stones of any composition may be safely treated via the robotic approach. Even infectious stones such as struvite or calcium phosphate may be treated provided sterile preoperative urine culture and appropriate antibiotic coverage (Table 12.1).

Electronic supplementary material: The online version of this chapter (doi:10.1007/978-3-319-45060-5_12) contains supplementary material, which is available to authorized users.

J.N. Lange, M.D. • A.K. Hemal, M.D. (✉)
Department of Urology, Wake Forest Baptist Health,
Winston-Salem, NC, USA
e-mail: ahemal@wakehealth.edu

M. Menon, M.D.
Department of Urology, Vattikuti Urology Institute,
Henry Ford Health System,
2799 W. Grand Blvd, Detroit, MI 48202, USA
e-mail: mmenon1@hfhs.org

© Springer International Publishing Switzerland 2017
L.-M. Su (ed.), *Atlas of Robotic Urologic Surgery*, DOI 10.1007/978-3-319-45060-5_12

Table 12.1 Various applications of robot-assisted procedures in treating stone disease in different locations

	Robotic procedure	Indication
Reconstructive + stone extraction	Pyeloplasty with pyelolithotomy	Ureteropelvic junction obstruction with secondary stones
	Ureteropyelostomy with pyelolithotomy	Duplex pelvicalyceal system with ureteropelvic junction obstruction in the lower moiety with secondary stone
	Ureteric reimplantation with stone extraction	Megaureter with ureteral stone
	Bladder diverticulectomy with stone	Stone in a bladder diverticulum
Primary stone removal	Ureterolithotomy	Impacted large ureteral calculus
	Extended pyelolithotomy	Partial staghorn renal calculus
	Nephrolithotomy	Inferior calyceal calculus with narrow infundibulum and thin overlying parenchyma
	Anatrophic nephrolithotomy	Staghorn calculus
Ablative	Simple nephrectomy	Non-functioning kidney with renal stone disease
	Nephroureterectomy with stone removal	Non-functioning kidney with impacted ureteric stone or with megaureter
	Lower pole partial nephrectomy with stone extraction	Non-functioning lower pole with inferior calyceal calculi

Preoperative Preparation

Urine Culture and Bowel Preparation

Patients must have documented sterile urine preoperatively, as there is considerable chance of spillage of urine into the abdomen or retroperitoneum intraoperatively. Perioperative antibiotics should be selected based on recent culture data, or, if cultures are negative, empiric broad-spectrum coverage should be provided against typical skin and urinary flora. Simple bowel preparation of clear liquids, the day prior to surgery, and an enema or suppository the evening prior to surgery help reduce colonic distension and facilitate dissection.

Informed Consent

Informed consent should address the potential complications of both laparoscopic renal surgery and traditional stone surgery. Risks of bleeding, infection, damage to kidney or abdominal viscera, loss of kidney, and conversion to open technique should be discussed. Further risks including failure to eradicate all stone fragments and stone recurrence should also be considered.

Operative Setup

Operating suite setup for REP is similar to other robotic renal surgery. Given the limited working space of most operating rooms, we prefer to have the operating table offset toward the side of the docked robot (patient's back). The robotic light source units and insufflators are in a common tower placed near the foot of the bed on the side of the patient's back. This allows ample room for a patient-side assistant, scrub nurse, and instrument table on patient's abdominal side. Additionally, the robotic console is placed remotely in the same room or adjoining room. This arrangement places all surgeons, assistants, and instruments in direct access to the working surface of the patient. Additional specialized equipment such as holmium laser units or ultrasonic/hydraulic lithotripters may be brought in as needed for fragmentation of stones if deemed necessary.

Patient Positioning and Preparation

Sequential compression devices are applied to the lower extremities and activated prior to induction of general anesthesia. An orogastric tube and an indwelling 16 French urethral catheter are inserted. For a transperitoneal approach, the patient is then placed in a modified (45°–60°) lateral decubitus position with minimal flexion of the operating table and kidney rest elevation. Slight reverse Trendelenburg is recommended with the daVinci S and Si model robots as the fourth arm and port may come close to iliac crest or collide with the patient's hip. We believe this minimizes arm collision when working in the pelvis. In contrast, with the da Vinci Xi model robot, this is not necessary.

For a retroperitoneal approach, the patient is placed in a full flank position. Care is taken to ensure adequate padding of all pressure points. An axillary roll is placed, and the patient is secured to the table with seatbelts, Velcro straps, and/or tape. Next, the urethral catheter is clamped to allow gradual distension of the urinary bladder. This facilitates antegrade placement of a double pigtail ureteral stent later in the operation, as a fuller bladder allows greater space for the distal end of the stent to coil. Additionally, the reflux of urine via the stent (seen as drops of urine emanating from the holes in the stent) provides reassurance regarding correct placement of the lower end of the stent in the bladder rather than in the distal ureter [8].

Trocar Configuration

We have performed REP via both transperitoneal and retroperitoneal approaches, but we now universally prefer a transperitoneal approach unless a compelling reason favors a retroperitoneal approach (i.e., prior extensive intraperitoneal surgery). The retroperitoneal approach, while theoretically superior in terms of reduced risk of peritoneal contamination with urine or stone fragments, remains an extreme technical challenge for REP, as the creation of the retroperitoneal space and appropriate placement of trocars to provide wide excursion is cumbersome. We have also found it difficult to employ a retroperitoneoscopic robotic approach in obese and short-statured patients. However, the design of the new Xi robot is more conducive to the retroperitoneal approach.

Transperitoneal Approach

Transperitoneal and retroperitoneal robotic pyelolithotomy were developed based on principles of laparoscopic management of stone disease [9–13]. The pneumoperitoneum is established using the Veress needle by placing it in the ipsilateral hypochondrium/iliac fossa. The remaining trocar placement and trocar configuration is mapped out after the pneumoperitoneum is established and is dependant upon the individual's physical features, the chosen surgical approach (i.e., transperitoneal or retroperitoneal), and the surgeon's preference of stereoscopic lens [14].

Port Placement for da Vinci S or Si Platform

If using a 0° or 30° down stereoscopic lens, a 12 mm camera trocar is placed through the lateral edge of the rectus muscle at the level of the umbilicus, while the two 8 mm robotic trocars are placed in such a manner to form a skewed wide isosceles triangle [14]. The cranial 8 mm robotic trocar is placed an inch away from the midline ipsilaterally between the xiphoid process and the umbilicus (almost at the level of the renal hilum), and the second more caudal 8 mm robotic trocar is placed in the ipsilateral iliac fossa along the anterior axillary line at least 7–8 cm away from the camera trocar, thus minimizing instrument collisions. A 12 mm assistant trocar in the mid-

Fig. 12.1 Trocar placement for transperitoneal robotic extended pyelolithotomy. A three-trocar configuration consisting of the camera trocar as well as cranial and caudal robotic trocars is the minimum recommended. Additional trocars such as a fourth arm robotic, 5 mm assistant, and 12 mm assistant may be placed as needed

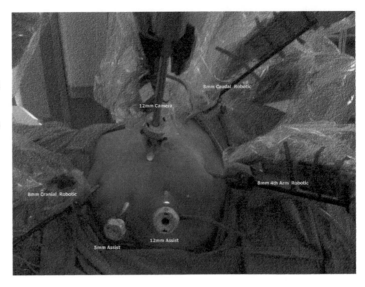

line allows for suction, retraction, and passage of suture materials and instruments such as the specimen retrieval bag and flexible nephroscope (Fig. 12.1). Another optional 5 mm assistant trocar in the midline allows for liver retraction during right-sided procedures. In general, we utilize a three-armed robotic technique; however, a four-armed robotic trocar can be added above the pubic symphysis in a paramedian location in line with the cranial robotic trocar for the purpose of retraction and dissection. This should only be utilized if felt to be necessary as it adds to the overall cost of the procedure.

Alternatively, when using a 30° up stereoscopic lens, the 12 mm camera trocar is placed at the level of umbilicus and lateral between the anterior axillary and mid-clavicular lines. The two 8 mm robotic trocars are placed alongside the rectus muscle, at a plane lower than the camera trocar and triangulated toward the renal pelvis [8, 14].

Port Placement for da Vinci Xi Platform

Pneumoperitoneum of 14 mmHg is achieved using a Veress needle in standard fashion. Trocars are placed linearly along the lateral border of rectus muscle. Port placement consists of an 8 mm camera port placed lateral and superior to the umbilicus and lateral to the rectus muscle. After placing this port, peritoneoscopy is performed, and the rest of the robotic ports are placed as dictated by the patient's intra-abdominal anatomy after inflation. The second robotic port is placed about 6 cm cranial to the camera port and lateral to the rectus muscle. The third 8 mm port is placed about 6 cm caudal to the camera port and lateral to the rectus muscle. For cost-saving purposes, stone surgery can be performed using three robotic ports inclusive of the camera port. A 12 cm AirSeal (SurgiQuest Inc, Milford, CT) assistant port is placed in the midline approximately 2–3 cm cranial to the umbilicus. For additional cost-reducing measures, AirSeal does not have to be used, and an alternative 12 mm port can be placed. The robot is docked perpendicular to the patient from the back on the ipsilateral side.

The illustrations of port placement for da Vinci Xi (Fig. 12.2) and da Vinci Si (Fig. 12.3) platform can be modified according to patient factors such as body mass index, previous surgeries, and disease factors such as large kidney and location of renal pelvis.

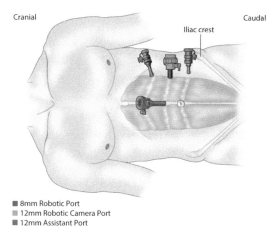

Fig. 12.2 Transperitoneal Ports for daVinci S or Si

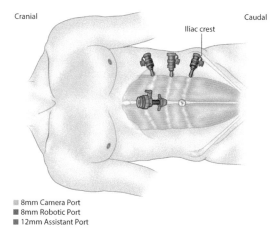

Fig. 12.3 Transperitoneal Ports for da Vinci Xi

Retroperitoneal Approach

In this approach, the patient is placed in the full lateral flank position. The bridge of the table is elevated to flatten the lumbar region. Initially tilting the table toward the anterior side allows the peritoneum and its contents to fall forward. This maneuver helps to avoid peritoneal transgression during trocar placement. A 1–1.5 cm incision is made 2 cm above the lateral apex of the anterior superior iliac crest traversing from skin through the thoracolumbar fascia and entering into the retroperitoneal space. During this step, there must be a deliberate effort made to prevent inadvertent dissection between the

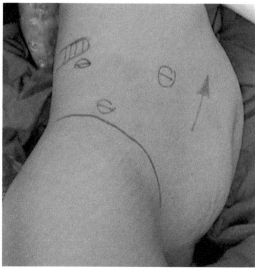

Fig. 12.4 Trocar configuration for retroperitoneal robotic pyelolithotomy. The 12 mm camera trocar is placed immediately above the iliac crest with the two more 8 mm robotic trocars 8–10 cm cephalad along the anterior and posterior axillary lines. Arrow points in the direction of the patient's head, and the tip of the 12th rib is indicated

subcutaneous and muscular planes, as gas extravasation can result. Blunt digital dissection can further develop this space.

A trocar-mounted pre-peritoneal dissection balloon (round OMS-PDB1000; kidney-shaped OMSPDBS2, Covidien, Minneapolis, MN) is introduced into the incision. With this balloon, the retroperitoneal space is created under direct vision, and the balloon is left inflated for 5 min to ensure adequate hemostasis. After verifying that an adequate working space has been created under laparoscopic vision, the balloon is deflated and replaced with a 12 mm blunt tip Hasson camera trocar (Covidien, Minneapolis, MN). Two additional 8 mm robotic trocars are subsequently placed under vision equidistant (approximately 8–10 cm) from the camera trocar at a right angle to each other along the anterior and posterior axillary lines, respectively (Fig. 12.4). A 5 mm assistant trocar is placed at the same level as the 12 mm camera trocar toward the anterior abdominal wall and equidistant from the 8 mm robotic trocar. The robot is docked and further extraperitoneal space is created as needed. Of note, the da Vinci Xi robot is more facile for this approach as it allows for swapping the camera among any of the ports. If you are using Xi system, the camera port is 8 mm, and you may want to use a home-made balloon by tying a finger stall over a rubber catheter.

Instrumentation and Equipment List

The robotic instruments required for the procedure include: Maryland bipolar or plasma kinetic forceps on the left-hand side and "hot" curved monopolar scissors on the right side which can be interchangeable with a needle driver. While using the da Vinci Xi, we use fenestrated or Maryland bipolar forceps as plasma kinetic forceps are currently not available with this platform. The instrument configuration may change according to dominant hand of the surgeon. Limiting the number of robotic instruments to three improves cost-effectiveness. Alternatively, two needle drivers for ease of suturing; a hook for blunt dissection of the Gil-Vernet's plane, and a ProGrasp™ forceps may be used.

Equipment
- da Vinci® Surgical System (S, Si, or Xi; three- or four-arm system; Intuitive Surgical, Inc., Sunnyvale, CA)
- EndoWrist® Maryland bipolar forceps or PK dissector (Intuitive Surgical, Inc., Sunnyvale, CA)
- EndoWrist® curved monopolar scissors (Intuitive Surgical, Inc., Sunnyvale, CA)
- EndoWrist® ProGrasp™ forceps (Intuitive Surgical, Inc., Sunnyvale, CA)
- EndoWrist® needle drivers suture cut (1) (Intuitive Surgical, Inc., Sunnyvale, CA)
- InSite® Vision System with 0° and 30° lens (Intuitive Surgical, Inc., Sunnyvale, CA)
- 5 mm Laparoscopic lens

The equipment needs are the same for the Xi model as for the S and Si except the camera is placed through an 8 mm port. Instrument names are the same other than PK dissector is not yet available for Xi.

Trocars
- 12 mm Blunt tip trocar (1)—alternatively 8 mm for Xi
- 8 mm Robotic trocars (2)
- 5 mm Trocar (1)—optional

Recommended Sutures
- 5-0 Poliglecaprone on an RB-1 needle cut to 10 cm in length

Instruments Used by the Surgical Assistant
- Laparoscopic scissors (not necessary if you are using suture cut needle driver)
- Blunt tip fenestrated grasper
- Suction irrigator device
- 17 French flexible cystoscope (optional)
- Nitinol stone basket or flexible stone graspers (optional)
- Pre-peritoneal distention balloon (round OMS-PDB 1000, kidney-shaped OMSPDBS2, Covidien, Minneapolis, MN)
- Blunt tip trocar with sealing device
- 10 mm Specimen entrapment bag
- 16 French urethral catheter
- Double pigtail ureteral stent
- 10 or 15 French Jackson–Pratt drain

Step-by-Step Technique (Video 12.1)

Step 1: Mobilization of the Ipsilateral Colon (Table 12.2)

The procedure is initiated using a Maryland bipolar forceps on the left side and a curved scissor on the right. Upon inspecting the abdominal cavity, if adhesions exist, these should be lysed sharply with minimal electrocautery in order to avoid inadvertent bowel injury. The electrocautery settings are 30 W for monopolar scissors and 25 W for bipolar forceps. In contrast, for the Xi robot, monopolar cut is set to 2–3 dry cut, monopolar coagulation is set to 2–3 forced coag, and bipolar cautery is set to 2–3 soft coag. The insufflation pressure used throughout the procedure is maintained at 15 mmHg. On the left side, a limited mobilization of the colon overlying the kidney

Table 12.2 Mobilization of the ipsilateral colon: surgeon and assistant instrumentation

Surgeon instrumentation		Assistant instrumentation
Right arm	Left arm	• Suction-irrigator
• Curved monopolar scissors	• Maryland bipolar grasper	
Endoscope lens: 0°, 30° down or 30° up depending on surgeon preference and trocar configuration		

and renal pelvis is performed by incising along the white line of Toldt. In a thin individual, sparse mesocolic fat may allow a trans-mesocolic approach wherein a window is created in the mesocolon overlying the renal pelvis. The renal pelvis may be identified as a bulge due to the presence of a stone within it with or without hydronephrosis. On the right side, an additional 5 mm liver retractor placed below the xiphoid may be required to elevate the right lobe of the liver and provide better visualization of the renal hilum and renal pelvis. The lateral peritoneal attachments of the hepatic flexure are incised to mobilize the ascending colon and duodenum providing access to the renal hilum. Contrary to the open technique, entire mobilization of the kidney (especially the lateral attachments) is avoided to prevent it from falling medially and hampering vision.

Step 2: Dissection of Ureter and Renal Pelvis

The next step is identification of the ureter. This is followed cranially in order to identify the renal pelvis (Fig. 12.5). It is important to dissect the renal pelvis free of its surrounding peripelvic fat, which may be adherent, especially, in patients who have undergone prior SWL or PCNL or have a history of pyelonephritis. This dissection is important to correctly develop the Gil-Vernet's plane which allows exposure of the infundibulae of the major calyces, especially in cases of intra-renal pelves. Due to a transperitoneal approach, the renal vessels (renal vein in particular) are found to lie abutting the cranial edge of the renal

pelvis. This tends to limit the superior extension of the pyelotomy to the superior infundibula. Correct dissection of the peripelvic fascia facilitates mobilization of the renal pelvis away from the vessels. Stone identification may be difficult given the presence of adhesions and inflammation, thus dissection of the renal pelvis should occur in a gentle, careful, and cautious manner. This allows for identification and preservation of the renal vessels, especially the anterior branch of renal artery or vein which may be closely abutting the renal pelvis, thus preventing vascular injury at the time of pyelolithotomy. Complete skeletonization of the main renal vessels is only performed in cases where entry into the renal parenchyma is required or when contemplating an anatrophic nephrolithotomy or extended pyelolithotomy.

Step 3: Pyelotomy, Infundibulotomy, and Removal of Stones (Table 12.3)

Once the pelvis is adequately dissected, a V-shaped pyelotomy is performed with or without extension into the inferior infundibulum (Fig. 12.6). However, depending upon the stone size and configuration, pyelotomy is extended into the superior or inferior infundibulum of the kidney to prevent inadvertent injury to the renal vessels. In addition, the laparoscopic assistant may carefully retract the vessels superiorly using a blunt suction tip. Once an adequate pyelotomy is created, the tip of the cold scissors is used to dissect the pelvic mucosa off of the stone, allowing it to be maneuvered into a position such that its smallest diameter aligns with the pyelotomy. This allows delivery of one end of the stone out of the pyelotomy first. This is followed by manipulation of the opposite end of the stone until the stone is fully delivered (Fig. 12.7). Secondary calyceal calculi are retrieved under direct vision as one has ability to move the camera into the pyelotomy incision and remove the stones using the Maryland bipolar forceps or by having the assistant use a laparoscopic grasper. Stones are then placed in the paracolic gutter for later retrieval.

Fig. 12.5 Right transperitoneal robotic extended pyelolithotomy: exposure of the renal pelvis. The perirenal fat is notably thickened, as is common with prior inflammation and scarring associated with large renal stones and prior procedures

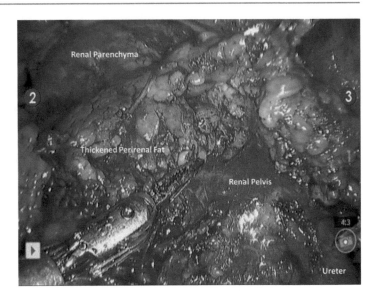

Table 12.3 Pyelotomy, infundibulotomy, and removal of stones: surgeon and assistant instrumentation

Surgeon instrumentation		Assistant instrumentation
Right arm	Left arm	• Suction-irrigator
• Curved monopolar scissors	• Maryland bipolar grasper	• Laparoscopic fenestrated grasper
Endoscope lens: 0°, 30° down or 30° up depending on surgeon preference and trocar configuration		

Step 4: Adjunctive Maneuver to Remove Calyceal Calculi (Table 12.4)

After retrieval of the pelvic stone, attention is directed at calyceal calculi. The camera is moved close to pelvicalyceal system allowing some calyceal calculi to be removed under direct vision. Next, the calyces are flushed with saline using the suction-irrigation device, further dislodging any remaining fragments. If needed, a flexible cystoscope can be used to assist with further extraction of calyceal calculi. The flexible cystoscope can be introduced into the abdomen through the cranial 8 mm robotic or midline assistant 12 mm trocar. To access different calyces, pressure irrigation is required. If needed, a nitinol basket or flexible graspers can be used for stone extraction. Small stone fragments may be immediately removed from the body, and any larger fragments can be left along the paracolic gutter for later retrieval.

Step 5: Antegrade Ureteral Stenting (Table 12.5)

Once the stones are removed, an antegrade double pigtail ureteral stent is placed over a guide wire introduced through the 5 mm assistant laparoscopic trocar. It is easily manipulated into the ureter with the robotic instruments (Fig. 12.8). This avoids the need for cystoscopy and ureteral stent placement and change in patient position prior to docking the robot. With the bladder now distended due to previous plugging of the urethral catheter, urine should emanate from the proximal end of the stent once it is in proper position within the bladder. The guide wire is removed, and the proximal end of the stent is then placed within the renal pelvis prior to closure.

Fig. 12.6 Right transperitoneal robotic extended pyelolithotomy. Incision of renal pelvis may be extended into an infundibulum to allow branches of a staghorn to be removed

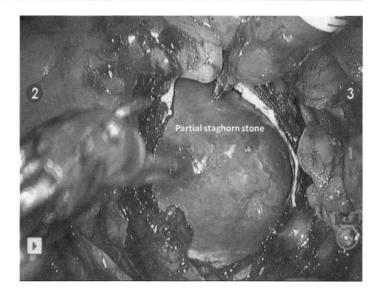

Fig. 12.7 Right transperitoneal robotic extended pyelolithotomy. The stone is grasped with robotic forceps and gently manipulated from the renal pelvis

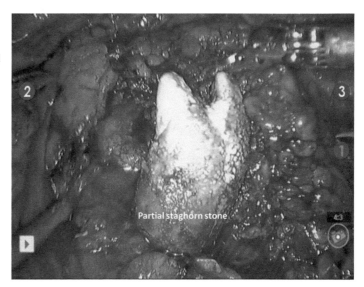

Table 12.4 Adjunctive maneuver to remove calyceal calculi: surgeon and assistant instrumentation

Surgeon instrumentation		Assistant instrumentation
Right arm	Left arm	• Suction-irrigator
• Curved monopolar scissors	• Maryland bipolar grasper	• Laparoscopic fenestrated grasper
		• 17 French flexible cystoscope
Endoscope lens: 0°, 30° down or 30° up depending on surgeon preference and trocar configuration		• Nitinol stone basket or flexible graspers

Table 12.5 Antegrade ureteral stenting: surgeon and assistant instrumentation

Surgeon instrumentation		Assistant instrumentation
Right arm	Left arm	• Suction-irrigator
• Needle driver	• Maryland bipolar grasper	• Laparoscopic fenestrated grasper
Endoscope lens: 0°, 30° down or 30° up depending on surgeon preference and trocar configuration		• Double pigtail ureteral stent

Fig. 12.8 Right transperitoneal robotic extended pyelolithotomy. A double pigtail ureteral stent is placed in an anterograde fashion over a guidewire through the assistant trocar

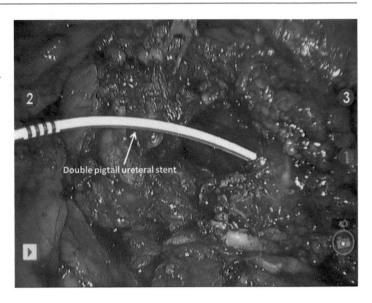

Double pigtail ureteral stent

Step 6: Repair of the Infundibular and Pyelotomy Incisions (Table 12.6)

The infundibular and pyelotomy incisions are sutured in a running fashion using 5-0 poliglecaprone on an RB-1 needle cut to 10 cm (Fig. 12.9). Moreover, the peripelvic fat is reapproximated to cover the repaired pyelotomy. Gerota's fascia is used to ensure that the perinephric space is closed off from the peritoneal cavity. An intraperitoneal 10 or 15 French Jackson-Pratt drain is placed through the 5 mm assistant trocar.

Step 7: Retrieval of Stones from the Body (Table 12.7)

The stone fragments are retrieved from the paracolic gutter using a 10 mm specimen entrapment bag inserted through the 12 mm assistant trocar (Fig. 12.10), taking caution not to risk losing fragments. The robotic instruments, camera, and robot are removed and undocked, and a 5 mm 30° laparoscope lens is placed through the 5 mm assistant trocar to provide laparoscopic vision. The specimen bag is retrieved by enlarging the 12 mm assistant trocar site. This avoids making another incision to remove the bag from the peritoneal cavity. Finally, the fascia along the 12 mm trocar is closed primarily, and subcuticular closures are performed at all skin incision sites.

Table 12.6 Repair of the infundibular and pyelotomy incisions: surgeon and assistant instrumentation

Surgeon instrumentation		Assistant instrumentation
Right arm	Left arm	• Suction-irrigator
• Needle driver	• Needle driver	• Laparoscopic fenestrated grasper
Endoscope lens: 0°, 30° down or 30° up depending on surgeon preference and trocar configuration		

Robotic Anatrophic Nephrolithotomy

The operative setup and technique for robotic anatrophic nephrolithotomy is similar to that used for REP. The procedure begins with mobilizing the kidney and exposing the renal hilum. Renal vascular control is obtained using bulldog clamps. A vertical incision is made along Brodel's line with cold monopolar scissors, and stones are identified and removed with robotic forceps. The collecting system is then closed in a running fashion with 3-0 Vicryl, and the renal parenchyma is closed with 2-0 V-Loc (Covidien, Mansfield, MA) suture in a horizontal mattress fashion. This technique was successfully described in seven patients [15]. The authors have also found use of barbed suture safe and effective in our experience [16]. Recently, indo-

Fig. 12.9 Right transperitoneal robotic extended pyelolithotomy. The pyelotomy is closed with 5-0 suture in a running or interrupted fashion. Care is taken to avoid inclusion of the proximal stent in the suture line

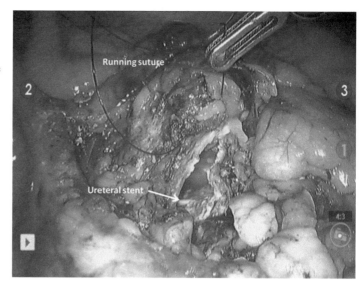

Table 12.7 Retrieval of stones from the body: surgeon and assistant instrumentation

Surgeon instrumentation		Assistant instrumentation
Right arm	Left arm	• Suction-irrigator
• Needle driver with suture cut	• Optional needle driver (Prograsp or bipolar forceps can be used to reduce cost)	• 10 mm specimen entrapment bag
Endoscope lens: 0°, 30° down or 30° up depending on surgeon preference and trocar configuration		

cyanine green has been used to visualize Brodel's avascular plane in a pig model for robotic anatrophic nephrolithotomy [17]. This may be an area of future exploration in robotic surgery.

Robotic Ureterolithotomy

The operative setup and technique for robotic ureterolithotomy is similar to that used for REP. Once the ureter is identified, it is traced to the site of the stone. Usually the calculus is large enough to be visually identified, appearing as a ureteral bulge. The portion of ureter containing

the stone is dissected with scissors and bipolar forceps, taking care not to skeletonize the ureter and compromise its blood supply. A longitudinal ureterotomy is performed with a cold curved scissors. At this stage, the stone is freed from the ureteral mucosa with the tip of the scissors or with bipolar forceps. After stone retrieval, the ureterotomy is closed with interrupted intracorporeal sutures of 5-0 poliglecaprone (Figs. 12.11 and 12.12). If double pigtail ureteral stenting is deemed necessary, it is performed in an antegrade fashion as described previously. The remaining steps are the same as for robotic pyelolithotomy.

Postoperative Management

After REP and robotic ureterolithotomy, patients are initially given clear liquids and advanced to regular diet as tolerated. Pain is usually well-controlled with scheduled ketorolac in addition to narcotics as needed for breakthrough pain. We routinely provide oral anticholinergics as needed for stent colic. Ambulation is encouraged as soon as tolerated. The surgical drain is left to gravity drainage rather than suction, and it is removed when there has been less than 30 cm³ drainage per 8 h, which is usually on postoperative day one. The urethral catheter is removed just prior to

Fig. 12.10 Right transperitoneal robotic extended pyelolithotomy. All stones are moved from the paracolic gutter into the specimen retrieval bag

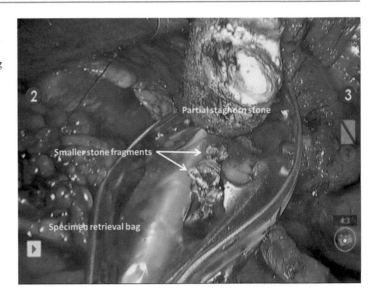

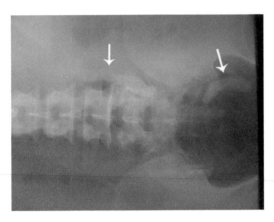

Fig. 12.11 Preoperative abdominal X-ray demonstrating multiple radiopaque large left ureteric stones (*arrows*)

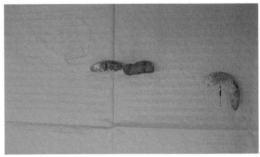

Fig. 12.12 Retrieved multiple ureteric stones by left robotic ureterolithotomy

discharge. With this regimen, most patients are generally able to go home within 24 h postoperatively (rarely 48 h later).

Special Anatomical Considerations

REP has been performed on patients with complex renal anatomy such as collecting system duplication, horseshoe kidney, and even crossed fused ectopia. These special cases are challenging regardless of approach and should be considered only after considerable experience with robotic surgery. More commonly, those with intrarenal pelves are encountered and represent about half of all REP patients in some series [6]. Retroperitoneal laparoscopic robotic pyelolithotomy has also been performed in select cases based on principles of retroperitoneal laparoscopy [18].

Current World Experience and Results

Presently, there are insufficient data to formulate specific usage of robotics for treating stone disease primarily. The combined world experience in published literature remains limited

Table 12.8 Current published world experience with robotic pyelolithotomy

	Number of patients (n)	Intra-renal pelvis configuration	Stone type		Mean stone size (cm)	Operative time (min)	Associated procedures
			Partial staghorn	Complete staghorn			
Badani et al. [6]	13	6	12	1	4.2	158	Lower polar nephrolithotomy-2
Nayyar et al. [8]	3	3	3	–	3.5	85	Secondary calculi in inferior and middle calyx-2
Lee et al. [7]	5	–	–	4		315.4	Open conversion-1 concurrent pyeloplasty-1
Hemal et al. [20]	50	–	6	–	3.5	106	–

(Table 12.8). Earlier series laid the ground work for feasibility and safety of performing REP [6]. The authors achieved a 100% clearance in cases of partial staghorn renal calculi, irrespective of the renal pelvis configuration with a mean robotic operative time of 108 min (range 60–193). None of the patients experienced postoperative fever or urine leak. In a later smaller series, we were able to further reduce operative time and incorporated modifications in cases that presented with intra-renal pelves [8]. An alternative trocar configuration was employed with a 30° downward viewing lens using the da Vinci S robot. Stone retrieval was performed using a homemade endobag or Endo Catch I bag (Covidien, Minneapolis, MN) via the robotic camera trocar (12 mm) by providing laparoscopic vision with a 5 mm laparoscope placed through the 5 mm trocar. Lee et al. reported their experience with robotic pyelolithotomy for staghorn calculi in four children (mean age 16.6 years) with cystine staghorn calculi [14]. Of these, three were rendered stone free, while one had a 6 mm residual lower pole stone. One patient required conversion to open surgery due to inability to retrieve the stone from the pyelotomy. In our experience, a flexible cystoscope through the robotic trocar or assistant trocar can be used to extract the stones from calyces; however, it is cumbersome and a tedious maneuver and can also lead to spillage of fluid into the peritoneal cavity.

An article was recently published in which 16 patients with large (>2 cm), impacted lower ureteral stones underwent robotic-assisted laparoscopic ureterolithotomy [19]. Stone-free rate was 100%, and there were no major postoperative complications. Mean follow-up time was only 13 months (longest 20 months), so long-term complications such as ureteral stricture formation could not be properly assessed.

Limitations of the Procedure

Robotic pyelolithotomy currently involves a transperitoneal approach in most cases, which is contrary to existing norms of treating urolithiasis. Due to this anterior approach, the renal vessels present a major limiting factor to superior infundibulotomy. The inherent position of the patient and the robot precludes the satisfactory use of intraoperative fluoroscopy to assess residual calculi. The lack of haptic feedback makes it difficult to perform a nephrolithotomy. We have performed retroperitoneoscopic robotic pyelolithotomy; however, we do not perform this routinely as it is challenging in morbidly obese patients and in those patients with unusual body habitus or stature.

Discussion

Although endoscopic techniques are the mainstay of treatment of large renal calculi, laparoscopic surgery is an acceptable minimally invasive alternative [1–5, 9–13]. Meria et al. compared PCNL and laparoscopic transperitoneal pyelolithotomy for renal pelvic stones >20 mm and found comparable results (82% vs. 88% 3-month stone-free rate) but significantly longer operative time and different postoperative morbidity [20, 21]. While bleeding was the predominant complication in the PCNL group, open conversion and urinary leakage were seen in the laparoscopic group. They concluded that, though PCNL remains the gold standard for most large pelvic stones, specific indications needed to be determined for each of the techniques. Transperitoneal laparoscopic pyelolithotomy was successfully utilized in children with large pelvic renal calculi with failed SWL therapy in whom a percutaneous access failed [22]. Laparoscopic management of stone disease has been described extensively in the literature [9–13].

REP is a feasible and safe technique for renal stone surgery [6]. It provides a combination of a minimally invasive technique and the surgical principles of renal parenchyma-sparing surgery [23, 24]. Clearly, bulky renal pelvic stones within an extrarenal pelvis are ideal candidates for the robotic approach; however, wristed instruments and magnification allow the procedure to be completed in intrarenal pelves as well. Despite transperitoneal access, no adverse sequelae of the inevitable minimal urine spillage have been reported [20]. The procedure attempts to replicate the principles of open stone surgery in a select group of patients (i.e., bulky renal pelvic stones) without transgression of the renal parenchyma, thus obviating its associated inherent complications [8]. REP may thus serve as an additional technique in the armamentarium of the urologist in treating large renal calculi [20, 25].

Patients on anti-platelet therapy and Jehovah's witnesses represent additional indications for robotic stone removal. This approach allows direct entry into the renal pelvis alleviating the need to traverse the renal parenchyma and thus minimizing chances of bleeding. This renal parenchyma-sparing approach may also prove useful in patients with bulky renal pelvic stone disease and impaired renal function with decreased renal functional reserve.

References

1. Menon M, Hemal AK. Vattikutti Institute prostatectomy: a technique of robotic radical prostatectomy: experience in more than 1000 cases. J Endourol. 2004;18(7):611–9.
2. Hemal AK, Abol-Enein H, Shrivastava A, Shoma AM, Ghoneim MA, Menon M. Robotic radical cystectomy and urinary diversion in the management of bladder cancer. Urol Clin North Am. 2004; 31(4):719–29.
3. Hemal AK, Kolla SB, Wadhwa P. Robotic reconstruction for recurrent supratrigonal vesicovaginal fistulas. J Urol. 2008;180(3):981–5.
4. Phillips CK, Taneja SS, Stifelman MD. Robot-assisted laparoscopic partial nephrectomy: the NYU technique. J Endourol. 2005;19:441–5.
5. Gettman MT, Neururer R, Bartsch G, Peschel R. Anderson–Hynes dismembered pyeloplasty performed with the daVinci robotic system. Urology. 2002;60:509–13.
6. Badani KK, Hemal AK, Fumo M, Kaul S, Shrivastava A, Rajendram AK, Yusoff NA, Sundram M, Woo S, Peabody JO, Mohamed SR, Menon M. Robotic extended pyelolithotomy for treatment of renal calculi: a feasibility study. World J Urol. 2006;24:198–201.
7. Lee RS, Passerotti CC, Cendron M, Estrada CR, Borer JG, Peters CA. Early results of robot assisted laparoscopic lithotomy in adolescents. J Urol. 2007;177(6):2306–9; discussion 2309–10.
8. Nayyar R, Wadhwa P, Hemal AK. Pure robotic extended pyelolithotomy: cosmetic replica of open surgery. J Robot Surg. 2007;1:207–11.
9. Hemal AK, Goel A, Kumar M, Gupta NP. Evaluation of laparoscopic retroperitoneal surgery in urinary stone disease. J Endourol. 2001;15(7):701–5.
10. Ramakumar S, Segura JW. Laparoscopic surgery for renal urolithiasis: pyelolithotomy, calyceal diverticulectomy, and treatment of stones in a pelvic kidney. J Endourol. 2000;14(10):829–32.
11. Gaur DD, Trivedi S, Prabhudesai MR, Gopichand M. Retroperitoneal laparoscopic pyelolithotomy for staghorn stones. J Laparoendosc Adv Surg Tech A. 2002;12(4):299–303.
12. Yagisawa T, Ito F, Kobayashi C, Onitsuka S, Kondo T, Goto Y, Toma H. Retroperitoneoscopic pyelolithot-

omy via a posterior approach for large impacted renal pelvic stone. J Endourol. 2001;15(5):525–8.

13. Goel A, Hemal AK. Evaluation of role of retroperitoneoscopic pyelolithotomy and its comparison with percutaneous nephrolithotripsy. Int Urol Nephrol. 2003;35(1):73–6.

14. Hemal AK, Eun D, Tewari A, Menon M. Nuances in the optimum placement of ports in pelvic and upper urinary tract surgery using the da Vinci robot. Urol Clin North Am. 2004;31(4):683–92.

15. King S, Klaassen Z, Madi R. Robot-assisted anatrophic nephrolithotomy: description of technique and early results. J Endourol. 2014;28(3):325–9.

16. Shah HN, Nayyar R, Rajamahanty S, Hemal AK. Prospective evaluation of unidirectional barbed suture for various indications in surgeon-controlled robotic reconstructive urologic surgery: Wake Forest University experience. Int Urol Nephrol. 2012;44(3):775–85.

17. Sood A, Rohde J, Van Winkle M, Assimos DG, Hemal AK, Peabody J, Menon M, Ghani K. Robotic anatrophic nephrolithotomy: idea, development, exploration, assessment and long-term monitoring (IDEAL) phase 0 study. Abstract. Accepted to American Urological Association Annual Meeting 2015.

18. Hemal AK. Laparoscopic retroperitoneal extirpative and reconstructive renal surgery. J Endourol. 2011; 25(2):209–16.

19. Dogra PN, Regmi SK, Singh P, Saini AK, Nayak B. Lower ureteral stones revisited: expanding the horizons of robotics. J Urol. 2013;82(1):95–9.

20. Hemal AK, Nayyar R, Gupta NP, Dorairajan LN. Experience with robotic assisted laparoscopic surgery in upper tract urolithiasis. Can J Urol. 2010;17(4):5299–305.

21. Meria P, Milcent S, Desgrandchamps F, Mongiat-Artus P, Duclos JM, Teillac P. Management of pelvic stones larger than 20 mm: laparoscopic transperitoneal pyelolithotomy or percutaneous nephrolithotomy? Urol Int. 2005;75(4):322–6.

22. Casale P, Grady RW, Joyner BD, Zeltser IS, Kuo RL, Mitchell ME. Transperitoneal laparoscopic pyelolithotomy after failed percutaneous access in the pediatric patient. J Urol. 2004;172(2):680–3; discussion 683.

23. Gil-Vernet J. New concepts in removing renal calculi. Urol Int. 1965;20:255–88.

24. Fitzpatrick JM, Sleight MW, Braack A, Marberger M, Wickham JEA. Intrarenal access: effects on renal function and morphology. Br J Urol. 1980;52: 409–14.

25. Badalato GM, Hemal AK, Menon M, Badani KK. Current role of robot-assisted pyelolithotomy for the management of large renal calculi: a contemporary analysis. J Endourol. 2009;23(10):1719–22.

Robot-Assisted Ureteral Reconstruction

13

Yuka Yamaguchi, Lee C. Zhao,
and Michael Stifelman

Patient Selection

Prior to bringing a patient to the operating room, the surgeon should determine if the ureteral pathology is extrinsic or intrinsic, document the length of the involved segment, and identify any surrounding pathology. Integral to the treatment of ureteral pathology is proper imaging to illustrate the disease process and allow for accurate planning of the surgical approach. We advise the use of a three-phase computed tomography scan or magnetic resonance image of the abdomen and pelvis, with dedicated arterial and urographic phases. Administration of a diuretic may be beneficial to obtain optimal ureteral imaging during the delayed urographic phase. Diuretic renal scans are useful to determine baseline function of the associated renal unit (in case nephrectomy is indicated) and to confirm obstruction in equivocal cases. When necessary, ureteroscopy with retrograde pyelography can be performed before or at the time of the reconstructive surgery to provide further anatomic information. The indications for each procedure will be discussed in the individual procedural sections that follow.

Preoperative Preparation

Patients receive an extensive informed consent regarding all possible options of ureteral reconstruction, which can include ileal ureter, Boari flap, psoas hitch, transureteroureterostomy, ureterocalicostomy, buccal ureteroplasty, ureteral reimplantation, autotransplant, and nephrectomy. All possible operative interventions, including open, endoscopic, laparoscopic, and robotic, are thoroughly discussed with and fully understood by the patient during the informed consent. In addition to bleeding, transfusion, and infection, patients undergoing robotic ureteral reconstruction must be aware of the potential for conversion to open surgery. The possibility of recurrence of ureteral obstruction from stricture should also be discussed, in addition to the need for long-term follow-up and the possible need for reoperation.

Electronic supplementary material: The online version of this chapter (doi:10.1007/978-3-319-45060-5_13) contains supplementary material, which is available to authorized users.

Y. Yamaguchi, M.D.
Department of Urology, Highland Hospital,
Oakland, 94602, CA, USA

L.C. Zhao, M.D., M.S.
Department of Urology, NYU Langone Medical Center, NYU Urology Associates, 150 East 32nd Street, 2nd Floor, New York, NY 10016, USA

M. Stifelman, M.D. (✉)
Department of Urology, Hackensack University Medical Center, Hackensack, NJ 07601, USA
e-mail: Michael.Stifelman@hackensackmeridian.org

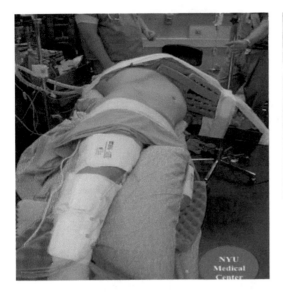

Fig. 13.1 Semi-lateral decubitus position

Operative Setup for Robotic Ureteral Surgery

The operating room setup depends on the location of the proposed reconstruction. For mid to upper ureteral reconstructions, we place the patient in a lateral or semi-lateral decubitus position with the operative side up (Fig. 13.1). Alternatively, a lateral decubitus position with the patient in a modified low-lithotomy can be employed if access to the bladder for ureteroscopy or antegrade stent placement is desired (Fig. 13.2). This position allows for simultaneous cystoscopy and ureteroscopy. The robot is docked at a 90° angle to the operating table with the robot in line with the camera trocars. For lower ureteral reconstructions, the patient is placed in a low-lithotomy position with steep Trendelenburg, similar to the positioning for a robotic prostatectomy. In these cases, the robot is docked in between the patient's legs (Fig. 13.3) or at the patient's side.

In all cases, we place the scrub nurse and assistant surgeon on the same side to facilitate the passing of instruments. It is important to note that the positioning of the table and robot can be changed intraoperatively to access other areas of pathology throughout the urinary tract. This may require placing an additional robotic trocar and

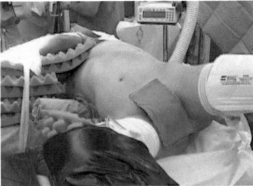

Fig. 13.2 Semi-lateral decubitus position with modified low-lithotomy

changing the position of the robotic arms. By no means is the surgeon restricted to the initial robotic setup, should a change in approach be required. Line drawings of possible operating room setups from an overhead perspective are shown in Figs. 13.4 and 13.5.

Ureterolysis and Omental Wrapping

Indications
We have performed robotic ureterolysis with omental wrap in patients with ureteral obstruction secondary to retroperitoneal fibrosis. This procedure can be done unilaterally or bilaterally as dictated based on the patient's clinical scenario.

Patient Positioning and Preparation
As most of our ureterolyses have involved the mid to upper ureter, we usually place the patient in a lateral or semi-lateral decubitus position. The patient's anterior superior iliac spine is placed directly over the flexion pivot of the operating table to allow for maximal patient flexion when desired. Two gel rolls are placed behind the patient, one at the upper back and the other at the lower back and buttocks, to help maintain a 45–60° angle. An axillary roll is placed under the patient's axilla to prevent brachial plexus injuries, and a rolled-up foam pad can be placed between the upper shoulder and neck for support. The patient's lower arm is

Fig. 13.3 Low-lithotomy
position

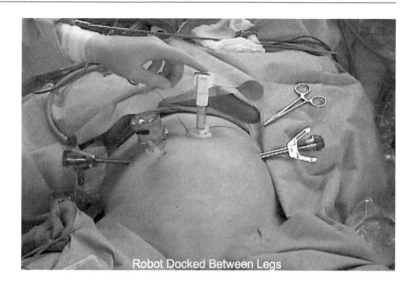

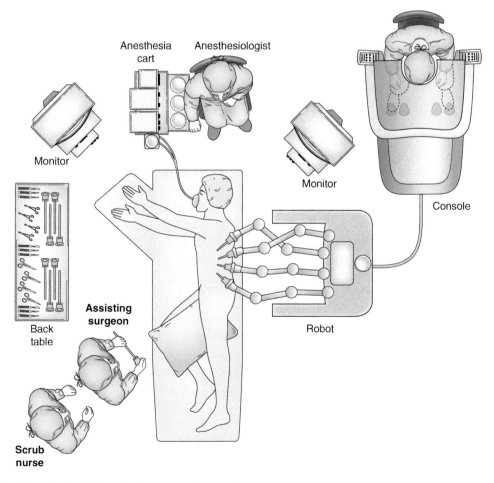

Fig. 13.4 Possible robotic ureteral reconstruction operating room setup

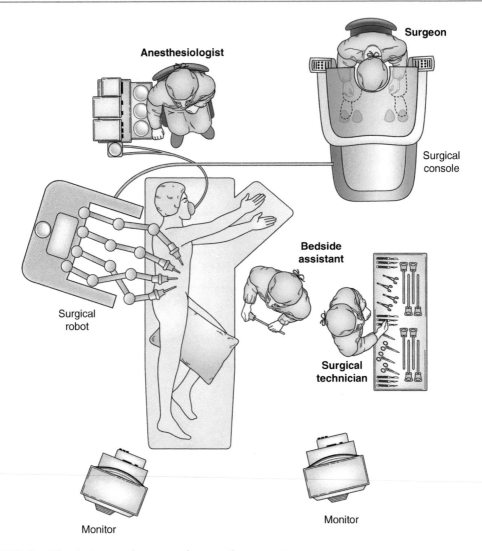

Fig. 13.5 Possible robotic ureteral reconstruction operating room setup

placed on an arm board, and foam pads are stacked on top of it to create a place for the patient's upper arm to rest comfortably. To improve access for the superior robotic trocar, instead of placing the upper arm across the body, the upper arm may be placed on the side of the body. The arm is placed on a neutral position, and a tape sling is placed under the elbow for support. The lower leg is flexed at the hip and knee while the upper leg is positioned straight; a pillow is placed in between the legs, and sequential compression boots are also employed for deep venous thrombosis prophylaxis. The patient is secured to the table with 3-in. silk or cloth tape. Attention is paid to

ensure that all pressure points are padded. Once docked, the table is maximally rotated to allow gravitational mobilization of the bowel.

Alternatively, a lateral decubitus position with the patient in a modified low-lithotomy can be employed, as described by Wong and Leveillee [1]. In this case, the patient's legs would be placed in low-lithotomy for access to the urethra in female patients. In male patients, for access to the urethra, the patient's penis is prepped into the field. It is very important that the legs are positioned so that the majority of the weight is supported by the feet and that adequate padding is used to prevent nerve compression. The advantage of this position is easier access to the bladder and ureter that does not require undocking the robot or changing patient position. The disadvantage is not being able to maximally flex the table to obtain increased working space along the ipsilateral flank.

In cases where bilateral ureteral surgery, we typically undock the robot, cover or close all trocar sites, move the robot to the contralateral side and reposition the patient with the contralateral side facing up. Our average repositioning time has been 20 min.

In patients who require ureterolysis of the distal ureter below the iliac vessels, requiring a ureteral reimplantation, it may be necessary to place the patient in a low-lithotomy position with steep Trendelenburg, similar to a robotic prostatectomy position. If using the modified flank low-lithotomy position, the table can be airplaned flat and robot moved inferior to the legs so it is in position for access to the bladder.

Trocar Configuration

We prefer to utilize four arms and one assistant trocar. For the Si robot, a 12 mm camera trocar is placed directly above the umbilicus and two 8 mm trocars are positioned 2–4 cm lateral and 8–10 cm away from the origin in either direction. These three trocars create a "V" shaped configuration (Fig. 13.6a). The fourth arm is in the lower quadrant 2 cm above pubic bone in the midclavicular line, and the assistant trocar is just below the umbilicus (Fig. 13.6b). We currently use an 8 mm AirSeal® Access Port (SurgiQuest, Milford, CT) which provides stable pneumoperitoneum as the assistant port. If AirSeal® is not available, a 5 mm trocar may be used instead. The robot is docked perpendicular to table. In terms of access, we use the Hasson technique and the Applied gel trocar (Applied Surgical, LLC, Birmingham, AL). For obese patients, this template is shifted laterally to ensure there is adequate access to the diseased ureter.

Fig. 13.6 Port configuration for robot-assisted lower ureteral reconstruction

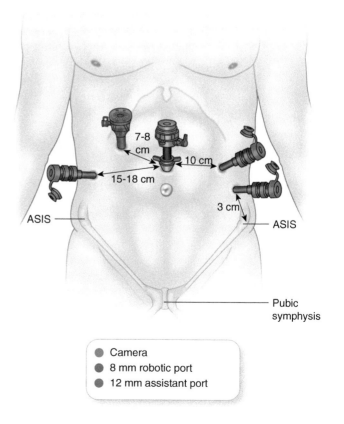

ASIS

7-8 cm

10 cm

15-18 cm

3 cm

ASIS

Pubic symphysis

● Camera
● 8 mm robotic port
● 12 mm assistant port

Instrumentation and Equipment List

Equipment
- da Vinci® Si or Xi HD Surgical System (Intuitive Surgical, Inc., Sunnyvale, CA)
- EndoWrist® PK dissector (Intuitive Surgical, Inc., Sunnyvale, CA)
- EndoWrist® Maryland bipolar forceps (Intuitive Surgical, Inc., Sunnyvale, CA)
- EndoWrist® curved monopolar scissors (Intuitive Surgical, Inc., Sunnyvale, CA)
- EndoWrist® Potts scissors (Intuitive Surgical, Inc., Sunnyvale, CA)
- EndoWrist® ProGrasp™ forceps (Intuitive Surgical, Inc., Sunnyvale, CA)
- EndoWrist® needle drivers (2) (Intuitive Surgical, Inc., Sunnyvale, CA)
- InSite® Vision System with 0° and 30° lens (Intuitive Surgical, Inc., Sunnyvale, CA)

Trocars
- 12 mm trocars (1)
- 8 mm robotic trocars (3)
- 5 mm trocar (1)
- 8 mm AirSeal® Access Port (SurgiQuest, Milford, CT)
- Applied Hasson balloon trocar (Applied Surgical, LLC, Birmingham, AL)

Instruments Used by the Surgical Assistant
- Laparoscopic needle driver
- Laparoscopic scissors
- Blunt tip bowel grasper
- Maryland dissector
- Genzyme retractor (Snowden Pencer, Genzyme; Tucker, GA)
- Laparoscopic Doppler ultrasound probe (Vascular Technology Inc. Laparoscopic Doppler System, Nashua, NH)
- 5 mm Ligasure device (for omental wrap) (Valleylab, Tyco Healthcare Group LP, Boulder, CO)
- Ethicon harmonic scalpel (for omental wrap) (Ethicon Endo-Surgery, Cincinnati, OH)
- Linear vascular stapling device (for omental wrap)
- Suction-irrigator device

- Hem-o-lok® clip applier (Teleflex Medical, Research Triangle Park, NC)
- Vessiloop (Getz Bros, Chicago, IL)

Step-by-Step Technique (Video 13.1)

Step 1: Cystoscopy and Ureteral Stent Placement

When cystoscopy, retrograde pyelography, and placement of an indwelling ureteral stent are initially performed we utilize the modified flank low-lithotomy position. Retrograde pyelography allows confirmation of the level and length of the compressed ureter, while placing the stent is mandatory in the event of inadvertent ureteral injury and may be helpful identifying the ureter with intraoperative ultrasonography in cases of severe fibrosis and inflammation.

Step 2: Trocar Placement

Trocar configuration is described in detail above. Prior to docking, the table is maximally rotated to full flank to allow gravitational mobilization of the intestines. The robot is then brought in perpendicular to the operating table.

Step 3: Exposure of Ureter (Table 13.1)

Exposure of the entire ureter is paramount, and this is accomplished on the left by medializing the colon to the aorta from the spleen to the blad-

Table 13.1 Exposure of ureter: surgeon and assistant instrumentation

Surgeon instrumentation		Assistant instrumentation
Right arm	Left arm	
• Curved monopolar scissors	• Gyrus bipolar dissector	• Suction-irrigator
Endoscope lens: 30° down		• Laparoscopic Doppler ultrasound probe

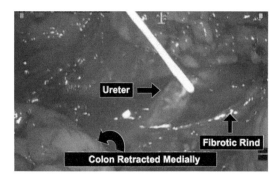

Fig. 13.7 Exposing ureter by medializing colon and using Vessiloop for retraction

Table 13.2 Ureterolysis: surgeon and assistant instrumentation

Surgeon instrumentation		Assistant instrumentation
Right arm	Left arm	
• Potts scissors	• Gyrus bipolar dissector	• Suction-irrigator
Endoscope lens: 30° down		• Maryland graspers
		• Genzyme retractor
		• Hem-o-lok® clip applier
		• Vessiloops

der, and, on the right, by medializing the colon and duodenum to the vena cava from the liver to the bladder (Fig. 13.7). Having the table rotated so that the patient is full flank helps with this exposure. The console surgeon utilizes the Gyrus PK bipolar graspers (ACMI/Olympus, Southborough, MA) in the left hand and the curved robotic scissors in the right, while the side surgeon assists with a suction-irrigator. Electrocautery settings include 50 W coagulation for the monopolar curved scissors, 50 W for Maryland bipolar graspers, and VP3-40 setting for the Gyrus PK bipolar graspers. Once the entire retroperitoneum is exposed landmarks such as the gonadal vessels, iliac vessels, and lower pole of the kidney become instrumental in identifying and locating the ureter. In some cases, intraoperative laparoscopic Doppler ultrasonography can help to identify the ureter (via imaging the course of the indwelling ureteral stent) and vascular structures, which may be obscured by the dense surrounding fibrosis.

Step 4: Ureterolysis (Table 13.2)

Once the ureter is identified, the healthy distal and proximal portions of the ureter are isolated with Vessiloops (Getz Bros, Chicago, IL), which are shortened and secured with a Hem-o-lok® clip (Fig. 13.8). To rule out the presence of lymphoma or other retroperitoneal malignancy, a frozen section of the retroperitoneal tissue is

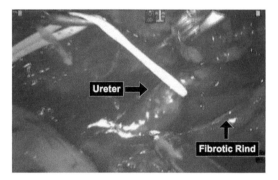

Fig. 13.8 Vessiloop with Hem-o-lok® clip used to isolate and retract ureter

routinely sent prior to proceeding with the ureterolysis. The diseased, entrapped ureteral segment is dissected free by splitting the fibrous capsule anteriorly so that the adventitia of the ureter is visible. For this, the console surgeon employs Gyrus PK bipolar graspers in the left hand and robotic Potts scissors in the right. The assistant uses a combination of laparoscopic Maryland graspers and the suction-irrigator to retract tissue and clear the field of blood and fluid. After identifying the anterior ureter, the remaining ureter is circumferentially released from the fibrous reaction using a combination of blunt and sharp dissection, avoiding the use of electrocautery around the ureter (Fig. 13.9). The ureter should bluntly peel out of the fibrotic rind once the correct plane is established. The fourth arm creates traction by advancing the Vessiloop and placing the ureter on stretch

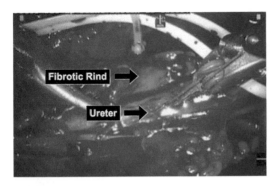

Fig. 13.9 Ureter being released circumferentially from fibrosis using sharp and blunt dissection

Table 13.3 Omental wrapping: surgeon and assistant instrumentation

Surgeon instrumentation		Assistant instrumentation
Right arm	Left arm	
• ProGrasp™ forceps	• Gyrus bipolar dissector	• Suction-irrigator
Endoscope lens: 30° down		• Atraumatic bowel grasper
		• 5 mm Ligasure
		• Ethicon harmonic scalpel
		• Hem-o-lok® clip applier
		• Laparoscopic needle driver

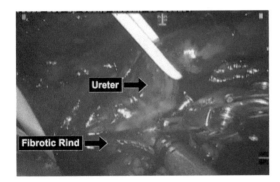

Fig. 13.10 Ureterolysis aided by traction provided on Vessiloop by side surgeon or fourth robotic arm

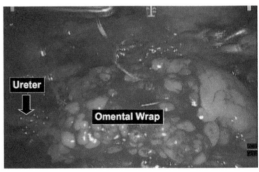

Fig. 13.11 Piece of omentum brought underneath ureter in preparation for wrapping

anteriorly (Fig. 13.10). The robotic surgeon places counter traction with a blunt dissector, and the Potts scissors are used to sharply release any adherent tissue and to sharply sweep the ureter out of the fibrotic reaction. It is important to completely mobilize the ureter from this dense tissue and be sure that healthy ureter is identified proximally and distally. It is not uncommon for the ureter to appear ischemic or congested once lysed.

Step 5: Omental Wrapping (Table 13.3)

Upon completing the robotic ureterolysis, attention is now paid to the omental wrapping. The surgeon uses Gyrus PK bipolar graspers in the left hand and ProGrasp™ forceps in the

right, while the assistant uses atraumatic graspers to expose and isolate the omentum. Once the omentum is identified, the assistant employs either a 5 mm Ligasure (Valleylab, Boulder, CO) or an Ethicon harmonic scalpel to harvest the omental pedicle. The most distal portion of the pedicle is brought underneath the ureter and tacked to the sidewall with either Hem-o-lok® clips or a 2-0 polyglactin suture (Fig. 13.11). Next, the lateral pedicle is tacked to the sidewall, allowing the entire omental flap to lay posterior to the ureter. The medial edge of the omentum, which is also medial to the ureter, is now wrapped anterior to the ureter and tacked to the sidewall (Figs. 13.12 and 13.13). At the end of the operation, a closed suction drain is placed near the omental wrap.

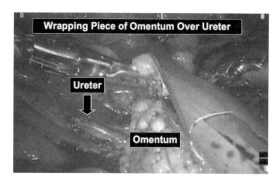

Fig. 13.12 Medial edge of omentum wrapped anterior to ureter and then tacked to side wall

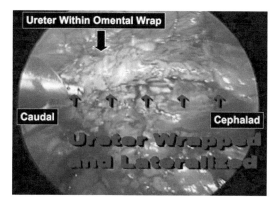

Fig. 13.13 Ureter wrapped and lateralized

Step 6: Exiting the Abdomen

The operative site and omentum are examined for bleeding under low insufflation pressure, and hemostasis is achieved. The trocars are then removed under laparoscopic view. The 8 mm and 5 mm trocars generally do not require fascial closure but are simply closed subcutaneously.

Postoperative Management

Patients typically remain in the hospital for 2 days. On the first postoperative day, patients begin a clear diet, aggressive ambulation, and oral pain medication. The urethral catheter is removed on postoperative day 2 for a trial of void, and 8 h later the output of the JP drain is sent for creatinine analysis to rule out a urine leak. If the JP fluid analysis is consistent with serum and not urine, the drain is removed. Diet is advanced, and the patient is discharged. The stent is removed with a local office cystoscopy in 4–6 weeks, and appropriate imaging studies are obtained thereafter.

Special Considerations

In the case of bilateral disease, we undock the robot, reposition the patient, and then redock the robot for patients undergoing bilateral robotic ureterolysis. In the event of an intraoperative ureteral injury, we prefer immediate primary closure. In addition, a closed suction drain is placed near the location of the injury to monitor for any urine leak in the postoperative period.

We routinely perform biopsies of the retroperitoneal tissue prior to ureterolysis to rule out lymphoma or other malignancies. We send the biopsies for frozen section, permanent section, and flow cytometry. If frozen section indicates that lymphoma may be present, we abort the procedure and wait for the results of the permanent sections before performing the ureterolysis at a later date.

Steps to Avoid Complications

Wide exposure is absolutely paramount to identify the transition of healthy to diseased ureter, as well adjacent organs and blood vessels that may be involved in the disease process. Athermal technique, via sharp dissection, is essential to avoid potential compromise of the blood supply to the already diseased ureter, which can develop into an ischemic urine leak. The judicious use of omentum is helpful in lateralizing the ureter and protecting it from the disease process, which is usually located more medially. As in all robotic ureteral reconstructive procedures, placing surgical drains at the end of the operation is important to help identify urine leaks (via fluid analysis for creatinine) in the postoperative period, which may alter when the urethral catheter and stent are removed.

Ureterocalicostomy

Indication

Robotic ureterocalicostomy is indicated in patients with a proximal ureteral stricture and a scarred renal pelvis who have failed prior antegrade or retrograde endoscopic management, or in patients with an inaccessible intrarenal pelvis.

Patient Positioning and Preparation

We prefer to have retrograde access to the bladder and ureter. For male patients, we use a flank position with the penis prepped into the field. In female patients, we prefer the semi-lateral decubitus with modified low-lithotomy.

Trocar Configuration

Trocar configuration is described in detail above. Prior to docking, the table is maximally rotated down to allow gravitational mobilization of the intestines. The robot is then brought in perpendicular to table.

Instrumentation and Equipment List

Equipment

- da Vinci® Si Surgical HD System (Intuitive Surgical, Inc., Sunnyvale, CA)
- EndoWrist® PK dissector (Intuitive Surgical, Inc., Sunnyvale, CA)
- EndoWrist® curved monopolar scissors (Intuitive Surgical, Inc., Sunnyvale, CA)
- EndoWrist® ProGrasp™ forceps (Intuitive Surgical, Inc., Sunnyvale, CA)
- EndoWrist® Potts scissors (Intuitive Surgical, Inc., Sunnyvale, CA)
- EndoWrist® needle drivers (2) (Intuitive Surgical, Inc., Sunnyvale, CA)
- InSite® Vision System with 0° and 30° lens (Intuitive Surgical, Inc., Sunnyvale, CA)

Trocars

- 12 mm trocars (1)
- 8 mm robotic trocars (2–3)
- 5 mm trocar (2)
- 8 mm AirSeal® Access Port (SurgiQuest, Milford, CT)
- Applied gel trocar (Applied Surgical, LLC, Birmingham, AL)

Recommended Sutures

- 3-0 polyglactin on RB-1 or SH needle for renal parenchyma
- 4–0 polyglactin suture on an RB-1 needle for anastomosis

Instruments Used by the Surgical Assistant

- Laparoscopic needle driver
- Laparoscopic scissors
- MicroFrance® grasper (Medtronic, Inc., Minneapolis, MN)
- Genzyme retractor (Snowden Pencer, Genzyme; Tucker, GA)
- Laparoscopic Doppler ultrasound probe (Vascular Technology Inc. Laparoscopic Doppler System, Nashua, NH)
- 10 mm LigaSure™ device (Covidien, Boulder, CO)
- Ethicon harmonic scalpel (Ethicon Endo-Surgery, Cincinnati, OH)
- Linear vascular stapling device
- Suction-irrigator device
- Vascular Bulldog Clamp
- Tissuelink Device (Tissuelink Medical Inc, Dover, NH)
- Flexible cystoscope/ureteroscope
- 1.9 Fr tipless Nitinol basket (Boston Scientific, Natick, MA)
- Vessiloop (Getz Bros, Chicago, IL)

Step-by-Step Technique

Step 1: Cystoscopy and Ureteral Stent Placement

Rigid cystoscopy, retrograde pyelography, and stent placement are performed at the outset of the case for the reasons outlined in the previous section. We place a guidewire to the level of the stricture. This allows the distal portion of the stricture to be identified by direct vision, via intraoperative ultrasound, or simultaneous ureteroscopy.

Step 2: Trocar Placement and Exposure of Ureter (Table 13.4)

Trocar placement and peritoneal access are performed as described for robotic ureterolysis. The ureter is exposed and isolated using a combination of sharp and blunt dissection, as has been described above. The main instruments employed by the console surgeon for this are the Maryland bipolar graspers, curved monopolar scissors, Potts scissors, and the Gyrus PK bipolar graspers. A Vessiloop (Getz Bros, Chicago, IL) is placed around the ureter to aid the side surgeon in applying atraumatic traction on the ureter during dissection. Careful dissection is continued to free the ureter up to the area of stricture, at which point any of the above-described maneuvers can be used to confirm the distal end of the stricture.

Step 3: Ureteral Transection (Table 13.5)

The ureter is then transected just below the level of the diseased segment using Potts scissors, and the proximal end of the stent is withdrawn below the area of transection (Fig. 13.14). The healthy ureter is spatulated laterally in preparation for the anastomosis with the lower pole calyx.

Table 13.4 Trocar placement and exposure of ureter: surgeon and assistant instrumentation

Surgeon instrumentation		Assistant instrumentation
Right arm	Left arm	
• Curved monopolar scissors	• Gyrus bipolar dissector	• Suction-irrigator
	• Maryland bipolar graspers	• Vessiloop
Endoscope lens: 30° down		• Laparoscopic Doppler ultrasound probe

Table 13.5 Ureteral transection: surgeon and assistant instrumentation

Surgeon instrumentation		Assistant instrumentation
Right arm	Left arm	
• Potts scissors	• Gyrus bipolar dissector	• Suction-irrigator
	• Maryland bipolar graspers	
Endoscope lens: 30° down		

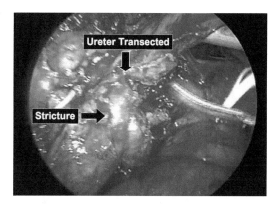

Fig. 13.14 Ureter transected below level of stricture

Step 4: Dissection of the Renal Hilum (Table 13.6)

Next, the renal hilum is isolated, the psoas muscle is identified, and the posterior surface of the kidney is dissected off the psoas. The kidney is then lifted anteriorly placing the renal hilum on stretch. This retraction is supplied by the assistant or the fourth arm using a ProGrasp™ forceps, allowing the console surgeon use two hands/instruments for the hilar dissection. A Doppler probe is used to identify the renal artery and vein, which is often encased in fibrotic tissue. The vessels are then dissected free from the surrounding tissue and isolated. A laparoscopic Doppler ultrasound probe is then introduced to identify the most dependent lower pole calyx. Gerota's fascia is cleared off this segment of kidney circumferentially (Fig. 13.15). Prior to clamping the artery, we ensure the patient is adequately volume resuscitated and administer 12.5 g of mannitol in an attempt to minimize ischemia-reperfusion injury.

Table 13.6 Dissection of the renal hilum: surgeon and assistant instrumentation

Surgeon instrumentation		Assistant instrumentation
Right arm	Left arm	
Curved monopolar scissors	• Gyrus bipolar dissector	• Suction-irrigator
	• Maryland bipolar graspers	• Laparoscopic Doppler ultrasound probe
Endoscope lens: 30° down		

Table 13.7 Renal hilar control, exposure of lower pole calyx and stone extraction: surgeon and assistant instrumentation

Surgeon instrumentation		Assistant instrumentation
Right arm	Left arm	
• Curved monopolar scissors	• Gyrus bipolar dissector	• Suction-irrigator
• Needle driver	• Maryland bipolar graspers	• Laparoscopic bulldog clamps
	• Needle driver	• TissueLink device
Endoscope lens: 30° down		• Flexible cystoscope/ureteroscope
		• 1.9 Fr tipless Nitinol basket

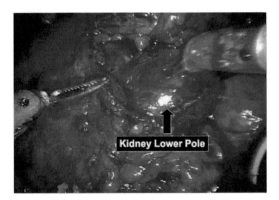

Fig. 13.15 Gerota's Fascia cleared off to expose kidney lower pole

Step 5: Renal Hilar Control, Exposure of Lower Pole Calyx and Stone Extraction (Table 13.7)

A laparoscopic vascular bulldog clamp is placed by the assistant on the renal artery. A separate clamp may be placed on the renal vein if there is excessive bleeding. The console surgeon utilizes robotic curved monopolar scissors to transect the renal lower pole to expose the calyx (Figs. 13.16 and 13.17). Vessels are suture ligated with 3-0 polyglactin sutures on either an RB-1 needle or SH needle by the console surgeon, and the renal cortex is cauterized with the TissueLink device (TissueLink Medical, Inc., Dover, NH) by the assistant, avoiding contact with the sutures or the calyceal opening. The bulldog clamp is now removed, any areas of bleeding are controlled with figure eight 3-0 polyglactin sutures, and another dose of 12.5 g of mannitol is administered. If stones are present, a flexible cystoscope or ureteroscope is

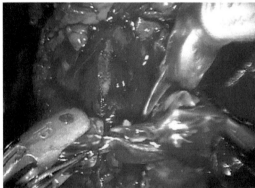

Fig. 13.16 Kidney lower pole transected to expose calyx

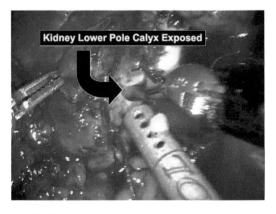

Fig. 13.17 Lower pole calyx exposed

introduced by the assistant through one of the trocars and then passed through the open lower pole calyx to examine the internal collecting system of the kidney. Any encountered stones are retrieved with a 1.9 Fr tipless Nitinol basket (Boston Scientific, Natick, MA).

Step 6: Ureterocalicostomy (Table 13.8)

Next, the anastomosis of the spatulated proximal healthy ureter to the lower pole calyx is performed using interrupted 4-0 polyglactin sutures on an RB-1 needle (Figs. 13.18 and 13.19). The mucosa of the lower pole calyx may be everted by placing sutures between the calyx and the renal capsule. Prior to completing the anastomosis, a wire is advanced through the open-ended stent into the pelvis. The double-J stent is placed in a retrograde fashion, under direct vision. We do not recommend antegrade stent placement since it creates significant tension on the anastomosis during the passage of the wire and stent. With the stent in position, the anastomosis is completed (Fig. 13.20). The proximal ureteral stump is

Table 13.8 Ureterocalicostomy: surgeon and assistant instrumentation

Surgeon instrumentation		
Right arm	Left arm	Assistant instrumentation
• Needle driver	• Needle driver	• Suction-irrigator
Endoscope lens: 30° down		• Flexible cystoscope/ ureteroscope

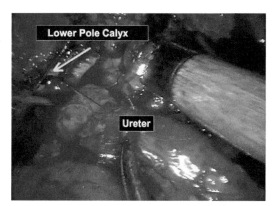

Fig. 13.18 Ureterocalycostomy anastomosis being performed

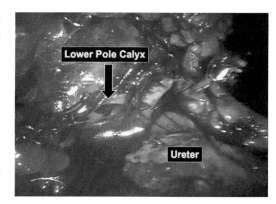

Fig. 13.19 Ureterocalycostomy anastomosis being performed

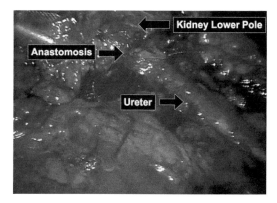

Fig. 13.20 Completed ureterocalycostomy anastomosis

suture ligated with a 2-0 polyglactin suture. We like to cover the anastomosis with either a vascularized pedicle of Gerota's fascia or omentum. We believe this improves healing, adds blood supply, and may protect from urine extravasation. As with all our ureteral reconstructions, a closed-suction drain is placed near the reconstruction to detect urine leakage in the postoperative period.

Step 7: Exiting the Abdomen

The operative site is examined for bleeding under low insufflation pressure and hemostasis achieved. The trocars are removed under direct vision. The 8 mm and 5 mm trocars generally do not require fascial closure but are simply closed subcutaneously. The fascia of the 12 mm assistant trocar also does not generally require formal closure if a non-bladed, self-dilating trocar is used.

Postoperative Management

Patients typically remain in the hospital for 2–3 days. On the first postoperative day, patients begin a clear diet, aggressive ambulation, and oral pain medication. The urethral catheter is removed on postoperative day 2 for a trial of void, and 8 h later the output of the JP drain is sent for creatinine analysis to rule out a urine leak. If the JP fluid analysis is consistent with serum and not urine, the drain is removed. Once passing flatus, a soft, regular diet is offered. The patient is discharged either the second or third postoperative day. The stent is removed with office cystoscopy in 4–6 weeks, and appropriate imaging studies are obtained thereafter.

Special Considerations

If ureteral length is preventing a tension-free anastomosis, there are some maneuvers that can help overcome this issue. A downward nephropexy may be performed to allow the ureter to reach the calyx more easily and without tension. If a tension-free anastomosis cannot be performed with this maneuver, the next step depends if salvaging the kidney is essential. If salvaging the kidney is essential, a renal autotransplant can be performed. Otherwise, a simple nephrectomy should be performed rather than creating a suboptimal anastomosis. Urine leaks or anastomotic stenosis can lead to significant morbidity and the need for further operations in the future. This decision highlights the importance of having an informed consent regarding all surgical possibilities with the patient.

Steps to Avoid Complications

Above all, ensuring a tension-free, secure anastomosis is paramount to the success of this operation. To that end, wide ureteral spatulation and apposition of ureteral and renal urothelium will help prevent stricture and urine leakage from the anastomosis. Furthermore, sharp dissection and athermal technique are essential to avoid poten-

tial compromise of the blood supply to the already diseased ureter, which can result in ischemia and urine leak. We also support the use of omentum or Gerota's fat to help protect the anastomosis, as mentioned above.

Ureteroureterostomy

Indications

This procedure should be performed in patients with proximal or mid-ureteral strictures that have been refractory to endoscopic treatments and in patients with ureteral obstruction secondary to a retrocaval ureter. The length of the stricture should be short enough for a tension-free anastomosis.

Patient Positioning and Preparation

The patient is positioned in semi-lateral decubitus or semi-lateral decubitus with modified low lithotomy to allow access to the urethra as has been previously described.

Trocar Configuration

Trocar configuration is described in detail above. Prior to docking, the table is maximally rotated down to allow gravitational mobilization of the intestines. The robot is then brought in perpendicular to the table.

Instrumentation and Equipment List

Equipment
- da Vinci® Si Surgical HD System (three- or four-arm system; Intuitive Surgical, Inc., Sunnyvale, CA)
- EndoWrist® PK dissector (Intuitive Surgical, Inc., Sunnyvale, CA)
- EndoWrist® curved monopolar scissors (Intuitive Surgical, Inc., Sunnyvale, CA)
- EndoWrist® ProGrasp™ forceps (Intuitive Surgical, Inc., Sunnyvale, CA)

- EndoWrist® Potts scissors (Intuitive Surgical, Inc., Sunnyvale, CA)
- EndoWrist® needle drivers (2) (Intuitive Surgical, Inc., Sunnyvale, CA)
- InSite® Vision System with 0° and 30° lens (Intuitive Surgical, Inc., Sunnyvale, CA)

Trocars
- 12 mm trocars (1)
- 8 mm robotic trocars (3)
- 5 mm trocar (1)
- 8 mm AirSeal® Access Port (SurgiQuest, Milford, CT)
- Applied gel trocar (Applied Surgical, LLC, Birmingham, AL)

Recommended Sutures
- 4-0 polyglactin suture on an RB-1 needle for anastomosis

Instruments Used by the Surgical Assistant
- Laparoscopic needle driver
- Laparoscopic scissors
- Genzyme retractor (Snowden Pencer, Genzyme; Tucker, GA)
- Suction-irrigator device

Step-by-Step Technique

Step 1: Cystoscopy and Ureteral Stent Placement
With the patient in lateral decubitus with modified low-lithotomy position, cystoscopy and retrograde pyelography are performed to delineate the ureteral stricture or point of obstruction. An open-ended ureteral catheter is inserted to the distal level of the stricture or obstruction and then secured to an indwelling urethral catheter.

Step 2: Trocar Placement and Exposure of Ureter (Table 13.9)
Trocar placement and peritoneal access are performed as have been described above. As previously described, the console surgeon reflects the colon medially, identifying and isolating the ureter using a combination of sharp and blunt dissec-

Table 13.9 Trocar placement and exposure of ureter: surgeon and assistant instrumentation

Surgeon instrumentation		Assistant instrumentation
Right arm	Left arm	
• Curved monopolar scissors	• Gyrus bipolar dissector	• Suction-irrigator
	• Maryland bipolar graspers	• Vessiloop
Endoscope lens: 30° down		• Laparoscopic Doppler ultrasound probe

Table 13.10 Transection of ureter and excision of diseased segment: surgeon and assistant instrumentation

Surgeon instrumentation		Assistant instrumentation
Right arm	Left arm	
Potts scissors	• Gyrus bipolar dissector	• Suction-irrigator
	• Maryland bipolar graspers	
Endoscope lens: 30° down		

tion. If required, the previously inserted open-ended ureteral catheter may be identified using an intraoperative ultrasound probe.

Step 3: Transection of Ureter and Excision of Diseased Segment (Table 13.10)
In the case of a ureteral stricture, the diseased portion of the ureter is excised with Potts scissors (Figs. 13.21 and 13.22). For a retrocaval ureter, the ureter proximal and distal to the retrocaval portion can be transected, leaving the retrocaval segment in situ. Alternatively, the ureter distal to the retrocaval portion can be transected while the proximal ureter is gently retracted to bring the retrocaval portion from under the vena cava; this should only be done if the retrocaval portion can be easily negotiated from under the vena cava. To avoid potential vascular injury, we prefer transecting the ureter twice as opposed to dissecting out the retrocaval ureteral segment. Prior to performing the anastomosis, the proximal ureter is spatulated laterally and the distal ureteral segment spatulated medially (Fig. 13.23). If there is any concern that the anastomosis will be under undue tension, the ureter can be further mobilized proxi-

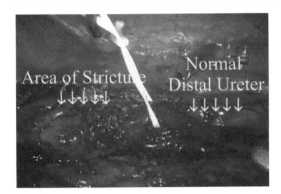

Fig. 13.21 Ureter with strictured segment

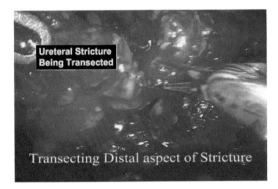

Fig. 13.22 Ureteral stricture excised with Potts scissors

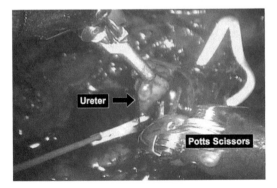

Fig. 13.23 Ureter being spatulated with Potts scissors

Table 13.11 Ureteroureterostomy: surgeon and assistant instrumentation

Surgeon instrumentation		Assistant instrumentation
Right arm	Left arm	
• Needle driver	• Needle driver	• Suction-irrigator
Endoscope lens: 30° down		

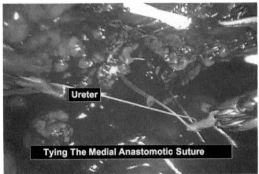

Fig. 13.24 Medial anastomotic suture being tied

4-0 polyglactin suture on an RB-1 needle. We anchor the dyed suture laterally and the undyed suture medially (Fig. 13.24). To perform the posterior wall anastomosis, we pass the medial undyed suture underneath the ureter to rotate the ureter 180° and present the posterior wall anteriorly. We run the undyed suture along the posterior wall and tie it to the dyed suture. Once the posterior wall is complete, the undyed suture is passed back underneath the ureter placing the ureter back into its anatomical position. A wire is now placed retrograde through the previously inserted 5 Fr open-ended ureteral catheter. Over this wire, the ureteral catheter is exchanged with a double-J stent, under direct visualization. The anterior anastomosis is then completed in a running fashion with the dyed suture, in a lateral to medial fashion (Fig. 13.25). We prefer to cover the anastomosis with a vascularized pedicle of omentum. As with all our ureteral reconstructions, a closed-suction drain is placed near the reconstruction to help detect urine leakage in the postoperative period.

mally and distally, the kidney can be mobilized inferiorly and pexed to the psoas muscle using a 2-0 nonabsorbable suture (i.e., Prolene).

Step 4: Ureteroureterostomy (Table 13.11)

Once it is confirmed that a tension-free anastomosis can be performed, we use a dyed and an undyed

Step 5: Exiting the Abdomen

The operative site is examined for bleeding under low insufflation pressure and hemostasis achieved. The trocars are removed under laparo-

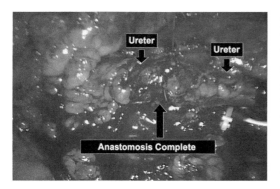

Fig. 13.25 Completed ureteroureterostomy anastomosis

scopic view. The 8 mm and 5 mm trocars generally do not require fascial closure but are simply
closed subcutaneously.

Postoperative Management

Patients typically remain in the hospital for 2 days.
On the first postoperative day, patients begin a clear
diet, aggressive ambulation, and oral pain medication. The urethral catheter is removed on postoperative day 2 for a trial of void, and 8 h later the output
of the JP drain is sent for creatinine analysis to rule
out a urine leak. If the JP fluid analysis is consistent
with serum and not urine, the drain is removed. The
patient is discharged and the stent is removed with a
local office cystoscopy in 4–6 weeks, and appropriate imaging studies are obtained thereafter.

Special Considerations

If ureteral length from either end is preventing a
tension-free anastomosis, maneuvers described
above can be employed to help overcome this issue.
One may also consider buccal mucosa graft ureteroplasty for long proximal ureteral strictures for which
a tension-free anastomosis is not possible. In cases
of a distal ureteral stricture, it may be more appropriate to perform a ureteral reimplantation.

   To preserve ureteral blood supply, it is important to minimize the use of thermal energy during
dissection and to preserve the periureteral adventitia. Furthermore, a "handle" of diseased ureter
can be left on each end of the ureter as the ureteral ends are spatulated and the anastomosis is

performed. This "handle" allows the manipulation of the ureter without having to grasp healthy
tissue and risk crush injury. Once the anastomosis has been started and the reconstruction is proceeding in a controlled fashion, both ureteral
"handles" can be excised and sent with the rest of
the excised specimen for pathologic analysis.

Steps to Avoid Complications

Above all, ensuring a tension-free, secure anastomosis is paramount to the success of this operation.
To that end, wide ureteral spatulation and apposition of ureteral urothelium will help prevent stricture and urine leakage from the anastomosis.
Furthermore, athermal technique, via sharp dissection is essential to avoid potential compromise of
the blood supply to the already diseased ureter,
which can develop into an ischemic urine leak. We
also support the judicious use of omentum to help
protect the anastomosis, as mentioned above.

Buccal Mucosa Graft Ureteroplasty

Indication

We have performed ureteroplasty using buccal
mucosa graft (BMG) in patients who have long or
multifocal proximal ureteral strictures not amenable
to ureteroureterostomy. Traditional surgical management options for this clinical scenario have
included autotransplantation or ileal ureter. We have
used robotic assistance to reconstruct the ureter in
these cases using buccal mucosa graft as an onlay as
previously described as an open technique [2–6].

Patient Positioning and Preparation

We prefer the semi-lateral decubitus position
(Fig. 13.1) with the affected side up. Practical considerations include adequate access to the patient's
mouth for buccal mucosa graft harvest as well as
access to the bladder for ureteral stent placement
and ureteroscopy. While in male patients, the semi-
lateral decubitus position allows for bladder access
using a flexible cystoscope, in female patients, a

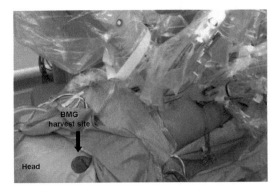

Fig. 13.26 The mouth is prepped and draped separately from the rest of the surgical field

semi-lateral decubitus position with modified low-lithotomy with legs secured in Allen stirrups (Fig. 13.2), is preferred to allow adequate bladder access. Both the modified lateral decubitus position and the modified lateral decubitus lithotomy positions are as discussed in detail above with slight modification for buccal mucosa graft harvest. The endotracheal tube is secured on the dependent side of the mouth to allow for BMG harvest from the contralateral cheek. The mouth is prepped and draped separately from the rest of the surgical field (Fig. 13.26). The patient generally will have a nephrostomy tube placed preoperatively for drainage of the affected collecting system; this nephrostomy tube is also prepped into the field to allow for intraoperative antegrade ureteroscopy as needed.

Trocar Configuration

Trocar configuration is described in detail above. Prior to docking, the table is maximally rotated to full flank to allow gravitational mobilization of the intestines. The robot is then brought in perpendicular to the operating table.

Instrumentation and Equipment List

Equipment
- da Vinci® Si Surgical System (Intuitive Surgical, Inc., Sunnyvale, CA)
- EndoWrist® PK dissector (Intuitive Surgical, Inc., Sunnyvale, CA)

- EndoWrist® curved monopolar scissors (Intuitive Surgical, Inc., Sunnyvale, CA)
- EndoWrist® Potts scissors (Intuitive Surgical, Inc., Sunnyvale, CA)
- EndoWrist® ProGrasp™ forceps (Intuitive Surgical, Inc., Sunnyvale, CA)
- EndoWrist® needle drivers (2) (Intuitive Surgical, Inc., Sunnyvale, CA)
- InSite® Vision System with 0° and 30° lens (Intuitive Surgical, Inc., Sunnyvale, CA)

Trocars
- 12 mm trocars (1)
- 8 mm robotic trocars (3)
- 5 mm trocar (1)
- 8 mm SurgiQuest AirSeal® Access Port
- Applied gel trocar (Applied Surgical, LLC, Birmingham, AL)

Recommended Sutures
- 4-0 polyglactin suture on an RB-1 needle for anastomosis

Instruments Used by the Surgical Assistant
- Laparoscopic needle driver
- Laparoscopic scissors
- Blunt tip bowel grasper
- Maryland dissector
- Linear vascular stapling device (for omental wrap)
- Suction-irrigator device
- Hem-o-lok® clip applier (Teleflex Medical, Research Triangle Park, NC)
- Vessiloop (Getz Bros, Chicago, IL)

Step-by-Step Technique

Step 1: Cystoscopy, Antegrade, and Retrograde Pyelography
We perform flexible cystoscopy and an open-ended ureteral stent is advanced up to the level of the stricture. A simultaneous retrograde pyelogram and antegrade nephrostogram is performed to delineate the length of the ureteral stricture. Then, a Sensor wire is advanced up the ureter to allow for easy access with a flexible ureteroscope.

Step 2: Trocar Placement, Exposure of Ureter, and Ureteroscopy (Table 13.12)

Trocar placement is performed as described for robotic ureterolysis. The colon is medialized, and the ureter is exposed and isolated. Careful dissection is continued to free the ureter proximal and distal to the area of stricture. Simultaneous ureteroscopy at the time of ureterolysis allows for identification of the distal extent of the stricture (Fig. 13.27). The near-infrared fluorescence modality of the da Vinci® Si™ allows visualization of the light of the ureteroscope [7]. If the ureteroscope can be maneuvered through the stricture, ureteroscopy can also identify the prox-imal extent of stricture. Otherwise, indocyanin green dye (ICG) can be injected intravenously, and the fluorescent lens can be used to evaluate ureteral perfusion to confirm the proximal margin of healthy tissue [8]. Both the proximal and distal ends of the ureteral stricture are marked with a stay suture (Fig. 13.28).

Step 3: Preparation of Graft Bed (Table 13.13)

The graft site is prepared by making an ureterotomy lengthwise through the previously demarcated stricture segment until healthy appearing normal caliber ureter is reached proximally and distally (Fig. 13.29a, b). We have performed both anterior and posterior ureterotomies for buccal mucosa graft onlay. It has not yet been determined whether one approach is advantageous over the other.

Step 4: Harvest of Buccal Mucosa Graft

BMG harvest from the ipsilateral cheek is performed in open fashion at the same time as the ureteral graft bed preparation. The size of the BMG harvest is generally 1–1.5 cm in width with the length specified by the length of the stricture. A self-retaining oral retractor is placed to maintain exposure of the cheek. Retraction sutures of 2-0 silk are placed inside the vermilion border, away from the lip and are lifted up by an assistant to expose the harvest site (Fig. 13.30). The intended graft site is marked with a marking pen, taking care to stay away from Stenson's duct near the second upper molar. The base of the site is infiltrated with 1% lidocaine with epinephrine for hydrodissection and hemostasis. The borders of the graft are incised with a scalpel, and the graft is raised using Dean or tenotomy scissors. Care is taken to leave the under-

Table 13.12 Trocar placement, exposure of ureter, and ureteroscopy: surgeon and assistant instrumentation

Surgeon instrumentation		Assistant instrumentation
Right arm	Left arm	
• Curved monopolar scissors	• Gyrus bipolar dissector	• Suction-irrigator
	• Maryland bipolar graspers	• Maryland graspers
Endoscope lens: 30° down		• Hem-o-lok® clip applier
		• Vessiloop

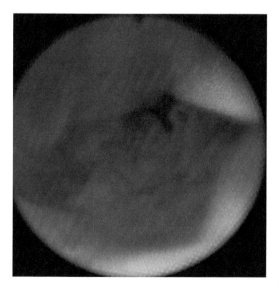

Fig. 13.27 Ureteroscopy is performed at the time of ureterolysis to identify the distal extent of stricture

Table 13.13 Preparation of graft bed: surgeon and assistant instrumentation

Surgeon instrumentation		Assistant instrumentation
Right arm	Left arm	
• Potts scissors	• Gyrus bipolar dissector	• Suction-irrigator
	• Maryland bipolar graspers	• Maryland graspers
Endoscope lens: 30° down		• Laparoscopic needle driver

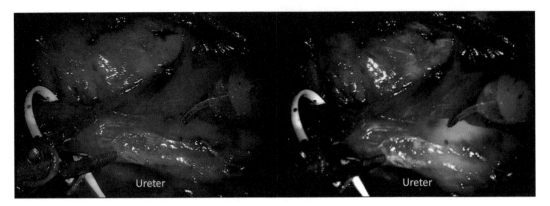

Fig. 13.28 The light of the ureteroscope is seen using the fluorescent lens of the da Vinci® Si™. The margins of the ureteral stricture are marked stay sutures

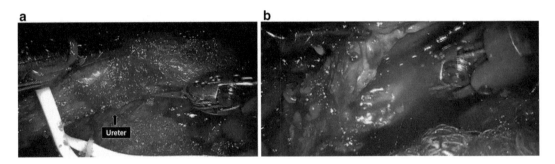

Fig. 13.29 (**a**, **b**) Ureterotomy is made with Potts scissors

lying tissue intact. A Yankauer suction is used to provide upward counter traction as the BMG is dissected down off the cheek. Once the BMG is harvested, the graft is thinned by removing the submucosal layer. The graft is then placed in normal saline until the recipient site is adequately prepared. Gauze is soaked with 1% lidocaine with epinephrine and placed into the cheek to assist with hemostasis. Prior to the end of the case, the graft harvest site is evaluated, and minimal cautery is used for hemostasis if necessary.

Step 5: Buccal Mucosa Graft Onlay and Omental Wrap

The BMG is then introduced into the abdomen through the assistant port (Fig. 13.31). The edges of the graft are sutured into the ureterotomy in running fashion using 4-0 polyglactin suture (Fig. 13.32a, b). Simultaneous evaluation with

the flexible ureteroscope allows visualization of the anastomosis from the ureteral lumen and allows for early recognition of misplacement of the suture into the back wall of the ureter. Once the anastomosis is complete, ureteroscopy confirms a patent and watertight anastomosis (Fig. 13.33). A guidewire is left in place in the ureter and a double J ureteral stent is placed in retrograde fashion. A urethral catheter is placed.

Step 6: Omental Wrap (Table 13.14)

Graft survival depends on adequate apposition of the graft to its blood supply. We frequently use a flap of omentum as the blood supply, as it is readily available, and easy to harvest. The omentum is prepared as previously described for omental wrap after ureterolysis. In patients with dorsal placement of the graft, an omental wrap is sutured in place dorsally, underlying the ureterotomy. In those with ven-

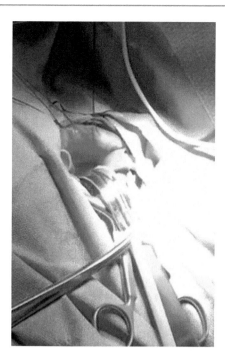

Fig. 13.30 Retraction sutures of 2-0 silk are placed inside the vermilion border, away from the lip and are lifted up by an assistant to expose the harvest site

Table 13.14 Omental wrap: surgeon and assistant instrumentation

Surgeon instrumentation		Assistant instrumentation
Right arm	Left arm	
• Curved monopolar scissors	• Gyrus bipolar dissector	• Suction-irrigator
	• Maryland bipolar graspers	• Atraumatic bowel grasper
Endoscope lens: 30° down		• Maryland graspers
		• Hem-o-lok® clip applier

Step 7: Exiting the Abdomen

The insufflation pressure is decreased and operative field is examined for bleeding. Hemostasis is obtained as needed. Instruments and trocars are removed under vision, and the port sites are closed with absorbable suture. The epinephrine soaked sponge is removed from the mouth and the buccal mucosa graft harvest site is reevaluated to ensure hemostasis.

Postoperative Management

An antiseptic mouthwash is administered postoperatively for improved donor site hygiene. Oral 20% benzocaine gel is used for analgesia of the buccal mucosa harvest site. The patient's diet is advanced as tolerated. If a nephrostomy tube is in place, this is left in place and capped. A drain creatinine is checked prior to Foley catheter removal at approximately 24–48 h postoperatively. If this is consistent with serum, the Foley catheter is removed. The drain creatinine is checked again after Foley removal and if it is consistent with serum, closed suction drain is removed prior to the patient's discharge home.

At 6 weeks after surgery, a retrograde or antegrade pyelogram is performed to confirm that there is no leak at the graft site prior to stent and nephrostomy tube removal. Subsequent surveillance includes renal ultrasound to evaluate for hydronephrosis after stent removal and diuretic renography at approximately 3 months to ensure the absence of obstruction.

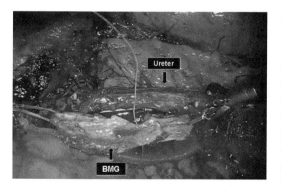

Fig. 13.31 The buccal mucosa graft is introduced into the abdomen

tral grafts, omentum or perirenal fat is sutured in placed over the graft after the graft is secured in the ureterotomy. The graft itself is also sutured to the omentum to maximize graft apposition to its new blood supply. A closed suction drain is placed adjacent to the anastomosis once omental or perirenal fat coverage is complete. If there is no omentum available, a flap of perirenal fat or the psoas muscle may be used to provide blood supply.

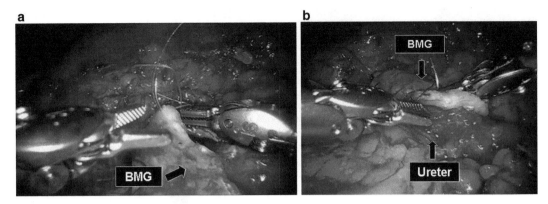

Fig. 13.32 (**a**, **b**)The buccal graft is sutured into the ureterotomy

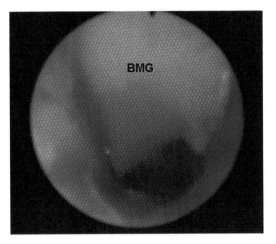

Fig. 13.33 Ureteroscopy demonstrates the anastomosis from the buccal mucosa graft to the ureter

Special Considerations

If there is an area of obliteration, excision of that segment may be performed as in a dismembered pyeloplasty. The posterior wall of the two segments then can be sutured together, leaving a diamond-shaped defect anteriorly onto which BMG can be placed as an onlay. This is analogous to the augmented anastomotic technique used in urethroplasty.

Steps to Avoid Complications

Wide spatulation to ensure the presence of healthy ureter at proximal and distal ends of the buccal mucosa graft onlay is important to avoid resteno-

sis of the ureter. Careful, watertight anastomosis of the graft to the graft recipient bed is needed to avoid urine leak which may cause inflammation and further scarring. Careful consideration of the blood supply to the graft and appropriate apposition of the graft to the blood supply must be achieved to allow for successful graft take.

Ureteral Reimplantation

Indications

We have performed this procedure in patients with congenital distal ureteral strictures, iatrogenic intraoperative distal ureteral injuries, and those requiring distal segmental resection for transitional cell carcinoma (TCC).

Patient Positioning and Preparation

The patient is positioned in a dorsal lithotomy position with steep Trendelenburg, similar to that of robotic prostatectomy.

Trocar Configuration

Five trocars are used as follows. A 12 mm trocar at the umbilicus, two 8 mm trocars to the left, one just lateral to the umbilicus in the midclavicular line and the other one, 2 cm superior to umbilicus in the anterior axillary line. To the right of the umbilicus we place an 8 mm trocar lateral to umbilicus in midclavicular line and a 5 mm assistant trocar above and between these two trocars (Fig. 13.3). The da Vinci® is then brought between the patient's legs.

Instrumentation and Equipment List

Equipment

- da Vinci® Si Surgical HD System (three- or four-arm system; Intuitive Surgical, Inc., Sunnyvale, CA)
- EndoWrist® PK dissector (Intuitive Surgical, Inc., Sunnyvale, CA)
- EndoWrist® curved monopolar scissors (Intuitive Surgical, Inc., Sunnyvale, CA)
- EndoWrist® ProGrasp™ forceps (Intuitive Surgical, Inc., Sunnyvale, CA)
- EndoWrist® Potts scissors (Intuitive Surgical, Inc., Sunnyvale, CA)
- EndoWrist® needle drivers (2) (Intuitive Surgical, Inc., Sunnyvale, CA)
- InSite® Vision System with 0° and 30° lens (Intuitive Surgical, Inc., Sunnyvale, CA)

Trocars

- 12 mm trocars (1)
- 8 mm robotic trocars (3)
- 5 mm trocar (1)
- 8 mm SurgiQuest AirSeal® Access Port
- Applied gel trocar (Applied Surgical, LLC, Birmingham, AL)

Recommended Sutures

- 3-0 polyglactin suture on RB-1 or SH needle
- 2-0 polyglactin suture on SH needle for psoas hitch
- 4-0 Monocryl suture for anastomosis on RB-1 needle

Instruments Used by the Surgical Assistant

- Laparoscopic needle driver
- Laparoscopic scissors
- Suction-irrigator device
- Hem-o-lok® clip applier (Teleflex Medical, Research Triangle Park, NC)

Step-by-Step Technique

Step 1: Patient Positioning and Trocar Configuration

The patient is positioned in a similar fashion to a robotic prostatectomy, in dorsal lithotomy with steep Trendelenburg. Five trocars are used as described above. A 12 mm trocar at the umbilicus, two 8 mm trocars to the left, one just lateral to the umbilicus in the midclavicular line and the other one, 2 cm superior to umbilicus in the anterior axillary line. To the right of the umbilicus we place an 8 mm trocar lateral to umbilicus in midclavicular line and a 5 mm assistant trocar above and between these two trocars. The da Vinci® is then brought between the patient's legs.

Step 2: Exposure of Ureter (Table 13.15)

The posterior peritoneum is incised longitudinally at the level of the iliac vessels, and the ureter is identified and isolated with a Vessiloop (Getz Bros, Chicago, IL). The peritoneum is then incised over the ureter until the diseased segment is identified (Fig. 13.34). In cases where a segmental distal ureterectomy is planned, the ureter must be dissected all the way to the posterior bladder wall. In male patients not concerned with fertility, the vas deferens can be sacrificed to improve exposure. In women, the peritoneum is incised to the level of the ovary. The ovary and ovarian ligaments are retracted anteriorly allowing the ureter to be dissected posteriorly to the level of the bladder.

Step 3: Division of Ureter and Excision of Diseased Segment (Table 13.16)

The ureter is then transected just proximal to the diseased segment with curved monopolar scissors

Table 13.15 Exposure of ureter: surgeon and assistant instrumentation

Surgeon instrumentation		Assistant instrumentation
Right arm	Left arm	
• Curved monopolar scissors	• Gyrus bipolar dissector	• Suction-irrigator
	• Maryland bipolar graspers	• Vessiloop
Endoscope lens: 30° down		

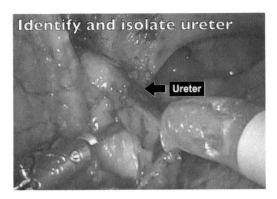

Fig. 13.34 Ureter is identified and isolated

Table 13.16 Division of ureter and excision of diseased segment: surgeon and assistant instrumentation

Surgeon instrumentation		Assistant instrumentation
Right arm	Left arm	
• Curved monopolar scissors	• Gyrus bipolar dissector	• Suction-irrigator
• Potts scissors	• Maryland bipolar graspers	• Vessiloop
• Needle driver	• Needle driver	• Laparoscopic Satinsky clamp
Endoscope lens: 30° down		• Hem-o-lok® clip applier

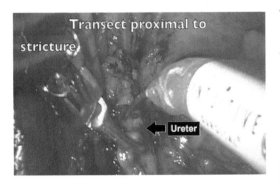

Fig. 13.35 Transecting ureter above diseased segment

and spatulated using a Potts scissors (Fig. 13.35). In patients undergoing distal ureterectomy for TCC, a Hem-o-lock® clip is placed to prevent spillage and the bladder cuff is isolated with a laparoscopic Satinsky clamp and oversewn with 3-0 polyglactin suture on either an RB-1 or SH needle.

Step 4: Mobilization of Bladder and Psoas Hitch (Table 13.17)

Next, the bladder is filled with 250 mL of normal saline, via the indwelling urethral catheter, and mobilized from the anterior abdominal wall, identical to the techniques used for robotic prostatectomy. The peritoneum is incised lateral to the medial umbilical ligament and the space of Retzius is entered and dissected to the pubic bone. The urachus is then transected allowing the space between the anterior abdominal wall and bladder to be developed (Fig. 13.36). Though rarely necessary, the contralateral superior bladder pedicle may be transected to increase bladder mobilization. Another technique to improve bladder mobilization is to incise the bladder horizontally and then stretch it vertically to the psoas muscle, similar to the Heineke-Mikulicz technique. In all cases, we perform a psoas hitch. We believe this minimizes tension at the anastomosis and keeps the path of the ureter lateral and away from bowel. We use 2-0 polyglactin suture on an SH needle to fix the posterior bladder wall to the psoas muscle

Table 13.17 *Mobilization of bladder and psoas hitch*: surgeon and assistant instrumentation

Surgeon instrumentation		Assistant instrumentation
Right arm	Left arm	
• Curved monopolar scissors	• Gyrus bipolar dissector	• Suction-irrigator
• Needle driver	• Maryland bipolar graspers	
	• Needle driver	
Endoscope lens: 30° down		

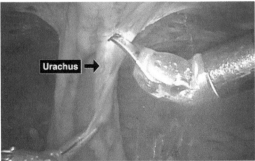

Fig. 13.36 Urachus being transected

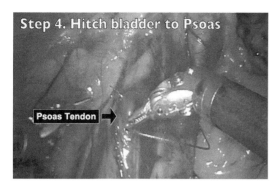

Fig. 13.37 Suture placed through psoas tendon

Table 13.18 *Creation of neocystostomy*: surgeon and assistant instrumentation

Surgeon instrumentation		Assistant instrumentation
Right arm	Left arm	
• Curved monopolar scissors	• Gyrus bipolar dissector	• Suction-irrigator
• Potts scissors	• Maryland bipolar graspers	
• Needle driver	• Needle driver	
Endoscope lens: 30° down		

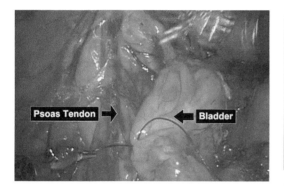

Fig. 13.38 Hitching bladder to psoas tendon

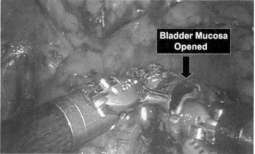

Fig. 13.39 Incision to open bladder mucosa

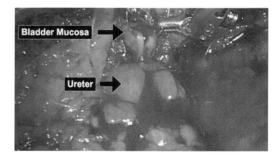

Fig. 13.40 Anastomosis between bladder and ureter

tendon after identifying and avoiding the genito-femoral nerve (Figs. 13.37 and 13.38).

Step 5: Creation of Neocystostomy (Table 13.18)

Next, a small area of the bladder is isolated at the lateral dome, and a 1.5 cm incision is made into the bladder wall and mucosa using Potts scissors (the bladder remains filled to help with this maneuver) (Fig. 13.39). With the bladder now opened and the ureter spatulated, an extravesical anastomosis is performed using 4-0 Monocryl sutures on an RB-1 needle in an interrupted fashion, ensuring proper mucosal apposition (Fig. 13.40). An ureteral stent is placed prior to completion of the anastomosis. After completing the mucosal anastomosis, the bladder is filled with 300 mL of normal saline, and the ureteral reimplantation site is assessed to verify that there is no leakage or tension. Additional sutures can be placed as necessary. A second anastomotic layer is performed with buttressing sutures between the serosa of the bladder and the adventitia of the ureter (Fig. 13.41). A closed-suction drain can be placed near the anastomosis through the most lateral trocars on the ipsilateral side (Fig. 13.42).

Step 6: Exiting the Abdomen

The operative site is examined for bleeding under low insufflation pressure and hemostasis achieved. The trocars are removed under laparoscopic view. The incisions are closed with absorbable suture.

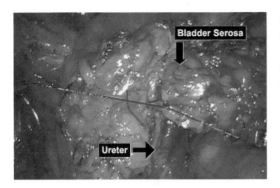

Fig. 13.41 Second closure layer of ureteral reimplantation

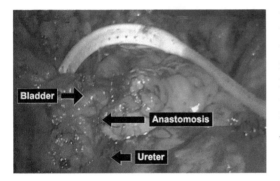

Fig. 13.42 Final anastomosis and drain placement

Postoperative Management

Patients typically remain in the hospital for 1–2 days. On the first postoperative day, patients begin a clear diet, aggressive ambulation, and oral pain medication. The JP fluid can be sent for creatinine analysis to rule out a urine leak, prior to removal. The patient is discharged, and the urethral catheter remains indwelling for 10–14 days and is removed in the office after a cystogram has documented no leak. The stent is removed with a local office cystoscopy in 4–6 weeks, and appropriate imaging studies are obtained thereafter.

Special Considerations

As discussed above, mobilizing the bladder to ensure a tension-free anastomosis is essential to ensuring a successful reconstruction. Either a refluxing or non-refluxing anastomosis can be made into the bladder. If a non-refluxing anasto-

mosis is desired, a longer submucosal tunnel can be made prior to reimplanting the ureter into the bladder mucosa. Non-refluxing anastomoses, however, are more technically challenging and have increased risk of stricture formation.

Steps to Avoid Complications

As has been discussed above for the other reconstructive procedures, ensuring a tension-free, secure anastomosis is paramount to the success of this operation. To that end, wide ureteral spatulation and apposition of ureteral and bladder mucosa will help prevent stricture and urine leakage from the anastomosis. Furthermore, athermal technique, via sharp dissection is essential to avoid potential compromise of the blood supply to the already diseased distal ureter, which can develop into an ischemic urine leak. We also support the judicious use of perivesical fat to help protect the anastomosis; this can be a third layer of closure.

References

1. Wong C, Leveillee RJ. Hand-assisted laparoscopic nephroureterectomy with cystoscopic en bloc excision of the distal ureter and bladder cuff. J Endourol Endourol Soc. 2002;16(6):329–32; discussion 332–3.
2. Naude JH. Buccal mucosal grafts in the treatment of ureteric lesions. BJU Int. 1999;83(7):751–4.
3. Agrawal V, Dassi V, Andankar MG. Buccal mucosal graft onlay repair for a ureteric ischemic injury following a pyeloplasty. Indian J Urol IJU J Urol Soc India. 2010;26(1):120–2.
4. Badawy AA, Abolyosr A, Saleem MD, Abuzeid AM. Buccal mucosa graft for ureteral stricture substitution: initial experience. Urology. 2010;76(4):971–5; discussion 975.
5. Kroepfl D, Loewen H, Klevecka V, Musch M. Treatment of long ureteric strictures with buccal mucosal grafts. BJU Int. 2010;105(10):1452–5.
6. Sadhu S, Pandit K, Roy MK, Bajoria SK. Buccal mucosa ureteroplasty for the treatment of complex ureteric injury. Indian J Surg. 2011;73(1):71–2.
7. Hockenberry MS, Smith ZL, Mucksavage P. A novel use of near-infrared fluorescence imaging during robotic surgery without contrast agents. J Endourol Endourol Soc. 2014;28(5):509–12.
8. Bjurlin MA, Gan M, McClintock TR, Volpe A, Borofsky MS, Mottrie A, et al. Near-infrared fluorescence imaging: emerging applications in robotic upper urinary tract surgery. Eur Urol. 2014;65(4):793–801.

Robot-Assisted Retroperitoneal Lymph Node Dissection

14

Haidar M. Abdul-Muhsin, J. Joy Lee,
James R. Porter, and Erik P. Castle

Abbreviations

IMA	Inferior mesenteric artery
IVC	Inferior vena cava
LN	Lymph nodes
RARPLND	Robot-assisted retroperitoneal lymph node dissection

Patient Selection

The indications for robot-assisted retroperitoneal lymph node dissection (RARPLND) are the same as those for open retroperitoneal lymph node dissection. In the modern era, RPLND is performed in patients with stage IIC or III non-seminomatous germ cell tumors (NSGCT) with a resectable residual mass ≥1 cm in the post-chemotherapy setting with normal serum tumor markers. The role of RPLND as primary treatment in stage I

Electronic supplementary material: The online version of this chapter (doi:10.1007/978-3-319-45060-5_14) contains supplementary material, which is available to authorized users.

H.M. Abdul-Muhsin, M.B., Ch.B.
E.P. Castle, M.D., F.A.C.S. (✉)
Department of Urology, Mayo Clinic Hospital,
5779 E. Mayo Blvd, Phoenix, AZ 85054, USA
e-mail: Castle.Erik@mayo.edu

J.J. Lee, M.D. • J.R. Porter, M.D.
Department of Urology, Swedish Medical Center,
Seattle, WA, USA

NSGCT, whether due to patient noncompliance or adverse pathologic features, as well as the timing of RPLND in stage IIA and IIB NSGCT, remains a source of active discussion. Regardless, the morbidity of open RLND with a "sternum to pubis" incision is a significant consideration for patients, many of whom are otherwise completely healthy active young men in their 20–30s. Initial series of laparoscopic RPLND were criticized for lower lymph node yields as well as higher utilization of adjuvant chemotherapy, but with more experience, subsequent series have demonstrated comparable lymph node counts. The refinement of minimally invasive RARPLND has allowed for equivalent oncologic efficacy, decreased blood loss, faster recovery, and shorter length of stay in the hospital compared to open RPLND.

Preoperative Preparation

All patients should undergo a thorough preoperative cardiopulmonary evaluation, especially for the post-chemo RARPLND patients who may have previously received bleomycin chemotherapy. A bowel preparation with one bottle of magnesium citrate can be given depending on surgeon preference (although in our practice we do not perform bowel preparation), and patients are asked to adhere to a clear liquid diet the day before surgery. Patients are counseled that despite the magnification afforded by the da Vinci operating system, complications such as nerve damage resulting in anejaculation, chylous ascites, vascular and bowel injuries may still occur. Perioperatively, subcutaneous heparin or low molecular weight heparin is given, and knee-high sequential compression devices are placed. A parenteral broad-spectrum antibiotic such as cefazolin is given 30 min prior to incision. An orogastric tube and urethral catheter are placed.

Operative Setup

The operating room setup during RARPLND is unique in that there will be bed movement and unconventional positioning of the robotic cart/platform. In general, the largest possible operating room is preferred. Our recommended room setup is demonstrated in Fig. 14.1. The assistant stands on the patient right side whereas as the scrub nurse stands on the left side. A Mayo stand is placed between patient legs to set up laparoscopic and robotic instruments. The robot is brought in from the patient head and docked over the left shoulder (please see patient positioning section). The anesthesia team will still be able to access the airway and patient lines from the right side of the body. At least two monitors are needed and placed in front of the assistant and the scrub nurse. Although vascular emergencies are not common in RARPLND, the whole surgical team should be ready for urgent open conversion and the open surgical instruments should be available inside the operating room. Open instruments to have immediately available should include a vascular set and appropriate retractors. The console should be placed inside the operating room itself rather than in a remote location outside the operating room in order to ensure direct and clear communication. The console surgeon should be ready to switch to laparoscopy or open surgery if needed.

Patient Positioning

Proper and safe patient positioning is of extreme importance in RARPLND. Most of these cases place the patient in a nonphysiological body position and can sometimes require a long operative times especially in post-chemotherapy patients. The patient is placed in low lithotomy, maximal Trendelenburg position with the left shoulder tilted downward (approximately 30°) as shown in Fig. 14.2. Placing the patient in this position will facilitate exposure as gravity will retract the bowel to the left upper quadrant of the abdomen. The patient should be secured to the table using 3-in. silk tape across the chest. The patient position should be tested prior to draping to ensure patient safety and stability on the table.

Si postition

With the new robotic platform, the nurse and the bed side assistant can stand on the right side of the patient and the robot come from the left side for side-docking where the boom can be rotated to direct the instruments towards the head.

Given the lengthy nature of the procedure it is of paramount importance to pay special attention to pressure point padding in order to decrease the chances of neuropraxia, rhabdomyolysis, and compartment syndrome. Padding can be done with gel pads, eggcrate foams, or rolled sheets and blankets. The head should be secured in a neutral position with a head rest on the left side in order to avoid neck flexion once the patient is tilted. Arms are tucked by the sides and the legs are spread and fixed. The peroneal nerve on the "down-side" is prone to compression and the surgical team should try to have the legs relatively extended without full extension. This area should be padded as well as the medial side of the right leg. This will provide space in between legs to place a Mayo stand as discussed above and more importantly will prevent clashing of the third robotic arm with the legs.

Trocar Configuration

The pneumoperitoneum is established using a Veress needle technique. However, a Hasson technique can be used if intra-abdominal adhesions are expected from previous surgery.

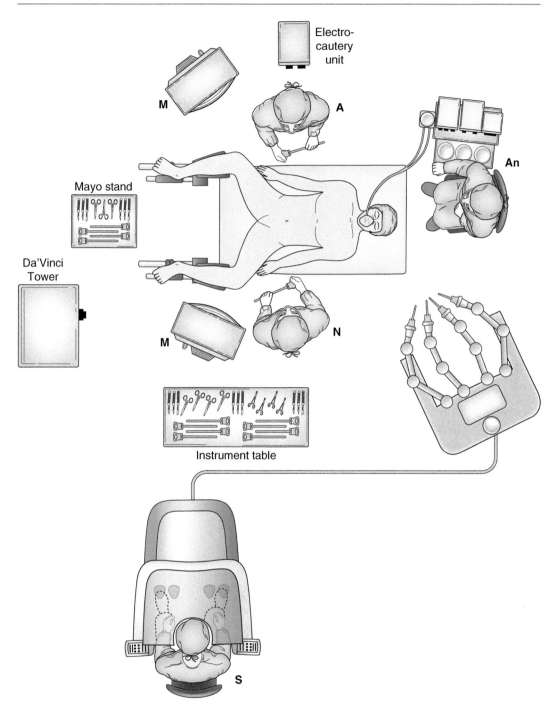

Fig. 14.1   Operating room setup

Establishing pneumoperitoneum can be performed while the patient is still in neutral position. However, trocar placement is best performed after changing to Trendelenburg position to move the bowel away and minimize the chances of injury. The trocar location varies based on surgical preference and several approaches have been described based on the template of dissection. However, when a full bilateral template is planned, we usually use the following template

Fig. 14.2 Patient positioning

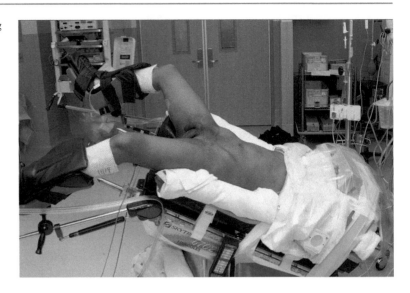

(Fig. 14.3) and trocar insertion takes place in the following order:

1. A 12-mm trocar is placed 3–4 cm below the umbilicus for the robotic camera. In order to avoid inadvertent injury in this infraumbilical access, the bladder should be actively drained. Once the trocar is inserted, a 0° camera should be used to visualize the peritoneal cavity and guide the rest of trocar placement under direct vision.
2. Two 8-mm robotic trocars are then placed under direct vision on either side of the camera trocar. These are placed along the same horizontal line and one hand breadth from the camera on each side. These will be used for the first and the second robotic arms on the right and left side, respectively. Extra-long (bariatric) trocars should always be used.
3. The third robotic arm trocar is then placed in the left upper abdomen approximately 1–2 cm above the level of the umbilicus at the left anterior axillary line.
4. A 15-mm assistant trocar is placed in the right lower abdomen approximately 2–3 cm supero-medial to the right anterior superior iliac spine.
5. An optional 5-mm assistant trocar is placed in a mirrored location to the third robotic trocar but in the right side of the abdomen.

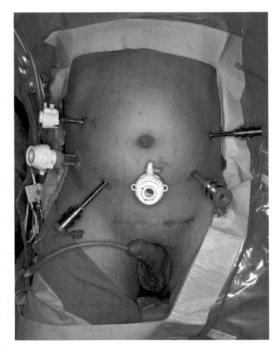

Fig. 14.3 Trocar locations

Instrumentation List (Table 14.1)

- 0 Polyglactin suture on a CT needle for retraction stitches
- Multiple 3-0 silk ties (4 in.) for lumbar vessel ligation

Table 14.1 Robot-assisted retroperitoneal lymph node dissection: surgeon and assistant instrumentation

Surgeon instrumentation			
Arm 1	Arm 2	Arm 3	Assistant Instrumentation
• Curved monopolar scissors	• Maryland bipolar grasper	• Prograsp dissector	• Laparoscopic Suction-Irrigator
• Needle driver	• Needle driver		• Laparoscopic blunt tip grasper
	• Hem-o-lock® clip applier		• Laparoscopic needle driver
			• Laparoscopic scissors
	• Robotic vessel sealer		• Laparoscopic vessel sealing device (LigaSure™)
			• Hem-o-lock® clip applier
			• Laparoscopic vascular stapler (Endo-GIA 30-2.5)
			• Reusable specimen retrieval bag

- Multiple 5-0 polypropylene on a c-1 needle sutures (6 in.) for vascular injury repairs
- Small abdominal laps/sponges to be used intra-abdominally
- Multiple vessel loops to retract and occlude vessels
- Multiple Hem-o-lock® clips of different sizes: ML (green), L (purple), and XL (gold)

Step-by-Step Technique (Videos 14.1, 14.2, 14.3, 14.4, 14.5, and 14.6)

We would like to highlight the following general principles:

- It is extremely important to be completely familiar with the patient's retroperitoneal anatomy.
- Meticulous examination of the preoperative imaging is important to ensure absence of congenital anomalies of the blood vessels or urinary system.
- The location and size of the retroperitoneal lymph nodes/masses should be taken into consideration to plan dissection.
- The rationale, merits, and indications of modified templates of dissection are beyond the scope of this chapter. However, familiarity with the boundaries of these templates is

extremely important. The boundaries of dissection are as follows:

1. Full bilateral template: This extends from the right to left ureters and from the level of renal vessels superiorly to the bifurcation of the common iliac vessels inferiorly (Fig. 14.4).
2. Right modified template: This template spares the lymphatic tissue below the level of the IMA on the contralateral side (Fig. 14.5).
3. Left modified template: This template spares the lymphatic tissue below the level of the IMA and lateral to the IVC (Fig. 14.6).
- During all the steps of vascular dissection the principles of vascular proximal and distal control with a vessel loop should be respected and applied as early as possible to promptly control bleeding early in the surgeon's experience. Once a vessel is circumferentially dissected, a vessel loop is passed around it twice and a Hem-o-lock® is applied at the free end of the loop. This will fix the loop in place. If bleeding is encountered in that vessel, the loop can be used to control the vessel. This is most commonly performed on the IVC and allows for retraction of the IVC and exposure of the posterior structures (Fig. 14.7). While lumbar veins can be controlled by a variety of ways including clips, we feel strongly that the best way to control the lumbar veins is with free silk ties as one would

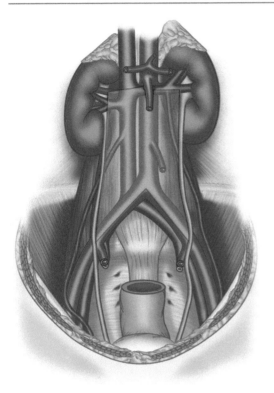

Fig. 14.4 Full bilateral templates

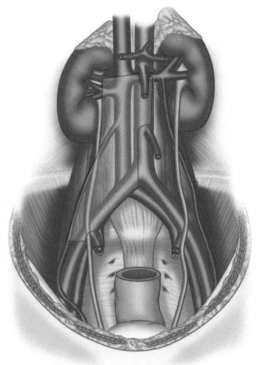

Fig. 14.5 Right modified template

do in open surgery. This avoids inadvertent dislodging of clips or delayed bleeding from a sealed vein. However, small branches can be controlled with the vessel sealing device.

- The assistant should be an experienced laparoscopic surgeon.
- An orogastric tube is inserted to completely deflate the stomach. A urethral catheter should be inserted to monitor urine output and to deflate the bladder. Of note, the mere insertion of a urethral catheter will not completely drain the bladder when the patient is in Trendelenburg. Thus, the bladder is actively drained with a 60 mL syringe to avoid any injury during trocar placement in the lower abdomen.

Step 1: Bowel Retraction and Suspension Stitches

One of the most helpful nuances that were developed during the evolution of this technique are the suspension stitches. Once the robot is docked,

the bowel is retracted toward the upper abdomen and a wide U shaped incision is made in the posterior peritoneum below the bifurcation of the great vessels. This incision is the same one that is performed during open RPLND and is started caudal to the cecum and appendix and extended medially to the root of the small bowel mesentery. The peritoneum is then lifted off the underlying great vessels and space is dissected as superiorly as possible. This will be done by lifting the peritoneum with the left hand and blunt dissection will be done with the back of the scissors on the right hand. It should be noted that the IMA can be divided with impunity without any sequelae in this young group of patients if this will facilitate para-aortic dissection. Ligation of the IMA is usually done in post-chemotherapy cases in order to perform a thorough para-aortic dissection; it greatly facilitates the mobilization of the peritoneum and retraction of the bowel and mesentery. The free edge of the peritoneum is then sutured to the anterior abdominal wall at multiple locations using 0 polyglactin on a CT needle, Fig. 14.8. This will help keep the bowel

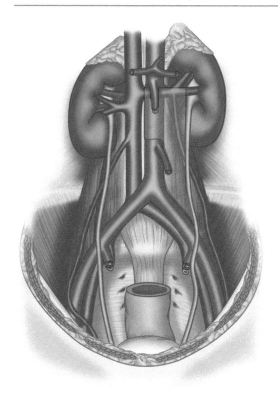

Fig. 14.6 Left modified template

artery is first identified along with the right ureter, which serves as the right and the lowermost border of the dissection. All LN tissue cephalad to the common iliac vessels is mobilized, "split," and "rolled" toward the head as we dissect toward the renal hilum (Fig. 14.10). The assistant will help retract the ureter laterally and maintains a dry field with suction. There is often a small vein (s) that comes off the anterior surface of the IVC just superior to the bifurcation and feeds into the lymph node packet. It can be controlled with a vessel sealer or suture ligated with a 5-0 polypropylene. The anterior surface of the IVC is devoid of nervous tissue and it is safe to use electrocautery to split the lymphatic tissue during this part of the dissection. However, care should be taken in any dissection posterolateral to the IVC since the ganglia and nerves may be encountered. During this step, the gonadal vessels are identified and ligated at their origin from the great vessels. The dissection is carried up to the right renal vessels where we carefully mobilize all tissue anterior to the right renal vein and posterior to the right renal artery.

retracted in the upper abdomen and prevent its fall in the surgical field during later dissection as shown in Fig. 14.9. Care should be taken to avoid injury to the bowel and the epigastric vessels when these sutures are placed. A small abdominal lap should be inserted and used to pack the uppermost part of the retroperitoneum where the duodenum is commonly encountered to avoid injury to the duodenum during retraction.

Step 2: Paracaval Lymph Node Dissection

The border of this LN packet extends from the right ureter laterally to an imaginary line along the middle of inferior vena cava (IVC) medially and from where the ureter crosses the common iliac artery inferiorly to the right renal vein superiorly. The dissection is carried out in a caudal to cephalic direction, using the "split and roll" technique. The bifurcation of the right common iliac

Step 3: Inferior Vena Cava Mobilization

One of the key steps to ensure completion of a good LN dissection is complete mobilization of the IVC. This will give access to lymphatic tissue behind the IVC which can harbor cancer and give access to the sympathetic trunk and postganglionic fibers that need to be spared in a nerve-sparing procedure. Once proximal and distal control is obtained as illustrated previously, mobilization should be carefully performed and all lumbar veins should be identified, controlled, and divided. We strongly recommend controlling these vessels as one would do in open surgery using permanent silk ties with surgical knots. The delicate wristed robotic instrument will allow the surgeon to do this rather than risk avulsion of a clip applied by the assistant. Hemorrhage from lumbar vessels can be bothersome and difficult to control. The IVC can be gently lifted using the

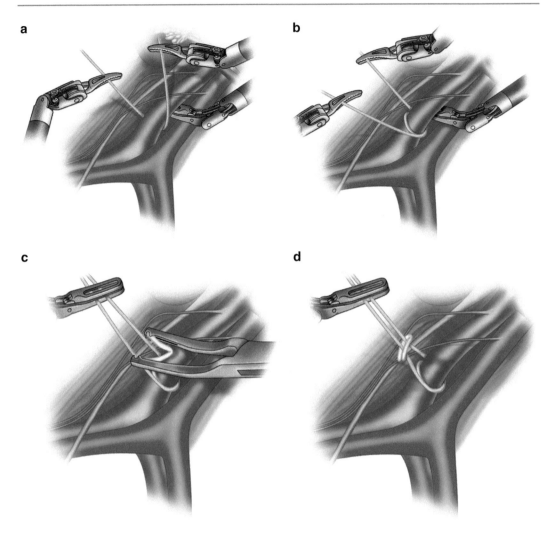

Fig. 14.7 (**a**) Passing loop behind a dissected vessel; (**b**) another pass to encircle the vessel; (**c**) applying a Hem-o-lock®; (**d**) sliding the Hem-o-lock® clip in case of bleeding

third robotic arm while these ties are placed (Fig. 14.11). Once all lumbar vessels are ligated, the IVC can be retracted using the vessel loop (Fig. 14.12). Retrocaval tissue is then completely mobilized and removed with the LN packet. The sympathetic chain is identified and preserved. Prior to removing the lymphatic tissue, the distal postganglionic fibers should have been identified in the interaortocaval region and below the IMA. By identifying this area the surgeon can appreciate the course of the fibers and avoid inadvertent division during dissection of the lymphatic tissue.

Step 4: Interaortocaval Lymph Node Dissection

This is located between two imaginary lines at the mid portions of the IVC on the right side and the aorta on the left side. The dissection during this step starts at the bifurcation of the aorta for a full template, or the IMA for a modified template. It is important to identify the nerve fibers at the aortic bifurcation first (where it is most easy to identify) and split and roll them in a cephalic direction. During this step of the procedure one should be mindful of the right gonadal artery

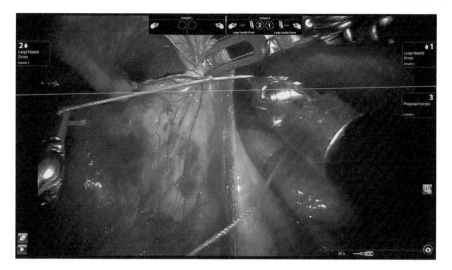

Fig. 14.8 Suspension stitches

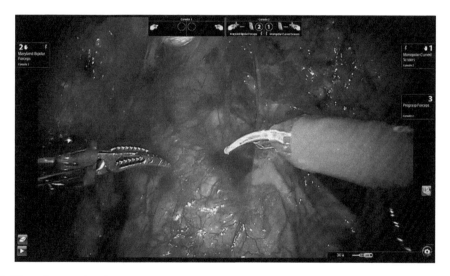

Fig. 14.9 View of retracted peritoneum

when working cephalad in the interaortocaval region where this artery crosses the interaortocaval field from its origin from the aorta toward the right internal ring (Fig. 14.13). The dissection then continues superiorly to the level of the right renal artery. It is important to use Hem-o-lock® clips while cutting lymphatic tissue in the upper most part of this field to prevent chylous ascites. The clips in this area should be applied by the robotic console surgeon using the robotic clip applier. Meticulous and accurate placement is key to avoid injury to the right renal artery and the surrounding nerve tissue.

Step 5: Para-aortic Lymph Node Dissection

We then move to the para-aortic LN packets. In some cases, the dissection can be carried to the left ureter and lateral to the aorta from the right side to the left side, especially if the IMA is ligated and divided. Similar to the paracaval dissection, the left ureter and common iliac vessels are identified and then split and rolled to free the LN tissue inferiorly. Using the left ureter as the lateral border, the dissection is carried superiorly and medially around the aorta to free up any

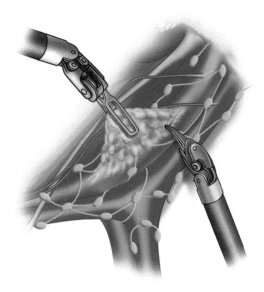

Fig. 14.10 Dissection of the paracaval lymph nodes

remaining retro-aortic tissue. The gonadal vessels are identified, traced to their origins at the aorta and left renal vein, and ligated. Lumbar vessels are ligated with silk ties and divided. The superior aspect of this dissection is the left renal vessels. It is important to remember that it has been reported that adequate dissection around the

left lumbar vein and renal vein has been a problem in laparoscopic and open series. Therefore, meticulous dissection by ligating and dividing the left lumbar vein and removing all lymphatic tissue here is critical. Locking clips should also be used superiorly to seal all lymphatics.

Step 6: Remnant of Cord Excision

The da'Vinci-Xi system allows operating on multiple abdominal quadrants and obviates the need to redock the robot to perform this step. If the new system is not available, the remnant of the cord can be resected either by redocking the robot between the patient legs or more easily through a simple laparoscopic approach to minimize reposition of the patient during the procedure. Redocking the robot should not be avoided if the surgeon feels that conducting a certain surgical step is better done robotically. This is specifically important if a vascular injury is encountered where it will be extremely challenging to control it laparoscopically.

The most distal part of the cord should be identified. If radical orchiectomy was properly

Fig. 14.11 Controlling lumbar vessels while the third arm retracts the IVC

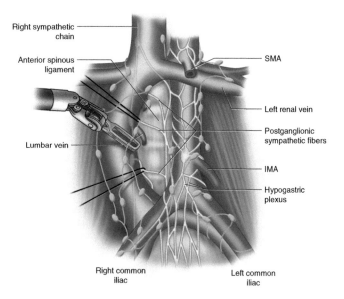

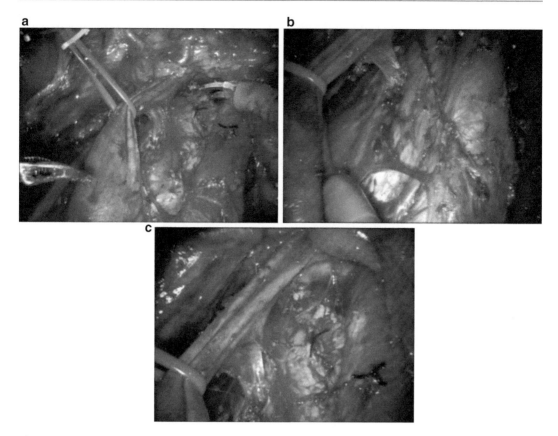

Fig. 14.12 (**a-c**) IVC retracted with the vessel loop

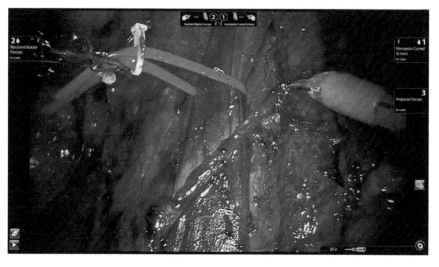

Fig. 14.13 Gonadal artery crossing the interaortocaval region

performed, there should be a permanent suture to mark the distal end of the resected cord. However, surgeons should not completely rely on this as sometimes it is absent and the cord should be dissected as far as possible. In some cases, a re-opening of the inguinal incision is required to completely remove the residual cord structures.

Special Considerations

Preoperative care

- Post-chemotherapy patients may have a compromised pulmonary function due to bleomycin administration. Preoperative medical evaluation to ensure fitness for surgery and pulmonary function testing can help better evaluate their risk. No bowel preparation is needed prior to surgery. Standard preoperative deep venous thrombosis prophylaxis with a single preoperative dose of low molecular weight heparin is given along with elastic stockings and sequential compression devices. A single intravenous dose of prophylactic antibiotic is given at time of induction. Two units of blood are typed and screened in the event bleeding is encountered.
- Postoperatively, autonomic dysreflexia is not uncommonly encountered especially in non-nerve-sparing RARPLNDs and this may result in confusion with postoperative tachycardia secondary to hypovolemia. This condition is usually short-lived and self-limited, and supportive care is all that is needed. Of note, assisted ambulation is important to avoid falls as patients may feel dizzy with autonomic dysreflexia. A β-blocker can be administered in severe cases.

If volume replacement is warranted, colloidal solutions such as blood and albumin can be used instead of crystalloids to avoid pulmonary edema. This is particularly important in patients who previously had chemotherapy and have compromised pulmonary function. However, this is all based on the open literature and has not been experienced in our series, as there are not significant needs for volume replacement from third-spacing since the abdomen was not opened. In most cases, the amount of intraoperative fluid administered is approximately 2 L. A high index of suspicion should be maintained for postoperative manifestations of vascular, bowel, and nerve injury as well as postoperative compartment syndrome. Early ambulation is of paramount importance and is generally not challenging for most of the patients in the immediate postoperative period. Required analgesics are usually minimal and most patients can be discharged home safely on the first postoperative day.

Common Complications and Steps to Avoid Them

- Vascular injuries are always a potential complication in any surgery around these structures. Certain steps can be undertaken to help control bleeding when a vascular injury is encountered. The pneumoperitoneal pressure can be increased to 20 mmHg which will decrease the venous bleeding and enable the surgeon to visualize and repair the injury. The insertion of a small abdominal lap can help apply pressure with the third arm to minimize blood loss. The assistant may play an important role in these situations. In order to avoid collapse of abdominal wall and complete loss of pneumoperitoneum, intermittent rather than continuous suction should be used. Vascular repair can be performed using 6 in. of 5-0 polypropylene sutures as indicated. This should be done carefully to avoid tears in the wall of the vein during the repair. It is important to examine the injury after repair with low pneumoperitoneal pressures.
- Neuropraxia is one of the most commonly encountered complications after any procedure with extreme positioning. It is extremely important to ensure careful and good padding of all pressure points. If the remnant of the cord is to be resected laparoscopically, the patient can be taken off lithotomy position to decrease the pressure applied to the calves and inner thighs. It is of paramount importance to be aware of the operating room time. The most common factors associated with compartment

syndrome or positioning complications are OR time and obesity. If the procedure has gone beyond 4 or 5 h, one should consider conversion or at least temporarily taking the patient out of Trendelenburg. Vigilant neurovascular checks of the lower and upper extremities are critical early in the surgeon's experience to promptly identify any compartment syndrome and avoid significant complications.

• Bowel injuries: Although not a common complication in RARPLND, bowel injuries can be devastating. The suspension stitches mentioned earlier can help retract bowel at the beginning of the case, but one should be careful with electrocautery application near the peritoneum and off-field movements as energy may be transmitted and result in delayed bowel injury.

• Ureteric injury: The ureter should be handled with care, and skeletonizing the ureter should be avoided as this can result in ischemic damage. If an intraoperative injury is identified, it should be primarily repaired and the ureter should be stented.

Complications and Management of Robotic Assisted Partial Nephrectomy

Brandon J. Otto and Li-Ming Su

Introduction

The rate of postoperative complications following robotic assisted partial nephrectomy (RAPN; Video 15.1) has been reported to range from 5.1 to 33% with major (Clavien ≥3) complications occurring in 1.6–8.2% of patients. The rate of intraoperative complications at the time of RAPN ranges from 0 to 6.5% [1–7]. Refer to Table 15.1 for additional information about published complication rates and grades. This chapter will aim to discuss the causes, prevention, and management of the more common types of intraoperative and postoperative complications of RAPN.

Intraoperative Complications

Hemorrhage from Resection Bed

One of the more common and challenging complications of RAPN is intraoperative hemorrhage from the resection bed. This complication arises

Electronic supplementary material: The online version of this chapter (doi:10.1007/978-3-319-45060-5_15) contains supplementary material, which is available to authorized users.

B.J. Otto, M.D. (✉) • L.-M. Su, M.D.
Department of Urology, University of Florida College of Medicine, 1600 SW Archer Road, 100247, Gainesville, FL 32610-2047, USA
e-mail: Brandon.otto@urology.ufl.edu
URL: http://Li-Ming.Su@urology.ufl.edu

from inadequate or improper control of the renal vessels, which can result in poor operative visualization, increased risk of tumor violation and positive margins, urine leak, and conversion to open surgery or radical nephrectomy. Hemorrhage can result from either arterial bleeding and/or venous back bleeding, each of which presents unique challenges in management.

Prior to performing a RAPN it is imperative to review all available cross-sectional imaging to study the details of both the renal artery and vein as well as duplicates when present. This includes reviewing both axial and coronal images as both sets of images can provide nuances of the renal vascular anatomy and proximity to surrounding structures such as the collecting system as well as the tumor. Approximately 25% of patients have more than one renal artery. These arteries may be duplicates that have a similar caliber or they may be an accessory artery with a smaller caliber. Accessory arteries usually arise from the aorta and supply the poles. Right renal vein duplication is found in approximately 15–20% of cases, and it is infrequently duplicated on the left. Accessory renal veins are uncommon [8].

We routinely identify and skeletonize all renal arteries in preparation for clamping prior to tumor resection. Having a thorough understanding of the renal arterial "road map" from careful review of preoperative cross-sectional imaging is imperative so as to avoid unexpected arterial bleeding from a missed arterial vessel at the time of tumor excision. The authors strongly advise

Table 15.1 Comparison of RAPN complication rates

Study	No Pts	Intra-op	Conversions	Complications	Low grade	High grade
Tanagho 2013	886	23 (2.6%)	7 (0.8%)	115 (13%)	107 (12%)	33 (3.7%)
Dulabon 2010	446	NR	10 (2.2%)	23 (5.1%)	16 (3.6%)	7 (1.6%)
Benway 2010	183	NR	2 (1.1%)	18 (9.8%)	3 (1.6%)	15 (8.2%)
Scoll 2010	100	NR	2 (2.0%)	11 (11%)	5 (5.0%)	6 (6.0%)
Ellison 2012	108	7 (6.5%)	NR	36 (33.3%)	40 (37%)	8 (7.4%)
Long 2012	199	6 (3.0%)	2 (1.0%)	64 (32.2%)	53 (26.6%)	11 (5.5%)
Benway 2009	129	0 (0%)	2 (1.6%)	11 (8.5%)	1 (0.8%)	10 (7.8%)

NR not reported

that a complete arterial clamping technique be used early in one's experience as segmental arterial clamping often leads to more bleeding from adjacent areas of the kidney that remain perfused. However, with experience, a segmental arterial clamping technique can be selectively utilized based upon tumor size, location (e.g., polar vs midpole; exophytic vs endophytic vs mesophytic), proximity to adjacent structures (e.g., collecting system, hilar vessels), and overall tumor complexity. Another potential reason for arterial bleeding during tumor resection is due to inadequate coaptation of the artery by the laparoscopic bulldog clamps. This may be from incorporation of nearby adipose and connective tissue within the clamp or renal ostial calcifications, both of which may lead to incomplete occlusion of the artery by the bulldog clamp. This emphasizes the importance of prospectively skeletonizing the arteries down to the renal arterial adventitia as well as looking for the presence of renal ostial calcifications on preoperative imaging and clamping the vessel in a portion absent of calcifications. Furthermore, studies in porcine and human cadaver models have shown that differences in occlusion capabilities exist both within and between different laparoscopic bulldog clamps. In general, occlusion pressures are highest at the most proximal position on the clamp and lowest at the distal tip of the clamp. In addition, occlusive forces may decrease with increased duration of use [9, 10]. As a result of this, we routinely place two bulldog clamps on each artery to ensure adequate occlusion of blood flow.

Venous bleeding can also complicate RAPN. The influence of clamping the artery alone or the artery and the vein on renal function remains controversial in the literature [11–13]. The authors do not routinely clamp the renal vein during RAPN based upon the theoretical benefit that retrograde venous blood flow may provide partial oxygenation to the kidney; however, if excessive venous back bleeding is noted, a subsequent bulldog clamp is placed on the vein at that time. In our experience, the need to clamp the renal vein is uncommon in peripherally located tumors versus those located near the larger venous branches in the renal hilum. Perhaps paradoxically, in cases where the renal vein is clamped from the start and there is excessive venous back bleeding, we routinely unclamp the renal vein to allow venous blood to drain from the kidney which often decreases the bleeding at the resection bed. Taken together, the authors strongly recommend that all arteries and veins to the affected kidney be identified and skeletonized in preparation for clamping prior to tumor excision as attempts at identification and dissection of these vessels once bleeding occurs from the resection bed can be time-consuming and hazardous. Vessel loops can be placed around each vessel for easy and quick identification and access in case of bleeding.

Adjacent Organ Injury

There are several potential intraoperative complications related to kidney exposure at the time of RAPN affecting the bowel, spleen, pancreas, liver amongst the many major organs adjacent to the kidney.

Bowel Injury

For left-sided RAPN the descending colon must be mobilized off the entire surface of the kidney. For right-sided RAPN the ascending colon requires less mobilization as it is usually displaced medially on the surface of the lower pole of the kidney; however, one often has to mobilize the duodenum to adequately expose the renal hilum. In a meta-analysis, colonic and small bowel injuries have been reported to occur in up to 1.5 and 0.6% of laparoscopic radical nephrectomies, respectively [14]. Tanagho and colleagues reported a 0.1% risk of bowel injury in their series of RAPN [1]. In order to reduce the risk of bowel injury either directly or through thermal spread, we routinely incised the line of Toldt two centimeters lateral to the edge of the colon during our initial dissection and subsequent mobilization. Additionally, bowel injuries can occur as instruments are passed into the abdomen. As such, it is important for the assistant to carefully pass instruments and to notify the surgeon of any issues with passage such as perceived resistance.

If an injury is noted intraoperatively, attempts can be made to repair the injury robotically. Small serosal injuries can often be managed with Lembert sutures as needed. A general surgery consultation should be considered for larger injuries. Fortunately, most injuries can be repaired by multilayer closure, rarely requiring bowel resection or diversion [15]. Missed bowel injuries often present in a delayed fashion and require multiple procedures to manage the injury [16]. As such having a heightened awareness of such injuries is prudent with immediate repair.

Splenic Injury

Splenic injury has been reported to occur in up to 1.3% of laparoscopic renal surgeries and up to 0.5% of RAPN series [1, 3, 14]. Prevention focuses on using gentle, blunt retraction of the spleen to minimize the risk of tearing the splenic capsule or injuring the spleen from direct, sharp injury. Complete mobilization of the spleen requires sharp dissection of its lateral attachments. The use of an oral gastric tube keeps the stomach decompressed which minimizes the risk of injury to the stomach while allowing the spleen to fall more medially as it is mobilized. Most capsular lacerations can be managed conservatively with the use of coagulation from a variety of energy sources (e.g., monopolar or bipolar electrocautery, argon beam electrocoagulation) or hemostatic agents [17, 18]. If the bleeding is not able to be controlled with the above methods and/or the injury is large, splenectomy may be necessary. However, the incidence of such an injury is rare as previously stated.

Pancreatic Injury

Pancreatic injuries are uncommon at the time of left-sided RAPN. They are reported to occur in <0.5% of left-sided laparoscopic upper tract procedures [19]. Prevention focuses on complete mobilization of the spleen and pancreas en bloc. If injury to the pancreas is recognized intraoperatively, a general surgery consultation should be obtained. Management usually consists of surgical repair of the injury if possible (e.g., laparoscopic stapling across the distal pancreas) and making the patient NPO, placing a nasogastric tube, total parenteral nutrition, somatostatin and percutaneous drainage. Delayed injuries often result in a patient presenting with abdominal pain, elevated serum amylase and lipase, and a fluid collection seen on imaging.

Diaphragmatic Injury

Diaphragmatic injuries have been reported in <1% of laparoscopic and robotic renal surgeries [1, 20]. During left-sided RAPN, the diaphragm can be injured during mobilization of the spleen or the upper pole of the kidney. For right-sided RAPN the diaphragm can be injured with mobilization of the liver. Judicious use of monopolar electrocautery while dissecting near the diaphragm is important as electrical transmission to the phrenic nerve can result in sudden contraction of the diaphragm with inadvertent sharp injury from nearby instrumentation. One should suspect an injury if they see billowing of the diaphragm. The anesthesiologist should be notified to monitor respiratory sounds and airway pressure. If recognized intraoperatively, the pleurotomy should be repaired with interrupted figure-of-eight sutures. Before final closure, air should be evacuated from the pleural cavity. This can be done with a laparoscopic suction device through the defect or by having anesthesia give a large inspiratory breath before securing the stitches [20]. A postoperative chest x-ray should be obtained to look for any evidence of a residual pneumothorax. If recognized postoperatively, a thoracostomy tube can be placed.

Hepatobiliary Injury

Hepatobiliary injuries have been reported in <1% of both laparoscopic upper tract surgeries and RAPN [1, 7, 21]. Minor tears of the capsule of the liver can either be observed or electrocautery can be used for hemostasis. Larger tears or injury to the parenchyma may require the argon beam coagulator to obtain hemostasis. Injuries to the gallbladder should prompt intraoperative consultation to a general surgeon for cholecystectomy. Similar to the spleen, the liver should be retracted with blunt force while using sharp dissection to release its lateral attachments.

Chylous Ascites

Chylous ascites is a rare but potential complication of predominately left-sided renal procedures as the ascending intestinal lymphatics that drain into the cisterna chyli travel in the para-aortic location. It occurs as a result of lymphatic leakage that usually results during dissection of the renal hilar vessels (in particular the renal artery) along the aorta. In the process of skeletonizing the left renal artery, perivascular lymphatics are often disrupted that may lead to lymphatic leak if not clipped and secured. If large lymphatics are encountered, they should be directly clipped as

electrocautery is generally insufficient at sealing lymphatic vessels. If chylous ascites develops postoperatively, it can usually be managed conservatively with a medium-chain triglyceride diet or total parenteral nutrition and somatostatin [22].

Vascular Injury

Vascular injuries can occur from inadvertent injury from Veress needle and trocar placement, sharp dissection, avulsion during dissection, thermal injury, and injury during robotic instrument exchange. Venous injuries are more common than arterial injuries.

For right-sided RAPN one should be aware of the location of the right gonadal vein and the right adrenal vein. The right gonadal vein drains directly into the inferior vena cava (IVC). Too much traction on the gonadal vein may cause it to tear at its junction with the IVC which can lead to copious venous bleeding. By keeping the dissection lateral to the right gonadal vein, this can help to minimize the chance of inadvertent injury. When performing a right-sided RAPN for an upper pole mass, it is important to be careful when dissecting near the adrenal gland as the right adrenal vein is short and drains directly into the posterolateral IVC. Such an injury can be difficult to control if the adrenal vein is avulsed flush with the IVC. Attempts at clipping or suturing the vena cava can be complicated. As such often applying pressure to the site of bleeding with prompt and temporary elevation of the intra-abdominal pressure can help the bleeding subside. Oxidized cellulose gauze may be placed as an adjunctive measure; however, prevention is the key to minimizing this complication. Finally, one must be careful when dissecting around the IVC as it is less robust than the aorta and more likely to be injured. In the event of a venotomy, the authors follow a stepwise algorithm. First the pneumoperitoneum is increased to 20 mmHg to assist with venous tamponade. Simultaneously, we apply pressure to the injury with a gauze or piece of oxidized cellulose. If bleeding persists in a small tear or for larger tears, the defect may be closed with a 4-0 or 5-0 prolene suture. This vascular suture or "rescue stitch" should be made readily available in the operating room when performing complex robotic renal procedures such as RAPN. This stitch can be cut to 4–5 in. with a Lapra Ty clip placed at the end to obviate the need for tying a knot. Although rare, the surgeon should be prepared for open conversion if the above measures fail to control the bleeding source.

For left-sided RAPN one should be aware of the location of the left gonadal vein, left gonadal artery, left adrenal vein, and lumbar veins. The left gonadal vein drains into the left renal vein. Injuries to the left gonadal vein can be controlled with bipolar electrocautery or clips. The left gonadal artery may be encountered as well as it courses from the aorta laterally to run parallel to the left gonadal vein. It is usually small and can be managed with either monopolar or bipolar electrocautery or clips as needed. The left adrenal vein is encountered on the superior aspect of the left renal vein. It usually inserts at a medial location compared to the insertion of the left gonadal vein. It can be controlled with bipolar electrocautery or clips as needed. Finally, injuries to lumbar veins can be difficult to control and one must be careful when dissecting near the hilum to avoid inadvertent injury. Often a left lumbar vein can be found at the base of the main left renal vein. This vein is prone to avulsion while retracting the renal vein superiorly to identify the renal artery lying posteriorly. This vein should be identified, clipped, and divided prospectively in efforts to gain better mobility of the renal vein and exposure of the left renal artery. Aortic injuries are rare and should prompt a conversion to an open procedure as they may be difficult to control by laparoscopic means.

Thermal injuries to vessels can occur due to failure of the insulation sleeve on the monopolar curved scissors. These failures occur most likely from accidental micropunctures in the insulation sleeve from grasping or clashing with the tips of another instrument. Vascular injuries can also occur during robotic instrument exchanges. The robotic arms are equipped with a safety mechanism to avoid "past pointing" of newly inserted instrument by ensuring that the new instrument tip returns to the original position of the previous instrument, less 1–2 mm from where the instrument tip was last positioned. This is called a guided instrument exchange. However, if the clutch button is inadvertently pressed, this will reset the instrument arm requiring a completely new instrument insertion, guided by the console surgeon under laparoscopic control. If not recognized by the bedside assistant, this can result in insertion of a new instrument with "past pointing" of the instrument into vital structures.

Tumor Violation and Positive Margins

Positive surgical margins are rare and have been reported in 1.0–5.7% of RAPNs [1–7]. Although the local recurrence free survival and metastatic progression free survival are similar in patients with and without microscopic positive surgical margins, every effort should be made to minimize the risk of a positive margin [23]. Simple enucleation is one method for performing RAPN; however, the authors feel that the risk of a PSM is greater with this approach [24]. To limit the risk of a PSM, the authors use an approach that relies on: (1) preoperative planning, (2) intraoperative ultrasound, (3) arterial ischemia, and (4) minimal cautery. Prior to performing a RAPN as well as intraoperatively the authors review the available cross-sectional imaging to establish visual landmarks to guide the depth of our planned incision. For example, if a tumor is close to, but not invading the renal sinus, dissection will be carried purposefully down to sinus fat to ensure a negative margin. Next, the authors rely upon intraoperative laparoscopic ultrasound using the "drop in" robotic ultrasound probe to plan and mark out a safe margin of incision along the tumor perimeter approximately 1 cm from the edge of the tumor. To reduce warm ischemia time, the periphery of the tumor margin can be safely incised circumferentially using monopolar electrocautery without renal hilar clamping. Next the authors rely upon artery-only ischemia as previously mentioned with plans to clamp the renal vein in cases of excessive venous back bleeding. Finally, dissection is carried out deep into the renal parenchyma based on knowledge from preoperative and intraoperative imaging as well as predetermined landmarks (i.e., collecting system, sinus fat). During tumor resection, the authors find that using minimal cautery but rather cold sharp excision is preferential as this allows for better differentiation between normal renal parenchyma and potential tumor surface. In the rare event that dissection is carried into or too close to the tumor, a separate incision is made 1–2 cm proximal to the leading edge of the original incision to achieve a negative margin.

Postoperative Complications

Urine Leak

Published urine leak rates following RAPN range from 1.1 to 2.3% as shown in Table 15.2. Urine leaks can present in either an early or delayed fashion. Early leaks are often evident immediately following surgery. Patients will have high drain output that persists for >48 h after surgery and their drainage creatinine will be elevated. They most likely reflect poor collecting system closure or unrecognized collecting system injury, thus again stressing the importance of proper renal vascular control and hemostasis during tumor excision. Conservative management includes replacement of a urethral catheter and placing the flank drain to gravity (i.e., off suction) after withdrawing the tip of the drain away from the repair. If high outputs persist beyond a

few days, placement of a double pigtail ureteral catheter may be required. Often this results in a prompt decline in the drain output. The urethral catheter is removed first followed by the flank over the ensuing days, followed by the ureteral stent in 3–4 weeks. Although imaging can be performed, it rarely changes overall management of a postoperative acute urine leak.

Delayed leaks tend to present days to weeks postoperatively and may become symptomatic. Risk factors for urine leak include warm ischemia time, blood loss, need for collecting system repair, tumor size, and nephrometry score. In a large multi-institutional review of urinary fistula following RAPN, Potretzke and colleagues found the median postoperative day of presentation was 13 days [25]. Patients commonly present with fever, gastrointestinal complaints, and flank pain. In the setting of fevers, a complete blood count and cultures of the blood and urine should be obtained prior to starting antibiotics. If the creatinine allows, a CT with intravenous contrast with delayed images should be obtained to look for urinary extravasation and a fluid collection. Once the diagnosis is confirmed, a percutaneous drain should be placed in cases of an infected urinoma. If the urine leak persists after percutaneous drain placement, a ureteral stent should be considered to maximize drainage. Additionally, placing the drain to gravity drainage (versus suction) may aid in antegrade urine flow. In the event that a ureteral stent is placed, it is important to also place a urethral catheter to limit the chance of urinary reflux back into the kidney, which may perpetuate the leak. Most leaks will close with prolonged drainage.

Table 15.2 Comparison of RAPN series conversion, positive margin, and common complication rates

Study	No Pts	Positive margin	Transfusion	Angioembolization	Urine leak
Tanagho 2013	886	NR	41 (4.6%)	10 (1.1%)	10 (1.1%)
Dulabon 2010	446	7 (1.6%)	18 (4.0%)	7 (1.6%)	7 (1.6%)
Benway 2010	183	7 (3.8%)	2 (1.1%)	3 (1.6%)	2 (1.1%)
Scoll 2010	100	5 (5.7%)	3 (3.2%)	1 (1.1%)	2 (2.1%)
Ellison 2012	108	6 (7.0%)	6 (6.0%)	NR	2 (1.9%)
Long 2012	199	2 (1.0%)	24 (12.1%)	1 (1%)	4 (2.0%)
Benway 2009	129	5 (3.9%)	1 (0.8%)	2 (1.6%)	3 (2.3%)

Arteriovenous Fistulas and Pseudoaneurysms

Delayed bleeding is usually the result of an arteriovenous (AV) fistula or a pseudoaneurysm. Published RAPN series report an AV fistula or pseudoaneurysm rate of 1–1.6% as shown in Table 15.2. Patients may present with gross hematuria and/or flank pain. The hematuria may be intermittent. In a laparoscopic partial nephrectomy series, patients presented at a median of 12 days [26]. For minor bleeding or hemodynamically stable patients imaging with CT angiography, magnetic resonance angiography or duplex ultrasound scan can be performed with a trial of conservative management and blood transfusions as necessary. In unstable patients or in cases of persistent bleeding, the authors recommend going straight to angiography for both diagnostic and therapeutic (i.e., selective angioembolization) purposes [26].

Conclusions

This chapter reviewed the more common intraoperative and postoperative complications of RAPN and their management. The authors feel that preoperative planning and attention to surgical technique can prevent most of these complications. However, complications can still occur and it is important to have a systematic plan when managing them. Below, we list our tips for minimizing complications at the time of RAPN.

- Build your robotics team (especially your bedside assistant and surgical technician)
- Gain experience with other robotic procedures first (e.g., RALP, pyeloplasty, nephrectomy)
- Begin your experience with low complexity renal tumors (i.e., small <4 cm, exophytic, anterior)
- Study your preoperative imaging thoroughly (all phases and cuts) to fully delineate the arterial anatomy and tumor location
- Avoid selective arterial or no ischemia technique in the beginning of your experience
- Develop a checklist of equipment and sutures and review both preoperatively and intraoperatively

- Perform a "time out"—rehearse each step of the operation (especially arterial clamping, resection, and repair) and develop a backup plan for adverse events
- Educate and inform your patient about the risks of RAPN
- Be prepared and expect the unexpected

References

1. Tanagho YS, Kaouk JH, Allaf ME, Rogers CG, Stifelman MD, Kaczmarek BF, et al. Perioperative complications of robot-assisted partial nephrectomy: analysis of 886 patients at 5 United States centers. Urology. 2013;81(3):573–9.
2. Dulabon LM, Kaouk JH, Haber GP, Berkman DS, Rogers CG, Petros F, et al. Multi-institutional analysis of robotic partial nephrectomy for hilar versus nonhilar lesions in 446 consecutive cases. Eur Urol. 2011;59(3):325–30.
3. Benway BM, Bhayani SB, Rogers CG, Porter JR, Buffi NM, Figenshau RS, et al. Robot-assisted partial nephrectomy: an international experience. Eur Urol. 2010;57(5):815–20.
4. Ellison JS, Montgomery JS, Wolf JS, Hafez KS, Miller DC, Weizer AZ. A matched comparison of perioperative outcomes of a single laparoscopic surgeon versus a multisurgeon robot-assisted cohort for partial nephrectomy. J Urol. 2012;188(1):45–50.
5. Long JA, Yakoubi R, Lee B, Guillotreau J, Autorino R, Laydner H, et al. Robotic versus laparoscopic partial nephrectomy for complex tumors: comparison of perioperative outcomes. Eur Urol. 2012;61(6): 1257–62.
6. Benway BM, Bhayani SB, Rogers CG, Dulabon LM, Patel MN, Lipkin M, et al. Robot assisted partial nephrectomy versus laparoscopic partial nephrectomy for renal tumors: a multi-institutional analysis of perioperative outcomes. J Urol. 2009;182(3):866–72.
7. Scoll BJ, Uzzo RG, Chen DY, Boorjian SA, Kutikov A, Manley BJ, et al. Robot-assisted partial nephrectomy: a large single-institutional experience. Urology. 2010;75(6):1328–34.
8. Klatte T, Ficarra V, Gratzke C, Kaouk J, Kutikov A, Macchi V, et al. A literature review of renal surgical anatomy and surgical strategies for partial nephrectomy. Eur Urol. 2015;68(6):980–92.
9. Lee HJ, Box GN, Abraham JB, Elchico ER, Panah RA, Taylor MB, et al. Laboratory evaluation of laparoscopic vascular clamps using a load-cell device—are all clamps the same? J Urol. 2008;180(4): 1267–72.
10. Tryon D, Myklak K, Alsyouf M, Conceicao C, Peplinski B, Arenas JL, et al. Renal vascular clamp placement: a potential cause of incomplete hilar control during partial nephrectomy. J Urol. 2015;195(3): 756–62.

11. Imbeault A, Pouliot F, Finley DS, Shuch B, Dujardin T. Prospective study comparing two techniques of renal clamping in laparoscopic partial nephrectomy: impact on perioperative parameters. J Endourol. 2012;26(5):509–14.

12. Funahashi Y, Kato M, Yoshino Y, Fujita T, Sassa N, Gotoh M. Comparison of renal ischemic damage during laparoscopic partial nephrectomy with artery-vein and artery-only clamping. J Endourol. 2014;28(3): 306–11.

13. Gong EM, Zorn KC, Orvieto MA, Lucioni A, Msezane LP, Shalhav AL. Artery-only occlusion may provide superior renal preservation during laparoscopic partial nephrectomy. Urology. 2008;72(4):843–6.

14. Pareek G, Hedican SP, Gee JR, Bruskewitz RC, Nakada SY. Meta-analysis of the complications of laparoscopic renal surgery: comparison of procedures and techniques. J Urol. 2006;175(4):1208–13.

15. van der Voort M, Heijnsdijk EA, Gouma DJ. Bowel injury as a complication of laparoscopy. Br J Surg. 2004;91(10):1253–8.

16. Schwartz MJ, Faiena I, Cinman N, Kucharczyk J, Meriggi JS, Waingankar N, et al. Laparoscopic bowel injury in retroperitoneal surgery: current incidence and outcomes. J Urol. 2010;184(2):589–94.

17. Biggs G, Hafron J, Feliciano J, Hoenig DM. Treatment of splenic injury during laparoscopic nephrectomy with BioGlue, a surgical adhesive. Urology. 2005; 66(4):882.

18. Canby-Hagino ED, Morey AF, Jatoi I, Perahia B, Bishoff JT. Fibrin sealant treatment of splenic injury during open and laparoscopic left radical nephrectomy. J Urol. 2000;164(6):2004–5.

19. Varkarakis IM, Allaf ME, Bhayani SB, Inagaki T, Su LM, Kavoussi LR, et al. Pancreatic injuries during laparoscopic urologic surgery. Urology. 2004;64(6): 1089–93.

20. Del Pizzo JJ, Jacobs SC, Bishoff JT, Kavoussi LR, Jarrett TW. Pleural injury during laparoscopic renal surgery: early recognition and management. J Urol. 2003;169(1):41–4.

21. Permpongkosol S, Link RE, Su LM, Romero FR, Bagga HS, Pavlovich CP, et al. Complications of 2,775 urological laparoscopic procedures: 1993 to 2005. J Urol. 2007;177(2):580–5.

22. Jairath A, Singh A, Ganpule A, Mishra S, Sabnis R, Desai M. Management protocol for chylous ascites after laparoscopic nephrectomy. Urology. 2015;86(3): 521–8.

23. Yossepowitch O, Thompson RH, Leibovich BC, Eggener SE, Pettus JA, Kwon ED, et al. Positive surgical margins at partial nephrectomy: predictors and oncological outcomes. J Urol. 2008;179(6): 2158–63.

24. Serni S, Vittori G, Frizzi J, Mari A, Siena G, Lapini A, et al. Simple enucleation for the treatment of highly complex renal tumors: perioperative, functional and oncological results. Eur J Surg Oncol. 2015; 41(7):934–40.

25. Potretzke AM, Knight BA, Zargar H, Kaouk JH, Barod R, Rogers CG, et al. Urinary fistula after robot-assisted partial nephrectomy: a multicentre analysis of 1 791 patients. BJU Int. 2016;117(1):131–7.

26. Singh D, Gill IS. Renal artery pseudoaneurysm following laparoscopic partial nephrectomy. J Urol. 2005;174(6):2256–9.

Part III

Robotic Surgery of the Lower Urinary Tract

Robot-Assisted Radical and Partial Cystectomy

David M. Golombos, Padraic O'Malley,
Gerald J. Wang, and Douglas S. Scherr

Patient Selection

Indications for robot-assisted radical cystoprostatectomy are identical to those of the open approach and the goal is surgical cure of disease. Indications include muscle-invasive bladder cancer and high-grade, non-muscle-invasive bladder cancer (CIS or T1) refractory to intravesical immunotherapy or chemotherapy. On rare occasions, palliative cystectomy is performed in patients with severe symptoms from disease as an adjunct to chemotherapy. All patients referred to our center with bladder cancer undergo an exam under anesthesia and restaging transurethral resection of bladder. There are no absolute contraindications to robotic cystoprostatectomy. However, level of difficulty must be balanced with surgeon comfort and experience, and one must always be prepared for open conversion, as oncologic efficacy and patient safety should not be compromised. Relative contraindications include history of extensive abdominal or pelvic surgery and radiation, as well as preoperative evidence of extensive local disease. We refer all patients with clinical T2 disease or higher to medical oncology in consultation for neoadjuvant platinum-based chemotherapy.

In our series, 36% of patients had prior abdominal surgery, 10% had prior abdominal or pelvic radiation, and 35% had undergone neoadjuvant platinum-based chemotherapy. All patients undergo pelvic lymphadenectomy at the time of cystectomy, with an average of 22 lymph nodes removed. Robotic cystectomy is certainly feasible in the setting of prior surgery or radiation, though again, the decision to proceed is determined primarily by surgeon experience. In patients with prior intra-abdominal surgery, extensive laparoscopic lysis of adhesions is sometimes needed to enable safe placement of all trocars. In cases of prior pelvic radiation, the posterior dissection can be particularly challenging and great care must be taken to avoid rectal injury. Classic determinants such as age and renal function drive our choice of optimal diversion, with about 58% of our patients receiving continent diversion. We have not found a significant difference in rates of diversion-related complications between those with and without a history of prior pelvic radiation. In over 350 robotic cystectomies, open conversion has occurred in eight patients (2–3%). Three were immediate conversions due to extensive abdominal adhesions

Electronic supplementary material: The online version of this chapter (doi:10.1007/978-3-319-45060-5_16) contains supplementary material, which is available to authorized users.

P. O'Malley, M.D. • D.M. Golombos, M.D.
D.S. Scherr, M.D. (✉)
Department of Urology, New York Presbyterian Hospital—Weill Cornell Medical College,
New York, NY, USA
e-mail: dss2001@med.cornell.edu

G.J. Wang, M.D.
Department of Urology, New York Presbyterian Queens, Flushing, NY, USA

or difficulty with ventilation, with the remaining occurring due to difficult dissection mostly as a result of locally advanced disease.

Patient Preparation

Prior to surgery, all patients are counseled extensively on the risks and benefits of radical cystoprostatectomy. Both the open and robotic approaches are explained, and patients are made fully aware that open conversion, while rare, is always a possibility. A great deal of time is spent explaining the different types of urinary diversions to patients and their families. Informed consent is obtained with the patient, family, and nursing staff present. For patients undergoing ileal conduit or orthotopic ileal neobladder, bowel preparation consists of 48 h of clear liquid diet prior to surgery, followed by one bottle of magnesium citrate (300 mL) at 3 p.m. and one tablespoon of mineral oil at bedtime on the day prior to surgery. For patients undergoing continent cutaneous diversion using right colon, bowel preparation begins with 48 h of clear liquids, followed by 1 gal of polyethylene glycol electrolyte solution (GoLYTELY®, Braintree Laboratories, Inc., Braintree, MA) on the day prior to surgery. Additionally, oral neomycin (1 g for three doses), erythromycin base (1 g for three doses), and one tablespoon of mineral oil are given the day before surgery for continent cutaneous diversions alone. Rectal enema is performed the evening before and the morning of surgery.

Operative Setup

Operative setup for robot-assisted radical cystectomy will in many cases be dictated by the specific characteristics of each surgeon's operating room. In Fig. 16.1, we provide a schematic overhead view of our preferred operative setup. Because of space constraints, any number of variations of operating room setup is possible as long as a few key principles are followed. (1) We currently use the four-arm da Vinci® Surgical System (Intuitive Surgical, Inc., Sunnyvale, CA)

and therefore employ a single assistant on the right hand side. We feel that at least three monitors are needed in this setting to allow for each team member to have optimum viewing of the operative steps. (2) The scrub nurse should be positioned on the side of the assistant with the 15 mm trocar to facilitate exchange of clip appliers, sutures, and Endo Catch™ (Covidien, Mansfield, MA) retrieval bags. (3) The console surgeon must have easy access to the operative table to scrub into the procedure at a moment's notice. The introduction of the most recent da Vinci robotic system allows for side-docking of the slave component. This also allows one to obviate the need for placing the patient in the lithotomy position.

Patient Positioning and Preparation

We place the patient in the dorsal lithotomy position using standard operative stirrups. With the table flat, we then tuck the patient's arms at the side. All pressure points are protected using standard eggcrate foam padding. Sequential compression stocking devices are placed on both legs and are activated. We also routinely administer 5000 units of subcutaneous heparin. Next, the patient is secured to the operating table using a cross-shoulder harness made by four strips of eggcrate foam padding. Each strip is 6 × 24 in., and two strips are used on each side of the patient creating an "X" configuration across the patient's chest. The pads are secured to the operating table using cloth tape. Care must be taken not to secure the lower portion of the pads below the costal margin, as this may interfere with subsequent lateral trocar placement. Once the patient is secured to the table, the leg attachment is lowered and the patient is placed in 30–40° steep Trendelenburg position (Fig. 16.2). Of note, the anesthesia team places an orogastric tube to low wall suction for the duration of the case, and a foam padding is placed over the patient's face to prevent injury from the camera, particularly when the 30°-down lens is being used. A urethral catheter is placed on the operative field.

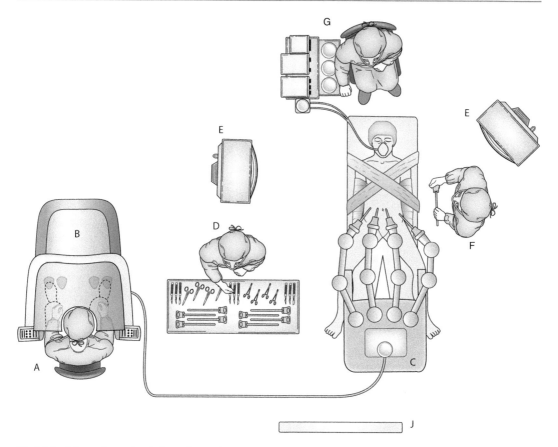

Fig. 16.1 Schematic overhead view of operative setup for robot-assisted radical cystectomy. (*A*) Surgeon, (*B*) Console, (*C*) da Vinci®, (*D*) Scrub nurse, (*E, J*) High-definition monitors, (*F*) Right assistant, (*G*) Anesthesia

Trocar Configuration

Our standard trocar configuration for robot-assisted radical cystectomy is shown in Fig. 16.3. Insufflation of the abdominal cavity is performed using a Veress needle to 15 mmHg, which in general is maintained throughout the operation. In particularly obese patients, communication with the anesthesia team is imperative as pneumoperitoneum can result in unacceptably high inspiratory pressure necessitating a lower abdominal insufflation pressure. Once the abdomen has been insufflated, we place a 10–12 mm, blunt, disposable trocar in the periumbilical location as our camera trocar. We mark a standard laparotomy incision at the beginning of the case and use the superior 1 cm of the curvilinear, periumbilical portion of the incision for our robotic camera tro-

car. The 30°-up lens is then passed through this trocar to aid in subsequent trocar placement. At this point, the left 8 mm robotic trocar is placed 10 cm lateral to, and 2 cm inferior to, the camera trocar. A second 8 mm robotic trocar is placed in the midaxillary line 3 cm superior to the ASIS. With the assistant on the left holding the camera, we then place our right 8 mm robotic trocar 10 cm lateral to, and 2 cm inferior to, the camera trocar. A Versaport™ Plus (Covidien, Mansfield, MA), 5–15 mm trocar, is then placed as the main right assistant trocar in the midaxillary line 3 cm superior to the anterior superior iliac spine (ASIS). A 5 mm AirSeal® Access Port (SurgiQuest, Milford CT) used primarily by the right-sided assistant for suction-irrigation is then placed midway between the camera trocar and the right robotic trocar. We place our suction trocar in the same axial plane as the camera trocar,

Fig. 16.2 Final patient positioning with the patient secured to the table with a cross-shoulder harness "X" configuration (A) and the arms tucked at the side (B)

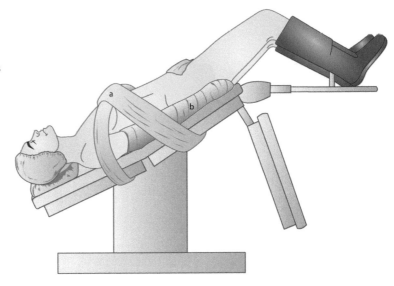

Fig. 16.3 Trocar configuration for robot-assisted radical cystectomy. *Top* figure demonstrates overhead view of trocar configuration and *bottom* figure demonstrates view from the patient's feet. (A) Main right-sided assistant trocar, (B) and (E) 8 mm robotic trocars, (C) secondary right assistant trocar, (D) camera trocar, (F) left-sided 8 mm robotic trocar

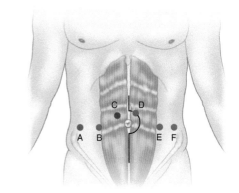

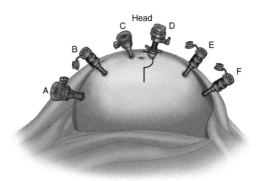

because placement of this trocar in a lower position can limit movement between the camera and right robotic arm. Because our suction is in a slightly higher position, we use the extra long suction tip adapter to reach the most dependent portions of the pelvis.

Instrumentation and Equipment List

Equipment

- da Vinci® Si or Xi Surgical System
- PreCise™ bipolar forceps (Intuitive Surgical, Inc., Sunnyvale, CA)
- EndoWrist® curved monopolar scissors (Intuitive Surgical, Inc., Sunnyvale, CA)
- EndoWrist® needle drivers (2) (Intuitive Surgical, Inc., Sunnyvale, CA)
- EndoWrist® Vessel Sealer (Intuitive Surgical, Inc., Sunnyvale, CA)
- InSite® Vision System with 0° and 30° lens (Intuitive Surgical, Inc., Sunnyvale, CA)

Trocars

- 5–15 mm trocar
- 10–12 mm blunt trocar (or standard 8 mm Xi robotic trocar for Xi system)
- 8-mm robotic trocars (3)
- A 5 mm AirSeal® Access Port (SurgiQuest, Milford CT)

Recommended Sutures (See Table 16.1)

Instruments Used by the Surgical Assistants

- MicroFrance® grasper (Medtronic, Inc., Minneapolis, MN)
- Laparoscopic scissors
- Hem-o-lok® clip applier (Teleflex Medical, Research Triangle Park, NC)

- Medium, Medium-Large, Large, and Extra-Large Hem-o-lok® clips (Teleflex Medical, Research Triangle Park, NC)
- Endo Clip™ 10 mm multifire titanium clip applier (Covidien, Mansfield, MA)
- 15 mm Endo Catch™ retrieval device (1) (Covidien, Mansfield, MA)
- 10 mm Endo Catch™ retrieval device (2) Suction-Irrigator device
- 15Fr round Jackson–Pratt drain
- 24Fr Malecot suprapubic tube
- 20Fr urethral catheter with 5 cm^3 balloon
- 7Fr single J ureteral catheter (2)
- Endo Close™ fascial closer device (Autosuture, Covidien, Mansfield, MA)

Step-by-Step Technique (Video 16.1)

Step 1: Identification and Dissection of the Ureter (Table 16.2)

Unless stated otherwise, robot-assisted radical cystectomy is performed using the 30°-down lens. For the majority of the operation, curved monopolar scissors are used in the right robotic arm and the PreCise™ bipolar forceps in the left, with the Prograsp forceps in the third arm. Electrocautery settings are 30 W for both monopolar and bipolar devices. The procedure begins by identification and dissection of the ureters. Identification of the left ureter (Figs. 16.4 and 16.5) begins with the right assistant retracting the sigmoid colon medially using a MicroFrance® grasper. The surgeon incises the posterior peritoneum along the white line of Toldt, sweeping the bowel medially and exposing the psoas muscle. The peritoneum overlying the external iliac artery is opened. The ureter is easily identified medially along the psoas and crossing the external iliac artery. The ureter should not be directly grasped by the surgeon or the assistants, and effective ureteral retraction can be accomplished by placing the left robotic grasper beneath the ureter and elevating it gently. The ureter is then dissected proximally as high as possible to the level above

Table 16.1 Recommended sutures

Suture	Length	Needle	Procedure	Note
0-polyglactin tie (secured to medium-large Hem-o-lok® clip)	Full length (24 in.)		Used to tag the ureter once it is transected	Dyed (right) and undyed (left)
0-polyglactin	8 in.	GS-21	Ligation of dorsal venous complex (DVC)	
2-0 Biosyn (undyed)	10 in.	GU-46	Urethral-neobladder anastomosis	
2-0 Monocryl (dyed)	10 in.	UR-6	Urethral-neobladder anastomosis	Sutures are tied together to create a double-armed suture
0-Maxon	Full length	GS-21	Fascial closure of periumbilical incision	
4-0 Biosyn	Full length	P-12	Skin closure	

Table 16.2 Identification and dissection of the ureter: surgeon and assistant instrumentation

Surgeon instrumentation			Assistant instrumentation
Right arm	Left arm	Third arm	
• Curved monopolar scissors	• PreCise™ bipolar forceps	• Prograsp™ forceps	• Suction-irrigator
Endoscope lens: 30° down			• MicroFrance® grasper

the level of the gonadal vessels. Distal dissection is performed to the level of the ureteral hiatus. During distal ureteral dissection, the vas deferens and the obliterated umbilical artery are encountered, clipped, and divided. The final portion of ureteral dissection is performed after division of the anterior pedicle.

Step 2: Development of the Anterior Bladder Pedicle

Development of the anterior bladder pedicle, shown in Figs. 16.5 and 16.6a, b on the patient's left side, begins with identifying the avascular plane located between the pelvic sidewall and the bladder. We begin developing this avascular plane by placing both robotic instruments in the space between the left pelvic sidewall and the bladder (Fig. 16.5). Then, using broad, horizontal sweeping movements with the robotic arms, the avascular plane is developed, as shown in Fig. 16.6a, b. The left obturator nerve and pelvic side-

wall are shown here as the lateral border of the avascular plane. The suction device is retracting the bladder and left ureter medially which reveals the fibrous connective tissue of the avascular plane.

Step 3: Transection of the Anterior Pedicle and Ureter (Table 16.3)

Development of the avascular plane between the left bladder and sidewall reveals the anterior bladder pedicle, shown on the patient's left side in Fig. 16.7a, b, just lateral to the ureteral hiatus. The anterior pedicle which contains the superior vesicle artery can be secured and divided using the Vessel Sealer. Prior to ureteral transection at the hiatus, a large Hem-o-lok® clip is applied distally and a second large Hem-o-lok® clip, which is attached to a long 0-polyglactin suture, is applied proximally on the ureter. The suture on the ureter facilitates subsequent ureteral identification during the later steps of urinary diversion.

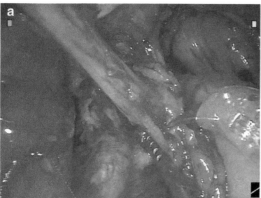

Fig. 16.4 (**a**, **b**) View of the left pelvic sidewall, iliac vessels, and left ureter (foreground) being dissected toward the bladder. Pertinent anatomy includes (*A*) pelvic sidewall and external iliac artery, (*B*) hypogastric artery, (*C*) left ureter, retracted anteriorly by left robotic arm, (*D*) bladder and ureteral hiatus, (*E*) rectum, (*F*) sigmoid colon, (*G*) right robotic arm, and (*H*) suction-irrigator

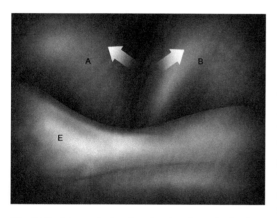

Fig. 16.5 Schematic drawing showing the early development of the avascular plane between the left side of the bladder (*B*) and left pelvic sidewall and iliac vessels (*A*). The arrows indicate the blunt horizontal sweeping motions used to develop the avascular plane. The peritoneal reflection is denoted by (*E*)

Step 4: Development of the Posterior Plane

Once the anterior pedicles are divided, we incise the posterior peritoneal reflection horizontally along the cul-de-sac, separating the bladder from the rectum along the midline (Fig. 16.8a, b). The third arm lifts the bladder anteriorly and the assistant retracts the posterior peritoneal edge. Using a combination of broad, sweeping motions and electrocautery with the monopolar scissors, we develop the posterior plane between the bladder and rectum beneath the posterior leaflet of Denonvilliers' fascia. This dissection is carried as distally as possible and well beyond the vasa deferentia and seminal vesicles (SVs) toward the prostatic apex.

Step 5: Identification and Transection of the Posterior Bladder Pedicles

Development of the plane between the bladder and rectum reveals the posterior bladder pedicle, shown on the patient's left side in Fig. 16.9a, b. The posterior bladder pedicle is located just distal to the previously divided anterior pedicle. Exposure of the left posterior bladder pedicle is

Additionally, we recommend using dyed and undyed polyglactin sutures to enable distinction between the right and left ureters. The left ureter, once divided, remains on the left side of the patient's body until after the cystectomy and lymph node dissection is performed to be passed by the assistant uses a MicroFrance® grasper to the right side. A similar dissection is carried out on the right side exposing the right anterior bladder pedicle, ureter, and pelvic sidewall.

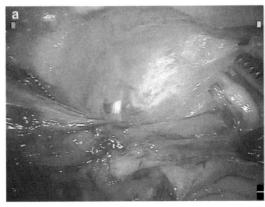 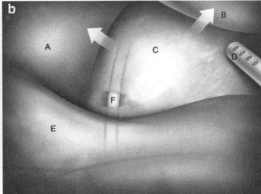

Fig. 16.6 (**a, b**) View of avascular plane between the left side of the bladder and pelvic sidewall with pertinent anatomy including (*A*) left pelvic sidewall and external iliac vessels, (*B*) bladder, (*C*) avascular plane, (*D*) suction-irrigator, (*E*) peritoneal reflection, and (*F*) left obturator nerve

Table 16.3 Transection of the anterior pedicle and ureter: surgeon and assistant instrumentation

Surgeon instrumentation			
Right arm	Left arm	Third arm	Assistant instrumentation
• Curved monopolar scissors	• PreCise™ bipolar forceps	• Prograsp™ forceps	• Suction-irrigator
• Vessel Sealer			• MicroFrance® grasper
Endoscope lens: 30° down			• LigaSure™ device
			• Hem-o-lok® applier

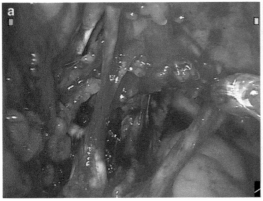 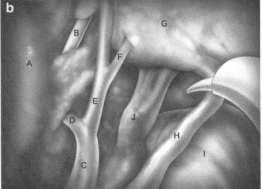

Fig. 16.7 (**a, b**) View of the left anterior bladder pedicle with pertinent anatomy including (*A*) pelvic sidewall, (*B*) obturator nerve, (*C*) hypogastric artery, (*D*) obturator artery, (*E*) superior vesical artery, (*F*) branch of superior vesical artery, (*G*) bladder, (*H*) left ureter, (*I*) sigmoid colon, and (*j*) posterior bladder pedicle

facilitated by the assistant providing superior and medial traction on the bladder, while the left arm provides posterior retraction of the rectum. In a non-nerve-sparing operation, we secure and divide the posterior pedicle using the Vessel Sealer device. In a nerve-sparing procedure, we use Hem-o-lok® clips to prevent thermal damage to the neurovascular bundle. Division of the pos-

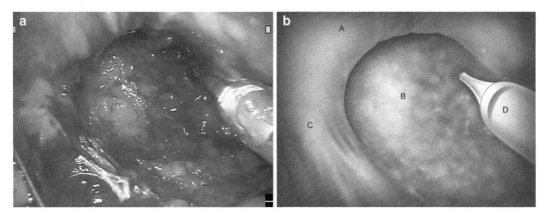

Fig. 16.8 (**a**, **b**) View of the posterior plane created between the bladder, (*A*) anteriorly and prerectal fat (*B*) posteriorly. The left posterior bladder pedicle (*C*) and right robotic arm with monopolar scissors (*D*) are also shown

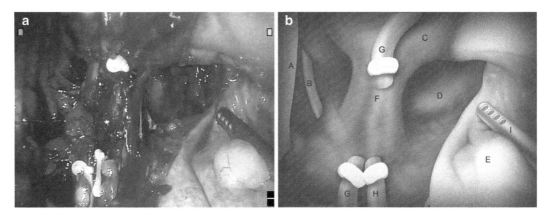

Fig. 16.9 (**a**, **b**) View of the left posterior bladder pedicle with relevant anatomy including (*A*) left external iliac vessel, (*B*) left obturator nerve, (*C*) bladder, (*D*) rectum, (*E*) sigmoid colon, (*F*) posterior bladder pedicle, (*G*) superior vesicle artery (clipped and cut), (*H*) branch of superior vesicle artery (clipped and cut), and (*I*) suction-irrigator

terior pedicle is complete when the endopelvic fascia is encountered.

Step 6: Exposure of the Endopelvic Fascia

The adipose tissue overlying the endopelvic fascia, shown on the patient's left side in Fig. 16.10a, b, is removed by the robotic instruments using blunt sweeping motions. The endopelvic fascia is sharply incised using the robotic scissors. This exposes the prostatic pedicles which are then secured and divided using the Vessel Sealer device in a non-nerve-sparing operation. Alternatively, Hem-o-lok® clips and titanium

clips can be used in a nerve-sparing procedure. To avoid injury to the rectum, the third arm can be used to retract the bladder and prostate superomedially while the Prograsp™ can be used to retract the rectum posteriorly. It is important to carry this dissection as distally as possible, because once the bladder is released from its anterior attachment, visualization of the posterior prostatic apex is quite limited.

Step 7: Anterior Dissection of the Bladder and Prostate (Table 16.4)

The 0° lens can be used at this point in the procedure to better visualize the anterior abdominal

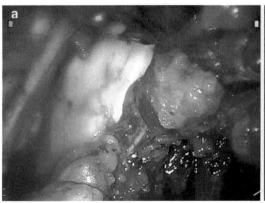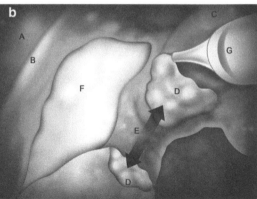

Fig. 16.10 (**a, b**) View of the left endopelvic fascia. Labeled structures include (*A*) pubic bone, (*B*) pectineal line, (*C*) bladder, (*D*) left posterior bladder pedicle (cut), (*E*) beginning of left prostatic pedicle, (*F*) left endopelvic fascia, and (*G*) right robotic arm

Table 16.4 Anterior dissection of the bladder and prostate: surgeon and assistant instrumentation

Surgeon instrumentation		Assistant instrumentation
Right arm	Left arm	
Curved monopolar scissors	• Maryland bipolar grasper	• Suction-irrigator
Endoscope lens: 0°		• Hem-o-lok® clip applier
		• Laparoscopic needle driver

wall, the dorsal venous complex (DVC), and the urethra. Similar to the oncologic principles in open radical cystectomy, we remove the urachus with the bladder en bloc taking wide peritoneal wings (Fig. 16.11a, b). The importance of placing the camera trocar several centimeters superior to the umbilicus at the beginning of the procedure is now revealed. If the camera trocar is not placed superiorly enough, then complete excision of the urachus will be compromised, as will the proximal extent of the subsequent pelvic lymphadenectomy. The medial umbilical ligament on each side is grasped by the assistant. Providing medial retraction, the monopolar scissors are then used to incise the anterior peritoneum which enables entrance into the space of Retzius. The peritoneum is incised widely, lateral to the medial umbilical ligaments and in an inferior direction until the pubic bone is exposed.

Step 8: Control of the Dorsal Venous Complex and Division of the Urethra (Table 16.5)

After dissecting the anterior attachments of the bladder and entering the space of Retzius, the visible landmarks include the anterior bladder, prostate, puboprostatic ligaments, and pubic bone (Fig. 16.12a, b). The puboprostatic ligaments are preserved for orthotopic urinary diversion. For nonorthotopic diversion, the urethra is not preserved and therefore we divide the puboprostatic ligaments for optimal distal dissection. A 0-polyglactin suture can be placed to secure the DVC. In a non-nerve-sparing cystoprostatectomy, we divide the DVC using electrocautery with the monopolar scissors. In nerve-sparing procedures, electrocautery is not used. The urethra is also divided without electrocautery for patients undergoing orthotopic neobladder. With the third arm providing superior traction on the bladder, the anterior one half of the urethra is divided and the urethral catheter is exposed and the catheter tip pulled in through the urethral opening. The catheter lumen is secured with a large Hem-o-lok® clip and is then divided using the scissors, preventing any possible spillage of tumor. The assistant provides superior retraction on the prostate and bladder by grasping the cut end of the urethral catheter. Remaining apical attachments are divided, and the bladder, pros-

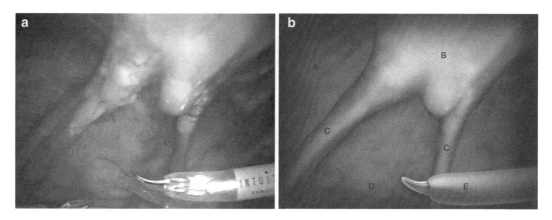

Fig. 16.11 (**a**, **b**) View of the anterior abdominal wall (*A*), urachus (*B*), bilateral medial umbilical ligaments (*C*), bladder (*D*), and right robotic monopolar scissors (*E*)

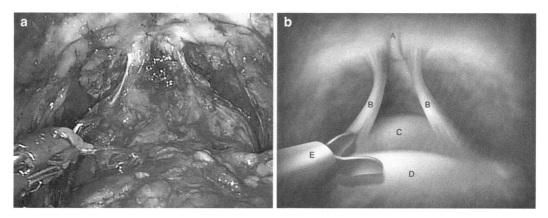

Fig. 16.12 (**a**, **b**) View of the pubic bone (*A*), puboprostatic ligaments (*B*), prostate (*C*), and anterior bladder (*D*), following release of the anterior bladder attachments and dissection of the space of Retzius. The left robotic bipolar forceps (*E*) is also shown

tate, and seminal vesicles are placed in a 15 mm Endo Catch™ retrieval device immediately.

Step 9: Pelvic Lymphadenectomy (Table 16.6)

At this time, the 0° lens should be replaced with the 30°-down lens. We begin our pelvic lymphadenectomy by completely denuding the external iliac artery of its surrounding lymphatic tissue, shown here on the patient's right side in Fig. 16.13a, b. The node packet is retracted medially with a MicroFrance® grasper and the packet is developed

proximally. Hem-o-lok® or titanium clips are applied liberally during pelvic lymphadenectomy to help minimize the risk of a postoperative pelvic lymphocele. The borders of our pelvic lymphadenectomy are Cooper's ligament inferiorly, the genitofemoral nerve laterally, and the sacral promontory medially, up to the level of the aortic bifurcation. All presacral, hypogastric, external iliac, obturator, and common iliac lymph node packets are removed en bloc and placed in a 10 mm Endo Catch™ retrieval device. The left and right pelvic lymph node packets are placed in separate bags and can be distinguished by placing a knot or Hem-o-lok® clip on one of the retrieval bags.

Table 16.5 Control of the dorsal venous complex and division of the urethra: surgeon and assistant instrumentation

Surgeon instrumentation		Assistant instrumentation
Right arm	Left arm	
• Curved monopolar scissors	• PreCise™ bipolar forceps	• Suction-irrigator
• Needle driver	• Needle driver	• Hem-o-lok® clip applier
Endoscope lens: 0°		• Laparoscopic needle driver
		• 15 mm Endo Catch™ retrieval device

Table 16.6 Pelvic lymphadenectomy: surgeon and assistant instrumentation

Surgeon instrumentation		Assistant instrumentation
Right arm	Left arm	
Curved monopolar scissors	PreCise™ bipolar forceps	• Suction-irrigator
Endoscope lens: 30° down		• MicroFrance® grasper
		• Hem-o-lok® clip applier
		• 10 mm titanium clip applier
		• 10 mm Endo Catch™ retrieval device

Step 10: Transposition of the Left Ureter (Table 16.7)

Prior to completion of the urinary diversion, the left ureter is transposed beneath the sigmoid colon mesentery to the right side of the pelvis. The assistant places a MicroFrance® grasper underneath the sigmoid colon. Exposure of the window for the placement is done by retraction of the colon to the left and creation of a window using the PreCise™ and monopolar scissors posterior to the sigmoid mesentery and superior to the aortic bifurcation just anterior to the great vessels. With the MicroFrance® in place the colon is then retracted to the right. The tie on the left ureter is then placed in the grasper and then delivered by the assistant to the right hand side (Figs. 16.14a, b and 16.15a, b).

Table 16.7 *Transposition of the left ureter*: surgeon and assistant instrumentation

Surgeon instrumentation		Assistant instrumentation
Right arm	Left arm	
• Curved monopolar scissors	• PreCise™ bipolar forceps	• Suction-irrigator
Endoscope lens: 30° down		• Maryland dissector

Step 11: Specimen Extraction (Table 16.8)

Before the robot is undocked, we place a 15Fr round Jackson–Pratt drain through the left 8 mm robotic trocar. For orthotopic neobladders, the drain is placed after the anastomosis has been completed robotically. Additionally, we use a 0-polyglactin tie on an Endo Close™ device to close the 5–15 mm right assistant trocar. After the robot has been undocked, the 1 cm periumbilical camera incision is extended inferiorly in a curvilinear fashion around the umbilicus (Fig. 16.16). Depending on the patient's body habitus, the periumbilical incision used for specimen extraction and extracorporeal urinary diversion ranges from 5 to 7 cm. The three separate Endo Catch™ retrieval bags containing the cystoprostatectomy specimen and the two separate lymph node packets are removed. If the surgeon plans to perform a completely intracorporeal urinary diversion in female patients, the specimens can be removed via the vagina. Urinary diversions including ileal conduit, continent cutaneous diversion, and orthotopic ileal neobladder and the bilateral ureteral anastomoses are performed in the standard open fashion [1, 2].

Step 12: Urethral-Neobladder Anastomosis (Table 16.9)

For patients undergoing orthotopic neobladder, the newly created neobladder is brought down into the pelvis. We then place a urethral catheter per urethra and into the opening created in the neobladder and the catheter balloon is inflated

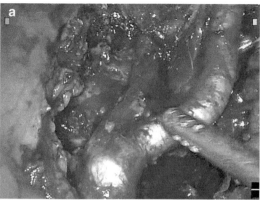

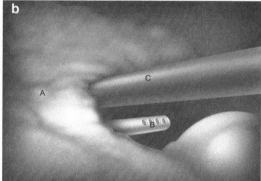

Fig. 16.13 (**a**, **b**) View of right pelvic lymph node dissection with the relevant anatomic landmarks including (*A*) posterior peritoneum (cut), (*B*) common iliac artery, (*C*) external iliac artery, (*D*) hypogastric artery, (*E*) external iliac lymph node packet, (*F*) hypogastric lymph node packet, (*G*) presacral lymph node packet, and (*H*) suction-irrigator

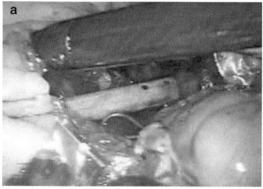

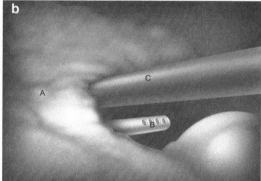

Fig. 16.14 (**a**, **b**) Preparing for transposition of the left ureter under the sigmoid colon mesentery. Labeled structures include (*A*) sigmoid colon, (*B*) suction-irrigator, passed posterior to the sigmoid mesentery from the patient's left to right side, and (*C*) right robotic arm, elevating sigmoid colon

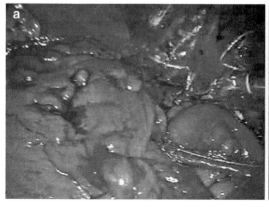

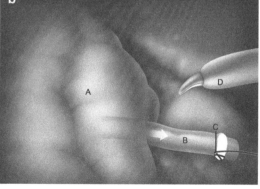

Fig. 16.15 (**a**, **b**) Final view following transposition of the left ureter underneath the sigmoid colon and mesentery. Labeled structures include (*A*) sigmoid colon, (*B*) left ureter, passed posterior to the sigmoid mesentery and delivered to the patient's right side, (*C*) Hem-o-lok® clip with 0-polyglactin tie attached to the cut end of the left ureter, and (*D*) right robotic arm

Table 16.8 Specimen extraction: surgeon and assistant instrumentation

Surgeon instrumentation		Assistant instrumentation
Right arm	Left arm	
Curved monopolar scissors	PreCise™ bipolar forceps	• Suction-irrigator
Endoscope lens: 30° down		• MicroFrance® grasper
		• 15Fr round Jackson–Pratt drain
		• Endo Close™ device

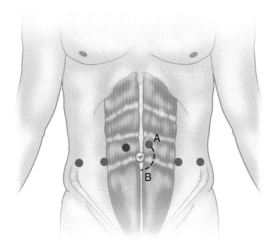

Fig. 16.16 Extraction of specimens is accomplished by extending the periumbilical camera trocar site (*A*) in a curvilinear fashion (*dotted line*) around the umbilicus. (*B*) The bladder, prostate, and bilateral pelvic lymph node specimens are removed through this incision

Table 16.9 Urethral-neobladder anastomosis: surgeon and assistant instrumentation

Surgeon instrumentation		Assistant instrumentation
Right arm	Left arm	
• Needle driver	• Needle driver	• Suction-irrigator
Endoscope lens: 0° or 30° down		• Laparoscopic needle driver
		• 15Fr round Jackson–Pratt drain

with 15 mL of sterile water and the catheter placed on mild traction to bring the neobladder in closer proximity to the urethra. Prior to redocking of the robot for the urethral-neobladder anastomosis, a suprapubic tube and ureteral stents are brought through a single stab wound in the right lower quadrant of the abdominal wall. This stabilizes the neobladder and facilitates the urethral-neobladder anastomosis. We then close the periumbilical anterior rectus fascia using a 0-Maxon suture in a simple interrupted fashion, leaving a 1 cm opening at the superior aspect of the wound for placement of the 10–12 mm robotic camera trocar. The robot is then redocked, pneumoperitoneum is reestablished, and the urethral-neobladder anastomosis is performed as shown in Fig. 16.17. Of note, Trendelenburg of approximately only 20° is useful here to facilitate the anastomosis.

Depending on the depth of the patient's pelvis, we use either the 30°-down or 0° lens for this portion of the procedure. We use a double-armed suture consisting of an undyed 2-0 Biosyn on a GU-46 needle cut to 10 in., which is then tied to a 10-in. segment of dyed 2-0 Monocryl on a UR-6 needle. We begin our anastomosis at the 6 o'clock position with the dyed 2-0 Monocryl suture. This suture is placed outside to in on the neobladder, then inside to out on the urethra. After five throws have been placed in a clockwise direction, the suture will be on the inside of the neobladder and the neobladder is brought down to the urethra. The third arm then grasps the dyed suture and places it on gentle traction to prevent the posterior anastomosis from distracting. The undyed 2-0 Biosyn suture is then placed outside to in on the urethra at the 5 o'clock position. This suture is run in a counterclockwise direction until the undyed 2-0 Biosyn is outside the bladder at the 2 o'clock position. The third arm is then switched to the undyed suture which is placed on gentle traction. The dyed 2-0 Monocryl suture is then run in a clockwise fashion until the suture is outside the urethra at the 12 o'clock position. The needle on the undyed suture is removed and the anastomosis is secured. The dyed suture is then used to fix and lift the anas-

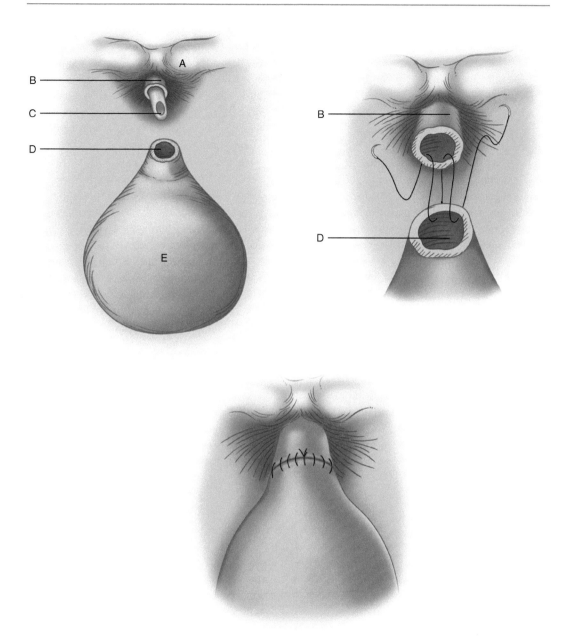

Fig. 16.17 Running vesicourethral anastomosis following creation of neobladder. Labeled structures are as follows: (A) pubic bone, (B) urethra, (C) urethral catheter, (D) everted mucosa of neobladder, (E) neobladder. Insets show the running anastomotic suture and the completed anastomosis

tomosis anteriorly to the pubic notch. A Hem-o-lok® clip is then placed on the two sutures crossed. The sutures are once again tied to one another to secure this lift. At this time, a 15Fr round Jackson–Pratt drain is placed through the 8 mm left-sided robotic trocar. We then undock the robot and remove the camera trocar to complete our fascial closure of the periumbilical incision. All wounds are copiously irrigated with sterile water. Skin closure is performed in a running subcuticular fashion using 4-0 Biosyn suture on a P-12 needle.

Postoperative Care

We use clinical pathways for routine postoperative care in our cystectomy patients, both open and robotic. Nasogastric tubes are not routinely used and bowel rest is maintained for 2–3 days postoperatively. Patients are aggressively ambulated and are closely followed by both physical and occupational therapy. If patients have not passed flatus by postoperative day 3, we then begin a promotility regimen consisting of metoclopramide 10 mg and erythromycin 125 mg intravenously every 6 h, and bisacodyl suppositories twice a day. Intravenous patient-controlled analgesia or epidural patient-controlled analgesia is used until patients are tolerating a liquid diet and patients routinely receive intravenous ketorolac to decrease narcotic requirement. Patients resume a regular diet after 1 day of clear liquids. Our median length of stay is 4–6 days, and we have found a decrease in our median length of stay with the use of clinical pathways.

We routinely place a self-contained suction drain at the completion of the robotic portion of the case and this is removed prior to discharge from the hospital. For ileal conduits, the stomal catheter is removed prior to discharge, and the bilateral ureteral stents are removed 2 weeks after surgery in the office. Intramuscular gentamicin and oral furosemide are administered at the time of ureteral stent removal. For continent cutaneous diversions, ureteral stents are removed prior to discharge. The stomal catheter is removed 2 weeks later in the office and patients begin a regimen of self-catheterization. If postvoid residuals are acceptable, the suprapubic tube is subsequently removed. For orthotopic diversions, ureteral stents are also removed prior to discharge. The urethral catheter is removed 2 weeks after surgery in the office and the suprapubic tube is subsequently removed if postvoid residuals are acceptable.

Special Considerations

1. To facilitate continent cutaneous urinary diversion through a small periumbilical incision, we use the 5 mm Ethicon™ Harmonic Scalpel™

after trocar placement to mobilize the right colon from the midtransverse colon to the ileo-cecal valve. This enables delivery of the right colon through the small periumbilical incision during extracorporeal urinary diversion.

2. In female patients, a sponge stick is placed in the vagina at the beginning of the case. The labia majora can be sutured together using a #1 Prolene to prevent loss of subsequent pneumoperitoneum through the vagina, although is rarely necessary. For most muscle-invasive bladder tumors, the anterior vaginal wall is excised en bloc with the bladder. This is done by anterior elevation of the sponge stick to define the vaginal apex which is then incised using the monopolar scissors. For anterior bladder tumors, the vagina can be spared by developing the avascular plane between the bladder and the anterior vaginal wall.

3. In female patients, prior to ureteral dissection, we divide the gonadal vessels using either Hem-o-lok® clips or the LigaSure™ device, and the ovaries and uterus are mobilized along with the bladder and are subsequently removed.

Steps to Avoid Complications

Posterior dissection should be performed beneath the posterior leaflet of Denonvilliers' fascia to ensure oncologic efficacy. Also, perirectal fat must always be visible during this portion of the dissection to decrease the risk of rectal injury, particularly at the apex where most rectal injuries occur. Posterior dissection should be carried as distally as possible, because once the bladder is released from the anterior abdominal wall, posterior visualization becomes quite limited.

The left ureter should be brought beneath the sigmoid mesentery as high as possible, preferably at the level of the aortic bifurcation or higher, to minimize kinking of the left ureter.

Robotic-Assisted Partial Cystectomy

A growing body of literature suggests partial cystectomy may represent a viable alternative to radical cystectomy [3]; however, appropriate patient selection is of paramount importance. Traditional indications include a solitary tumor in a favorable location and absence of carcinoma in situ. Robotic partial cystectomy is our preferred approach to organ-sparing surgery, although again this decision must be balanced with surgeon comfort and experience. In our series, perioperative complications are rare (<10%), estimated blood loss is modest (median 50 cc), and most patients are able to be discharged home the day after surgery. Urethral catheter is removed in the clinic about 10 days post-op, with a cystogram prior at the discretion of the surgeon.

For patients undergoing robotic partial cystectomy, bowel preparation consists of 24 h of clear liquid diet prior to surgery, followed by one bottle of magnesium citrate (300 mL) at 3 p.m. Operative setup and patient positioning, including dorsal lithotomy position and utilization of steep Trendelenburg position to allow small bowel contents to fall out of the pelvis, is similar to that described for radical cystectomy. Our standard trocar configuration for robot-assisted radical cystectomy is also used for partial cystectomy, as shown previously in Fig. 16.3.

Once the patient is positioned and the ports are placed, but prior to docking the robot, the operating surgeon should begin with a flexible or rigid cystoscopy. While the surgeon performs the cystoscopy, the bedside assistant manually controls the robotic camera, which is pointed into the pelvis. The light on the robotic camera within the abdominal cavity should be dim to allow for better visualization of the cystoscopic light within the bladder. Once the involved area of the bladder is identified cystoscopically, the bedside assistant uses monopolar laparoscopic scissors and electrocautery to outline the necessary area of resection on the outside of the bladder, using the light from the cystoscope as a guide. The area of resection should be wide enough to ensure adequate margins, but not too wide to compromise bladder capacity. Once this is complete, the cystoscope is removed, a urethral catheter is placed, and the robot is docked.

The bladder can be filled with approximately 200–300 cm^3 of sterile water to better define the anatomy. The location of the tumor within the bladder will dictate the extent of necessary dissection for exposure, which can usually be achieved using broad, horizontal sweeping movements with the robotic arms. Ideally, the surgeon should leave the bladder attached to the anterior abdominal wall to maximize visualization and exposure. Using electrocautery, full thickness dissection of the previously demarcated area is performed. Wide peritoneal "wings" are removed en block with the bladder resection to ensure adequate resection. Initial entry into the bladder should be a longitudinal incision in the most cephalad portion of the demarcated area (anterior to the tumor). This allows for intravesical inspection under direct vision, helping to ensure adequate margins and avoidance of the ureteral orifices. Of note, if the bladder was previously filled to facilitate dissection, it should be emptied prior to dividing the mucosa to avoid gross spillage into the abdominal cavity.

Once excised, the specimen should be immediately placed in an Endo Catch™ retrieval bag and removed from the field. The bladder is then closed using a 0-polyglactin suture on a GS-21 needle in a running and interrupted double layer closure. A bilateral pelvic lymphadenectomy, as previously described, is then performed with node packets sent in separate Endo Catch™ retrieval bags. A 15Fr round Jackson–Pratt drain is left in place, and port sites and skin are closed as previously described.

References

1. Rowland RG, Mitchell ME, Bihrle R, Kahnoski RJ, Piser JE. Indiana continent urinary reservoir. J Urol. 1987;137:1136–9.
2. Hautmann RE, Egghart G, Frohneberg D, Miller K. The ileal neobladder. J Urol. 1988;139:39–42.
3. Knoedler JJ, Boorjian SA, Kim SP, Weight CJ, Thapa P, Tarrell RF, et al. Does partial cystectomy compromise oncologic outcomes for patients with bladder cancer compared to radical cystectomy? a matched case-control analysis. J Urol. 2012;188(4):1115–9.

Transperitoneal Robot-Assisted Laparoscopic Radical Prostatectomy: Anterior Approach

17

David I. Lee

Patient Selection

Patients who are candidates for open radical prostatectomy are generally also good candidates for robot-assisted laparoscopic radical prostatectomy (RALP). We do not select patients based on weight or prostate size although these patients are certainly more challenging and should be cautiously approached early in a particular surgeon's learning curve. Patients with prior abdominal surgery or prior prostate surgery can also be quite difficult; however, these are also not strict contraindications to a robotic approach. We have performed RALP for patients with prior laparoscopic hernia repairs, J pouches, renal transplants, and colectomy.

Preoperative Preparation

Patients are typically screened preoperatively with an EKG, complete blood count, chemistries, coagulation profile, and urinalysis with culture if

Electronic supplementary material: The online version of this chapter (doi:10.1007/978-3-319-45060-5_17) contains supplementary material, which is available to authorized users.

D.I. Lee, M.D. (✉)
Department of Surgery/Urology, University of Pennsylvania, 51 N. 39th St., MOB Ste 300, Philadelphia, PA 19104, USA
e-mail: David.lee@uphs.upenn.edu

indicated. In patients who have intermediate to high-risk disease we routinely order a multiparametric MRI of the prostate. We recommend a clear liquid diet commencing the afternoon before surgery and then nothing by mouth after midnight. A laxative is self administered the night before surgery. Upon arrival to the operating room, parenteral antibiotics are administered prior to skin incision. Sequential compression boots are routinely used in all patients. In patients who are at high risk for deep venous thrombosis, a single dose of 5000 U of subcutaneous heparin may be administered preoperatively.

Operative Setup

Selection of the operating room and subsequent organization of the equipment is critical for rapid patient setup, robot docking, and room turnover. A consistent preoperative approach and setup that involves the entire surgical team will minimize wasted time and maximize utilized operating room space. Our operating room setup is shown in Fig. 17.1. For transperitoneal robot-assisted laparoscopic radical prostatectomy (RALP), the robot must be brought in from the patient's feet and so this pathway must be unobstructed.

Our preference is to place the tableside surgical assistant on the patient's left side such that his or her dominant hand (usually right) can manipulate the suction device. The scrub nurse is on the

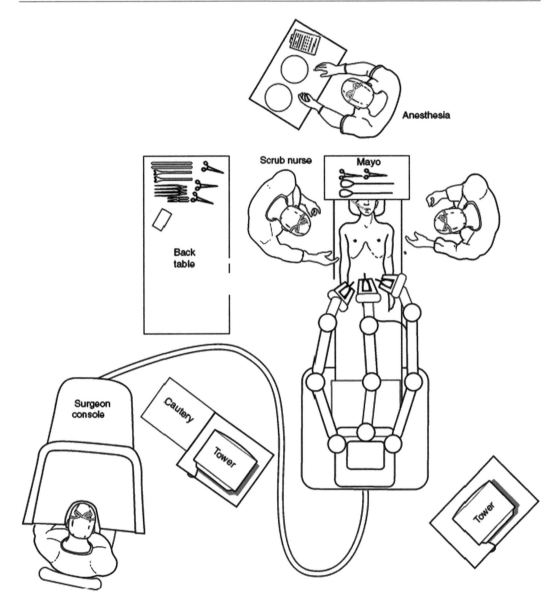

Fig. 17.1 Typical operating room setup for transperitoneal robot-assisted laparoscopic radical prostatectomy (RALP). Adequate room for rolling the robot to and away from the table is necessary. If a fourth arm is utilized, it can be placed on either side of the patient depending on surgeon preference

patient's right side. We make use of a Mayo stand placed over the patient's face as an instrument stand. It should be lowered as far as the ET tube will allow and thus will protect the tube from inadvertent dislodgement from the camera movement. If the Mayo stand is not low enough, the patient might need to be raised upward to create sufficient camera clearance.

Patient Positioning and Preparation

Lower extremity compression stockings are placed. After induction of general anesthesia, the legs are split 30° away from each and then extended at the hip 30° using either split leg positioners (preferable) (Amsco Surgical, San Antonio, TX) or alternatively using stirrups (Fig. 17.2).

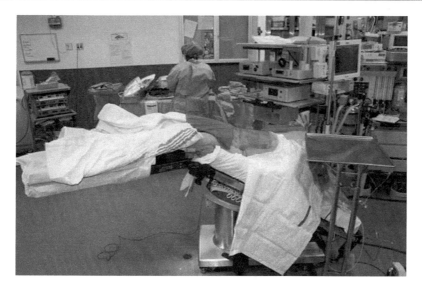

Fig. 17.2 Patient is positioned with legs on spreader bars and in the steep Trendelenburg position

This positioning facilitates docking of the robot. We loosely wrap each leg with a blanket. We then tuck the arms to the patient's side after wrapping each arm with a gel pad and remove the arm boards. The bed is then placed into a 30° Trendelenburg position. Eye protection is routinely used for the patient to prevent corneal abrasion. We do not routinely use shoulder rolls or foam padding because we feel that simply tucking the arms and lowering the legs sufficiently anchors most patients from sliding. Once the patient is prepped and draped, we place an 18 Fr urethral catheter and place it to gravity drainage. An intraoperative oral-gastric tube is placed at the outset and then removed at the completion of the procedure.

Trocar Configuration

We typically use a Veress needle to obtain pneumoperitoneum; alternatively, use a Hasson approach, if desired. We place the Veress through the belly of the rectus muscle infraumbilically. Once adequate insufflation has been obtained, trocars are placed as shown in Fig. 17.3, beginning with the midline supraumbilical trocar. Insert the camera, with a 0° lens and inspect the abdomen for any adhesions or injury as a conse-

quence of Veress needle or primary trocar placement. Meticulously place the remaining trocars under laparoscopic vision. The robot trocar sites should be no more than 18 cm from the pubis because the robotic instruments have a maximum working length of 25 cm [2].

We standardly use a total of six trocars: three Intuitive 8 mm metal robotic trocars for the robotic working arms, a 5 mm and a 12 mm trocar for the tableside assistant, and one 12 mm trocar for the camera. When working with the Xi robot, the 12 mm trocar is substituted with another 8 mm metal robotic trocar.

We feel that it is critical to precisely measure, rather than estimate by hand width, the distances for each trocar, especially in patients that are very small or large. Initially, we use a marking pen to identify the top of the pubis. We then place a 12 mm mark just above the umbilicus for the camera trocar. Once the abdomen is insufflated, a midline mark is made 14.5 cm cephalad from the pubis. Then, the robot trocar sites are triangulated such that they are 14.5 cm from the pubis and 8 cm from the lower midline mark. This ensures sufficient working room between the arms of the robot as well as adequate reach such that the tips of the instruments will reach to the membranous urethra. Difficulty with robot arm collisions can become greatly magnified if the

Fig. 17.3 A midline, periumbilical, point 15 cm from the pubic symphysis is marked. The two medial robotic trocars are placed 14.5 cm from the pubic symphysis and 8 cm from the periumbilical mark. The two lateral trocars are placed in a straight line 8 cm lateral from the medial trocars. The camera is placed in a 12 mm trocar placed superior to the umbilicus

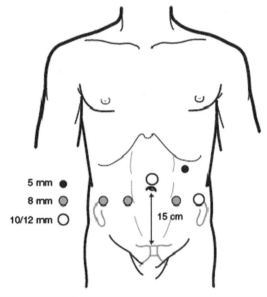

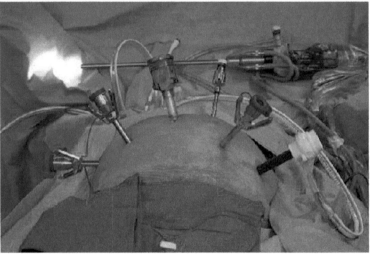

trocar sites are too close together. The straight line that is created by the first two robot trocars then delineates placement of the fourth arm trocar and the assistant's 12 mm trocar. These trocars are placed 8 cm lateral to the two robotic trocars. Finally, place a 5 mm trocar 8 cm on a diagonal line cephalad and lateral to the camera trocar. This trocar site can lie very close to the costal margin on smaller patients. This high position is essential, however, to provide working room for the hand of the assistant; placing this trocar too low can trap the assistant's hand between the robotic arms.

Once the trocars are placed, move the robot into position between the legs of the patient. When using the da Vinci® S or Si system, all arms are brought over the top of the patient and docked. The fourth arm once docked should be checked to ensure sufficient mobility such that its instrument tip can easily touch the anterior abdominal wall. This ensures that adequate upward retraction can be performed. When using the da Vinci Xi system, the robot may be side docked, that is, the side cart may be brought in across the side of the patient. This may be useful in patients with limited mobility of the lower extremities. We have also used this configuration to perform work in the upper abdomen if necessary before beginning the prostate portion of the operation. Be sure the previously placed mayo stand does not inhibit the fourth arm's and camera arm's mobility.

Instrumentation and Equipment List

Equipment

- da Vinci® S, Si or Xi Surgical System (four-arm system; Intuitive Surgical, Inc., Sunnyvale, CA)
- EndoWrist® Maryland bipolar forceps or PK dissector (Intuitive Surgical, Inc., Sunnyvale, CA)
- EndoWrist® curved monopolar scissors (Intuitive Surgical, Inc., Sunnyvale, CA)
- EndoWrist® Spatula Electrocautery (Intuitive Surgical, Inc., Sunnyvale, CA)
- EndoWrist® ProGrasp™ forceps (Intuitive Surgical, Inc., Sunnyvale, CA)
- EndoWrist® needle drivers (2) (Intuitive Surgical, Inc., Sunnyvale, CA)
- InSite® Vision System with 0º and 30º lens (Intuitive Surgical, Inc., Sunnyvale, CA)

Trocars

- 12 mm trocars (1 or 2)
- 8 mm robotic trocars (3 or 4)
- 5 mm trocar (1)

Recommended Sutures

- Vesicourethral anastomosis: 3-0 Quill stitch (Surgical Specialties Corporation, Wyomissing, PA).

- Modified Rocco stitch: 3-0 V-lok suture on an SH needle (Covidien, Mansfield, CT)
- Anterior bladder neck closure (if necessary): 3-0 polyglactin suture on an SH needle cut to 6 in.

Instruments Used by the Surgical Assistant

- Laparoscopic needle driver
- Laparoscopic scissors
- Blunt tip grasper
- Suction irrigator device
- 10 mm specimen entrapment bag
- Hem-o-lok® clip applier (Teleflex Medical, Research Triangle Park, NC)
- Small, Medium-Large, and Extra Large Hemo-lok® clips (Teleflex Medical, Research Triangle Park, NC)
- Endo-GIA linear stapling device (Covidien, Mansfield, MA) with a 45 mm cartridge length and purple Tristapler cartridge.
- EnSeal® device 5 mm diameter, 45 cm shaft length (SurgRx®, Redwood City, CA) (optional)
- SURGICEL® hemostatic gauze (Ethicon, Inc., Cincinnati, OH)
- 18 Fr urethral catheter

Step-by-Step Technique (Video 17.1)

Step 1: Entering the Space of Retzius (Table 17.1)

Our lens preference is a 0° lens at the outset. The monopolar scissors (right hand) and bipolar grasper (left hand) are the primary working instruments at this stage. The ProGrasp™ forceps is

Table 17.1 Entering the space of Retzius: surgeon and assistant instrumentation

Surgeon instrumentation			
Right arm	Left arm	Fourth arm	Assistant instrumentation
• Curved monopolar scissors	• Maryland bipolar grasper	• ProGrasp™ forceps	• Suction-irrigator
Endoscope lens: 0°			

used with the fourth robotic arm for grasping and retraction of tissues. The electrocautery generator settings used throughout the operation are 35 W for both monopolar and bipolar electrocautery. Once abdominal access is achieved, inspect the peritoneum for bowel adhesions and identify the internal inguinal rings, urachus, and the medial umbilical ligaments. Lyse adhesions as is necessary. We also prefer to mobilize the sigmoid colon so that it is fairly mobile. On occasion, the sigmoid is bunched and adhered to the peritoneum posterior to the bladder. We always mobilize these attachments as the colon in this position may greatly limit the working space in the pelvis once the bladder is dropped.

We prefer the anterior transperitoneal approach and thus drop the bladder to enter the space of Retzius as our initial step of the operation. Incise the peritoneum just lateral to the medial umbilical ligaments and carry the dissection laterally to the level of the vas deferens. We prefer to keep the incision just medial and anterior to the internal inguinal ring. Keep the incisions superficial so as not to injure the epigastric vessels. The assistant can use the suction device to prevent camera fogging by evacuating smoke during this dissection. Bladder irrigation via the urethral catheter can help define the limits of the bladder; however, incisions created lateral to the medial ligaments obviate the likelihood of bladder injury. Carry the incisions medially and anteriorly until they are joined at the midline at the urachus, which is then divided. We prefer to incise as cephalad as possible to avoid redundant

tissue obscuring the view of the camera throughout the case. As the bladder flap is created, the whitish fibers of the transversalis fascia come into view. Follow these fibers caudally; once these thin out, follow the contour of the abdominal wall inferiorly until the pubis is seen. Clean the pubis of connective tissue. We thoroughly sweep all periprostatic fat toward the midline. This move also cleans off the endopelvic fascia. The superficial dorsal vein is usually contained within this fat; use bipolar electrocautery to seal this vessel. After the vein is divided, roll the fat away from the apical portion of the prostate toward the base. We excise the large fat bundle and send it for pathologic examination due to the possible presence of lymph nodes that may harbor metastatic disease [3].

Step 2: Incision of the Endopelvic Fascia

Sharply incise the fascia laterally so that the underlying prostate and levator muscles are seen (Fig. 17.4). We prefer cold sharp incision with scissors; this prevents the "jumping" of the pelvic floor muscles that can be seen with electrocautery. Initiate this incision in the region of the prostatovesical junction and then carry it toward the apex of the prostate. This helps avoid bleeding from the vessels that are consistently present at the prostatic apex. We prefer to create a small separation of the levator muscles from the prostate; too much separation at this point is

Fig. 17.4 The right endopelvic fascia has been opened. The levator muscle is seen to the right. This dissection is through a mostly avascular plane and can be carried proximally as far as the bladder neck (Reproduced by permission of Saunders, 2007 [1])

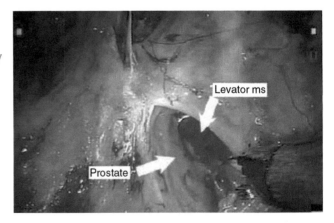

not necessary and may lead to inadvertent injury of the neurovascular bundle (NVB). Inferolateral to apex of the prostate, a band of muscle is often present that usually encases a vein, artery, or both. Using a small amount of bipolar electrocautery to seal these vessels prior to incising this tissue close to the prostate can limit blood loss and as such preserve visibility (Fig. 17.5). To better define the dorsal venous complex (DVC), we coldly incise the puboprostatic ligaments. With the prostate apex clearly in view, thin the fascia overlying the lateral aspect of the DVC in order to better define the junction between the vein and the urethra.

Step 3: Ligation of the Dorsal Venous Complex (Table 17.2)

The DVC can be handled by one of several methods; the most common methods are suture ligation or stapling. If suturing is to be performed, a 0-Polyglactin or PDS suture on a CT-1 needle is typically used to place a figure of eight around the DVC. We have used a figure-of-eight suture that is pexed into the pubic periosteum. This helps elevate the urethra after division of the prostatic apex which helps to visualize the urethra during the anastomosis and may be associated with recovery of urinary continence. Often, a back-bleeding suture is also placed toward the prostate base. Once tied, the DVC can be divided at this point, but many surgeons leave this intact temporarily until the urethra is approached later during the case. Alternatively as of late we have on occasion cold cut across the DVC and then used a 3-0 V-lok suture to oversew the bleeding vessels after all vascular structures are divided. Some theorize that this may help limit compression damage that the preplacement of a suture may create.

We prefer to staple the DVC using the laparoscopic Tri stapler (Covidien, Mansfield, MA) with a 45 mm cartridge length and purple load. The assistant introduces the stapler into the field through the lateral 12 mm assistant trocar. From this angle, place the anvil portion of the stapler on the contralateral side so that the black lines just

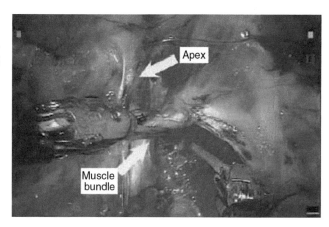

Fig. 17.5 Apical vessels traversing between the levator muscle and prostatic apex are usually cauterized with bipolar energy before division from the prostate to help minimizing bleeding (Reproduced by permission of Saunders, 2007 [1])

Table 17.2 Ligation of the dorsal venous complex: surgeon and assistant instrumentation

Surgeon instrumentation			
Right arm	Left arm	Fourth arm	Assistant instrumentation
• Curved monopolar scissors	• Maryland bipolar grasper	• ProGrasp™ forceps	• Suction-irrigator
• Needle driver (if suturing DVC)	• Needle driver (if suturing DVC)		• Laparoscopic scissors
Endoscope lens: 0°			• Endo-GIA linear stapling device (if stapling DVC)

pass the edge of the DVC (Fig. 17.6). The console surgeon can bunch up the prostate apex to aid in the assistant's visualization of the DVC. Clamp the stapler to the locked position and fire the stapler very slowly. This provides tissue compression, which improves staple formation and hemostasis. Once divided, there should be a small line of stapled tissue left, which can be easily divided later during the apical dissection. If there is any bleeding or if the staple line separates, use a small figure-of-eight stitch with a 3-0 polyglactin suture to stop the remaining bleeding.

Step 4: Division of the Prostatovesical Junction (Table 17.3)

The endoscope lens is switched to a 30° down lens to provide a more familiar downward view of the prostatovesical junction. Our preference is to utilize the monopolar electrocautery spatula in the right hand during this step as this instrument has a very atraumatic tip which can be used for gentle blunt dissection. To help visualize the bladder neck, the bedside assistant slowly pushes in and withdraws the urethral catheter. The prior removal of superficial fat from the prostate usually allows easy visualization of the catheter balloon. Lateral deviation of the urethral catheter during this "wiggle" maneuver is a clue for the presence of the median lobe. Once the location of the prostatovesical junction is firmly in mind, use small bursts of electrocautery alternating with blunt dissection to define the superficial layer of the bladder just proximal and lateral to the junction (Fig. 17.7). If this plane is developed carefully, the large superficial veins coursing from the prostate to the bladder can be lifted off the underlying structures thereby minimizing bleeding. The lateral junction between the prostate and the bladder can then be identified by a visible drop-off around the edge of the bladder. From this point, carry the dissection toward the prostate along this drop off paying close attention to the consistency of the tissue. With practice the bladder tissue can be easily differentiated from the firmer prostate tissue. The prostate will then be identified and from this point the attachment

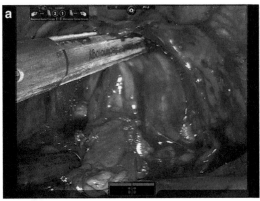
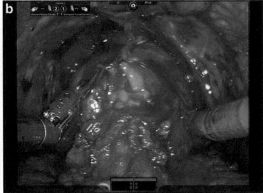
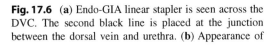

Fig. 17.6 (**a**) Endo-GIA linear stapler is seen across the DVC. The second black line is placed at the junction between the dorsal vein and urethra. (**b**) Appearance of the transected dorsal vein after stapling showing the urethra beneath (Reproduced by permission of Saunders, 2007 [1])

Table 17.3 Division of the prostatovesical junction: surgeon and assistant instrumentation

Surgeon instrumentation			
Right arm	Left arm	Fourth arm	Assistant instrumentation
• Monopolar electrocautery spatula	• Maryland bipolar grasper	• ProGrasp™ forceps	• Suction-irrigator
Endoscope lens: 30° down			

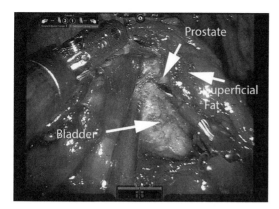

Fig. 17.7 Movement of the urethral catheter balloon (inflated to 10 mL) in (**b**) and out (**a**) greatly aids in the visual identification the prostatovesical junction. If an eccentric movement of the catheter balloon is noted, then the presence of a median lobe is likely (Reproduced by permission of W. B. Saunders, 2007 [1])

fibers should be divided from lateral to medial. This will help drop the lateral edges of the bladder from the prostate creating an increasingly defined bladder neck. This dissection essentially grooms the prostatovesical junction so that it is easily visualized. Key aspects of this dissection are the technique; short bursts of electrocautery followed by sweeping of the tissue helps to maintain excellent vision of the tissue planes. Too much electrocautery and the tissue will become charred; not enough and the tissue will bleed. The table-side assistant during this dissection is providing downward countertraction with the suction irrigator against the upward pull or lift of tissues by the console surgeon. Careful dissection usually allows excellent vision of the entire junction and the bladder neck can be spared or taken widely at the surgeon's discretion.

Enter the bladder neck medially, and deflate the balloon of the urethral catheter. Grasp the catheter through its eye with the fourth arm Prograsp™ forceps and pull the catheter anteriorly. We ensure that the catheter tip is lifted far above cranially to the pubis to provide optimal visualization of the posterior bladder neck margin. This holds the fourth arm well out of the way of the other two robot working arms minimizing arm collisions. The table-side assistant then provides tension on the urethral catheter outside the patient thereby lifting the prostate

upward facilitating the posterior dissection. The catheter can be secured to the draped outside the patient to maintain steady retraction. Once the bladder is opened, great care must be taken to visualize the posterior bladder neck for the presence of a median lobe. Also, inspect the bladder neck to ensure that there is sufficient distance from the ureteral orifices for later suturing and any need for later bladder neck reconstruction. We do not typically use indigo carmine to identify the ureteral orifices; however, this can be a useful adjunct. Finally, completely divide the bladder neck by reestablishing the lateral aspects of the bladder. Dissection at these points should define adipose tissue laterally thus confirming the plane between the bladder and the prostate and more posteriorly should reveal a whitish longitudinal plane of fibers extending from the bladder to the prostate known as the retrotrigonal plane. We prefer to drop the bladder from the prostate along this plane.

Step 5: Dissection and Ligation of the Seminal Vesicles and Vas Deferens

Once the retrotrigonal plane has been well visualized, this layer should be divided sharply to reveal a layer of fat that in turn overlies the ampulla of the vas. It is helpful at this point of the dissection to observe the general size of the prostate (Fig. 17.8). If the prostate is very large or has a significant median lobe component, then the angle at which this layer is divided is much steeper than if the prostate is small. If this is not appreciated, for example, in the case of large prostate, a portion of the prostate may easily be shaved off as one is searching for the vasa if too shallow a plane is taken.

Once one of the vasa is identified, gentle dissection should be used to enable grasping with the Prograsp™ forceps. The fourth arm is then used to lift the vas of interest upward and away from the rectum. Careful dissection should reveal an anterior plane on top of this structure that allows easy blunt sweeping of all surrounding tissues. Lateral dissection along the vas will reveal its paired seminal vesicle (SV). The assistant's downward pres-

Fig. 17.8 (a) Large prostates require a much steeper plane (*arrow*) to find the ampulla of the vas. (b) Smaller prostates require a much shallower plane

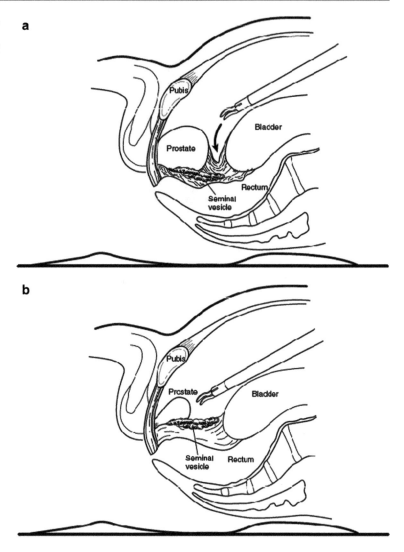

sure with the suction device opens this space and significantly aids the dissection. Blunt dissection along the medial edge of the SV will allow this structure to roll up away from its bed (Fig. 17.9). Spot bipolar electrocautery or clips can control small feeding vessels. Continuous and minor repositioning of the fourth arm can provide subtle retraction that can greatly facilitate this dissection. The use of electrocautery lateral to the SVs should be avoided to prevent thermal energy damage to the NVB [4]. One can excise a piece of vas for later use as a pledget during the anastomosis. If a pledget is not used, simply clip and transect the vas and leave them in situ. Once the vasa are divided and the SVs are rotated medially, very little lateral dissection is necessary to complete the dissection.

Step 6: Posterior Prostate Dissection (Table 17.4)

Grasp the stumps of the vasa with the fourth arm and use them to pull the prostate upward toward the pubis (anteriorly) and out of the pelvis (cranially) to gain optimal retraction. Once proper traction is obtained, note the posterior contour of the prostate which can be appreciated very nicely with the three-dimensional vision provided by the (Fig. 17.10). Incising Denonvillier's fascia precisely at this point helps to minimize any chance of injuring the rectum or incising into the prostate. Divide the Denonvillier's fascia horizontally along the posterior surface of the prostate, and gently push down the fat overlying the rectum, away from the prostate. Definitively identify the posterior capsule of the prostate, and carry the dissection along this plane toward the apex and laterally as far as can be reached. We feel that a key point in the dissection proper use of the left hand to push upward on the prostate so that the capsule can be clearly seen while the right hand gently pushes along the edge of the prostate to drop the rectum. In men with smaller prostates, the fibers of the rectourethralis can often be identified. Once the rectum has been definitively mobilized posteriorly, either excise

or spare the cavernous nerves based on clinico-pathologic findings.

Step 7: Neurovascular Bundle and Prostatic Pedicle Dissection (Table 17.5)

For a non-nerve-sparing procedure, the plane adjacent to the rectum can be continued laterally. This provides as large a margin as possible around the base and lateral portion of the prostate

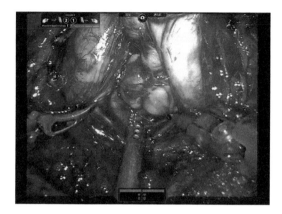

Fig. 17.9 (**a**) The Prograsp instrument in the fourth arm acts as an excellent retractor especially during the course of the vas dissection. As movement of the fourth arm is performed, one must be aware to not strike the pubic arch with the wrist of the instrument resulting in unwanted bleeding. (**b**) Elevation of the SV allows identification of its insertion into the prostate completing the SV dissection (Reproduced by permission of Saunders, 2007 [1])

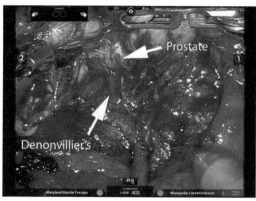

Fig. 17.10 (**a**) Grasping both vas stumps and retracting anteriorly helps to delineate the posterior plane on the prostate. (**b**) Incision directly on the curve demonstrated is a reproducible landmark if proper anterior traction of the prostate is obtained (Reproduced by permission of Saunders, 2007 [1])

Table 17.4 Posterior prostate dissection: surgeon and assistant instrumentation

Surgeon instrumentation			
Right arm	Left arm	Fourth arm	Assistant instrumentation
• Curved monopolar scissors	• Maryland bipolar grasper	• ProGrasp™ forceps	• Suction-irrigator
Endoscope lens: 30° down			

Table 17.5 Neurovascular bundle and prostatic pedicle dissection: surgeon and assistant instrumentation

Surgeon instrumentation			
Right arm	Left arm	Fourth arm	Assistant instrumentation
• Curved monopolar scissors	• Maryland bipolar grasper	• ProGrasp™ forceps	• Suction-irrigator
Endoscope lens: 30° down			• Linear stapling device (for non-nerve-sparing cases)
			• Hem-o-lok® clip applier (for nerve-sparing cases)

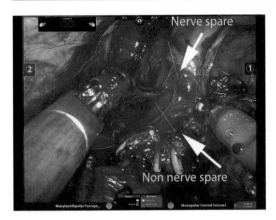

Fig. 17.11 Once the rectum has been dropped away from the posterior aspect of the prostate, the NVB can be either spared or resected. *Arrows* indicate the plane of dissection for a nerve-sparing (NS) and non-nerve-sparing (NNS) approach (Reproduced by permission of Saunders, 2007 [1])

(Fig. 17.11). Use of electrocautery, a bipolar sealing device or even a laparoscopic stapler, is acceptable and can be expedient if a non-nerve-sparing procedure is planned. Wide resection can be difficult especially when approaching the apex as the NVBs must be once again divided just past the apex of the prostate. Careful use of clips or bipolar energy can be helpful. Care must be exercised to not injure the rectum in this region with careful dissection and clear visualization. In the small number of rectal injuries that we have encountered, they have been in patients in whom wide resections were performed near the apex.

For a nerve-sparing procedure, our preference is to use an interfascial technique, where the lateral prostatic fascia is entered and a small amount of tissue is left covering the prostate capsule. In patients with very low-risk disease, a very close plane on the capsule may be utilized (intrafascial technique). We prefer to start this nerve sparing by performing an early anterior release of the lateral prostatic fascia beginning at the apex to mid portion of the prostate. The lateral prostatic fascia is identified and incised with scissors. Sweeping of the fascia posterolaterally releases the NVB from the prostate. We continue to separate the posterolateral portion of the NVB from the prostate so that the prostatic pedicles are clearly defined and then return to the antegrade

dissection for control of the pedicles. The pedicles of the prostate are secured athermally with large Hem-o-lok® clips (Teleflex Medical, Research Triangle Park, NC). Once the bulk of the pedicle has been divided, the remainder of the posterolateral plane opens up rather easily and the remaining bundle can be teased away from the prostate with very little difficulty. Small perforators are commonly encountered along this dissection and these vessels are usually allowed to bleed. These will stop spontaneously the majority of the time. If not, they can be individually clipped or suture ligated. However, electrocautery should be avoided so as to avoid damage to the nearby cavernous nerves.

Several different methods have been described to control bleeding around the pedicle, including bipolar electrocautery and sharp dissection, hemostatic clips, and placement of bulldog clamps on the pedicles with later oversewing [5]. Intuitively, minimizing energy discharge in the region of the pedicles seems the most prudent; this idea has been supported by experimental work in the canine model [6]. However, clinical outcomes are awaited to support the optimal method for sparing the NVB.

Step 8: Prostatic Apex Dissection

Once the apex is reached during the NVB dissection, the anterior urethra is dissected and exposed. If staples were used to ligate the DVC, a short burst of monopolar electrocautery expeditiously divides the tissue, allowing the underlying urethra to come into view. The remainder of the apical dissection is completed without thermal devices to avoid injury to the nerves or striated sphincter. After maximizing its length with gentle blunt dissection, the urethra is entered with scissors; the urethral catheter is withdrawn until it is just visible in the stump of the urethra. The fourth arm is then used to pull the prostate away from the pelvic floor. Gradually rocking the prostate back and forth provides exposure for division of the posterior urethra, remaining rectourethral, and posterior rhabdosphincter attachments.

Step 9: Entrapment of Specimen (Table 17.6)

Once freed, the prostate is placed into an entrapment sac and left in upper abdomen until the anastomosis is complete. A careful inspection of the bed of the prostate is performed to ensure no significant bleeders are present that might need attention. If there are arterial pumpers noted our preference is to bipolar these vessels if the stalk can be individually grasped; if the stalk is not visible a figure of eight suture will efficiently ligate the vessel.

Step 10: Reconstruction of Posterior Rhabdosphincter (Table 17.7)

In order to reduce time to continence by restoring urethral length and posterior support, we reconstruct the posterior rhabdosphincter as described in 2006 in both open and laparoscopic RRP by Rocco [7, 8]. During radical prostatectomy, the posterior prostatic musculofascial plate is transected. The Rocco maneuver serves to restore the plate's original anatomy and hence its functional support. To perform this, we use a single 3-0 V-lok suture. We have found that use of the barbed suture during this step greatly simplifies the process. The first pass is through the cut edge of Denonvilliers' where the suture is anchored down. Next, the suture is passed through the posterior edge of the rhabdosphincter lying immediately beneath the urethra. The next passes on the blad-der side then incorporate the cut edge of the retrotrigonal plane. This move effectively pulls the bladder toward the urethra without deformation of the bladder neck which then greatly facilitates the later anastomosis. The urethral catheter can be placed so as to be visible in the urethra at this time to ensure proper stitch placement. This is repeated in a figure-of-eight fashion, pulling gentle traction at each pass. The suture is then tied down, rejoining the musculofascial plate to continuity. We feel that this stitch is also a significant aid to hemostasis along the prostatic bed. Smaller venous oozing will often subside after this stitch is completed.

Step 11: Vesicourethral Anastomosis

For the anastomosis, we prefer to use the Van Velthoven stitch [9]. This running, double-armed suture has many benefits, including minimizing knot-tying and providing a water-tight anastomosis. We use a 3-0 Quill suture which is a pre-formed barbed suture that comes in a variety of monofilaments and needles but is barbed in a bidirectional fashion with a needle on either end. The configuration that we prefer is the 18 cm length with an SH type needle. The UR-6 or RB-1 needles can alternatively be utilized.

We start the anastomosis by placing both arms of the suture outside-in at the 4 and 5 o'clock positions along the posterior bladder neck. Place the sutures in the urethra inside-out at the corresponding positions. We then use the 5 o'clock

Table 17.6 Entrapment of specimen: surgeon and assistant instrumentation

Surgeon instrumentation			
Right arm	Left arm	Fourth arm	Assistant instrumentation
• Curved monopolar scissors	• Maryland bipolar grasper	• ProGrasp™ forceps	• Suction-irrigator
Endoscope lens: 30° down			• Specimen entrapment bag

Table 17.7 Reconstruction of posterior rhabdosphincter: surgeon and assistant instrumentation

Surgeon instrumentation			
Right arm	Left arm	Fourth arm	Assistant instrumentation
• Needle driver	• Needle driver	• ProGrasp™ forceps	• Suction-Irrigator
Endoscope lens: 30° down			• Laparoscopic scissors
			• Needle driver

stitch to move in a clockwise running fashion by going to the 6 and 7 o'clock positions. This creates a firm back wall to the anastomosis; the catheter is then passed in and the integrity of that back wall confirmed. This clockwise stitch is then run to the 11 o'clock position to complete the left side of the anastomosis. To ensure coaptation as the anastomosis progresses, we pull on the stitch with one needle driver and use the other as a "pulley" that anchors the delicate urethral tissue by placing the jaws of the instrument just below the stitch. By doing this, we have found that a large amount of force can be applied to the stitch serving to bring the bladder to the urethra without tearing the urethra.

Once the left side is completed then complete the right hand side of the anastomosis by placing the 4 o'clock stitch through the bladder and then the 3 o'clock in the urethra. We then ensure that no slack exists after these throws and then complete the anastomosis to the 12 o'clock position. Pass the transition suture at 12 o'clock outside-in on the urethra and pass it inside-out on the bladder neck. Pass the catheter into the bladder. Ensure that all passes through the urethra have been sufficiently pulled taught in order to avoid a gap in the anastomosis. Tie the two sutures together across the anastomosis. We irrigate the bladder with 120 mL of saline and then push down on top of the bladder to ensure a water tight anastomosis. If there is a small leak, a figure-of-eight stitch can be used to close the defect. We have not, in general, been leaving pelvic drains in place even with very small leaks.

Step 12: Exiting the Abdomen

The assistant places the drawstring from the specimen retrieval bag into the abdomen under laparoscopic vision. The console surgeon then grasps the end of the string in the right hand needle driver and then lines up the camera trocar directly to the string. Then, the camera is placed into the lateral 12 mm assistant trocar. The assistant places a laparoscopic needle driver into the camera trocar site and removes the drawstring from the grasp of the right hand needle driver. The tail of the drawstring is clamped externally with a hemostat to

prevent the drawstring from slipping back into the abdomen. The robot is then undocked and the trocars removed under laparoscopic vision to check for any bleeding. The specimen is then removed by extending the incision of the camera trocar site. The fascia is opened with electrocautery until the specimen can be retrieved and then closed with #1 Maxon suture following extraction of the specimen. The remaining trocar sites are closed with a subcuticular stitch of 4-0 monocryl, and the skin reapproximated with a skin adhesive or stitches and steristrips.

Postoperative Management

Remove the orogastric tube in the operating suite. Patients are prescribed ketorolac around the clock and morphine as needed for pain. Patients are encouraged to ambulate as soon as possible, usually within 6 h of the returning to their hospital room. A clear liquid diet is instituted that is advanced to a regular diet by the patient's next meal. Discharge is planned for the morning of postoperative day 1. Patients are seen back in 1 week for catheter removal.

Special Considerations

Some surgeons may utilize adjustments in trocar configuration for obese patients; however, we typically use the same configuration for even very large patients. Other patients that may also present difficulty are those with very large prostates or large median lobes, prior prostate or abdominal surgery, and those with relatively small bony pelvises. These more complex patient scenarios will be the subject of a later chapter entitled "Robot-Assisted Radical Prostatectomy: Management of the Difficult Case."

Steps to Avoid Complications

All complications related to laparoscopic surgery readily apply to robot-assisted laparoscopic radical prostatectomy (RALP). Intraoperative complications include bleeding, injury to adjacent organs, and conversion to open surgery. Rectal injury is an ever-present danger, especially in patients with a history of preoperative androgen ablation. In cases of small rectal tears, consideration can be given to primary closure in two layers with interrupted sutures in patients who have been given a preoperative bowel preparation. Copious irrigation of the pelvis and broad-spectrum intravenous antibiotics should be instituted. Large injuries may be handled by conversion to an open procedure with primary rectal repair and consideration of a diverting ileostomy. Postoperative hematuria may be troublesome for some patients. Instruct patients to seek immediate attention for problems involving catheter obstruction related to clot retention. Late complications such as incontinence and impotence are beyond the scope of this chapter but are explained in detail in other sources.

References

1. Lee DI. Robotic prostatectomy. Atlas of Laparoscopic Retroperitoneal Surgery. In: Bishoff J, editor. Philadelphia: WB Saunders; 2007. p. 273–81.

2. Pick DL, Lee DI, Skarecky DW, et al. Anatomic guide for port placement for daVinci robotic radical prostatectomy. J Endourol. 2004;18:572.

3. Finley DS, Deane L, Rodriguez E, et al. Anatomic excision of anterior prostatic fat at radical prostatectomy: implications for pathologic upstaging. Urology. 2007;70:1000.

4. Tewari A, Rao S, Martinez-Salamanca JI, et al. Cancer control and the preservation of neurovascular tissue: how to meet competing goals during robotic radical prostatectomy. BJU Int. 2008;101:1013.

5. Ahlering TE, Eichel L, Chou D, et al. Feasibility study for robotic radical prostatectomy cautery-free neurovascular bundle preservation. Urology. 2005;65:994.

6. Ong AM, Su LM, Varkarakis I, et al. Nerve sparing radical prostatectomy: effects of hemostatic energy sources on the recovery of cavernous nerve function in a canine model. J Urol. 2004;172:1318.

7. Rocco B, Gregori A, Stener S, et al. Posterior reconstruction of the rhabdosphincter allows a rapid recovery of continence after transperitoneal video-laparoscopic radical prostatectomy. Eur Urol. 2007;51:996.

8. Rocco F, Carmignani L, Acquati P, et al. Restoration of posterior aspect of rhabdosphincter shortens continence time after radical retropubic prostatectomy. J Urol. 2006;175:2201.

9. Van Velthoven RF, Ahlering TE, Peltier A, et al. Technique for laparoscopic running urethrovesical anastomosis: the single knot method. Urology. 2003;61:699.

Transperitoneal Robot-Assisted Radical Prostatectomy: Posterior Approach

18

Jennifer Kuo, Jason Joseph, and Li-Ming Su

Patient Selection

The indications for robot-assisted laparoscopic radical prostatectomy (RALP) are identical to that for open surgery, that is, patients with clinical stage T2 or less with no evidence of metastasis either clinically or radiographically (computed tomography and bone scan). Absolute contraindications include uncorrectable bleeding diatheses or the inability to undergo general anesthesia due to severe cardiopulmonary compromise. Patients who have received neoadjuvant hormonal therapy or who have a history of prior complex lower abdominal and pelvic surgery such as partial colectomy, inguinal mesh herniorrhaphy, or prior transurethral resection of the prostate (TURP) pose a greater technical challenge due to distortion of normal anatomy and adhesions. Morbidly obese patients pose additional challenges due to the potential respiratory compromise encountered when placing these patients in a steep Trendelenburg position as well as the relatively limited working space and limitations of trocar size and instrumentation length. Patients with large prostate volumes (e.g., >70 g) are often associated with longer operative times, blood loss, and hospital stay than those with smaller glands. Salvage surgery after failure of primary treatment (e.g., radiation, brachytherapy, cryotherapy, high-intensity focused ultrasound) has been successfully reported in properly selected patients, but should be approached with caution due to the higher attendant risks and complications [1, 2]. These more complex patient scenarios should be avoided in a surgeon's early experience with RALP. However, these patient features are not by themselves absolute contraindications.

Preoperative Preparation

Bowel Preparation

One bottle of citrate of magnesium can be provided the day before surgery in order to evacuate bowel contents and prepare the colon in the event of a rectal injury. However, with experience, the authors no longer utilize any formal oral bowel preparation. The patient's diet is limited to clear liquids the day prior to surgery. A Fleet Enema (C.B. Fleet Company, Inc., Lynchburg, VA) is administered the morning of surgery. A broad-spectrum antibiotic such as cefazolin is administered intravenously 30 min before surgery. Ideally, aspirin and other anticoagulants should be held at least 7–10 days prior

Electronic supplementary material: The online version of this chapter (doi:10.1007/978-3-319-45060-5_18) contains supplementary material, which is available to authorized users.

J. Kuo, M.D. • J. Joseph, M.D. • L.-M. Su, M.D. (✉)
Department of Urology, University of Florida College of Medicine, 1600 SW Archer Road, 100247, Gainesville, FL 32610-2047, USA
e-mail: Li-Ming.Su@urology.ufl.edu

to surgery; however, the authors have noticed no significant difference in complications or blood loss in those patients where aspirin could not be safely held.

Informed Consent

In addition to bleeding, transfusion, and infection, patients undergoing RALP must be aware of the potential for conversion to open surgery. As with open surgery, patients must be counseled on the risk of impotence, incontinence, incisional hernia, and adjacent organ injury (e.g., ureter, rectum, bladder, small bowel). The risks of general anesthesia must also be presented to the patient as RALP cannot be performed under regional anesthesia.

Obtaining a baseline assessment of the patient's preoperative urinary and sexual function are critical in guiding preoperative counseling in providing a realistic forecast of return of urinary and sexual function following surgery even despite efforts at preserving the neurovascular bundles. Use of a validated questionnaire such as the Sexual Health Inventory for Men and International Prostate Symptom Score allow for an objective evaluation of baseline function.

Operative Setup

At our institution, we use the da Vinci® Si HD Surgical System (Intuitive Surgical, Inc., Sunnyvale, CA) with a four-armed technique. As such, only one assistant is required and is placed on the patient's right side. Across from the assistant is the scrub technician with video monitors placed for easy viewing by each team member. A Mayo stand is placed next to the assistant for commonly used instrumentation. After the patient is placed in the steep Trendelenburg position, the patient-side surgical robotic cart is positioned between the patient's legs. The final operating room setup is as shown in Fig. 18.1. Having a large operating room, ideally dedicated solely to robotic surgery, is important as these surgeries require significant equipment that is large as well as delicate. Moving this equipment from one operating room to another risks damage and may delay surgery.

Patient Positioning and Preparation

Having a dedicated team versed in robotic surgery helps to ensure a smooth and efficient surgery. Preoperative briefings allows for the entire team including the surgeon, circulating nurse, scrub technician, and anesthesiologist to identify the patient and planned procedure as well as verbalize any concerns so that these may be addressed and resolved before beginning the surgery. This includes communication with the anesthesiologist, making them aware of surgical expectations and anticipated challenges such as placement of an orogastric tube, intravenous access, fluid administration, and end-tidal carbon-dioxide monitoring especially with the patient placed in the steep Trendelenburg position.

Once in the operating room, the patient is placed in a supine position. After induction of general endotracheal anesthesia, the patient's arms are tucked to the sides using two draw sheets and egg-crate padding (Fig. 18.2a–d). To secure the patient's arms, one draw sheet is left below the arm, while the second draw sheet is held taught against the patient's abdomen. The arm is placed on an egg-crate padding to provide additional cushion (Fig. 18.2a). The first draw sheet is then brought over the arm and tucked below the patient while using the second draw sheet to slightly lift and roll the patient to aid in tucking (Fig. 18.2b). The second draw sheet is then brought down and tucked under the patient while an assistant gently lifts the ipsilateral hip to aid in securing the second draw sheet. Alternatively, arm sleds padded with egg-crate padding may be used. Finally, the hand and wrist are protected using an additional egg-crate padding, keeping the thumb directed upward (Fig. 18.2c). The patient's legs are abducted and placed in a gently flexed position on a split leg table to allow for access to the rectum and perineum. The patient's legs are secured to the split leg supports with egg-crate padding and adhesive tape.

Fig. 18.1 Operating room setup for transperitoneal robot-assisted laparoscopic radical prostatectomy (RALP) demonstrating standard configuration of operating room personnel and equipment (© 2009 Li-Ming Su, M.D., University of Florida)

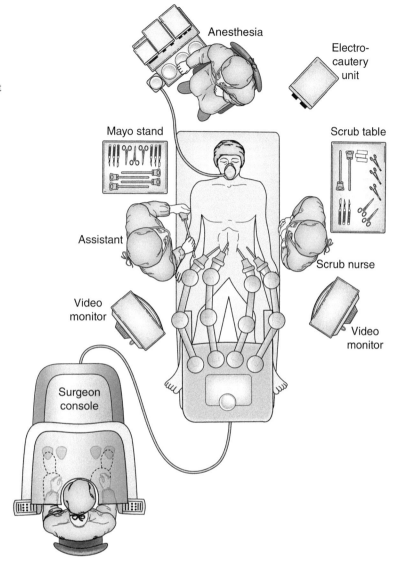

Alternatively, yellow fin stirrups may be used; however, docking of the fourth arm can at times be compromised by the relatively wide profile of the stirrups as compared to the more narrow split leg supports. Sequential compression stocking devices are placed on both legs and activated. Fixed shoulder pad supports to prevent the patient from cephalad migration in the Trendeleburg position should be avoided as this can result in compression and neuropraxic injury. Instead, the patient is secured to the operating room table above the xyphoid process with egg-crate pad-

ding and a band of heavy cloth tape across the chest or in a criss-cross pattern. A gel pad can be placed beneath the patient to minimize slippage during the steep Trendelenburg position. The patient is placed in steep Trendelenburg and is ready for shaving and prepping (Fig. 18.2d). An orogastric tube is inserted to decompress the stomach and a 16 Fr urethral catheter is placed under sterile conditions so that it can be accessed throughout the surgery by the bedside assistant.

The prostate biopsy pathology is again reviewed on the day of surgery to help guide the

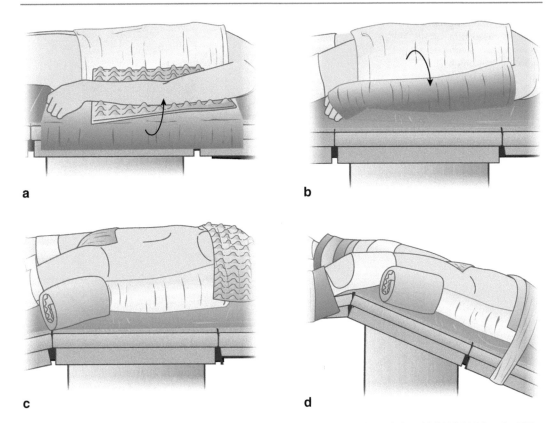

Fig. 18.2 Patient positioning including padding along the patient's arms, hands, and chest (© 2009 Li-Ming Su, M.D., University of Florida)

intraoperative surgical approach. By mapping the approximate site-specific locations of cancer based upon sextant biopsy findings, a surgeon can begin to formulate a tentative plan for bilateral vs. unilateral vs. incremental neurovascular bundle (NVB) preservation. If high-risk features (i.e., high-grade disease, high percent core involvement, palpable disease) are present, plans for a non-nerve-sparing approach may be prudent. A digital rectal examination can be performed with the patient now under general anesthesia as this is the best opportunity to examine the prostate, while the patient is fully relaxed. This is the only time during the surgery that the surgeon has true tactile feedback to assess the size, shape, and abnormalities of the patient's prostate, especially along the posterolateral border adjacent to the location of the NVB.

Trocar Configuration

In total, six trocars are placed transabdominally (Fig. 18.3). The first trocar is a 12 mm trocar for the endoscope and camera and is placed 15–17 cm superior to the pubic symphysis and generally just above the umbilicus. Two 8 mm pararectus trocars are placed 8–9 cm lateral and 2–3 cm caudal to camera trocar on the left and right sides. These accommodate the second and third robotic arms. An additional 8 mm trocar is placed 8–9 cm lateral to the left pararectus trocar in the left lumbar region high above the iliac crest and accommodates the fourth arm of the robot, allowing for intraoperative retraction among other uses. For the surgical assistant, a 12 mm trocar is placed 8–9 cm lateral to right pararectus trocar in the right lower quadrant above the anterior iliac spine

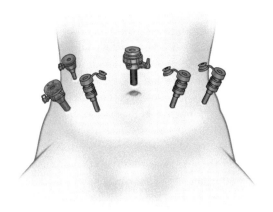

Fig. 18.3 Trocar configuration for transperitoneal robot-assisted laparoscopic radical prostatectomy (RALP) (© 2009 Li-Ming Su, M.D., University of Florida)

at the same level as the pararectus trocars. An additional 5 mm assistant trocar is placed in the right upper quadrant at the apex of a triangle made between the assistant trocar and the right pararectus trocar.

Instrumentation and Equipment List

Equipment

- da Vinci® Si HD Surgical System (four-arm system; Intuitive Surgical, Inc., Sunnyvale, CA)
- EndoWrist® Maryland bipolar forceps or PK dissector (Intuitive Surgical, Inc., Sunnyvale, CA)
- EndoWrist® curved monopolar scissors (Intuitive Surgical, Inc., Sunnyvale, CA)
- EndoWrist® ProGrasp™ forceps (Intuitive Surgical, Inc., Sunnyvale, CA)
- EndoWrist® needle drivers (2) (Intuitive Surgical, Inc., Sunnyvale, CA)
- EndoWrist® Mega™ SutureCut™ needle driver (1) (Intuitive Surgical, Inc., Sunnyvale, CA)
- InSite ®Vision System with 0° and 30° lens (Intuitive Surgical, Inc., Sunnyvale, CA)

Trocars

- 12 mm trocars (2)
- 8 mm robotic trocars (3)
- 5 mm trocar (1)

Recommended Sutures

- Ligation of the deep dorsal vein complex (DVC): 0 PDS suture on a CT-1 needle cut to 10 in. and 4-0 polyglactin suture on an RB1 needle cut to 6 in. (if necessary)
- Modified Rocco stitch and vesicourethral anastomosis: double armed 2-0 Quill Monoderm™ (Quill Medical, Inc., Research Triangle Park, NC) barbed suture (16 × 16 cm) on taper point needles (17 mm, half-circle)
- Anterior bladder neck closure (if necessary): 2-0 polyglactin suture on a UR-6 needle cut to 6 in.
- Anterior bladder neck intussusception suture: 2-0 PDS suture on an SH needle cut to 6 in.

Instruments Used by the Surgical Assistant

- Laparoscopic needle driver
- Laparoscopic scissors
- Blunt tip grasper
- Suction irrigator device
- Hem-o-lok® clip applier (Teleflex Medical, Research Triangle Park, NC)
- Small, Medium-Large and Extra Large Hemo-lok ® clips (Teleflex Medical, Research Triangle Park, NC)
- 10 mm specimen entrapment bag
- Sponge on a stick
- SURGICEL® hemostatic gauze (Ethicon, Inc., Cincinnati, OH)
- 18 Fr silicone urethral catheter
- Hemovac or Jackson-Pratt closed suction pelvic drain

Step-by-Step Technique (Videos 18.1, 18.2, 18.3, 18.4, 18.5, 18.6, 18.7, 18.8, 18.9, 18.10, 18.11, 18.12, 18.13, 18.14, 18.15, and 18.16)

Step 1: Abdominal Access and Trocar Placement

For a transperitoneal RALP approach, pneumoperitoneum is established using a Veress needle inserted at the base of the umbilicus. Alternatively, an open trocar placement with a Hasson technique can be used. The insufflation pressure is maintained at 15 mmHg. A 12 mm trocar is placed immediately above the umbilicus (approximately 15–17 cm from the pubic symphysis) under direct visualization using a visual obturator. Occasionally, this trocar is placed infraumbilical if the distance from the umbilicus and pubic symphysis is more than 15 cm. Secondary trocars, as mentioned above, are then placed under laparoscopic view. The da Vinci® robot is then positioned between the patient's legs and the four robotic arms are docked to their respective trocars.

Once intraperitoneal access and a pneumoperitoneum are established, the camera is inserted through the 12 mm supraumbilical trocar. The console surgeon controls camera movement by depressing the foot pedals and using brief arm movements to affect camera and instrument positioning. Stereo endoscopes with either angled (30°) or straight ahead (0°) viewing are available and interchangeable at various portions of the procedure. However, our preference is to use the 0° lens throughout the entire operation. Under direct visualization, the robotic arms are then loaded with instruments and positioned within the operative field at which point the console surgeon takes control. The curved monopolar scissors are placed in the second robotic arm ("right hand" of the console surgeon) while Maryland bipolar forceps are inserted into the third robotic arm ("left hand"). Finally, the fourth arm is used to control a ProGrasp™ forceps (Intuitive Surgical, Inc., Sunnyvale, CA). Once the bedside-assistant advances these instruments into proper position within the operative field, the robotic arms, in general, do not require any further adjustment for the remainder of the case. When instruments are exchanged, the robot will retain "memory" of the precise location of the removed instrument within the body, and therefore the new instrument will return to a few millimeters short of the last position automatically, reducing the risk for accidental injury to intra-abdominal and pelvic structures. The electrocautery settings used during the operation are 30 W for both monopolar and bipolar electrocautery.

Step 2: Dissection of Seminal Vesicles and Vas Deferens (Table 18.1)

Upon initial inspection of the operative field, the relevant landmarks include the bladder, median (urachus) and medial umbilical ligaments, vas deferens, iliac vessels, and rectum (Fig. 18.4). Frequently, adhesions are encountered within the pelvic cavity especially between the sigmoid colon and the left lateral pelvic side wall, which are released using sharp dissection. During transperitoneal-posterior approach, the initial step is retrovesical dissection of the vas deferentia and seminal vesicles (SVs) following the same principles described by the Montsouris technique [3]. After using the ProGrasp™ forceps to retract the sigmoid colon out of the pel-

Table 18.1 Dissection of seminal vesicles and vas deferens: surgeon and assistant instrumentation

Surgeon instrumentation			
Right arm	Left arm	Fourth arm	Assistant instrumentation
• Curved monopolar scissors	• Maryland bipolar grasper	• ProGrasp™ forceps	• Suction-irrigator
Endoscope lens: 0°			• Hem-o-lok® clip applier

Fig. 18.4 Anatomic
landmarks within the pelvis.
Upon initial inspection of
pelvis, the bladder, urachus,
medial umbilical ligaments,
vas deferens, and iliac vessels
as well as the rectum should be
identified to serve as
anatomical landmarks to aid in
dissection

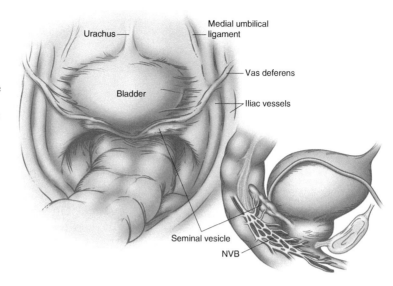

vic cavity, the vas deferens is identified laterally coursing over the medial umbilical ligaments. The peritoneum overlying the vas deferens is incised sharply and the vas is traced medially to its coalescence with the ipsilateral SV. The contralateral vas is then dissected. Hemoclips are placed on the vasa superior to their coalescence into the ejaculatory ducts, and the vasa are freed anteriorly off of the posterior aspect of the bladder to aid in later identification of the vasa during division of the bladder neck. The vasa are transected near the coalescence so as to not leave long vasal ends that may become a hindrance later in the operation.

Next the SVs are dissected. The assistant provides counter traction by lifting the bladder at the 12 o'clock position to improve exposure to the SVs. The posterior dissection of the SV is carried out first as very few blood vessels are encountered along this relatively avascular plane. Next, the anterior dissection of the SV is performed using gentle, blunt dissection to define and isolate the two to three vessels that often course along the anterolateral surface of the SV. Hemoclips are judiciously applied to these vessels along the lateral surface of the SV starting from the tip and traveling toward the base. These vascular packets are divided using cold scissors, and use of thermal energy is avoided if possible during this dissection in efforts to avoid injury to the nearby NVBs (Fig. 18.5).

Step 3: Posterior Dissection of the Prostate

The SVs and vasa are lifted anteriorly with the ProGrasp™ forceps and a 2–3 cm horizontal incision is made through the posterior layer of Denonvillier's fascia approximately 0.5 cm below the base of the SVs (Fig. 18.6). In patients with low-volume, nonpalpable disease, the posterior dissection plane is developed between Denonvillier's fascia posteriorly and the prostatic fascia anteriorly to help facilitate later release of the NVB located along the posterolateral surface of the prostate. In the case of high volume or palpable disease, this posterior dissection should be carried out one layer deeper, between Denonvillier's fascia and the prerectal fat plane, thus maintaining additional tissue coverage along the posterior aspect of the prostate. In addition, in cases of prior acute prostatitis, this prerectal fat plane if often preserved with few adhesions and may be a safer plane of dissection in these unique cases.

The assistant provides counter traction by applying gentle pressure at the 6 o'clock position using a suction-irrigator, retracting Denonvillier's fascia and the rectum posteriorly. The surgeon elevates the posterior aspect of the prostate with the Maryland bipolar forceps (left hand) using blunt dissection with the curved monopolar scissors (right hand) to develop this avascular plane

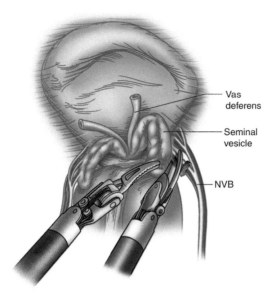

along the posterior aspect of the prostate. Using gentle sweeping motions, all posterior attachments are released as far as possible toward the prostatic apex. Thorough and wide dissection of the rectum off of the posterior prostate is critical in order to minimize the risk of rectal injury during subsequent steps such as division of the urethra and dissection of the prostatic apex. Once again, thermal energy should be minimized especially along the medial aspect of the NVBs.

Step 4: Developing the Space of Retzius

The bladder is dissected from the anterior abdominal wall by dividing the urachus high above the bladder and incising the peritoneum bilaterally just lateral to the medial umbilical ligaments (Fig. 18.7). Prior to dividing the medial umbilical ligaments, the obliterated umbilical vessels must be controlled with bipolar electrocautery prior to

Fig. 18.5 Seminal vesicle dissection. Anterolateral dissection of the SV is performed using Hem-o-lok® clips and cold scissors. Electrocautery should be avoided if possible during this step due to the close proximity of the NVBs (© 2009 Li-Ming Su, M.D., University of Florida)

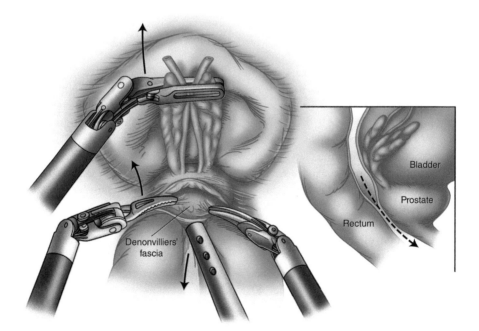

Fig. 18.6 Posterior dissection of the prostate. During the posterior dissection of the prostate, the fourth robotic arm is used to lift the SVs anteriorly. Denonvillier's fascia is incised horizontally 0.5 cm below the base of the SVs and the dissection is carried caudally toward the prostatic apex (© 2009 Li-Ming Su, M.D., University of Florida)

Fig. 18.7 Entering the space of retzius. The bladder is dissected from the anterior abdominal wall by dividing the urachus and medial umbilical ligaments laterally. The presence of fatty alveolar tissue ensures the correct plane that is extended down to the pubic symphysis (© 2009 Li-Ming Su, M.D., University of Florida)

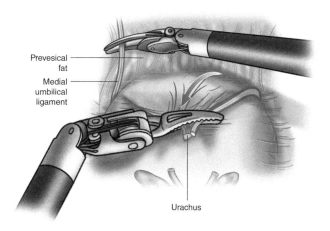

Prevesical fat

Medial umbilical ligament

Urachus

division so as to avoid unwanted bleeding. The presence of fatty alveolar tissue confirms the proper plane of dissection within the space of Retzius. Applying posterior traction on the urachus, the prevesical fat is identified and bluntly dissected, exposing the pubic symphysis. The dissection is maintained within the pelvic brim in order to avoid injury to the iliac vessels laterally. The bladder is released laterally to the point where the medial umbilical ligament crosses the vas deferens. This ensures that the bladder is optimally mobilized from the pelvic side wall so as to avoid tension at the vesicourethral anastomosis during the later steps of the operation.

The fat overlying the anterior prostate is then removed to improve exposure of the prostate. Using mainly blunt dissection, this fat pad is dissected from a lateral to medial direction, which simultaneously helps to isolate the superficial DVC. These vessels travel anterior to the prostatic apex and through the anterior prostatic fatty tissue and are coagulated with bipolar electrocautery prior to division. The fat pad is rolled off of the prostate in a cephalad direction from apex to base. The distal branches of the superficial DVC are then coagulated with bipolar electrocautery prior to division allowing for the fat pad to be removed as a single specimen. Upon removal of the anterior fat, visible landmarks include the anterior aspect of the bladder and prostate, puboprostatic ligaments, endopelvic fascia, and pubis (Fig. 18.8). Using the ProGrasp™ forceps to grasp and retract the bladder, the endopelvic fascia and

puboprostatic ligaments are sharply divided exposing the levator muscle fibers attached to the lateral and apical portions of the prostate. The endopelvic fascia is first divided from the mid prostate dissecting toward the base. The endopelvic fascia at the apex is left to the end as often there are small vessels travesing between the sidewall and the prostatic apex that can bleed, obscuring the operating field. The levator muscle fibers are meticulously and bluntly dissected from the surface of the prostate and preserved, exposing the prostatic apex, DVC, and urethra.

Step 5: Ligation of the Deep Dorsal Venous Complex (Table 18.2)

The ProGrasp™ forceps is used to bunch the deep DVC along the anterior prostatovesical junction while simultaneously applying slight cephalad traction. This provides optimal exposure of the DVC and pubis. A 0-PDS suture on a CT-1 needle is passed by the assistant to the surgeon using a laparoscopic needle driver and the DVC is suture ligated using a slip knot or figure-of-eight suture (Fig. 18.9). The needle is passed beneath the DVC from right to left and anterior to the urethra. Securing the DVC as far away from the prostatic apex as possible can help minimize iatrogenic entry into the prostatic apex during later division of the DVC. A second DVC stitch is placed distal to the first and used to suspend the DVC to the inferior pubic symphysis. The DVC

Fig. 18.8 View of the anterior prostate. The fat overlying the anterior prostate is dissected in a lateral to medial direction and removed in a single packet by rolling the tissue from the apex toward the base of the prostate. Bipolar electrocautery is used to transect the superficial DVC. This helps to better expose the anterior prostate and bladder, puboprostatic ligaments, and endopelvic fascia (© 2009 Li-Ming Su, M.D., University of Florida)

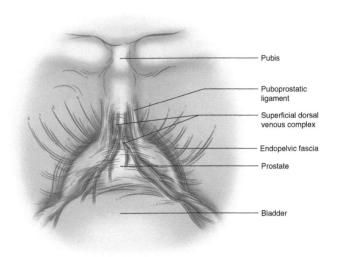

Pubis

Puboprostatic ligament

Superficial dorsal venous complex

Endopelvic fascia

Prostate

Bladder

Table 18.2 Ligation of the deep dorsal venous complex: surgeon and assistant instrumentation

Surgeon instrumentation			
Right arm	Left arm	Fourth arm	Assistant instrumentation
• Mega™ SutureCut™ needle driver	• Needle driver	• ProGrasp™ forceps	• Suction-irrigator
Endoscope lens: 0°			• Laparoscopic needle driver

is not divided until later in the operation and immediately prior to prostatic apical dissection and division of the urethra. An additional 0-PDS suture may be placed along the anterior bladder neck to prevent venous back bleeding and to help identify the contour of the prostate for subsequent bladder neck transection. The authors prefer the use of the Mega™ SutureCut™ needle driver when suturing as this facilitates suture cutting by the operative surgeon and obviates the need for the assistant to change instruments to perform this task.

Step 6: Anterior Bladder Neck Transection (Table 18.3)

The anterior bladder is divided using monopolar electrocautery. With experience, the proper plane of dissection can be visualized by simply inspecting the contour of the prostate and bladder neck [4]. Several maneuvers are used to better delineate this plane of dissection. First,

visual inspection of the prevesical adipose tissue as it transitions to the bare anterior prostate gland often defines the bladder neck. Second, lifting the dome of the bladder in a cephalad direction with the ProGrasp™ forceps often reveals a "tenting" effect that defines the point at which the bladder connects to the less mobile base of the prostate. Third, performing a "bimanual pinch" by compressing the tissues of the bladder and prostate between the two robotic instruments allows the surgeon to gain a sense of where the plane lies. Using this technique and visual cues, the surgeon will note that the bladder tissue easily coapts between the two instruments while the prostate tissue remains more substantive and more "stiff." Finally, having the bedside assistant provide traction on the urethral catheter, bringing the balloon to the bladder neck, also provides a visual cue to the proper plane of dissection. Use of all four of these maneuvers is advised during one's early experience with RALP so as to avoid inadvertent entry into the base of the prostate resulting in a posi-

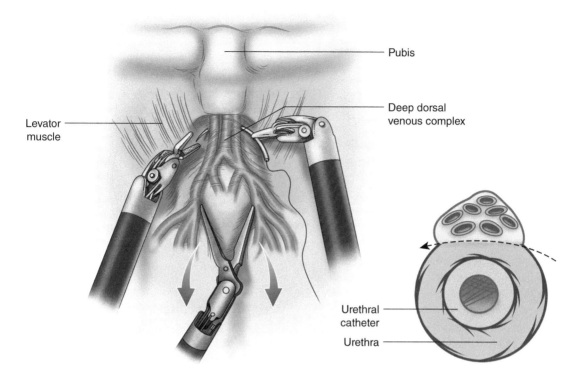

Fig. 18.9 Ligation of the deep dorsal venous complex. The DVC is secured by passing the needle below the venous complex and anterior to the urethra, ligating the DVC as distal to the apex as possible (© 2009 Li-Ming Su, M.D., University of Florida)

Table 18.3 Anterior bladder neck transection: surgeon and assistant instrumentation

Surgeon instrumentation			
Right arm	Left arm	Fourth arm	Assistant instrumentation
• Curved monopolar scissors	• Maryland bipolar grasper	• ProGrasp™ forceps	• Suction-irrigator
Endoscope lens: 0°			• Hem-o-lok® clip applier

tive bladder neck margin. When in doubt, a more proximal plane of dissection at the bladder neck is advised with later bladder neck reconstruction, if necessary, to correct for any discrepancy between the bladder neck opening and urethra.

The anterior bladder neck is divided horizontally staying close to the midline. Carrying the dissection too laterally can result in unwanted bleeding from the lateral bladder pedicles. Once the anterior bladder neck is transected, the ure-thral catheter is exposed. The catheter balloon is decompressed and the catheter tip is advanced through the anterior bladder defect. The ProGrasp™ is then used to grasp the catheter tip and provide traction by pulling superiorly toward the anterior abdominal wall. The proximal end of the catheter is cinched by the assistant at the penile meatus thus creating a "hammock" effect, suspending the prostate anteriorly. This maneuver provides improved exposure to the posterior bladder neck.

Step 7: Posterior Bladder Neck Transection

The posterior bladder wall is inspected to identify the presence or absence of a median lobe as well as the location of the ureteral orifices (Fig. 18.10). If a median lobe is encountered, dissection of the posterior bladder neck is performed beneath the protruding median lobe by lifting the median lobe anterior with the Maryland forceps or ProGrasp™ forceps. Similar to the anterior bladder neck, the posterior bladder neck is divided horizontally along the midline avoiding the lateral pedicles. Once the mucosa is incised, the posterior bladder neck is divided from the base of the prostate with monopolar electrocautery by taking an approximately 45° downward angle of dissection. This angle helps to avoid inadvertent entry into the prostate as well as excessive thinning of the posterior bladder neck. If excessive bleeding is encountered, one should be concerned about the possibility of inadvertent entry into the prostate gland. When dividing the posterior bladder neck, one should ensure that the posterior bladder wall thickness remains uniform with the anterior bladder neck thickness.

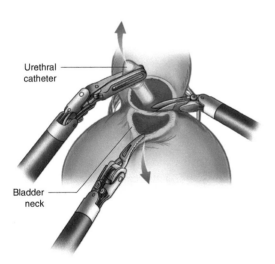

Fig. 18.10 Posterior bladder neck division. Horizontal dissection is carried out through the posterior bladder neck in a 45° downward angle to prevent entry into the prostate base and excessive thinning of the posterior bladder neck (© 2009 Li-Ming Su, M.D., University of Florida)

Upon entering the retrovesical space, the SVs and vas deferentia that have been previously dissected are grasped and brought through the opening created between the bladder neck and prostate. This is one of the unique advantages of the transperitoneal posterior approach to RALP as since the SVs and vasa have been already dissected in previous steps, these structures are now easily identified and do not require extensive dissection especially in cases of a median lobe where visualization is compromised. The bladder pillars (i.e., remaining anterolateral attachments between the bladder and prostate base) are divided either between hemoclips as the terminal branches from the DVC travel through this tissue.

Step 8: Lateral Interfascial Dissection of the Neurovascular Bundles

The NVB travels between two distinct fascial planes that surround the prostate, namely the levator fascia and prostatic fascia (Fig. 18.11). For select patients with low-risk disease (i.e., low-grade, low-volume, nonpalpable disease), a more aggressive approach to NVB preservation may be taken, preserving the NVB along with a generous amount of periprostatic fascia containing accessory nerves, which have been suggested by some to improve postoperative erectile function [5]. This high anterior release of the periprostatic fascia and NVB entails a longitudinal incision of the levator fascia along the more anteromedial border of the prostate. For patients with intermediate-risk disease, a more conservative approach to NVB preservation may be taken so as to avoid an iatrogenic positive margin from dissecting too close to the surface of the prostate. In such cases, a standard release of the NVB may be chosen by incising the levator fascia along the 5 and 7 o'clock position along the posterolateral surface of the prostate.

In preparation for the lateral release of the NVBs, the base of the prostate or tip of the urethral catheter is grasped with the ProGrasp™ and retracted medially, exposing the lateral surface of the prostate. An opening in the levator fascia is

Fig. 18.11 Schematic cross section of the periprostatic fascial planes and NVBs. Anatomically, the NVBs run between the levator fascia and above the prostatic fascia (i.e., interfascial plane). The high anterior release of the NVB is begun by making a higher incision of the levator fascia along the anteromedial border of the prostate as compared to a more posterolateral incision made for a standard nerve-sparing procedure (© 2009 Li-Ming Su, M.D., University of Florida)

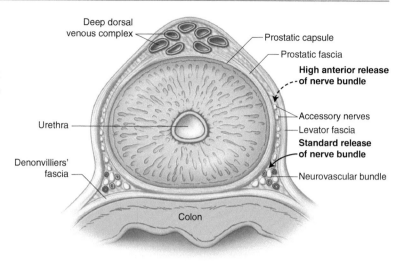

made by sharp incision and carried out toward the apex and base (Fig. 18.12). The interfascial plane (i.e., between the levator and prostatic fascia) is developed gently using blunt dissection. A groove between the NVB and prostate (i.e., the lateral NVB groove) is created by progressively developing this interfascial plane toward the posterolateral aspect of the prostate. Dissection continues in close approximation to the surface of the prostatic fascia in efforts to optimize quantitative cavernous nerve preservation. If bleeding occurs from periprostatic vessels, insufflation pressure can be temporarily increased and pressure applied to the source of bleeding with SURGICEL® hemostatic gauze. Hemostasis with electrocautery should be avoided if possible during dissection near the NVBs as these energy sources have been shown to be harmful to cavernous nerves function in both canine and human studies [6, 7]. Proximal dissection of the NVB is carried to the level of the prostatic pedicles.

Step 9: Ligation of the Prostatic Pedicles

The SVs and vasa are lifted anteriorly with the ProGrasp™ forceps defining the proximal extent of the prostatic pedicles located at the 5 and 7 o'clock positions. Having already accomplished the lateral release of the NVB and established

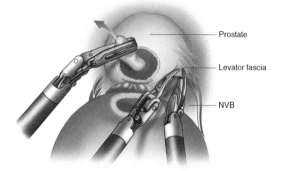

Fig. 18.12 Incising the levator fascia. Using the fourth robotic arm to provide countertraction on the prostate, the levator fascia is incised longitudinally along the anteromedial border of the prostate to perform the high anterior release. The sharp dissection is carried out toward the apex and base, developing the lateral NVB groove (© 2009 Li-Ming Su, M.D., University of Florida)

the lateral NVB groove, this helps to define the distal limit of the prostatic pedicles (Fig. 18.13). The assistant provides further exposure of the pedicles by applying posterior and cephalad counter traction on the bladder neck. The surgeon creates tissue packets within the prostatic pedicles and two to three medium-large Hem-o-lok® clips are applied to control the prostatic vessels in lieu of electrocautery. Great care must be taken so as to avoid past pointing with the hemoclips resulting in potential entrapment of the nearby NVB.

Fig. 18.13 Ligation of the prostatic
pedicles. Countertraction is again provided
by use of the fourth robotic arm to help
display the prostatic pedicles. The
previously formed lateral NVB groove helps
to identify the precise location of the NVB
in reference to the prostatic pedicle, thus
minimizing nerve injury during clip
placement (© 2009 Li-Ming Su, M.D.,
University of Florida)

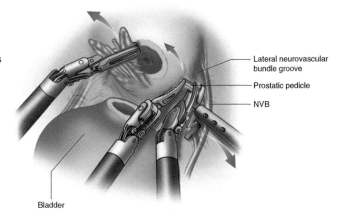

Lateral neurovascular
bundle groove

Prostatic pedicle

NVB

Bladder

Fig. 18.14 Antegrade preservation of the
neurovascular bundle. Combined blunt and
sharp dissections are used to free the final
prostatic attachments from the NVB as far
distally toward the apex as possible (© 2009
Li-Ming Su, M.D., University of Florida)

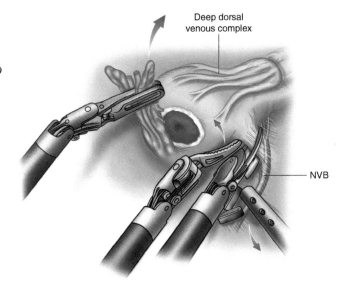

Deep dorsal
venous complex

NVB

Step 10: Antegrade Neurovascular Bundle Preservation

After division of the prostatic pedicles, dissection is carried out toward the previously defined lateral NVB groove in an "antegrade" or "descending" manner (Fig. 18.14). As the posterior dissection between the rectum and prostate has already been completed, the medial border of the NVB is already visibly defined. Both the medial border of the NVB and lateral NVB groove serve as critical landmarks to help guide the proper angle and direction of dissection to optimize antegrade NVB preservation. The remaining attachments between the NVBs and

prostate are gently teased off of the posterolateral surface of the prostate using a combination of blunt and sharp dissection. When small vessels coursing between the NVB and prostate are encountered, small hemoclips may be used. Antegrade dissection of the NVBs is carried out as far distally toward the apex as possible. The use of electrocautery and direct manipulation of the NVB is minimized to avoid injury to the cavernous nerves. If adhesions are encountered between the NVB and prostate, slightly wider dissection may be carried out in efforts to avoid an iatrogenic positive surgical margin, especially in locations at risk for extraprostatic extension of cancer. As such, incremental preservation of cavernous nerves can often be achieved without having to sacrifice the entire NVB (i.e., wide excision of NVB).

Step 11: Division of the Deep Dorsal Venous Complex

The DVC is divided sharply just proximal to the previously placed DVC suture. Great care must be taken to avoid inadvertent entry into the prostatic apex, resulting in an iatrogenic positive apical margin. Spot electrocautery may be required for minor arterial bleeding from the DVC. If adequate dissection of the NVBs has been accomplished in previous steps, the NVBs should be visible immediately adjacent and lateral to the DVC. Attention should be paid to avoid the use of electrocautery specifically at this location. Occasionally, additional 4-0 polyglactin DVC sutures may be required if large venous sinuses are encountered that were not adequately secured or if the original DVC suture becomes dislodged. After complete division of the DVC, a notch representing the anterior aspect of the prostatourethral junction should be visible.

Step 12: Prostatic Apical Dissection and Division of Urethra

As the distal portion of the NVBs lie in intimate association with the lateral aspect of the prostatic apex, the remaining attachments between the NVB and prostatic apex are gently and meticulously dissected free using sharp dissection without electrocautery (Fig. 18.15). The anterior urethra is divided sharply, taking care to preserve the NVBs coursing along the posterolateral surface of the urethra. With the urethral catheter now exposed, the tip of the catheter is withdrawn by the assistant into the urethral stump. Prior to division of posterior urethra, great care must be taken to inspect the contour of the posterior prostatic apex. In some patients, the posterior prostatic apex can protrude beneath and beyond the posterior urethra resulting in an iatrogenic positive margin if not identified and cut across. Having already completed the posterior prostatic dissection, little additional dissection is often required to free the prostate in its entirety once the posterior urethra and posterior rhabdosphincter is divided.

Fig. 18.15 Division of prostatic apex. After transecting the DVC, the anterior urethra is divided sharply, taking care to preserve the NVBs coursing along the posterolateral surface of the urethra. The posterior urethra is also divided sharply after carefully inspecting for the presence and contour of the posterior prostatic apex (© 2009 Li-Ming Su, M.D., University of Florida)

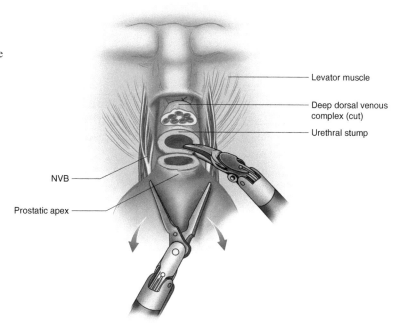

Levator muscle

Deep dorsal venous complex (cut)

Urethral stump

NVB

Prostatic apex

Fig. 18.16 Pelvic lymph node dissection. Anatomic landmarks during pelvic lymph node dissection include the external iliac vein, obturator nerve, pubic symphysis, and bifurcation of the iliac vessels (© 2009 Li-Ming Su, M.D., University of Florida)

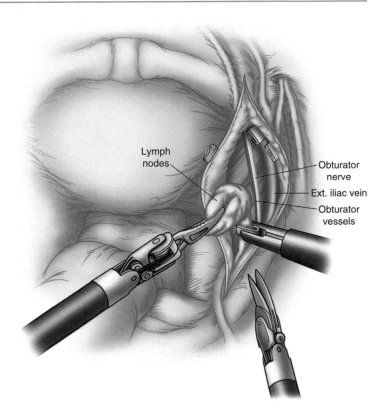

Lymph nodes

Obturator nerve

Ext. iliac vein

Obturator vessels

Step 13: Pelvic Lymph Node Dissection

With the prostate now removed and prior to completion of the vesicourethral anastomosis, a pelvic lymph node dissection is completed. As with an open approach, a key initial step is separation of the nodal packet from the external iliac vein. The lymph node packet is grasped, retracted medially, and a relatively avascular plane between the lymph node packet and lateral pelvic sidewall is identified and dissected using blunt dissection and spot monopolar electrocautery. Dissection is carried out proximally to the iliac bifurcation and distally to the pubis, thus defining the lateral extent of the lymph node packet. By retracting the lymph node packet medially, the precise course of the obturator nerve and vessels can be identified and protected (Fig. 18.16). After securing the distal extent of the lymph node packet with hemoclips, the packet is then retracted cranially to separate it from the obturator vessels and nerves. The proximal extent of the lymph node packet is then secured with hemoclips at the

bifurcation of the iliac vessels. The lymph nodes can usually be removed as a single packet and are extracted in the specimen entrapment bag along with the prostate specimen. For identification purposes, a single Hem-o-lok®clip is applied to the left packet to distinguish it from the right pelvic lymph nodes.

Step 14: Laparoscopic Inspection and Entrapment of the Prostate Specimen (Table 18.4)

Prior to entrapment of the specimens, the margins of the prostate are closely inspected by laparoscopic means. If a close margin is noted, excision of site-specific tissue for frozen section analysis may be performed along the bed of the prostate; however, with experience this should be a rare occurrence. The prostate specimen along with the pelvic lymph nodes are placed in an entrapment bag and stored in the right lower quadrant of the abdomen until completion of the operation.

Table 18.4 Laparoscopic inspection and entrapment of the prostate specimen: surgeon and assistant instrumentation

Surgeon instrumentation			
Right arm	Left arm	Fourth arm	Assistant instrumentation
• Curved monopolar scissors	• Maryland bipolar grasper	• ProGrasp™ forceps	• Suction-irrigator
Endoscope lens: 0°			• 10 mm specimen entrapment bag

Table 18.5 Posterior support of the vesicourethral anastomosis (modified Rocco stitch): surgeon and assistant instrumentation

Surgeon instrumentation			
Right arm	Left arm	Fourth arm	Assistant instrumentation
• Mega™ SutureCut™ needle driver	• Needle driver	• ProGrasp™ forceps	• Suction-irrigator
Endoscope lens: 0°			• Laparoscopic needle driver
			• Sponge on a stick

Step 15: Posterior Support of the Vesicourethral Anastomosis (Modified Rocco Stitch) (Table 18.5)

To help reduce tension at the vesicourethral anastomosis and provide support to the bladder neck, reapproximation of the remnant Denonvillier's fascia, posterior detrusor, and posterior rhabdosphincter located below the urethra is performed [8]. A double-armed 2-0 barbed Monoderm™ suture is passed by the assistant to the surgeon using a laparoscopic needle driver and the remnant Denonvillier's fascia and superficial detrusor from the posterior bladder is brought together with the posterior rhabdosphincter located below the urethra using a running continuous suture (Fig. 18.17). A total of two bites on both the right and left sides are often sufficient to reapproximate these layers. Use of a urethral catheter and perineal pressure to visualize the urethral lumen allows for easier identification of the posterior rhabdosphincter lying just posterior to the urethra. In theory, this stitch also helps to bring the sphincteric complex into the peritoneal cavity, restoring its natural positioning and therefore promoting earlier return of urinary continence.

Step 16: Vesicourethral Anastomosis

A critical first step in accomplishing the vesicourethral anastomosis is the establishment of secure posterior tissue approximation. The posterior anastomosis is typically the site of greatest tension. It is at risk for disruption and subsequent urinary leakage during passage of the urethral catheter if mucosa-to-mucosa approximation of the posterior anastomosis is not established. To avoid this complication, the assistant can apply pressure to the perineum using a sponge stick to better reveal the posterior urethra during placement of the posterior urethral bites. The previously placed 2-0 barbed Monoderm™ suture used for the modified Rocco stich is also used for the vesicourethral anastomosis. The suture is transitioned from the Rocco stich to the anastomosis by passing the needle outside-in at the 5 and 7 o'clock positions at the bladder neck and then inside-out on the urethra (Fig. 18.18). A urethral catheter is passed and withdrawn repeatedly to identify the urethral opening during the urethral bites of the anastomosis. Once the two sutures are run up to the 3 and 9 o'clock position, respectively, ending

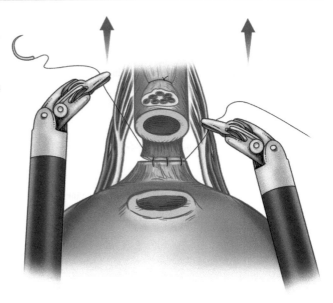

Fig. 18.17 Modified Rocco stitch. The remnant Denonvillier's fascia and superficial detrusor from the posterior bladder is brought together with the posterior rhabdosphincter located below the urethra using a running continuous 2-0 barbed suture (© 2009 Li-Ming Su, M.D., University of Florida)

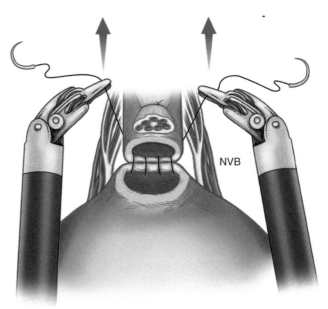

Fig. 18.18 Running vesicourethral anastomosis. The vesicourethral anastomosis is accomplished in a running continuous fashion. The anastomosis is begun by starting each suture at the 5 and 7 o'clock positions, outside-in along the posterior bladder neck. Corresponding inside-out bites are taken of the urethra at the 5 and 7 o'clock positions. A urethral catheter is passed and withdrawn repeatedly to identify the urethral opening during the urethral bites of the anastomosis (© 2009 Li-Ming Su, M.D., University of Florida)

inside-out on the urethral side of the anastomosis, the two ends of the sutures are lifted *anteriorly*, cinching the bladder neck down to the urethra. Great care must be taken not to lift back or in a cephalad direction as this will result in applying excessive forces on the urethral bites resulting in tearing of the urethral tissues. The anterior portion of the anastomosis is completed by running the right arm of the suture to the 12 o'clock position while tension is maintained on the left arm of the suture using the ProGrasp™ device to lift the suture anteriorly. Next, the ProGrasp™ is used to apply tension on the right suture while the left suture is used to complete the anastomosis, reversing the suture outside-in on the urethral bite to allow for the two sutures to be tied across the anastomosis. If any remaining redundancy in the bladder opening is noted as compared to the urethral opening, an anterior bladder neck closure suture can be placed using 2-0 polyglactin suture on a UR6 needle in an interrupted figure of eight closure. Additionally, a bladder neck intussusception suture can be placed using 2-0 PDS suture on an SH needle in a horizontal figure of eight closure anterior and 2 cm proximal to the bladder neck in order to increase bladder funneling and resistance for optimal restoration of postoperative continence.

Following completion of the anastomosis, a final 18 F urethral catheter is placed by the assistant and the balloon inflated with 20 ml of sterile water. The integrity of the anastomosis is tested by filling the bladder with approximately 120 mL of saline through the urethral catheter. Any visible leaks at the anastomosis may be repaired with additional sutures as necessary. A closed suction pelvic drain is placed exiting the left lower quadrant fourth arm 8 mm robotic trocar site and secured to the skin with 2-0 nylon suture.

Step 17: Delivery of the Specimens and Exiting the Abdomen

The entrapment bag containing the prostate and lymph node specimens is delivered via extension of the supraumbilical incision and fascia. The fascia is closed primarily with 0-PDS interrupted sutures to prevent incisional hernia. The 8 mm and 5 mm robotic trocars generally do not require fascial closure but are simply closed subcutaneously. The fascia of the 12 mm assistant trocar also does not generally require formal closure if a nonbladed, self-dilating trocar is used.

Postoperative Management

Intravenous narcotics are provided for postoperative pain. Alternatively, ketorolac may be administered if the risk of bleeding and renal insufficiency is low. Patients are provided liquids on the day of surgery and advanced to regular diet on postoperative day 1 as tolerated. Hospital stay is in general 1–2 days. The pelvic drain is removed prior to discharge if outputs are low. However, if a urine leak is suspected, the fluid may be sent for creatinine and the drain maintained for an additional few days to a week off of suction if an anastomotic leak is confirmed. A cystogram can be performed on postoperative day 7 to ensure a water tight vesicourethral anastomosis prior to removal of the urethral catheter if the integrity of the anastomosis is in question.

Special Considerations

A large-size prostate gland and/or presence of a median lobe may dictate a more proximal incision of the bladder neck, leaving a large bladder neck opening and the ureteral orifices at close proximity to the edge of the bladder neck. Either an anterior or posterior tennis racquet closure of the bladder neck using 2-0 polyglactin suture on a UR-6 needle may be required if there is significant discrepancy between the bladder neck opening and urethra. If the ureteral orifices are located along the immediate edge of the posterior bladder neck, a 5 and 7 o'clock figure-of-eight suture may be placed using 2-0 monocryl suture to imbricate the ureteral orifices and keep them out of harm's way prior to completion of the vesicourethral anastomosis.

On occasions, a subclinical inguinal (direct or indirect) hernia is identified during RALP. It is the authors' opinion that these hernias be fixed if possible at the time of surgery so as to avoid symptoms or strangulation down the road. Our practice is to apply a polypropylene mesh to cover the hernia defect after fully reducing the hernia and tack the mesh into place using either a laparoscopic hernia stapler or 2-0 PDS suture. The mesh is then covered with either a peritoneal flap or the bladder to avoid direct contact with the bowels and minimize the chance of bowel fistulization.

In the rare event of a rectal injury, prompt identification and repair is paramount. Large defects may be identified by the assistant by transrectal digital inspection of the rectum. Smaller injuries may be missed by this maneuver and therefore insufflation of the rectum with air in a saline-filled pelvis (through a catheter placed transrectally) can identify bubbles at the site of a small rectal defect. Once identified, the edges of the defect are clearly delineated and the injury closed in multiple layers with 2-0 silk suture. An omental flap may be brought beneath the bladder to cover the repair as an additional layer and interpose between the rectum and vesicourethral anastomosis in efforts to avoid a rectovesical fistula.

Other more complex patient scenarios will be the subject of a later chapter entitled "Robot-Assisted Laparoscopic Radical Prostatectomy: Management of the Difficult Case."

Steps to Avoid Complications

For novice robotic surgeons, establishing a consistent operative schedule with at least 1–2 RALPs per week can help promote consistency and standardization of surgical approach by the surgeon and surgical team alike. The use of a skilled surgical assistant knowledgeable in laparoscopic and robotic surgery and equipment is perhaps one of the most important steps to gaining consistency in technique, improving operative efficiency, and avoiding complications. Such an individual can aid in obtaining optimal and timely exposure and visualization during each step of the operation as well as troubleshoot instrumentation issues such as instrument exchanges and clashing of robotic arms at the bedside.

It is our practice to achieve meticulous hemostasis throughout all steps of the surgical dissection where the risk of electrocautery effect on the NVB is negligible. By maintaining hemostasis, tissue planes, important anatomic structures, and landmarks remain well visualized. This helps to facilitate a cleaner and more precise dissection, which in turn can lead to improved patient outcomes. When working in close proximity to the anatomic course of the NVB, electrocautery is

avoided as much as is possible and instead hemoclips or superficial absorbable (e.g. 4-0 polyglactin) sutures are applied to small arteries and veins. In addition to this, direct manipulation of the NVBs as well as traction is minimized in efforts to maintain the integrity of the cavernous nerves as well as optimize postoperative recovery of erectile function. In terms of optimizing postoperative incontinence, the length of the urethral stump is optimized and integrity of the surrounding supportive tissues of the urethra is maintained.

Ureteral and rectal injuries are rare events during RALP and by in large avoidable if proper steps are followed. Ureteral injury can occur during three steps of a transperitoneal posterior approach to RALP. First, the ureter may be encountered during dissection of the vas deferens. Maintaining close dissection to the adventitia of the vas will help prevent inadvertent compromise to the nearby ureter traveling lateral and posterior to the vas. Second, the ureter may be injured during completion of the vesicourethral anastomosis especially in cases of a large bladder neck opening where the ureteral orifices are in close proximity to the posterior bladder neck. In such cases, imbrication of the ureteral orifices prior to performing the anastomosis may reduce compromise to the ureters as mentioned previously. Lastly, the ureter may in theory be encountered during dissection of the pelvic lymph nodes. During dissection of the proximal extent of the lymph node packet at the iliac bifurcation, use of thermal energy should be minimized as this may compromise the ureter as it passes over the iliac vessels. Rectal injuries, in general, can be avoided by thorough and dissection of the rectum and overlying Denonvillier's off of the posterior aspect of the prostate. With inadequate dissection of the rectum, the prostate remains adherent posteriorly to the rectum, making these attachments difficult to visualize and safely dissect free once the bladder neck and urethra are divided. Therefore, wide dissection of the rectum off of the entire posterior border of the prostate is strongly recommended early in the operation as is the case with the posterior approach to RALP.

References

1. Kaouk JH, Hafron J, Goel R, Haber GP, Jones JS. Robotic salvage retropubic prostatectomy after radiation/brachytherapy: initial results. BJU Int. 2008;102(1):93–6.
2. Boris RS, Bhandari A, Krane LS, Eun D, Kaul S, Peabody JO. Salvage robotic-assisted radical prostatectomy: initial results and early report of outcomes. BJU Int. 2009;103(7):952–6.
3. Guillonneau B, Vallancien G. Laparoscopic radical prostatectomy: the Montsouris experience. J Urol. 2000;163(2):418–22.
4. Smith JA. Robotically assisted laparoscopic prostatectomy: an assessment of its contemporary role in the surgical management of localized prostate cancer. Am J Surg. 2004;188(4A Suppl):63S–7.
5. Kaul S, Savera A, Badani K, Fumo M, Bhandari A, Menon M. Functional outcomes and oncological effi- cacy of Vattikuti Institute prostatectomy with Veil of Aphrodite nerve-sparing: an analysis of 154 consecu- tive patients. BJU Int. 2006;97(3):467–72.
6. Ong AM, Su LM, Varkarakis I, Inagaki T, Link RE, Bhayani SB, Patriciu A, Crain B, Walsh PC. Nerve sparing radical prostatectomy: effects of hemostatis energy sources on the recovery of cavernous nerve function in a canine model. J Urol. 2004;172(4 Pt 1):1318–22.
7. Ahlering TE, Eichel L, Chou D, Skarecky DW. Feasibility study for robotic radical prostatec- tomy cautery-free neurovascular bundle preservation. Urology. 2005;65(5):994–7.
8. Rocco F, Carmignani L, Acquati P, Gadda F, Dell'Orto P, Rocco B, Bozzini G, Gazzano G, Morabito A. Restoration of posterior aspect of rhab- dosphincter shortens continence time after radical retropubic prostatectomy. J Urol. 2006;175(6): 2201–6.

Extraperitoneal Robot-Assisted Radical Prostatectomy

19

Jean V. Joseph, David Horovitz, and Matthew Lux

Patient Selection

During RARP, one may gain access to the prostate transperitoneally or extraperitoneally, and certain patient and/or disease factors may favor a given approach. With similar safety profiles, surgeons are encouraged to add both techniques to their armamentarium in order to most effectively individualize patient care [1, 2].

In patients who have had extensive prior intra-abdominal surgery, a transperitoneal RARP often requires early adhesiolysis, risking visceral injury. Such an injury may occur in the surgical field or away from the operative site during blind passage of instruments through an assistant trocar. Thus, an extraperitoneal approach can be quite advantageous in this setting. Further, this approach risks the development of de novo intra-abdominal adhesions, which can cause mechanical bowel obstruction and complicate future intra-abdominal surgery.

With the extraperitoneal approach, the peritoneum serves as a natural retractor of the bowels such that steep Trendelenburg may be avoided. This can be quite beneficial, especially in the obese, and in patients with chronic obstructive pulmonary disease [3, 4]. Urine leaks and bleeding become less of a concern after extraperitoneal RARP as an intact peritoneum can limit their spread and hasten their resolution. This technique may also decrease postoperative ileus [5, 6].

In the patient with a history of prior extraperitoneal surgery, particularly mesh herniorrhaphy, an inflammatory reaction may ensue and obliterate the extraperitoneal space. This can make both the RARP and concomitant lymph node dissection difficult, if not impossible when performed extraperitoneally [7, 8]. Patients who have had prior abdominal surgery with incisions extending to the pubic symphysis might also be best served with a transperitoneal RARP as the extraperitoneal space may be scarred or obliterated. Other noted challenges with the extraperitoneal approach include a limited working space and difficulty creating space laterally to use the fourth arm. The confined space keeps the specimen bag in the operative field, potentially impairing visibility during the vesicourethral anastomosis stage [2, 9]. Moreover, lymphocele formation after pelvic lymphadenectomy may be more common

Electronic supplementary material: The online version of this chapter (doi:10.1007/978-3-319-45060-5_19) contains supplementary material, which is available to authorized users.

J.V. Joseph, M.D. (✉)
D. Horovitz, M.D., F.R.C.S.C.
Department of Urology, Strong Memorial Hospital, University of Rochester Medical Center, 601 Elmwood Ave, Rochester, NY 14642, USA
e-mail: jean_joseph@urmc.rochester.edu

M. Lux, M.D.
Department of Urology, Kaiser Permanente Medical Center, San Diego, CA, USA

with extraperitoneal RARP [10]. Inadvertent peritoneotomies made during the procedure may cause transperitoneal insufflation, further compressing the extraperitoneal space and rendering the procedure more difficult.

Preoperative Preparation

All patients receive a bowel preparation consisting of one bottle of magnesium citrate, doses of neomycin, metronidazole, and an enema the day before surgery. They are admitted to the hospital 2 h prior to surgery. Broadspectrum intravenous antibiotics and 5000 U subcutaneous heparin are administered 1 h before incision. We do not recommend routine donation of autologous blood since our transfusion rate is insignificant.

Operative Setup

The location of the surgical console, bedside surgical cart, and the assistants are as shown (Fig. 19.1).

Patient Positioning

The patient is placed supine on a split-leg bed on top of a surgical bean bag. The legs are abducted slightly and secured to the table. The arms are internally rotated, placed parallel to the long axis of the patient, and secured in foam to avoid pressure sores or neuropraxia. Any hair on the patient's abdomen within the surgical field is trimmed with an electrical shaver. The surgical bean bag is manually molded to conform to the patient's body shape and air is suctioned from the device to secure the patient in place (Fig. 19.2). A digital rectal examination is performed for intraoperative clinical staging and to help with planning for subsequent nerve sparing. An Opium and Belladonna rectal suppository is administered to help prevent bladder spasms postopera-

tively. Orogastric tube and sterile urethral catheter placement are done prior to trocar insertion. Trendelenburg positioning is generally at about 10°. The patient's abdomen, genitals, and perineum are prepped and draped to provide a sterile field.

Trocar Configuration

Once the extraperitoneal space is developed and insufflated (see step 1 below), additional trocars are placed laparoscopically. A total of six trocars are used in a "W" shaped configuration as shown (Fig. 19.3). An 8 mm camera trochar is placed in the paraumbilical location and a 12 mm assistant trochar is placed 5 cm cephalad and just medial to the right anerior superior iliac spine. Three 8 mm trochars are placed under direct vision: one approximately 5 mm cephalad and just medial to the left anterior superior iliac spine, two in the middle of each rectus belly about 3 cm caudad to the umbillicus (taking great care to avoid injuring the epigastric vessels). A 5 mm assistant trochar is placed between the umbilicus and the right 8 mm trochar, approximately 3 cm cephalad to the umbillicus. The following technique will be based upon this operative arrangement and personnel.

Instrumentation and Equipment List

Equipment

- da Vinci® S Surgical System (4-arm system; Intuitive Surgical, Inc., Sunnyvale, CA)
- EndoWrist® Maryland bipolar forceps or (Intuitive Surgical, Inc., Sunnyvale, CA)
- EndoWrist® curved monopolar scissors (Intuitive Surgical, Inc., Sunnyvale, CA)
- EndoWrist® ProGrasp™ forceps (Intuitive Surgical, Inc., Sunnyvale, CA)

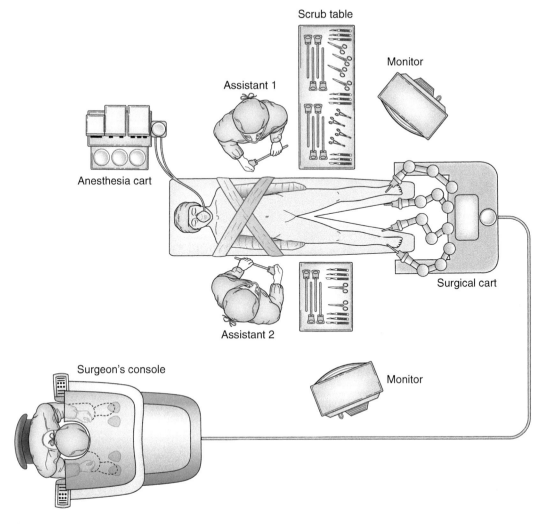

Fig. 19.1 View of operative setup

- EndoWrist® needle drivers (2) (Intuitive Surgical, Inc., Sunnyvale, CA)
- InSite® Vision System with 0° and 30° lens (Intuitive Surgical, Inc., Sunnyvale, CA)

Trocars

- 12 mm trocar (1)
- 8 mm robotic trocars (4)
- 5 mm trocar (1)

Recommended Sutures

- Ligation of the deep dorsal vein complex (DVC): 2-0 Covidien V-Loc™ barbed suture (Medtronic, Minneapolis, MN) cut to 9 in., and 2-0 polyglactin suture on a RB1 needle cut to 6 in. (if necessary)
- Vesicourethral anastomosis: 2 (2-0 polyglactin) sutures (9 in. each) on a RB1 needle
- Posterior reconstruction stitch: 2-0 polyglactin suture on a RB1 needle cut to 9 in.

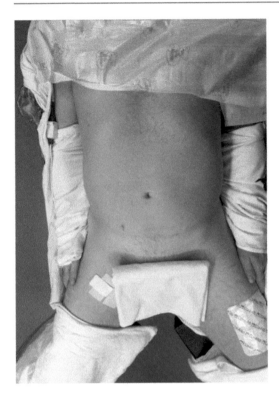

Fig. 19.2 The patient is secured to the table with a surgical bean bag and placed in mild Trendelenburg. The legs are taped below the knees to the abducted limbs of the split-leg surgical bed

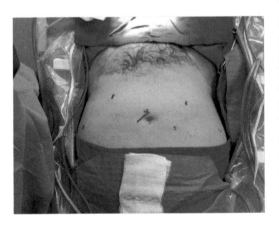

Fig. 19.3 "W" configuration of trocars are shown. Numbers marked on patient's abdomen refer to size of trocar size (in French units) placed after insufflation

- Anterior bladder neck closure (if necessary): 2-0 polyglactin suture on a RB1 needle cut to 9 in.

Instruments Used by the Surgical Assistant

- Laparoscopic scissors
- Blunt tip grasper
- Suction irrigator device
- Hem-o-lok® clip applier (Teleflex Medical, Research Triangle Park, NC)
- Large Hem-o-lok® clips (Teleflex Medical, Research Triangle Park, NC)
- 10 mm specimen entrapment sac
- EnSeal® device 5 mm diameter, 45 cm shaft length (SurgRx®, Redwood City, CA) (optional)
- SURGICEL® hemostatic gauze (Ethicon, Inc., Cincinnati, OH)
- 20 Fr silicone urethral catheter
- Jackson–Pratt closed suction pelvic drain

Step-by-Step Technique (Videos 19.1, 19.2, 19.3, 19.4, 19.5, 19.6, 19.7, 19.8, and 19.9)

Step 1: Creation of Extraperitoneal Space

The initial step of extraperitoneal robot-assisted laparoscopic radical prostatectomy (RALP) is creation of the extraperitoneal space. A 2.5 cm paraumbilical skin incision is made down to the level of the anterior rectus sheath. A 1 cm incision is made in the latter to expose the rectus muscle. A 0-polyglactin suture is placed through the two apices of this incision and the free ends are secured with a snap (Fig. 19.4). The muscle fibers are pushed laterally using a clamp, exposing the posterior rectus sheath. A balloon dilator (Extra View™ Balloon, OMS-XB 2, Tyco Healthcare, Norwalk, CT) is inserted just above the posterior sheath and advanced down to the pubic symphysis in the midline (Fig. 19.5). A 0° scope is placed in the balloon trocar to allow direct visualization of the space being created. Care should be taken not to overstretch or tear the epigastric or iliac vessels from overinflation. Once the space is created, the balloon dilator is replaced by a 10/12 mm Dilating Tip Ethicon

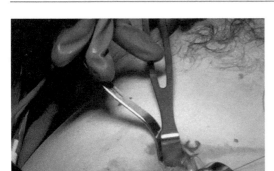

Fig. 19.4 A 2.5 cm paraumbilical skin incision is made down to the level of the anterior rectus sheath. A 1 cm incision is made through the anterior rectus sheath and a 0-polyglactin suture is placed through the two apices and secured with a snap

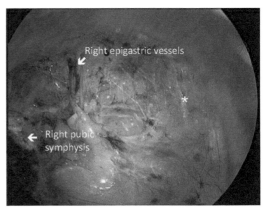

Fig. 19.6 View of right pelvis following balloon dilation of extraperitoneal space. *Asterisk* denotes loose alveolar connective tissue where blunt dissection is carried out in an anterior cephalad direction to push the peritoneum away and expose the transversus abdominis muscle

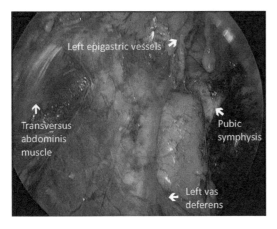

Fig. 19.5 View of left pelvis following balloon dilation of extraperitoneal space

Endopath 512XD (Ethicon Inc. US, LLC., Somerville, NJ) trocar. It is necessary to use a transparent trocar such as this so that the retropubic space can be developed under direct vision. The retroperitoneum is insufflated up to 12–15 mmHg. The beveled tip of the trocar is used to further create the extraperitoneal space laterally, facilitating placement of the assistant trocars as mentioned above. The loose areolar tissue is swept laterally and cephalad, bluntly pushing the peritoneum off the abdominal wall. The epigastric vessels are left attached to the anterior abdominal wall to avoid bleeding from branches

entering the rectus muscle (Fig. 19.6). If a da Vinci® Xi Surgical System is used, the 12 mm paraumbilical Ethicon Endopath 512XD trocar must be replaced with a 12 mm da Vinci® trocar with a reducer placed on its hub to accommodate an 8 mm, 0° laparoscopic camera. A petroleum jelly-impregnated gauze is wrapped around the trocar at the level of the anterior rectus sheath and the previously placed 0-polyglactin is tied tightly around the trocar to avoid leakage of CO_2. The additional trochars are then placed under direct vision as described above.

Step 2: Endopelvic Fascia Dissection (Table 19.1)

A 0° lens is used throughout the entire operation. Monopolar and bipolar electrocautery settings are set to 90 and 30 W, respectively. Accessing the retropubic space by the extraperitoneal approach described above eliminates the bladder "takedown" step required during the transperitoneal approach, and allows rapid visualization and access to the prostate, endopelvic fascia, and puboprostatic ligaments (Fig. 19.7). The fatty tissue overlying the endopelvic fascia is easily swept away exposing the prostate. We routinely incise the endopelvic fascia, freeing the prostate from its lateral attachments. Accessory pudendal vessels, if

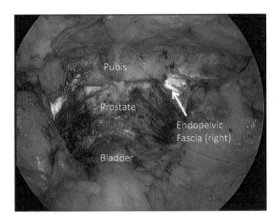

Fig. 19.7 Complete view of the pelvis including the pubis, prostate, bladder, and endopelvic fascia following balloon dilation of the extraperitoneal space

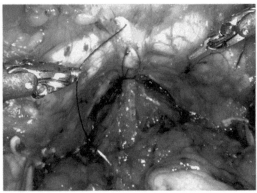

Fig. 19.8 Control of the DVC with a 2-0 Covidien V-Loc™ barbed suture

present, are identified and preserved. We routinely incise the puboprostatic ligaments to allow adequate mobilization of the prostatic apex. Superficial vessels encountered are cauterized.

Step 3: Dorsal Vein Ligation (Table 19.2)

A 2-0 Covidien V-Loc™ barbed suture is used to ligate the dorsal venous complex (DVC). With medial retraction of the prostatic apex, a groove is visualized between the DVC and the anterior urethra. We routinely pass the needle three times through this plane and suspend the complex to periosteum of the pubic symphysis after the first and third pass. A Hem-o-lok® clip is applied to the distal end of the suture and used to further cinch it to the pubic symphysis (Fig. 19.8).

Step 4: Bladder Neck Dissection (Table 19.3)

With cephalad tension on the bladder, the loose areolar connective tissue crossing the bladder neck is removed allowing identification of the bladder neck (Fig. 19.9). With the magnification afforded by the da Vinci® robot, the plane between the prostate and bladder neck is easily identified. A combination of electrocautery and blunt dissection

allows separation of the bladder from the prostate. Judicious use of electrocautery is necessary to avoid excessive charring and obliteration of the tissue planes. Given the lack of tactile feedback, following the tissue planes allows an accurate anatomical dissection, without violation of the prostate capsule. Once the longitudinal urethral fibers are identified, the bladder neck is transected (Fig. 19.10). The previously placed urethral catheter is removed allowing access to the posterior bladder neck. The transection is done sharply, with no significant bleeding encountered. If a bleeding vessel is present, it can be selectively cauterized avoiding the bladder neck mucosa. The anatomical groove between the bladder and prostate is further dissected, pushing the bladder cephalad. The bladder neck dissection is completed with the identification of the longitudinal muscle fibers coursing posterior to the bladder, covering the seminal vesicles (SVs) (Fig. 19.11).

Step 5: Seminal Vesicle Dissection (Table 19.4)

Once the longitudinal fibers are transected, the ampullae of the vasa and attached SVs are identified. These fibers need to be incised transversely in the midline allowing identification of both vasa. Once the ampullae are fully identified, the fourth arm can also be used to elevate the attached SVs. Optimal traction is achieved by pulling the vas toward the contralateral pubic bone. The dissec-

Fig. 19.9 View of bladder neck (*dashed line*) following control of distal DVC, with traction placed on the perivesical fat

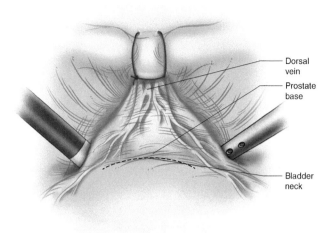

Dorsal vein

Prostate base

Bladder neck

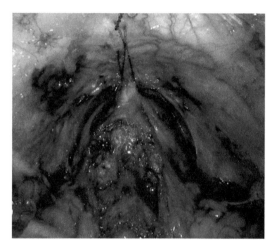

Fig. 19.10 View of longitudinal urethral fibers prior to bladder neck transection

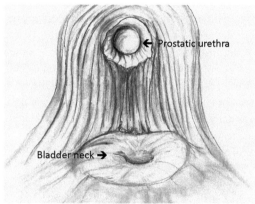

Prostatic urethra

Bladder neck →

Fig. 19.11 View of bladder neck following transection

Table 19.1 Endopelvic fascia dissection: surgeon and assistant instrumentation

Surgeon instrumentation			Assistant instrumentation
Right arm	**Left arm**	**Fourth arm**	• Suction-irrigator
• Curved monopolar scissors	• Maryland bipolar grasper	• ProGrasp™ forceps	
Endoscope lens: 0°			

Table 19.2 Dorsal vein ligation: surgeon and assistant instrumentation

Surgeon instrumentation			Assistant instrumentation
Right arm	**Left arm**	**Fourth arm**	• Suction-irrigator
• Needle driver	• Needle driver	• ProGrasp™ forceps	• Laparoscopic scissors
			• Laparoscopic needle driver
Endoscope lens: 0°			

Table 19.3 Bladder neck dissection: surgeon and assistant instrumentation

Surgeon instrumentation			Assistant instrumentation
Right arm	**Left arm**	**Fourth arm**	• Suction-irrigator
• Curved monopolar scissors	• Maryland bipolar grasper	• ProGrasp™ forceps	
Endoscope lens: 0°			

Table 19.4 Seminal vesicle dissection: surgeon and assistant instrumentation

Surgeon instrumentation			Assistant instrumentation
Right arm	**Left arm**	**Fourth arm**	• Suction-irrigator
• Curved monopolar scissors	• Maryland bipolar grasper	• ProGrasp™ forceps	• Hemoclip applier
Endoscope lens: 0°			

tion should be carried cephalad to the tip of the SVs. Dissecting in a caudal direction will inadvertently enter the posterior aspect of the prostate. It is helpful to avoid directly grasping or traumatizing the SVs, since that will alter the dissection plane. Instead, leaving the SVs attached to their respective ampullae helps with retraction of both structures by grasping only the ampulla. The artery to the vas located between the SVs and the vas deferens is clipped en bloc. When performing a nerve-sparing procedure, electrocautery is avoided to prevent damage to the nerve plexus traveling near the tip of the SVs.

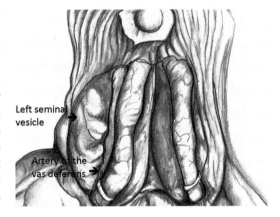

Fig. 19.12 Seminal vesicles with clipped ampulla

Step 6: Posterior Prostate Dissection

Once the SVs are completely dissected, both ampullae are retracted anteriorly exposing Denonvilliers' fascia (Fig. 19.12). The latter is incised transversely, exposing the yellow perirectal fat. The assistant uses the suction to gently retract the rectal wall in a cephalad direction. The rectal wall is pushed bluntly from the posterior aspect of the prostate all the way to the prostate apex. If the latter is not possible due to a very enlarged gland, this step can be carried out once the posterior prostate pedicles are mobilized. It is important to note that the rectal wall is being pulled anteriorly with the traction on the prostate or SVs. The caudad dissection should be carried out parallel to the posterior prostate to avoid injury to the rectal wall. A rectal bougie or

an assistant's finger can be used to help delineate the rectal wall if necessary. This dissection is carried out primarily in the midline, avoiding trauma to the laterally located neurovascular bundles (NVBs).

Step 7: Neurovascular Bundle Dissection

The ampullae and SVs are pulled medially in the opposite direction from the side being dissected. Using the suction, the assistant can place traction on Denonvilliers' fascia posterior to the bladder, allowing better visualization of the bundles. In patients selected for nerve sparing, the prostate capsule is exposed bluntly using graspers to push off the overlying fat and periprostatic fascia. With further lateral dissection, arterial pulsations from the cavernous vessels within the NVBs are easily noted. These vessels are preserved by gently pushing them posterolaterally toward the rectum. Dissecting in a cephalad direction helps identify the main neurovascular trunks, bifurcating in anterior branches entering the prostate, and the posteriorly located NVBs coursing toward the pelvic diaphragm and toward the corpora cavernosum.

Prior to clipping the prostatic branches, the levator fascia is incised allowing improved identification of the lateral aspects of the NVBs. As for the posterior dissection, this can be carried out bluntly with minimal bleeding encountered. Dissection in a medial direction leads to the previously dissected anterior rectal space, with the NVBs mobilized posteriorly. Clips can be selectively applied, in lieu of electrocautery, to the vascular branches of the prostatic pedicles prior to their transection (Fig. 19.13). Once the prostatic pedicles are transected, the periprostatic fascia encompassing the NVBs can be detached bluntly from the prostate, in a caudal direction all the way to the prostatic apex.

In non-nerve-sparing cases, the periprostatic fascia is incised next to levator ani. The bundles and their investing fascia are left attached to the prostate capsule, allowing for wide excision of the NVBs along with the prostate.

Step 8: Apical Dissection

With the prostate retracted in a postero-cephalad direction, the DVC is transected (Fig. 19.14). A urethral catheter should be inserted in the urethra to facilitate identification of the urethral stump. Electrocautery should be avoided in order not to damage the NVBs coursing lateral to the prostatic apex. Care should be taken not to enter the prostate at this point. This is best achieved by following the normal curvature of the apex, transecting the vein in a caudal direction. A perpendicular dissection plane inevitably will enter the prostate gland. If bleeding is encountered or the previously placed DVC suture is dislodged, additional sutures are placed on the DVC, using 2-0 polyglactin suture on a RB1 needle, to achieve hemostasis. Temporary increase in intra-abdominal pressure up to 20 mmHg facilitates completion of the DVC transection when profuse bleeding from venous sinuses is present.

Step 9: Urethral Transection

With the urethral catheter in place, the longitudinal anterior urethral fibers can be identified. The urethra is dissected cephalad, close to the prostate and transected. Urethral length should be preserved without compromising cancer control

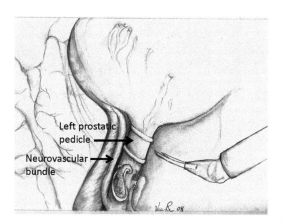

Fig. 19.13 Hem-o-lok® clips used to control the prostatic pedicle, while leaving the NVBs intact, coursing posterior to the prostate to enter the pelvic diaphragm

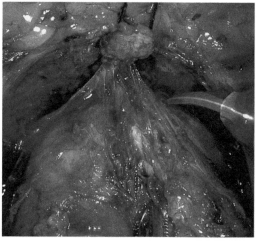

Fig. 19.14 View of prostatic apex following DVC transection, prior to urethral transection

at the apex. Once the urethral catheter is exposed, it is retracted by the assistant, facilitating visualization and transection of the posterior urethra (Fig. 19.15). We prefer cutting the urethra sharply to avoid ischemic mucosal injury that can occur with the use of electrocautery.

The prostate is then retracted in an anterior and cephalad direction to allow visualization of the posterior apex. The NVB should be thoroughly dissected, pushed in a posterolateral direction prior to transecting the remaining posterior apical attachments. The prostate is placed in a 10 mm ENDO CATCH™ bag (Covidien, Mansfield, MA), which is pulled out of the pelvis and stored out of the operative field in the abdomen until the end of the operation. The prostate fossa is irrigated and inspected for hemostasis and integrity of the rectal wall. When arterial bleeding is noted from the NVB, the bleeding vessel is selectively controlled using 2-0 polyglactin suture ligatures. If a rectal injury is suspected, a finger or rectal bougie is placed to tent the rectal wall to allow a thorough examination.

Step 10: Posterior Reconstruction (Table 19.5)

A posterior reconstruction is routinely performed prior to completing the vesicourethral anastomosis. In one step, the posterior layer of the rhabdosphincter is sewn to Denonvilliers' fascia and the posterior aspect of the bladder using two interrupted Covidien V-Loc™ barbed sutures. The posterior bladder tissue encompassed is the longitudinal fibrous layer which previously covered the anterior aspect of the SVs (Fig. 19.16). The insufflation pressure in the retroperitoneum is lowered to 8–10 mmHg, while pressure is applied to the perineum to facilitate tying of these two interrupted sutures. This reconstructed layer helps bring the bladder and urethra in close proximity in preparation for the vesicourethral anastomosis. After cinching these sutures, the bladder is brought in close proximity to the transected urethra, greatly reducing tension on the anastomosis. The needle ends of the two Covidien V-Loc™ barbed sutures are left loose and temporarily tucked away lateral to the bladder for later use.

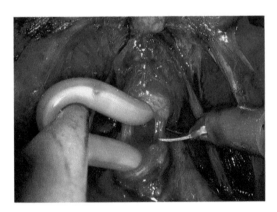

Fig. 19.15 View of the posterior urethra prior to transection

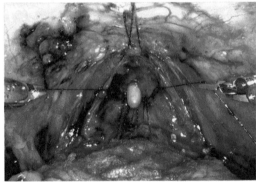

Fig. 19.16 The bladder is pulled towards the transected urethra using as part of the posterior reconstruction

Table 19.5 Posterior reconstruction: surgeon and assistant instrumentation

Surgeon instrumentation			Assistant instrumentation
Right arm	**Left arm**	**Fourth arm**	• Suction-irrigator
• Needle driver	• Needle driver	• ProGrasp™ forceps	• Laparoscopic scissors
			• Laparoscopic needle driver
Endoscope lens: 0°			

Step 11: Vesicourethral Anastomosis

The anastomosis is completed using two separate sutures (2-0 polyglactin suture on an RB1 needle). The first suture is placed at the 5 o'clock position approximating the bladder neck and urethra using the right hand (forehand on both bladder and urethra). Urethral sutures are placed while the assistant withdraws the urethral catheter exposing the urethral mucosa. Initially, the anastomosis is carried out in a clockwise fashion to the 7 o'clock position when the needle placement is done using right hand (backhand) on the urethra, and left hand (forehand) on the bladder. This suture is tied to itself at the 11 o'clock position. The second suture is carried out in a counterclockwise direction completing the anterior wall of the anastomosis. The 5–1 o'clock locations are done using the right hand (forehand) on the bladder, and the left hand (backhand) on the urethra. The anterior-most aspect of the anastomosis (1–11 o'clock) is accomplished using the right hand (backhand) on the bladder, and the left hand (backhand) on the urethra. The second suture is also tied at the 11 o'clock position. Bladder neck mucosa is encompassed into every suture to facilitate mucosal apposition. Care should be taken for the suture not to pass through the posterior bladder neck mucosa, while placing the anterior bladder sutures. Once the anastomosis is completed, a new 20 Fr urethral catheter is inserted into the bladder under direct vision, prior to cinching the second counterclockwise anastomotic suture (Fig. 19.17). When cinching this suture, it is best to pull on the urethral side of the anastomosis, in a direction perpendicular to the longitudinal urethral fibers. This maneuver avoids shearing the urethral wall, while achieving water tightness of the anastomosis. The urethral catheter is irrigated verifying absence of anastomotic leakage. Once the vesicourethral anastomosis is complete, the catheter is flushed both to confirm the absence of a significant leak and to irrigate clots from the bladder. Attention is then turned to the two needle ends of the previously placed posterior reconstruction Covidien V-Loc™ barbed sutures. These needles are passed through the pectineal ligament, approximately 3 cm lateral to the midline, the sutures are

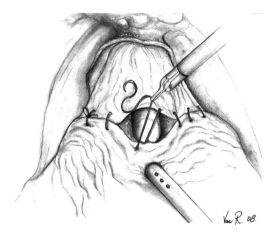

Fig. 19.17 View of the vesicourethral anastomosis. Final urethral catheter is passed into the bladder prior to cinching the anterior anastomotic suture

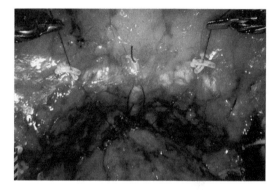

Fig. 19.18 After completion of the vesicourethral anastomosis, the two previously placed posterior reconstruction sutures are passed through the pectineal ligaments bilaterally and cinched with Hem-o-lok® clips

held with a moderate amount of tension and two Hem-o-lok® clips are applied to the distal ends of both in order to cinch them down firmly (Fig. 19.18). Our group believes that this step may aid in the prevention of postoperative urinary incontinence by acting as a prophylactic male urinary sling.

Step 12: Delivery of the Specimens and Exiting the Abdomen

The surgical cart is disconnected from the trocars and wheeled away from the patient. The specimen bag is retrieved from the periumbilical camera tro-

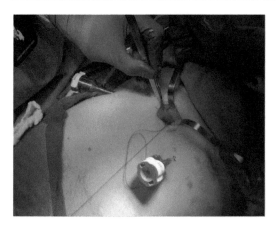

Fig. 19.19 Specimen retrieval through the previously created periumbilical incision

car at the end of the procedure (Fig. 19.19). A 19 Fr Jackson-Pratt (JP) drain is placed in the retropubic space via the 10 mm lateral assistant trocar site and subsequently secured to the skin. The robotic trocars are removed under vision, verifying hemostasis from the exit sites. The anterior rectus sheath adjacent to the midline fascia is incised to allow withdrawal of the bag. The anterior rectus fascia opening is closed using absorbable sutures. All skin openings are later closed in a similar manner. With the extraperitoneal approach, no other fascial closure is necessary. In conditions where air is trapped into the peritoneal cavity, it is evacuated with a small opening in the posterior sheath and peritoneum, which is later closed.

Postoperative Management

Postoperative pain management consists of ketorolac, and morphine sulfate for breakthrough pain. We do not use ketorolac in patients with bleeding diathesis or abnormal renal function. Two additional doses of 5000 U of subcutaneous heparin are administered postoperatively following the initial preoperative dose. Patients are ambulated and fed once they fully recover from anesthesia. They are generally discharged within 23 h of surgery. Jackson–Pratt drains are removed before discharge if the output remains low with less than 30 cm^3 in an 8 h shift. The urethral catheter is removed in the outpatient setting 7–10

days after surgery. We perform cystograms only in patients with gross hematuria, or prolong JP drainage, to verify the integrity of the anastomosis prior to instituting a void trial.

Special Considerations

Obesity

In the obese patient, we favour an extraperitoneal approach to RARP for a variety of reasons. The peritoneum serves as an excellent natural retractor which keeps the bowels out of the operative field. Furthermore, the steep Trendelenburg position, which may be associated with anesthetic complications in an obese patient due to diaphragmatic splinting, is not necessary Laryngeal and facial edema associated with the steep Trendelenburg position may otherwise lead to delayed extubation and a prolonged recovery.

Large Prostate Gland

A large gland may be difficult to manipulate during extirpation, especially when associated with a narrow pelvis. The posterior apical dissection may be challenging due to inability to lift the prostate anteriorly to reach the posterior aspect of the prostate apex. Anterior mobility of the prostate is limited by the pubic symphysis. In such cases, the posterior dissection is best completed following dissection of the apex and transection of the urethra.

Steps to Avoid Complications

Bleeding is the most common complication encountered during the development of the extraperitoneal space. Balloon insufflation should be carried out under direct vision to avoid stretching or tearing of the epigastric or iliac vessel. The epigastric vessels give off several perforators entering the rectus muscles which can be injured during creation of the extraperitoneal space. Occasionally this may result in tearing of a branch of the epigastric artery which may necessitate clipping. Increasing the pressure in the preperitoneal space may help decrease the bleeding until an additional trocar is inserted to allow clipping of the bleeding vessel. If mild venous bleeding is encountered, which can be from perforating veins or vessels behind the pubic symphysis, it is easily controlled with preperitoneal insufflation. Overcompression of the iliac vessels, impairing flow from the lower extremities, should be avoided.

References

1. Ghazi A, Scosyrev E, Patel H, Messing EM, Joseph JV. Complications associated with extraperitoneal robot-assisted radical prostatectomy using the standardized Martin classification. Urology. 2013;81(2):324–31.
2. Erdogru T, Teber D, Frede T, Marrero R, Hammady A, Seemann O, et al. Comparison of transperitoneal and extraperitoneal laparoscopic radical prostatectomy using match-pair analysis. Eur Urol. 2004;46(3):312–9; discussion 20.
3. Dogra PN, Saini AK, Singh P, Bora G, Nayak B. Extraperitoneal robot-assisted laparoscopic radical prostatectomy: initial experience. Urol Ann. 2014;6(2):130–4.
4. Boczko J, Madeb R, Golijanin D, Erturk E, Mathe M, Patel HR, et al. Robot-assisted radical prostatectomy in obese patients. Can J Urol. 2006;13(4):3169–73.
5. Akand M, Erdogru T, Avci E, Ates M. Transperitoneal versus extraperitoneal robot-assisted laparoscopic radical prostatectomy: a prospective single surgeon randomized comparative study. Int J Urol. 2015.
6. Brown JA, Rodin D, Lee B, Dahl DM. Transperitoneal versus extraperitoneal approach to laparoscopic radical prostatectomy: an assessment of 156 cases. Urology. 2005;65(2):320–4.
7. Katz EE, Patel RV, Sokoloff MH, Vargish T, Brendler CB. Bilateral laparoscopic inguinal hernia repair can complicate subsequent radical retropubic prostatectomy. J Urol. 2002;167(2 Pt 1):637–8.
8. Cook H, Afzal N, Cornaby AJ. Laparoscopic hernia repairs may make subsequent radical retropubic prostatectomy more hazardous. BJU Int. 2003;91(7):729.
9. Joseph JV, Rosenbaum R, Madeb R, Erturk E, Patel HR. Robotic extraperitoneal radical prostatectomy: an alternative approach. J Urol. 2006;175(3 Pt 1):945–50; discussion 51.
10. Porpiglia F, Terrone C, Tarabuzzi R, Billia M, Grande S, Musso F, et al. Transperitoneal versus extraperitoneal laparoscopic radical prostatectomy: experience of a single center. Urology. 2006;68(2):376–80.

Robotic Radical Prostatectomy: Complex Case Management

20

Hariharan Palayapalayam Ganapathi,
Gabriel Ogaya-Pinies, Vladimir Mouraviev,
and Vipul R. Patel

Introduction

Prostate cancer is the second most common malignancy among men in the United States and the second leading cause of cancer death [1]. With early screening and prostate biopsy more than 90% of the cases identified have organ-confined disease and are potentially curable [2]. In general, radical prostatectomy (RP) is the treatment of choice for patients with clinically localized prostate cancer and life expectancy >10 years [3]. More than 80% of RPs in the United States are performed with robotic assistance [2]. The feasibility and safety of the procedure has been well documented. As more RALPs are performed, procedural difficulties will be more widely encountered and, hopefully, better understood. Surgeons may face challenges during any step of RALP starting from patient positioning, trocar placement, bladder neck identification, dissection of surgical planes, and urethrovesical anastomosis. Many of these challenges are due to difficult access or anatomical variation of prostate and bladder neck. Some common etiologies inherent to patients are obesity, large prostate, and large median lobe; otherwise altered surgical anatomy following prior intervention (TURP, abdominal surgery, or hernia repair). In this chapter, we discuss the commonly encountered difficulties during RALP (Videos 20.1, 20.2, 20.3, 20.4, 20.5, 20.6, 20.7, 20.8, and 20.9).

Obesity

Obesity represents a major healthcare problem that is significantly affecting people of all ages in developed countries. Obese (body mass index [BMI] > 30) and morbidly obese (BMI > 40) patients require special consideration from the surgical and anesthesia teams when undergoing RALP. National Health and Nutrition Examination Survey (NHANES) reported that 35.7% adult population in the USA were obese during year 2009–2010. The same data showed obesity prevalence of 37.2% for men aged 40–60 years and 36.6% for those aged ≥60 years [4]. So, it is likely that every third patient undergoing radical prostatectomy in the USA is obese.

Traditionally, some urologists have postponed surgical intervention until after weight loss or recommended alternative forms of treatment for morbidly obese men presenting with prostate cancer. During the past decade, the application of robot-

Electronic supplementary material: The online version of this chapter (doi:10.1007/978-3-319-45060-5_20) contains supplementary material, which is available to authorized users.

H.P. Ganapathi, M.D. • G. Ogaya-Pinies, M.D.
V. Mouraviev, M.D., Ph.D.
V.R. Patel, M.D., F.A.C.S. (✉)
Global Robotics Institute, Florida Hospital
Celebration Health, 410 Celebration Place, Suite 200,
Celebration, FL 34747, USA
e-mail: hari.uro@gmail.com

assisted technology has evolved and its advantages and disadvantages in obese patients have been examined. Many studies have compared the clinical, pathological, and functional outcomes of robot-assisted radical prostatectomy (RARP) in obese and nonobese patients [5, 6]. One of the largest studies comparing morbidly obese patients was published by our group. This study did not show any significant difference in perioperative complication rate, pain scores, length of stay, indwelling catheter duration, and oncological outcome while operated by a single highly experienced surgeon [7]. Obviously, these outcomes can be different in less experienced hands.

In obese men who elect to undergo robotic radical prostatectomy, body habitus can present a challenge to even an experienced surgeon. These patients are more prone to venous thromboembolism and compression nerve injuries by faulty positioning. These patients may also be difficult to ventilate in the Trendelenburg position. From a technical viewpoint, the large amount of intraperitoneal fat and the difficult working angles create unique operative challenges.

Careful positioning with padding of all pressure points is important. We use a modified lithotomy position securing the patient on a bean bag covered with a gel foam mattress. Extra foam padding is used at the shoulders, elbows, and hands. The patient and bean bag are also secured to the operating table with tape. We recommend using both mechanical and pharmacological deep venous thrombosis (DVT) prophylaxis in these patients due to the increased risk of thromboembolism (Fig. 20.1).

Following positioning, correct trocar placement is crucial. After establishing a pneumoperitoneum, there may be abnormal protuberance of abdominal wall in obese patients. Then, instruments tend to have a more vertical angle, whereby their path may be obstructed by the pubic symphysis and pelvic brim [8]. Thus, in patients with a large abdomen, the ports must be placed at a greater distance from the pubic symphysis. Typically measured on the body surface after insufflation, a distance of 15 cm increased into 17–18 cm from the pubic symphysis. This may

vary according to protuberance of abdominal wall. Additionally, robotic trocars may need to be inserted deeper into the abdominal cavity and the arms deflected laterally to flatten the working angle of the robotic arm as they reach deep into the pelvis under the pubic bone. The use of an extra-long da Vinci® robotic trocar (Intuitive Surgical, Sunnyvale, CA) is helpful in this situation. Ideally, the trocar should be inserted into the abdomen completely perpendicular to the abdominal wall and fascia. There is a relatively long distance between the skin and the fascia; correct angulation of the trocar during insertion through the skin is essential.

Following trocar insertion, due to the increased fat content, the urachal remnant often hangs from the anterior abdominal wall and obstructs the camera-port field of view. Thus, we recommend releasing the bladder's anterior and lateral attachments further cephalad than with a nonobese patient. During apical dissection or urethrovesical anastomosis, the instruments may occasionally be unable to reach their desired points. In these cases, it is helpful to reduce the pressure to 10 mmHg and to deepen the position of the robotic trocars within the abdominal wall. Our institution does not exclude surgical candidates for RALP based on BMI although some reports suggest higher complication rates, longer operation times for urethral dissection and urethrovesical anastomosis, and longer convalescence in obese patients (Fig. 20.2).

Steps to Facilitate Vesicourethral Anastomosis and Posterior Reconstruction in Obese Patients

The following maneuvers help to maximize the vision in operative field: Increasing Trendelenburg position. This should be done with all precautions during positioning to prevent sliding of the patient by usage of the gel pads with bean bag and fixing the patient. The usual angle of the table is around 25°, and it may be extended to 30°. After establishing a pneumoperitoneum in overweight patients, the instrument's path may

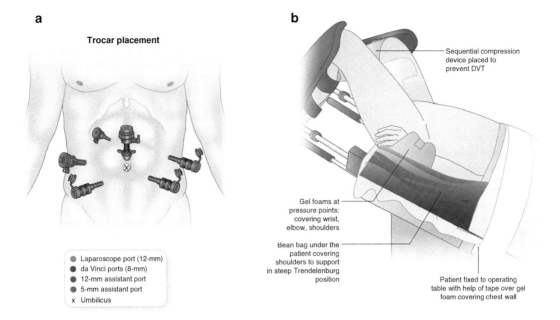

Fig. 20.1   (a, b) Proper patient positioning for robot-assisted laparoscopic radical prostatectomy

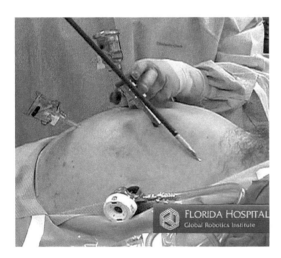

Fig. 20.2   The lax abdominal wall in obese patients insufflates like a dome raising the height of the trocars. This creates difficult working angles when dissecting about the apex of the prostate as collision with the pubis limits access to the apex. Moving the trocars lower on the abdomen (i.e., toward the pubic bone) will worsen these angles and increase clashes with the pubic symphysis

be obstructed by the pubic symphysis and the pelvic brim due to a more vertical angle. Depressing the robotic arms to prevent the instruments from hitting the pelvic brim can help avoid

this. If it is difficult to visualize the bladder neck and posterior sphincter complex, the scope is switched from 30° to 0°. Two instruments are used to retract the fat and the bladder and to prevent fat from falling into the operative field. High flow insufflator (Airseal® technology) [9] has been a useful new addition to the armamentarium for laparoscopic procedures, reducing the number of episodes of pressure loss <8 mmHg. This helps in maintaining already compromised working space in these populations. Barbed suture has shown to decrease the anastomotic time but did not affect the urinary extravasation or long-term continence rates.

Adhesions Due to Prior Abdominal Surgery

It is not uncommon for a radical prostatectomy patient to have had prior abdominal or inguinal surgery. A large RALP series reported prior history of abdominal or inguinal surgery in 27% of patients [10]. Appendectomy was the most common previous surgery identified (11%); but patients with a previous history of colectomy had the highest incidence of adhesiolysis. They have reported five bowel injuries in a cohort of 3950 patients; of these three patients had a history of prior abdominal surgery [10].

Patients with prior midline laparotomies have unpredictable amounts of adhesions. With prior abdominal surgery, consideration must be given not only to the location of the incision, but also to the procedure that was performed. Anticipating area of likely adhesions in the parietal wall, position of each trocar should be marked. A favorable initial access position that corresponds to an intended trocar site should be determined. The spleen and the left lobe of the liver are almost always above the costal margin. Therefore, in the case of a prior midline incision where there are no other compelling factors to dictate the location of initial peritoneal access, the left upper quadrant is the ideal position for initial access. Patient positioning can be used to take advantage of gravity to shift peritoneal contents away from the region of the initial trocar insertion. In our institute, initial insufflation is done with Veress needle. Then, the first trocar is placed in the right or left upper quadrant by the direct visualization entry method using a transparent port. Very careful attention should be paid to the flow of CO_2 when insufflation is initiated. Once the initial trocar has been placed, all other trocar placement must be under direct visualization, taking care of adhesions. Laparoscopic adhesiolysis is performed to create clear entry points for all trocars. Once the robot is docked, adhesions in the lower abdomen and pelvis can be released robotically (Fig. 20.3).

Prior Inguinal Hernia Repair

Prior inguinal hernia repair either open or laparoscopic distorts the operative anatomy during RALP. Despite this, RALP can be performed safely and effectively in these patients [11]. The key is early identification of anatomical landmarks to provide spatial orientation prior to dis-

secting in the area of hernia repair and scarring. The mesh is often readily apparent during the initial laparoscopy. We begin by dividing the urachus and medial umbilical ligaments. The retropubic space is entered in the midline and the posterior aspect of the pubic symphysis is identified. Dissection deep in the true pelvis is usually unaltered by hernia repairs. The superior pubic rami can be exposed and the dissection continues below this level within the pelvis to expose the endopelvic fascia bilaterally. Hence prior to approaching the region of hernia repair/mesh, several valuable anatomical landmarks have been identified and can be used to maintain correct spatial orientation as the dissection proceeds laterally. The peritoneal incisions are then extended laterally to the medial border of the vas deferens. In this method, prior mesh in place is not disturbed. If the mesh is seen, it is essential to keep the plane of dissection deep to the mesh at all times. In patients with prior laparoscopic preperitoneal hernia repairs, the scarring is typically more extensive. Again the same principles are followed. The midline dissection is usually less affected and the retropubic space and pelvic dissection can be approached in the midline with little difficulty. Again early exposure of anatomical landmarks in the pelvis will provide the necessary spatial orientation prior to dissecting further laterally beneath the mesh (Fig. 20.4a, b).

Difficulties in Individuals with Narrow Pelvis

Several authors have reported various degrees of difficulties both in extraperitoneal and transperitoneal robotic prostatectomy in patients with a narrow pelvis. Two technical issues in patients with a narrow pelvis are decreased intrapelvic working space and clashing of robotic instruments externally. Clashing between the third and fourth arm is common in patients with a smaller BMI and narrow pelvis. A minimum distance of 8 cm will negate the instrument clashing exter-

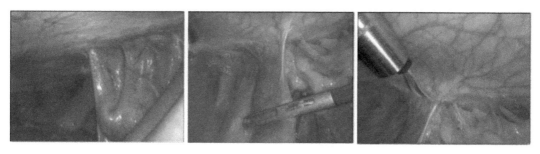

Fig. 20.3 Adhesions following midline laparotomy performed 20 years ago for appendicular abscess. Conventional laparoscopic lysis of adhesion through robotic ports before docking robot for RALP

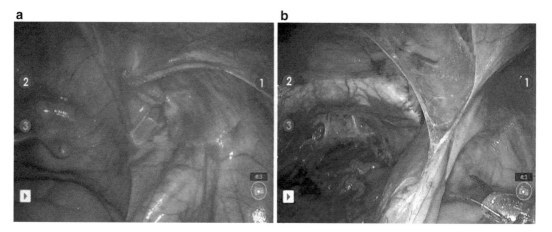

Fig. 20.4 (**a**) synthetic hernia mesh can be seen overlying the right internal ring. (**b**) the true pelvis has been dissected along the midline, displaying the superior pubic ramus, which serves as an important anatomic landmark when dissecting the bladder away from the mesh

nally. Additional maneuvers of depressing the fourth arm, elevating the third arm, and medially rotating the third arm help to prevent clashing. Further intraoperative clashing can be avoided with experience (Figs. 20.5 and 20.6).

Large Prostate

The enlarged prostate offers technical challenges that make radical prostatectomy more difficult regardless of surgical technique. For initial cases, selecting a prostate size of 30–40 g is generally recommended, as a large prostate often occupies much of the pelvis, making maneuverability and exposure of the prostate difficult during dissection. Moreover, there is a tendency for the presence of a coexistent median lobe and increased vascularity with a wide vascular pedicle, further increasing the difficulty and possibly operative time and blood loss. A large prostate also displaces the neurovascular bundle posteriorly, thereby obscuring it from view. These drawbacks can result in significant differences in intra- and postoperative outcomes. Identification of the BN in patients with a large prostate is perhaps the most challenging aspect of the procedure, as the large prostate requires a technically precise dissection in the correct plane to

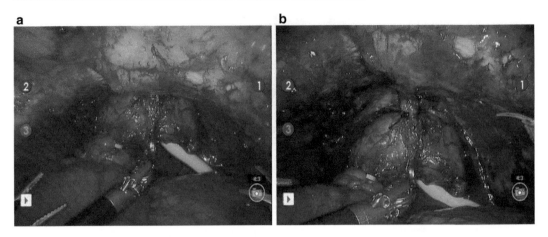

Fig. 20.5 Apical visualization improved: Same view with toggling of camera angle from 30 down to 30 up with Da Vinci Xi® Surgical Robot

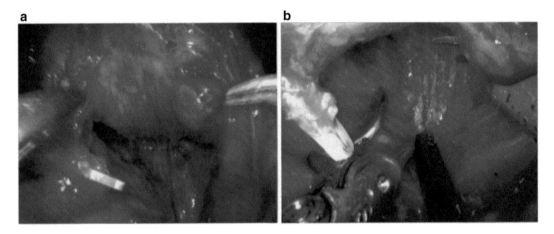

Fig. 20.6 Posterior dissection and early neurovascular bundle release visualization improved: Same view with toggling of camera angle from 30 down to 30 up with Da Vinci Xi® Surgical Robot

avoid leaving prostate tissue in the bladder. However, defining the BN by traction of an inflated Foley catheter may be misleading in cases of a concomitant median lobe. In this circumstance, the fat insertion line can be reliably utilized for defining the BN, as the bladder fat stops at the prostatovesical junction. The contour of the lateral prostate also provides an additional clue for identifying the BN. By employing gentle compression on the lateral aspect of the prostate with both robotic arms, the prostatovesical junction is revealed as a dimpling point due to the consistency of the prostate. The published results on large prostates are promising, and authors have commonly reported no clinical differences in terms of operative and pathologic outcomes in the

robotic era, even though there were trends toward higher blood loss and longer operative time in patients with larger prostates (Fig. 20.7) [12, 13]

Large Median Lobe of Prostate

The larger protrusion of the median lobe of the prostate into the urinary bladder represents a significant surgical challenge. The planes of dissection may be distorted; vascularity is also increased with a median lobe. In a study from a high volume center, median lobe was identified in 19% of 1693 patients who underwent RALP [14]. The same study reported that the estimated blood loss, length of hospital stay, pathologic

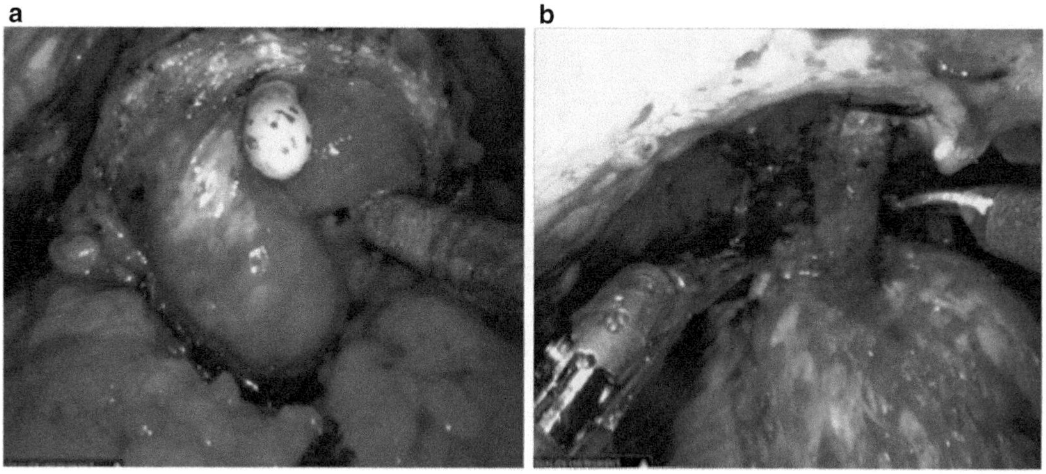

Fig. 20.7 Bladder neck and apical dissection in a case of large prostate weighing 90 g

stage, complication rates, anastomotic leakage rates, overall positive surgical margin (PSM) rates, and PSM rate at the bladder neck were not influenced by the presence of a median lobe [14].

The first step for managing a middle lobe is identifying its presence. Preoperative ultrasound or cystoscopy usually diagnoses the presence of a significant median lobe. Magnetic Resonance Imaging (MRI) provides information not only on the clinical tumor stage, but reconstructed images provide the surgical anatomy of the prostate, including the presence of a median lobe and shape of the apex and seminal vesicles. The proximity between the urethral orifices and the bladder neck (BN) should be considered together.

If not diagnosed preoperatively, several intraoperative signs can assist with recognizing the presence of a median lobe. Prior to beginning the bladder neck dissection, the urethral catheter balloon may be seen deviating to one side. This typically indicates the presence of a middle lobe or other complicated bladder neck anatomy (i.e., prior TURP). The next sign to look for is an elevated bladder when the urethral catheter is retracted upwards with the fourth arm after dividing the anterior bladder neck. The most definitive observation, however, is absence of the "drop-off" sign. When the urethral catheter is elevated and the bladder neck is spread with the bipolar

forceps, the vertical drop-off of the mucosa of the posterior bladder neck should be observed in the case of normal prostate anatomy. If the bladder is seen continuing cranially, however, a middle lobe is almost certainly present.

In this situation, the lateral bladder neck fibers should be carefully divided to increase exposure at the bladder neck and visualization within the bladder. With retraction on the anterior bladder neck, the middle lobe can be delivered out of the bladder neck and elevated with the fourth arm. If unable to do this despite releasing the lateral bladder attachments, the bladder can be opened further with a midline anterior cystotomy to gain definitive visualization and assessment of the bladder neck anatomy. Once the middle lobe is elevated, time is taken to ensure that the location of the ureteral orifices is confirmed with certainty. If doubt exists as to their precise location, intravenous methylene blue or indigo carmine may be administered to look for blue efflux from the ureteric jets. It is vital that the posterior bladder neck is not incised until the location of the ureteral orifices is confirmed so as to avoid inadvertent ureteral injury or compromise. With large middle lobes they can lie in close proximity to the intravesical adenoma.

The posterior dissection begins laterally releasing the corners of the bladder first. The bladder is then incised full thickness below the

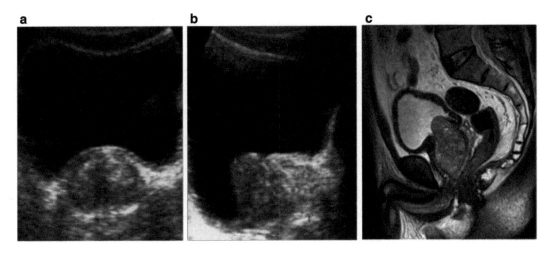

Fig. 20.8 Ultrasound and sagittal MRI reveals large median lobe protruding into the bladder neck

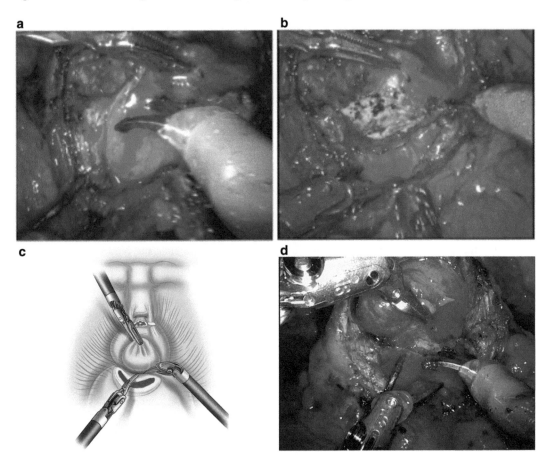

Fig. 20.9 (a–d) Incision on the posterior BN in a patient with a large median lobe. After delivery of the median lobe by the robotic fourth arm, the incision on the posterior BN is made directly inferior to the base of the median lobe, dividing the posterior BN with full thickness

level of the median lobe. The plane between the adenoma and bladder is identified and followed anteriorly. As the bladder neck is released and traction on it decreases, the ureteral orifices drift closer to the plane of dissection. The surgeon must remain cognizant of their location throughout this portion of the dissection.

Following the plane of the median lobe adenoma is useful during the initial dissection. The surgeon must be aware, however, that once under the middle lobe, the dissection will turn more posteriorly to follow the plane of the bladder. If one were to continue on the plane of the adenoma, they risk inadvertently creating a plane between it and the peripheral zone of the prostate. Zooming out for a global view of the anatomy, judging the thickness of the posterior bladder neck, moving the bladder on the base of the gland, and following the detrusor fibers all aid in identifying the correct plane. Keeping a broad dissection and a relatively bloodless field are valuable during these challenging dissections. Provided the anatomy of the prostate is followed, complications can be avoided.

The impact of the presence of a median lobe has been addressed in the current literature, noting similarity in outcomes in terms of margin positivity, resumption of continence, and complication rates with a slight increase in total operative time and blood loss (Figs. 20.8 and 20.9).

Post-Transurethral Resection of Prostate (TURP)

Given the prevalence of benign prostatic hyperplasia and that the gold standard surgical approach for treatment of this condition is transurethral resection of the prostate (TURP), many patients presenting with a diagnosis of prostate cancer have had a prior TURP or were diagnosed following TURP. In the early postoperative period, the prostate may be inflamed. Due to adhesive changes induced by heat or energy-based resections, the tissue planes between the prostate fascia and surrounding fascial structure tend to be adhered. The normal planes of dissection of the prostate may be obliterated, necessitating a greater use of sharp dissection. When judging the position of the vesicoprostatic junction, the most reliable signs are cessation of vesical fat at the junction between the bladder and prostate gland and assessing the contour of the prostate. Observing the position of the urethral catheter balloon while applying traction on the catheter is a misleading sign, as the balloon will often descend into the prostatic fossa in these patients. The anterior bladder is again approached in the midline to enter the bladder quickly and elevate the urethral catheter with the fourth robotic arm. The bladder neck anatomy can then be surveyed from within. Identification of the posterior bladder neck is usually complicated by either reurothelialization or regrowth of adenoma. Again in these cases, identification of the ureteral orifices is essential prior to proceeding with the posterior bladder neck incision. Once the ureteral orifices have been identified, the posterior bladder neck is incised full thickness. The normal tissue planes are replaced by scar tissue complicating the dissection. Careful assessment of bladder thickness while dissecting posteriorly is usually the best approach.

Published data shows compromised oncological and continence outcome for RALP following TURP (Higher PSM and poor continence results) [15]. These results are attributed to altered surgical anatomy (Fig. 20.10).

Table 20.1 lists a summary of troubleshooting suggestions in difficult scenario related to robotic-assisted laparoscopic radical prostatectomy.

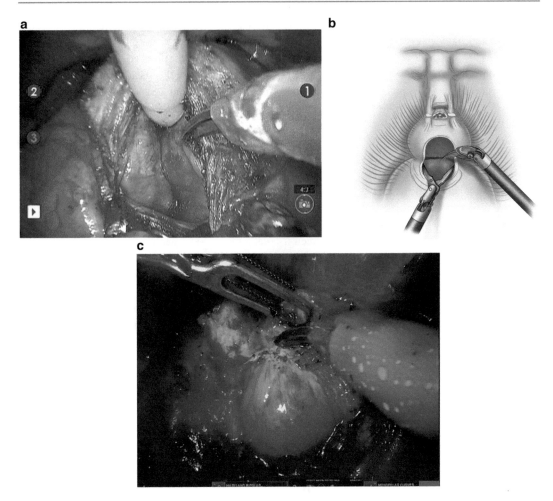

Fig. 20.10 (a–c) Incision on the posterior BN in a patient with a widened BN due to prior TURP. Surgeons should beware of re-urothelialized prostatic tissue that causes the prostatic urethra to resemble bladder urothelium. Application of indigo carmine at the beginning of the incision to aid in identification of the ureteral orifice may be helpful

Table 20.1 Summary of troubleshooting suggestions in difficult scenario of robotic assisted laparoscopic radical prostatectomy

Problem	Surgical challenge	Troubleshooting suggestions
Large median lobe	• Distorted bladder neck anatomy	– Anticipation and early identification
	• Increased vascularity and blood loss	– Retraction of median lobe with fourth arm/ retraction stich
	• Wider bladder neck	– Ureteric orifice identification (use dye if required)
		– Proper bladder neck reconstruction
Prior surgical scar	• Adhesions and difficult access	– Left hypochondrial insufflation
		– Entry with direct visualization
		– Laparoscopic adhesiolysis
Obesity	• Positioning	– Bean bag, padding, fixing
	• DVT	– Mechanical and pharmacological prophylaxis
	• Difficult access	– Proper trocar placement
		– Extra-long trocars
		– High flow insufflators (AirSeal®)
		– 30′ scope up and down toggling for better visualization during apical dissection
Narrow pelvis	• Arms clashing	– Appropriate trocars placement
		– 30′ scope up and down toggling for better visualization during apical dissection
Large prostate	• Poor visualization and maneuverability	– Experience-based case selection
		– Transperitoneal approach
	• Wide DVC	– Double ligation with CT1 needle
		– Suspension stitch
		– Staple device
	• Difficult to identify BN	– Foley traction
		– Fat insertion line
		– Prostate contour
	• Difficult visualization in apical dissection	– 30′ scope up and down toggling for better visualization during apical dissection
Prior TURP	• Difficult to identify BN	– Fat insertion line
		– Visualize ureteric orifice
	• Difficult neurovascular bundle dissection	– 30′ scope up and down toggling for better visualization during apical dissection

References

1. Siegel R, Naishadham D, Jemal A. Cancer statistics, 2012. CA Cancer J Clin. 2012;62:10–29.
2. BillAxelson A, Holmberg L, Ruutu M, Garmo H, Stark JR, Busch C, et al. Radical prostatectomy versus watchful waiting in early prostate cancer. N Engl J Med. 2011;364:1708–17.
3. Froehner M, Litz R, Manseck A, Hakenberg OW, Leike S, Albrecht DM, et al. Relationship of comorbidity, age and perioperative complication in patients undergoing radical prostatectomy. Urol Int. 2001;67:283.
4. Ogden CL, Carroll ME, Kit BK, Flegal KM. Prevalence of obesity in the United States, 2009–2010. NCHS Data Brief. 2012;82:1–8.
5. Zilberman DE, Tsivian M, Yong D, Ferrandino MN, Albala DM. Does body mass index have an impact on the rate and location of positive surgical margins following robot assisted radical prostatectomy? Urol Oncol. 2012;30:790–3.
6. Ahlering TE, Eichel L, Edwards R, Skarecky DW. Impact of obesity on clinical outcomes in robotic prostatectomy. Urology. 2005;65:740–4.
7. Muhsin HA, Giedelman C, Samavedi C, Schatloff O, Coelho R, Rocco B, et al. Perioperative and early oncological outcomes after robot-assisted radical

prostatectomy (RARP) in morbidly obese patients: a propensity score-matched study. BJU Int. 2014;113:84–91.

8. Mikhail AA, Stockton BR, Orvieto MA, et al. Robotic assisted laparoscopic prostatectomy in overweight and obese patients. Urology. 2006;67:774–9.

9. Horstmann M, Horton K, Kurz M, Padevit C, John H. Prospective comparison between the AirSeal® System valve-less Trocar and a standard Versaport™ Plus V2 Trocar in robotic-assisted radical prostatectomy. J Endourol. 2013;27:579–82.

10. Siddiqui SA, Krane LS, Bhandari A, Patel MN, Rogers CG, Stricker H, Peabody JO, Menon M. The impact of previous inguinal or abdominal surgery on outcomes after robotic radical prostatectomy. Urology. 2010;75:1079–82.

11. Laungani RG, Kaul S, Muhletaler F, et al. Impact of previous inguinal hernia repair on transperitoneal robotic prostatectomy. Can J Urol. 2007;14: 3635–9.

12. Link BA, Nelson R, Josephson DY, Yoshida JS, Crocitto LE, Kawachi MH, Wilson TG. The impact of prostate gland weight in robot assisted laparoscopic radical prostatectomy. J Urol. 2008;180: 928–32.

13. Levinson AW, Ward NT, Sulman A, Mettee LZ, Link RE, Su LM, Pavlovich CP. The impact of prostate size on perioperative outcomes in a large laparoscopic radical prostatectomy series. J Endourol. 2009;23: 147–52.

14. Coelho RF, Chauhan S, Guglielmetti GB, Orvieto MA, Sivaraman A, Palmer KJ, Rocco B, Coughlin G, Hassan RE, Dall'oglio MF, Patel VR. Does the presence of median lobe affect outcomes of robot-assisted laparoscopic radical prostatectomy? J Endourol. 2012;26:264–70.

15. Gupta NP, Singh P, Nayyar R. Outcomes of robot-assisted radical prostatectomy in men with previous transurethral resection of prostate. BJU Int. 2011; 108:1501–5.

Carlos Eduardo Schio Fay, Sameer Chopra, and Monish Aron

Abbreviations

BPH	Benign prostatic hyperplasia
CBI	Continuous bladder irrigation
DRE	Digital rectal exam
IPSS	International prostate symptom score
JP	Jackson–Pratt
LUTS	Lower urinary tract symptoms
OSP	Open simple prostatectomy
PSA	Prostate-specific antigen
RSP	Robotic simple prostatectomy
SHIM	Sexual health inventory for men
TRUS	Transrectal ultrasound
TURP	Transurethral resection of the prostate
UTI	Urinary tract infection

Electronic supplementary material: The online version of this chapter (doi:10.1007/978-3-319-45060-5_21) contains supplementary material, which is available to authorized users.

C.E.S. Fay, M.D. • S. Chopra, M.D., M.S
M. Aron, M.D. (✉)
Catherine & Joseph Aresty Department of Urology, USC Institute of Urology, Keck School of Medicine, University of Southern California, 1441 Eastlake Ave. STE 7416, Los Angeles, CA 90089, USA
e-mail: monish.aron@med.usc.edu

Introduction

Surgical treatment for BPH is indicated in patients with moderate-to-severe lower urinary tract symptoms (LUTS), who have failed medical therapy or desire a more effective treatment option, and for patients who develop BPH-related complications such as acute urinary retention, recurrent urinary tract infection (UTI), renal insufficiency, gross hematuria, and bladder stone(s) secondary to BPH. Bladder diverticulum associated with recurrent UTI and bladder dysfunction is also an indication for surgical intervention [1].

The type of surgery recommended to the patient will depend on patient and prostate anatomy, patient comorbidities, surgeon's experience and training. Transurethral resection of the prostate (TURP) remains the gold standard for the treatment of prostates less than 80 g, and open simple prostatectomy (OSP) has been the gold standard for the treatment of prostates larger than 80 g [2]. However, OSP is associated with a significant risk for complications [3, 4].

In 2002, laparoscopic simple prostatectomy was first described as a minimally invasive alternative to OSP to reduce perioperative complications, especially blood loss, blood transfusions, reoperation, and to decrease the length of hospital stay [5–7]. Robotic simple prostatectomy (RSP) was first described in 2008 and since then its role for surgical treatment of BPH is increasing [8, 9].

Using robotics has demonstrated benefit in providing stereoscopic magnified 3-D vision, tremor filtration, seven degrees of freedom wristed instruments, and enhanced ergonomics. The benefits of these have resulted in a shorter learning curve for RSP than for laparoscopic simple prostatectomy [4]. We have previously reported on our experience of using the transperitoneal approach [4, 10]. The transperitoneal approach is usually preferred, which is reflective of the surgeon's background experience with robotic radical prostatectomy.

Preoperative Preparation

Preoperative Evaluation

Preoperative evaluation includes history, physical examination, digital rectal exam (DRE), and laboratory testing including kidney function tests, urinalysis, reflex culture, and prostate-specific antigen (PSA). We also administer the International Prostate Symptom Score (IPSS) and Sexual Health Inventory for Men (SHIM) questionnaires, and obtain uroflowmetry with peak flow rate (Qmax) measurement, transrectal ultrasound to estimate prostate size, and perform a bladder scan to assess post-void residual volume. A transrectal prostate biopsy is performed, to rule out prostate cancer, if the patient has an elevated PSA or abnormal DRE, if clinically indicated.

Patients are counseled as to all treatment alternatives and surgical options. Risks and benefits, potential complications, and the possibility of conversion to open surgery are discussed. Informed consent is obtained.

Antiplatelet and anticoagulant medications are discontinued or bridged before surgery, as clinically indicated. Medical and anesthesia clearance are obtained if necessary. No bowel preparation is usually required unless the patient is habitually constipated, and the patient is made NPO after midnight on the day of surgery. Prophylactic intravenous antibiotics are administered at induction of anesthesia prior to skin incision and are usually discontinued 24 h after surgery.

Operative Room Setup

For RSP, we use a four-arm robotic technique. The additional arm allows for the need of only one assistant who is positioned on the patient's left side. The scrub technician is positioned on the patient's left side as well with video monitors on both sides of the patient for easy viewing by the surgical team. A Mayo stand is placed next to the assistant where frequently used instruments are placed. The da Vinci® Surgical System (Intuitive Surgical, Inc., Sunnyvale, CA) will be docked in between the patient's legs for the Si robot (Fig. 21.1) or on the right side of the patient for the Xi robot.

Patient Positioning

Under general endotracheal anesthesia, the patient is placed in a modified lithotomy position (Fig. 21.2) over a nonskid foam pad. The patient is secured using the Yellofin® stirrups and an upper-body warming blanket is applied. Care is taken to adequately pad all pressure points to avoid positioning injuries. The abdominal skin is shaved with clippers, and the patient is prepped and draped in standard sterile fashion for a transperitoneal pelvic robot-assisted surgery. An 18-French urethral catheter is inserted and an orogastric tube is placed. A standard time-out is called prior to incision.

Instrumentation and Equipment List

Equipment
- Si or Xi da Vinci®
- 0° robotic scope (Intuitive Surgical, Inc., Sunnyvale, CA)
- Monopolar Scissors (Intuitive Surgical, Inc., Sunnyvale, CA) × 1
- ProGrasp™ Forceps (Intuitive Surgical, Inc., Sunnyvale, CA) × 2
- Needle Drivers (Intuitive Surgical, Inc., Sunnyvale, CA) × 2
- Clip Appliers (Intuitive Surgical, Inc., Sunnyvale, CA) × 2
- Tenaculum Forceps (Intuitive Surgical, Inc., Sunnyvale, CA) × 1

Trocars
- 12 mm trocars × 2 (1 for the Xi)
- 8 mm trocars × 3 (4 for Xi)

Fig. 21.1 Operating room setup for robotic simple prostatectomy. Schematic demonstrating the typical operating room setup for robotic simple prostatectomy utilized at our institution

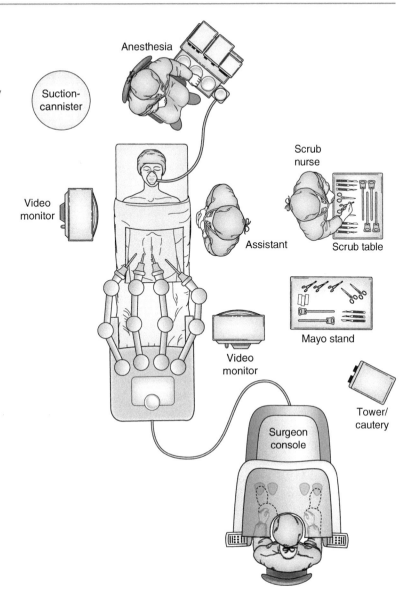

Assistant Instruments

- Suction irrigator device (Bariatric length)
- Laparoscopic spoon forceps
- Hem-o-lok applier (Teleflex Medical, Research Triangle Park, NC)
- Medium (purple) Hem-o-lok clips (Teleflex Medical, Research Triangle Park, NC)
- Laparoscopic needle driver
- Laparoscopic scissor
- 10 mm specimen entrapment bag

Step-by-Step Technique (Videos 21.1, 21.2, 21.3, 21.4, 21.5, 21.6, 21.7, 21.8, and 21.9)

Step 1: Pneumoperitoneum and Trocar Placement

The first incision is made approximately 1–2 finger-breadths above the umbilicus. Through this incision we establish pneumoperitoneum to 15 mmHg with

Fig. 21.2 Patient positioning. For robotic simple prostatectomy, the patients are positioned in lithotomy and modified Trendelenburg

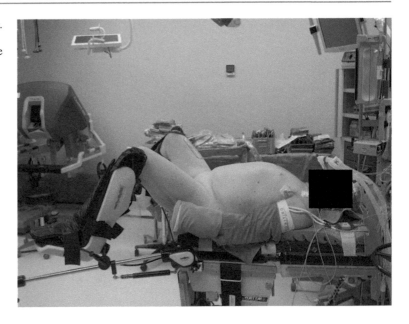

a Veress needle. A 12-mm port (8 mm for the Xi) is inserted through this incision into the peritoneal cavity. The peritoneal cavity is then inspected using the 0° scope to ensure absence of any intra-abdominal injury from the Veress needle or the trocar. Four additional trocars are then inserted under direct vision. The 8-mm da Vinci® working trocars are all placed at the horizontal level of the umbilicus with a separation of 8–10 cm between trocars. We prefer to keep the fourth robotic arm on the right side of the patient. A 12-mm assistant trocar is placed in the left upper quadrant in the midclavicular line taking care to avoid being too close to the camera trocar or the left robotic arm. Thus, a 4-arm, 5-trocar transperitoneal approach is employed (Fig. 21.3).

At this point, the patient is placed in Trendelenburg position, and the da Vinci® is docked (Fig. 21.4) between the legs for the Si or from the right side of the patient for the Xi. The instruments are inserted into the peritoneal cavity under direct vision. We initially start with a ProGrasp™ in the left and fourth arm and a monopolar scissor in the right arm.

Step 2: Cystotomy (Table 21.1)

The sigmoid colon is initially mobilized out of the pelvic cavity for better exposure of the target anatomy (Fig. 21.5a–d). The bladder is filled with approximately 200 mL of saline through the urethral catheter and a vertical midline cystotomy is created with monopolar scissors gaining access to the bladder lumen (Fig. 21.6a, b).

Step 3: Deploying Stay Sutures (Table 21.2)

All the fluid is suctioned out and 2–4 stay sutures are deployed to keep the edges of the cystotomy widely retracted. These stay sutures are 2-0 Polyglactin sutures, 6-in. long, on a CT-1 needle with a medium Hem-o-lok clip tied into the end of the suture. The stay suture is passed outside-in through the bladder wall at the edge of the cystotomy, anchored laterally to the abdominal wall, then pulled taut and secured with an additional Hem-o-lok clip (Fig. 21.7a, b).

Typically, a large prostatic adenoma that bulges into the bladder is immediately apparent. A 2-0 Polyglactin suture on a CT-1 needle stay suture is placed in the median lobe to provide traction and countertraction during the procedure using the ProGrasp forceps in the fourth robotic arm (Fig. 21.8). Bilateral ureteral orifices are then carefully identified and care is taken to keep them safe throughout the procedure.

If simultaneous bladder diverticulectomy is to be performed, or if the intravesical adenoma is

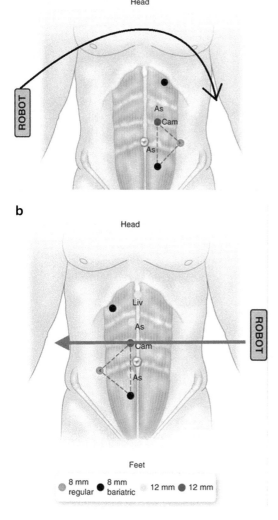

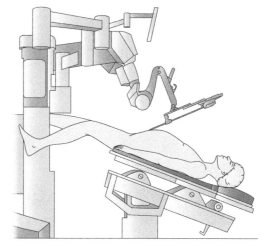

Fig. 21.4 Robot docking. With the patient placed in lithotomy position and modified Trendelenburg, the da Vinci® Si is docked in between the patient's legs

Fig. 21.3 Trocar placement. For transperitoneal robotic simple prostatectomy, a five-trocar placement is utilized. This placement is identical to that for robotic radical prostatectomy

extremely large and very close to the ureteral orifices, ureteral double J stents can be placed using a 2 mm mini-port deployed in the suprapubic area. A 0.035-in. guide wire is inserted through the mini-port, floppy end first, and then a 4.8–6 French ureteral stent is advanced over the wire (Fig. 21.9a–d).

Step 3: Adenoma Dissection (Table 21.3)

The urethral catheter is pulled back into the urethra after deflating the balloon, and a stay suture is used to elevate the median lobe using the fourth robotic arm. With the median lobe retracted anteriorly, a mucosal incision is made at the junction between the median lobe and the trigone using hot monopolar scissors. This incision is deepened to reach the plane of the adenoma at the junction between the adenoma and the compressed peripheral zone and capsule of the prostate (Fig. 21.10).

After a plane of dissection has been established posteriorly, the surgeon progresses both laterally and distally using a combination of blunt and sharp dissection (Fig. 21.11a). Bleeding vessels are coagulated concurrently using monopolar electrocautery. Once the posterior aspect of the adenoma has been separated from the compressed peripheral zone and prostate capsule, the dissection proceeds along the lateral surface of the prostate adenoma, mobilizing the lateral aspect of the adenoma (Fig. 21.11b). The plane of dissection should hug the pearly white surface of the adenoma. Care should be taken to avoid transgressing the compressed peripheral zone and the prostate capsule. Once enough of the adenoma has been freed up, the previously placed stay suture in the median lobe is removed and the adenoma is grasped with a robotic tenaculum forceps brought in under vision through the fourth robotic arm. The tenaculum provides an excellent grip on the adenoma, and allows excellent trac-

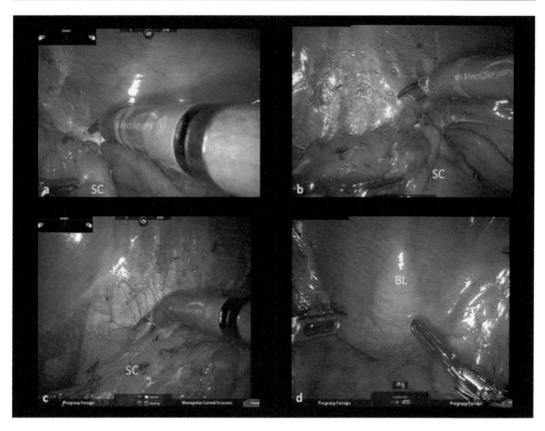

Fig. 21.5 (**a–d**) Mobilization of the sigmoid colon. The sigmoid colon (SC) is mobilized to allow for better exposure of the bladder (BL)

Table 21.2 Instrumentation required for deploying stay sutures

Surgeon instrumentation			Assistant instrumentation
Left arm	**Right arm**	**Fourth arm**	• Hem-o-lok applier
• Needle driver	• Needle driver	• ProGrasp™ forceps	• Laparoscopic scissors
• **Endoscope lens**: 0°			

tion and countertraction to aid in the dissection of the adenoma. During dissection of the adenoma, we maintain a ProGrasp™ in the left arm and the monopolar scissors in the right arm. As the dissection of the lateral aspect of the adenoma progresses distally, the previously made posterior mucosal incision is carried laterally in a circumferential fashion. The lateral aspect of the adenoma is mobilized down towards the apical tissue where the lateral shoulders of the adenoma start tapering medially towards the membranous urethra. The anterior aspect of the adenoma mobilization is done last and the anterior bladder neck

mucosa is incised with hot scissors at the 12 o'clock position and the dissection progresses distally along the anterior surface of the adenoma (Fig. 21.11c, d).

The dissection continues distally to the point the urethra is visualized (Fig. 21.12). The urethra is then sharply transected using cold scissors. The adenoma is completely released from the prostate and then placed in a 10-mm specimen entrapment bag. The prostate fossa is examined for any residual adenoma, which can be excised separately and removed with a laparoscopic spoon forceps.

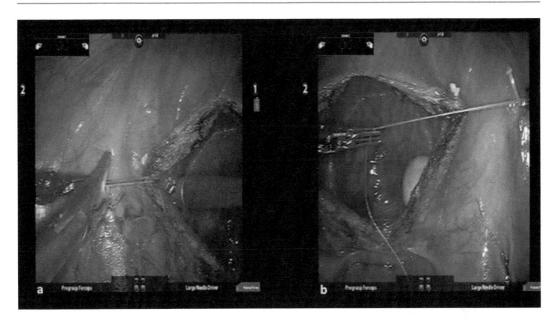

Fig. 21.7 (**a, b**) Exposing the operative space of the bladder. A 2-0 Polyglactin suture on a CT-1 needle stitch with a Hem-o-lok at the end is passed through the bladder, anchored laterally to the abdominal wall, then pulled and secured with a Hem-o-lok to expose the bladder and keep open the operative space

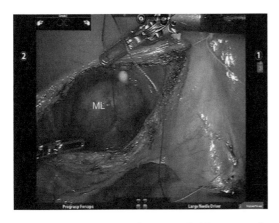

Fig. 21.8 Prostatic median lobe control. A large prostatic adenoma is identified from within the bladder and a 2-0 Vicryl on a CT-1 needle stay suture is placed within the median lobe (ML) to provide traction and countertraction during the procedure

Step 4: Hemostasis (Table 21.4)

The key to excellent hemostasis is being in the correct plane during enucleation of the adenoma and obtaining concurrent hemostasis while the adenoma is being enucleated. This will significantly decrease the amount of time spent in obtaining hemostasis after the adenoma has been enucleated. Post-enucleation hemostasis is obtained using a combination of electrocautery and sutures. Discrete arterial bleeders can be point coagulated with the monopolar scissors while venous bleeding is best secured with sutures. We use either 2-0 V-loc™ sutures or figure-of-eight, 2-0 Polyglactin sutures for hemostatic suturing in the prostatic fossa (Fig. 21.13a–d). Small bleeders near the sphincter are suture ligated with 4-0 Polyglactin sutures. The suturing is done with robotic needle drivers in the left and right robotic arm. The fossa is thoroughly irrigated to ensure excellent hemostasis.

Step 5: Retrigonization

We do not routinely retrigonize the prostatic fossa. If retrigonization is considered appropriate, we do this after carefully obtaining perfect hemostasis and a clean prostatic fossa. This is accomplished using a 2-0 V-loc™ suture on a GS-21 needle placed at the 6 o'clock position in the bladder neck mucosa and advancing it into the prostatic fossa at a convenient location, usually in the midfossa. The stitch is then advanced

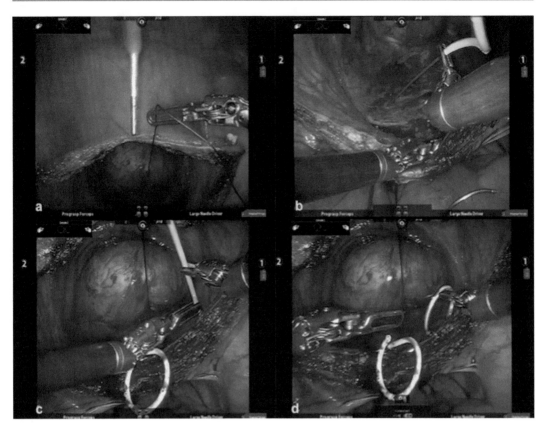

Fig. 21.9 Insertion of bilateral ureteral stents. (**a**) A 2-mm mini-port is inserted into the suprapubic area. (**b**) Guide wire insertion and left ureteral stent placement. (**c**) Right ureteral stent placement. (**d**) Final aspect showing bilateral ureteral stents

Table 21.3 Instrumentation required for step 3: adenoma dissection

Surgeon instrumentation			Assistant instrumentation
Left arm	**Right arm**	**Fourth arm**	• Laparoscopic suction irrigator
• ProGrasp™ forceps	• Monopolar scissors	• ProGrasp™ forceps	
		• Tenaculum forceps	
• **Endoscope lens**: 0°			

along the left side of the bladder neck to advance the lateral mucosa down into the prostatic fossa. An additional 2-0 V-loc™ suture on a GS-21 needle is used for the advancement of the right-sided bladder neck mucosa. The goal of retrigonization is to cover the raw surface of the prostatic fossa and theoretically decrease the risk of postoperative hemorrhage and irritative symptoms. Retrigonization is done with robotic needle drivers in the left and right robotic arm.

Step 6: Bladder Closure (Table 21.5)

A 22-French 3-way hematuria catheter is inserted into the bladder via the urethra and 30 mL of sterile water is used to inflate the balloon. The previously placed stay sutures are now cut and removed. The Hem-o-lok clips on the stay sutures, on the bladder wall and the abdominal wall, are removed by the assistant using a laparoscopic spoon forceps. The midline cystotomy is now closed in two layers; the first is an inner full thickness layer using 2-0 V-loc™ sutures on a GS-21 needle (Fig. 21.14) and the second layer is also a full thickness layer using the same sutures (Fig. 21.15). After the first layer is complete, the bladder is filled with 200 mL of saline to ensure the closure is watertight and also to avoid hitting the urethral catheter balloon with the second layer closure.

To confirm a watertight closure, the bladder is now distended with 300 mL of saline and continuous bladder irrigation (CBI) is now commenced after irrigating out any clots. CBI is titrated to ensure a clear return of irrigant.

Hemostasis is now confirmed in the peritoneal cavity and a 19-French Jackson–Pratt (JP) drain is placed in the retrovesical space and brought out through the right lateral 8-mm trocar site and affixed to the skin using 2-0 Nylon. Robotic instruments are now removed under vision and the robot is undocked.

The midline camera trocar incision is now enlarged as needed to allow extraction of the ade-

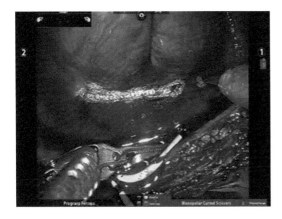

Fig. 21.10 Bladder mucosa incision. With traction stitch retracted with fourth arm, bladder mucosa is incised between median lobe and bladder trigone

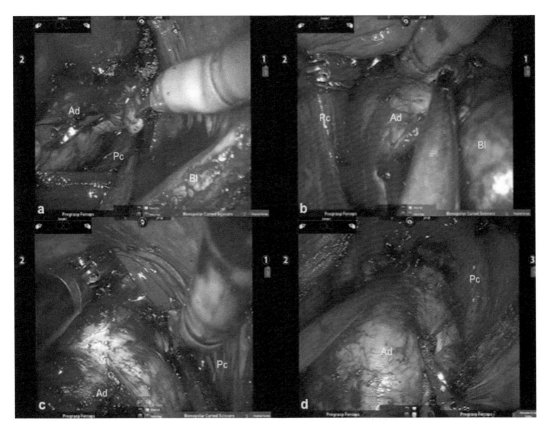

Fig. 21.11 Adenoma dissection. (**a**) Posterior dissection (**b**) Dissection of the lateral aspect of the adenoma (**c**, **d**). Anterior dissection. *Pc* prostate capsule, *Bl* bladder, *Ad* adenoma

noma specimen within the specimen entrapment bag. The fascia of the extraction site is closed using 0 PDS figure-of-eight stitches. The 12-mm assistant trocar site is closed using the Carter-Thomason Port Closure System® and 0 Polyglactin sutures. Subcutaneous tissue is re-approximated using 3-0 Polyglactin suture and the skin is closed using 4-0 Monocryl® in subcuticular fashion. Dermabond® is applied over the incisions. The patient is then extubated and transferred to recovery room.

Special Considerations

Potential Bladder Tumor

To rule out a potential bladder tumor in smokers or patients with a history of hematuria, a flexible cystoscopy is performed either at the time of preoperative office visit or at the start of the case. The presence of a bladder tumor is a contraindication to opening the bladder.

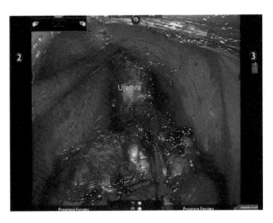

Fig. 21.12 Urethral exposure. The urethra is exposed

Previous Open Abdominal Surgery

In a patient with a prior midline abdominal incision from an open procedure, pneumoperitoneum is obtained either with a Veress needle away from the incision, or with the open (Hasson) technique. The cavity is carefully inspected, and adhesions, if present, are taken down laparoscopically prior to docking the robot.

Bladder Diverticulum

A bladder diverticulectomy can be performed at the same time as a RSP. We prefer to place a JJ stent on the side of the diverticulum to protect the ipsilateral ureter during dissection of the diverticulum. Also the vertical cystotomy is moved slightly off center away from the side of the diverticulum to avoid having the two suture lines very close together.

Bladder Calculi

Bladder calculi can be easily and expeditiously removed at the time of RSP since the bladder is wide open.

Potential Complications

The most common complication from this procedure is ongoing hematuria. This can lead to prolonged CBI, prolonged length of stay, and even potential clot retention and possible bladder rupture. The best way to avoid this is to spend the necessary amount of time in the

Table 21.4 Instrumentation required for step 4: hemostasis

Surgeon instrumentation			Assistant instrumentation
Left arm	**Right arm**	**Fourth arm**	• Laparoscopic suction irrigator
• Needle driver	• Needle driver	• ProGrasp™ forceps	• Laparoscopic needle driver
	• Monopolar scissors (for pinpoint coagulation)		
• **Endoscope lens**: 0°			

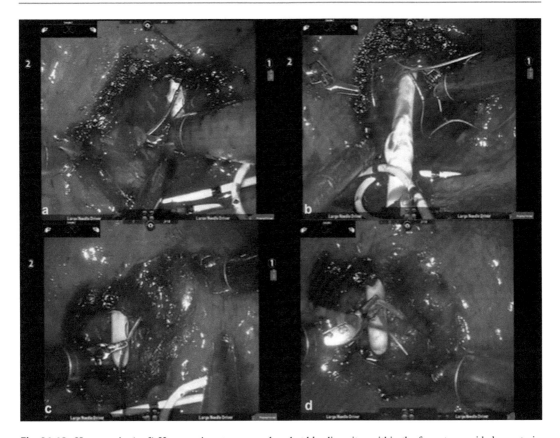

Fig. 21.13 Hemostasis. (**a–d**) Hemostatic sutures are placed at bleeding sites within the fossa to provide hemostasis. 4-0 Vicryl sutures and spot coagulation are performed to complete this step

Table 21.5 Instrumentation required for step 5: bladder closure

Surgeon instrumentation			Assistant instrumentation
Left arm	**Right arm**	**Fourth arm**	• Laparoscopic suction irrigator
• Needle driver	• Needle driver	• ProGrasp™ forceps	• Laparoscopic spoon—to remove Hem-o-lok clips from stay sutures
			• Laparoscopic needle driver
• **Endoscope lens**: 0°			

operating room to get perfect hemostasis prior to bladder closure.

If there is persistent ongoing hematuria which looks arterial, it may become necessary to take the patient back to the operating room. Often it is a simple matter to address this cystoscopically and fulgurate the arterial bleeder with a resectoscope loop.

Rarely, if the urethral catheter gets blocked and is not recognized in a timely fashion, the bladder closure may give way and there can be an intraperitoneal leak. In this situation, the best

approach is to go back robotically, open the bladder, wash it out, get hemostasis, and close the bladder again.

Transient incontinence and erectile dysfunction can occur rarely, in less than 5% of patients. Some patients have symptoms of overactive bladder and dysuria for a few weeks to months after surgery. Most of these are self-limiting and resolve spontaneously.

Rarely, if residual adenoma is left behind at the apex, patients may not be able to void well

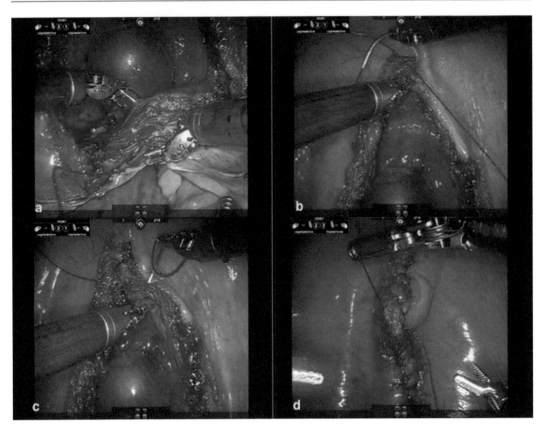

Fig. 21.14 First layer of bladder closure. (**a–c**) First layer of bladder closure. A 2-0 V-loc suture on a GS-21 needle is used to perform the first layer of bladder closure. (**d**) Final aspect of the first layer of bladder closure

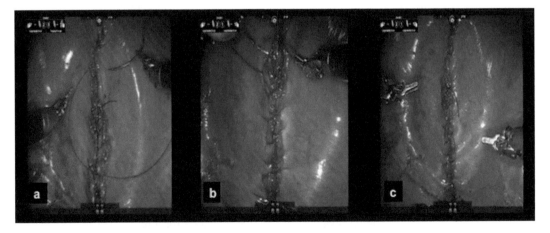

Fig. 21.15 Second layer of bladder closure. (**a, b**) Second layer of bladder closure. A 2-0 V-loc suture on a GS-21 needle is used to perform the second layer of bladder closure. (**c**) Final aspect of the second layer of bladder closure

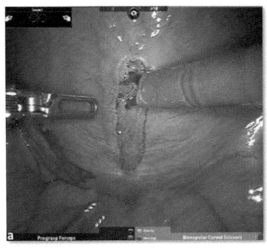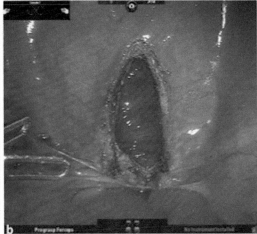

Fig. 21.6 (**a, b**) Midline vertical cystostomy. A midline vertical cystostomy is created to gain access to the anterior portion of the bladder

Table 21.1 Instrumentation required for step 2: cystotomy

Surgeon instrumentation			Assistant instrumentation
Left arm	**Right arm**	**Fourth arm**	• Laparoscopic suction irrigator
• ProGrasp™ forceps	• Monopolar scissors	• ProGrasp™ forceps	
• **Endoscope lens**: 0°			

postoperatively. This can be diagnosed at the 3-month visit and confirmed with an office cystoscopy. Residual adenoma at the apex associated with poor flow and high IPSS score can be treated with a TURP directed at this residual tissue.

Follow-up

Intermittent compression stockings and subcutaneous heparin are used during the hospital stay to prevent thromboembolic events. Continuous bladder irrigation is stopped on the first postoperative day if the urine is clear or light pink. The JP drain is removed prior to discharge after confirming absence of urine leak. The median length of hospital stay in our experience is 3 days. The urethral catheter is removed on postoperative day 7 with a voiding trial. A follow-up visit is scheduled at 3 months for symptom check, uroflowmetry, postvoid residual urine measurement, and administration of IPSS and SHIM questionnaires.

References

1. McVary KT, Roehrborn CG, Avins AL, Barry MJ, Bruskewitz RC, Donnell RF, et al. Update on AUA guideline on the management of benign prostatic hyperplasia. J Urol. 2011;185(5):1793–803.
2. Oelke M, Bachmann A, Descazeaud A, Emberton M, Gravas S, Michel MC, et al. EAU guidelines on the treatment and follow-up of non-neurogenic male lower urinary tract symptoms including benign prostatic obstruction. Eur Urol. 2013;64(1):118–40.
3. Parsons JK, Rangarajan SS, Palazzi K, Chang D. A national, comparative analysis of perioperative outcomes of open and minimally invasive simple prostatectomy. J Endourol. 2015;29(8):919–24.
4. Autorino R, Zargar H, Mariano MB, Sanchez-Salas R, Sotelo RJ, Chlosta PL, et al. Perioperative outcomes of robotic and laparoscopic simple prostatec-

tomy: a European-American multi-institutional analysis. Eur Urol. 2015;68(1):86–94.

5. Mariano MB, Graziottin TM, Tefilli MV. Laparoscopic prostatectomy with vascular control for benign prostatic hyperplasia. J Urol. 2002;167(6):2528–9.

6. Matei DV, Brescia A, Mazzoleni F, Spinelli M, Musi G, Melegari S, et al. Robot-assisted simple prostatectomy (RASP): does it make sense? BJU Int. 2012;110(11 Pt C):E972–9.

7. Patel ND, Parsons JK. Robotic-assisted simple prostatectomy: is there evidence to go beyond the experimental stage? Curr Urol Rep. 2014;15(10):443.

8. Sotelo R, Clavijo R, Carmona O, Garcia A, Banda E, Miranda M, et al. Robotic simple prostatectomy. J Urol. 2008;179(2):513–5.

9. Pariser JJ, Pearce SM, Patel SG, Bales GT. National trends of simple prostatectomy for benign prostatic hyperplasia with an analysis of risk factors for adverse perioperative outcomes. Urology. 2015;86(4): 721–5.

10. Leslie S, Abreu AL, Chopra S, Ramos P, Park D, Berger AK, et al. Transvesical robotic simple prostatectomy: initial clinical experience. Eur Urol. 2014;66(2):321–9.

Nishant D. Patel and Christopher J. Kane

Introduction

Robotic pelvic lymphadenectomy is a routine staging procedure performed at the time of robotic radical prostatectomy for men at risk for nodal metastases. The procedure is safe and reproducible with limited complications and provides important risk stratification information that helps stratify patients by risk of biochemical and clinical progression. Patients with limited lymph node metastases may do well after surgery alone and be observed closely. Those with higher volume lymph node metastases or N1 disease and biochemical recurrence may benefit from androgen deprivation therapy or radiation therapy or the combination.

Traditionally pelvic lymphadenectomy has been limited to the obturator and external iliac lymph nodes; however, more modern series suggest that with a more extended lymphadenectomy a much greater proportion of men will be recognized with lymph node metastases. The extended dissection should incorporate the internal iliac lymph nodes along with the obturator and external iliac lymph nodes to the common iliac artery. Some authors include presacral lymph nodes as well.

We perform extended lymphadenectomy for all D'Amico high-risk patients. The technique involves a peritoneal incision over the common iliac artery, identification, and medial reflection of the ureter to identify the iliac artery bifurcation. We begin the dissection at the bifurcation, dissecting the nodal tissue from the bifurcation distally along the external iliac artery and vein to the node of Cloquet medially and the ilioinguinal nerve laterally. The nodal tissue along the distribution of the internal iliac artery is then removed. The obturator lymph nodes are then dissected from the obturator nerve proximally to the internal iliac artery. Lymphostasis is obtained with small hemo-lock or titanium clips and monopolar electrocautery.

The extended lymphadenectomy takes 10–30 min of operative time per side and yields 10–20 lymph nodes per side. The risk of lymphocele formation is 1–5%. Major complications are exceedingly rare; however, lymphadenectomy may increase the risk of thromboembolic events and therefore may warrant greater DVT prophylaxis.

We believe extended lymphadenectomy is an important staging procedure for men undergoing radical prostatectomy for high-risk prostate cancer; that the procedure can be done safely and efficiently robotically, with similar oncologic outcomes to an open pelvic lymph node dissection.

N.D. Patel, M.D.
Department of Urology, Cleveland Clinic Foundation, 9500 Euclid Avenue, Q10-1, Cleveland, OH 44195, USA
e-mail: pateln10@ccf.org

C.J. Kane, M.D. (✉)
Department of Urology, University of California San Diego Health System, 200 W Arbor Drive, MC 8897, San Diego, CA 92103, USA
e-mail: ckane@ucsd.edu

© Springer International Publishing Switzerland 2017
L.-M. Su (ed.), *Atlas of Robotic Urologic Surgery*, DOI 10.1007/978-3-319-45060-5_22

Patient Selection

Indications

In the PSA era, 1–3% of men will have positive lymph nodes (LN) at the time of radical prostatectomy and, of those, 50% will have a clinical recurrence within 10 years of prostatectomy [1]. Traditionally, the indication for pelvic lymph node dissection (PLND) in prostate cancer was that of a staging procedure, as CT or MRI preoperative imaging has low sensitivity (39–42%) for detecting nodal metastases if <11 mm [2]. However, more recent data suggest that a more extended pelvic lymphadenectomy can improve staging accuracy and potentially provide a therapeutic benefit in biochemical recurrence-free survival and prostate cancer-specific mortality [1, 3]. Extended PLND (E-PLND) is thought to confer a therapeutic benefit by decreasing the burden of histologically undetectable metastatic disease, i.e., micrometastatic disease.

Per NCCN guidelines, pelvic lymphadenectomy is recommended in low and intermediate risk categories (Table 22.1) when the predicted probability of nodal metastases is >2%. Several nomograms are available to calculate this risk including the MSKCC Kattan nomogram, UCSF CAPRA score, and the updated Partin Tables [4].

The EAU and NCCN recommend performing PLND using an extended template. The AUA 2013 Guidelines state that PLND "may not be necessary" in low-risk patients with PSA ≤10 ng/mL, clinical stage T1 or T2, and Gleason score ≤6 with no Gleason pattern 4 or 5. The AUA mentions the extended template as an option. At our institution, very low and low-risk patients do not receive a PLND, intermediate-risk patients receive a standard PLND (S-PLND) if the risk of LN metastases is ≥2%, and all high-risk and very high-risk patients receive E-PLND. The paradox is that although intermediate-risk patients have a relatively low risk of lymph node metastases at PLND, in order to adequately determine if LN metastases are present a more extended node dissection is required. So many authors now recommend extended node dissections for intermediate-risk patients as well. Compared to open or laparoscopic PLND, robotic PLND can be performed with a comparable nodal yield [5, 6].

Imaging

As stated earlier, preoperative CT and MRI imaging has poor sensitivity for detecting LN mets <11 mm. New technologies are emerging

Table 22.1 Risk categories

Very low risk[a]	PSA < 10		Gleason ≤ 6		
	PSAD < 0.015	&	No pattern 4 or 5	&	Clinical stage T1c
			< 50% cancer/core		
			≤ 2 positive cores[b]		
Low risk	PSA < 10	&	Gleason ≤ 6	&	Clinical stage T1 or T2a
Intermediate risk	PSA 10–20	or	Gleason = 7	or	Clinical stage T2b or T2c
High risk	PSA > 20	or	Gleason ≥ 8	or	Clinical Stage T3a
Very high risk	Any PSA	&	Primary Gleason	or	Clinical Stage T3b–T4
			Pattern 5	or	
			> 4 cores with		
			≥ Gleason 8		

PSA prostate-specific antigen, *PSAD* PSA density (PSA/prostate volume)
[a]All criteria are required
[b]Two or less cores that show cancer using a biopsy template taking ≥ 10 cores

that may improve the accuracy of MRI including restriction spectrum imaging (RSI), in addition to diffusion weighted imaging (DWI) [7]. Novel methods are emerging to preoperatively detect LN metastases and subsequently detect these LNs intraoperatively. In one study, fluorescent-labeled tilmanocept was injected into male dogs, a pelvic PET/CT scan was performed for sentinel lymph node mapping, and robotic-assisted sentinel lymph node dissection using a fluorescence-capable camera system was completed [5].

Preoperative Preparation

The same preoperative preparation instruction and orders used for robotic-assisted laparoscopic prostatectomy are given for pelvic lymph node dissection. One important consideration is the administration of pharmacologic venous thromboembolism (VTE) prophylaxis prior to surgery. VTE rates following robotic-assisted radical prostatectomy range from 0.2 to 8%. In a large series of 2572 robotic-assisted prostatectomies, a 0.7% prevalence of VTE was observed; however, the addition of a pelvic lymph node dissection increased the risk of deep venous thrombosis (DVT) and pulmonary embolism (PE) by eight- and six-fold, respectively [8]. Pelvic lymphocele is thought to be a contributing factor to VTE because compression of large pelvic veins can worsen lower extremity stasis and associated pain may result in immobility. While lymphocele formation may be related to surgical technique and extent of PLND, there is some evidence to suggest that pharmacological VTE prophylaxis may increase the risk of lymphocele formation—anticoagulation may increase the drainage of lymph by preventing lymphatic coagulation. For the surgeon, the decision to administer preoperative VTE prophylaxis should be based on patient risk factors for VTE and need for PLND, as well as its extent. At our institution, we do not routinely administer preoperative VTE prophylaxis beyond sequential compression devices and early ambulation unless the patient is high risk (i.e., previous history of VTE) and we routinely use hemo-lock or titanium clips extensively to occlude lymphatic vessels and minimize the risk of lymphocele formation.

Operative Setup and Patient Positioning

At the time of PLND, the patient will already be positioned appropriately in steep Trendelenburg and the same trocar configuration for transperitoneal robotic-assisted laparoscopic prostatectomy is utilized.

Instrumentation and Equipment List

Equipment

- da Vinci® Si HD Surgical System (4-arm system; Intuitive Surgical, Inc., Sunnyvale, CA)
- EndoWrist® ProGrasp™ forceps (Intuitive Surgical, Inc., Sunnyvale, CA)—left robotic arm and third arm (left)
- EndoWrist® curved monopolar scissors (Intuitive Surgical, Inc., Sunnyvale, CA)—right robotic arm
- InSite® Vision System with 0° lens (Intuitive Surgical, Inc., Sunnyvale, CA)

Trocars

- 12 mm trocar (1—assistant)
- 8 mm robotic trocars (3)

Instruments Used by the Surgical Assistant (Table 22.2)

- Blunt tip grasper
- Suction irrigator device
- 5-mm Small Hem-0-lok® clip applier and clips (Teleflex Medical, Research Triangle Park, NC)
- 10 mm Reusable Endo Catch™ specimen retrieval bag

Table 22.2 Surgeon and assistant instrumentation

Surgeon instrumentation			Assistant instrumentation
Arm 1 (right)	Arm 2 (left arm)	Arm 3	• Suction irrigator
• Curved monopolar scissors	• Prograsp dissector	• Prograsp dissector	• Blunt tip grasper
			• Clip applier
			• Endo Catch™ bag

Step-by-Step Technique

Step 1: Port Placement and Radical Prostatectomy

We use a *five-port technique with a single 12 mm assist port* and four 8.5 mm robotic trocars (for the Xi robot) or three 8 mm trocars with a 12 mm camera port (for the Si robot). The access and camera trocar is supraumbilical. The right 8.5 mm trocar is 15–18 cm to the right of the umbilicus with the 12 mm assist port 7–8 cm to the right of the umbilicus (between the right robotic arm and the camera trocar). We place two left-sided robotic trocars, one about 3 cm medial and superior to the left anterior superior iliac spine and one about 10 cm to the left of the umbilicus (Fig. 22.1).

We then perform the robotic prostatectomy. The peritoneal incision to release the bladder anteriorly is brought laterally to the edge of the bladder and brought down to the level where the vas deferens crosses the external iliac artery. I also routinely reflect the sigmoid colon left lateral peritoneal attachments so the peritoneum overlying the left common iliac artery is free of sigmoid attachments.

At the end of the prostatectomy and prior to the vesicourethral anastomosis, we perform the pelvic lymphadenectomy. The reasoning for that timing is that performing the prostatectomy exposes the obturator fossa and distal iliac vein well. If the PLND is performed prior to prostatectomy, medial retraction is required on the medial edge of the peritoneum. Finally, I prefer to perform the PLND prior to the anastomosis so that any required retraction isn't placing tension on the anastomosis. So I prefer the PLND after the prostatectomy and prior to the vesicourethral anastomosis.

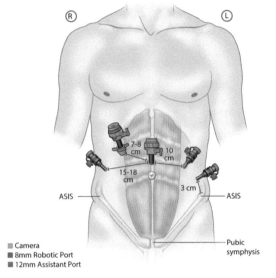

Fig. 22.1 Five-port placement and a single 12 mm assist port. Camera place is supraumbilical. The 8 mm right robotic port is 15–18 cm laterally from the camera port and along the level of the umbilicus. The 12 mm assist port is inserted superiorly and 7–8 mm right lateral to the camera port. The 8 mm left robotic port is placed 10 cm laterally from the camera port along the level of the umbilicus. The fourth arm robotic port is placed 3 cm superomedially to the left anterior superior iliac spine

Step 2: Peritoneal Incisions and Retraction

For the purpose of this chapter, we will describe the right-sided dissection. The incisions, landmarks, and surgical steps are identical for the left-sided dissection. We identify the right ureter, which can usually be seen under the peritoneum at the level of the common iliac artery. I make a longitudinal incision in the peritoneum with monopolar electrocautery, just lateral to the ureter. With the prograsp forceps in my left-handed instrument, I retract the peritoneum medially and continue the incision in the peritoneum up in the direction of the vas deferens as it is crossing the external iliac vein (Fig. 22.2). When the peritoneum is completely incised, I commit my third robotic arm to medical retraction on the peritoneum and bladder.

Step 3: Identification and Medial Displacement of the Ureter to Identify the Common Iliac Artery Bifurcation

Medial retraction of the peritoneum allows the ureter to be easily visualized as it will typically move medial with the peritoneum. The ureter can also be visualized by placing superior traction on

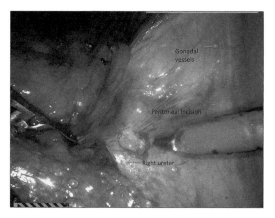

Fig. 22.2 A peritoneal incision is made just lateral to the ureter with medial retraction by the left robotic arm of the bladder

the obliterated umbilical artery at the edge of the bladder peritoneal junction and the ureter passes medial to the obliterated umbilical artery. At this point the external and internal iliac artery junction is visualized. I then pick up the nodal tissue over the external iliac artery and split it with monopolar cautery identifying the adventitial surface of the artery. I then dissect this nodal tissue medially off the edge of the artery and the proximal portion of the external iliac vein (Fig. 22.3).

Step 4: Dissection of the External Iliac Artery Lymph Nodes

I then continue the dissection of the nodes over the external iliac artery distally to the inferior epigastric artery. I remove the nodal tissue lateral to the external iliac artery to the level of the genitofemoral laterally (Fig. 22.4).

Step 5: Dissection of the Internal Iliac Artery Lymph Nodes

We then dissect the nodes from the surface of the internal iliac artery. Typically the obliterated umbilical artery will be visualized first, then the obturator artery, and then the superior vesical artery. The nodal tissue lateral to the internal iliac artery is swept medially exposing the artery and its branches (Fig. 22.5).

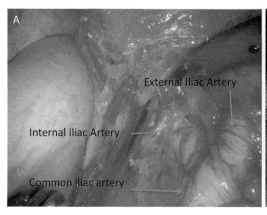

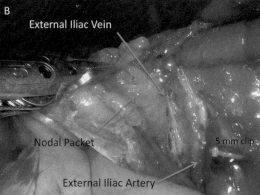

Fig. 22.3 (**a**) Junction of the internal and external iliac artery (**b**) Nodal tissue dissected off the medial edge of the external iliac artery and external iliac vein

Step 6: Dissection of the External Iliac Vein and Obturator Lymph Nodes (Standard or Limited Dissection)

I then move distally to perform the external iliac vein dissection taking the nodal tissue off the medial portion of the external iliac vein and dissecting distally to the inguinal canal (Fig. 22.6). The circumflex iliac artery is visualized and preserved. There are often medial veins coming from the external iliac vein and joining the obturator vein. I clip the distal limit of the node of Cloquet. I then retract the nodal tissue medially and superiorly and clip and divide the small lymphatics that go to the pelvic sidewall, and the obturator nerve is visualized and protected (Fig. 22.7).

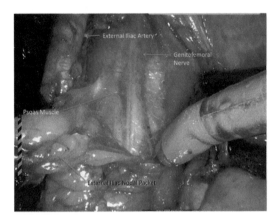

Fig. 22.4 Dissection of the external iliac artery nodal packet away from the psoas muscle with the genitofemoral nerve seen coursing laterally

Fig. 22.5 Internal iliac nodal dissection with the first branch of the internal iliac artery, the obliterated umbilical artery

At the proximal limit of this dissection, the previously dissected internal iliac lymph nodes and artery will be visualized. The final clips typically go on lymphatics that are just medial to the obturator nerve and adjacent to the internal iliac vein.

Step 7: Lymph Node Dissection Specimen Retrieval

The lymph node packet is typically in one or two large pieces. I favor using a reusable Endo Catch™ bag to remove the specimen through the 12 mm assist port (Fig. 22.8). The assistant may need to expand the incision and remove and replace the trocar as the specimen is often quite large. The other option is to remove the specimen with grasping forceps through the assist port; however, this typically fractures the specimen and may diminish the pathologic assessment.

Step 8: Vesicourethral Anastomosis and Prostate Specimen Retrieval and Close

These portions of the procedure proceed as usual practice. If a reusable Endo Catch™ bag was used for lymph node specimen retrieval, it can also be used for prostate specimen removal.

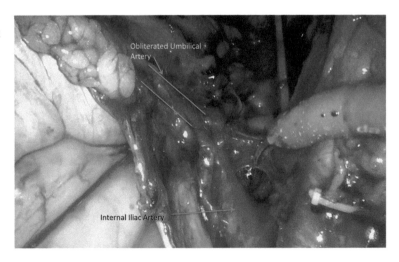

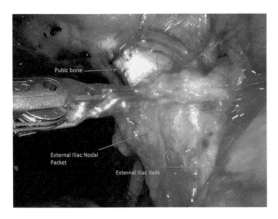

Fig. 22.6 External iliac nodal tissue dissected directly from the surface of the external iliac vain

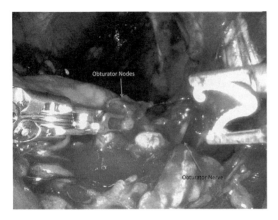

Fig. 22.7 Obturator nodes retracted medially to allow for lymphostasis with 5-mm Small Hem-0-lok® clip

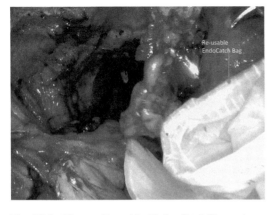

Fig. 22.8 10 mm Reusable Endo Catch™ specimen retrieval bag

Postoperative Management

The postoperative management for PLND is the same as for RALP. Our institution has moved away from placement of JP drains and 90% of our patients are discharged postoperative day 1. The Foley catheter remains in place for 7 days prior to removal and a voiding trial is performed in clinic—no cystogram is performed.

Common Complications and Steps to Avoid Them

In order to avoid injuries to surrounding key structures, a thorough understanding of pelvic anatomy is requisite. The median umbilical ligament should be identified and dissection carried laterally to avoid injury to the ureter, which enters the pelvis in the region of the bifurcation of the common iliac artery. Repair of a ureteral injury proceeds with mobilization of the proximal end of the cut ureter with reimplantation into the bladder over a ureteral stent. To avoid vascular injury, separation of nodal packets should be directly between the plane of the nodes and vessels to prevent unnecessary traction. Injuries to the major vessels (external and internal iliac artery and vein) are rare events. Small lacerations to the external iliac vein may be repaired with increase in insufflation pressure and nonabsorbable suture (4-0 polypropylene), while larger injuries may require vascular surgery consultation, and possibly open conversion.

The most common nerve injury during PLND is the obturator nerve (reported rates 0–1.8%), which provides sensory cutaneous innervation of the medial thigh and motor innervation of the adductor muscles, responsible for adduction of the thigh [9]. When the injury is recognized intraoperatively, an epineural approximation can be performed with fine nonabsorbable suture (5-0 or 6-0 polypropylene or nylon). Alternatively, for larger defects an interposition nerve graft may be necessary. Postoperatively, intensive physical therapy should be instituted to regain and maintain function.

Lymphoceles are lymph fluid-filled collections without a distinct epithelial lining. They comprise the majority of postoperative complications following PLND and are caused by disruption of the efferent lymphatics during dissection. Reported rates of symptomatic lymphocele formation vary from 2.6 to 15% [10]. Contributing factors to lymphocele include excessive use of diathermy, extent of PLND (extended > limited), disruption of the lymphatics overlying the external iliac artery, prior radiation, and subcutaneous heparin (see Preoperative Preparation). We advocate minimizing use of thermal injury and placing 5-mm Small Hem-0-lok® clips to ensure thorough hemostasis and lymphostasis. Symptomatic lymphoceles may present with pelvic pain, lower extremity pain or edema, fevers from infected lymph fluid, or storage lower urinary tract symptoms from mass effect upon the bladder. A lower extremity ultrasound should be performed to rule out deep venous thrombosis. Simple aspiration by interventional radiology colleagues can provide symptomatic relief, although fluid reaccumulation may occur. We advocate for aspiration and temporary drain placement, especially in the setting of suspected infection. Sclerotherapy has been described using various chemical agents including povidone–iodine, ethanol, bleomycin, talcum, and doxycycline with varied results. Surgical treatment involves marsupialization or unroofing of the lymphocele into the peritoneal cavity. Our approach has been laparoscopic marsupialization when approaching persistent or bilateral lymphoceles.

References

1. Bivalacqua TJ, Pierorazio PM, Gorin MA, et al. Anatomic extent of pelvic lymph node dissection: impact on long-term cancer-specific outcomes in men with positive lymph nodes at time of radical prostatectomy. Urology. 2013;82:653–8.
2. Briganti A, Abdollah F, Nini A, et al. Performance characteristics of computed tomography in detecting lymph node metastases in contemporary patients with prostate cancer treated with extended pelvic lymph node dissection. Eur Urol. 2012;61:1132–8.
3. Joslyn SA, Konety BR. Impact of extent of lymphadenectomy on survival after radical prostatectomy for prostate cancer. Urology. 2006;68:121–5.
4. Chun FK, Karakiewicz PI, Briganti A, et al. Prostate cancer nomograms: an update. Eur Urol. 2006;50:914–26; discussion 926.
5. Liss MA, Stroup SP, Qin Z, et al. Robotic-assisted fluorescence sentinel lymph node mapping using multimodal image guidance in an animal model. Urology. 2014;84:982.e9–14.
6. Cooperberg MR, Kane CJ, Cowan JE, et al. Adequacy of lymphadenectomy among men undergoing robot-assisted laparoscopic radical prostatectomy. BJU Int. 2010;105:88–92.
7. Rakow-Penner RA, White NS, Parsons JK, et al. Novel technique for characterizing prostate cancer utilizing MRI restriction spectrum imaging: proof of principle and initial clinical experience with extraprostatic extension. Prostate Cancer Prostatic Dis. 2015;18:81–5.
8. Tyritzis SI, Wallerstedt A, Steineck G, et al. Thromboembolic complications in 3,544 patients undergoing radical prostatectomy with or without lymph node dissection. J Urol. 2015;193:117–25.
9. Loeb S, Partin AW, Schaeffer EM. Complications of pelvic lymphadenectomy: do the risks outweigh the benefits? Rev Urol. 2010;12:20–4.
10. Liss MA, Palazzi K, Stroup SP, et al. Outcomes and complications of pelvic lymph node dissection during robotic-assisted radical prostatectomy. World J Urol. 2013;31:481–8.10.

Robotic-Assisted Inguinal Lymphadenectomy: The University of Texas M.D. Anderson Cancer Center Approach

Isuru S. Jayaratnam, Surena F. Matin, and Curtis A. Pettaway

Patient Selection

Robotic-assisted inguinal lymphadenectomy (RAIL) was developed for the surgical staging of the inguinal region for squamous cell carcinoma of the penis in the clinically node negative setting, although this technique can be applied to any genital or lower extremity malignancy that has drainage to the inguinal lymph nodes (vulvar carcinoma, melanoma). This technique has been developed to minimize the morbidity associated with the standard open approach, which includes both infectious complications and lymphedema. Despite the minimally invasive approach, standard oncologic principles are maintained, including adherence to the dissection limits and complete removal of lymph nodes within the dissection template.

RAIL is best suited to remove the inguinal nodes in patients with stage T1b or greater penile tumors (which increases the risk of occult lym-

phatic metastasis in the groin), but have an otherwise negative inguinal lymph node examination. The primary tumor should be adequately controlled, with tumor-free margins if treated surgically. Occasionally, patients may receive definitive radiotherapy for control of the primary tumor. In this setting, RAIL can be performed after primary tumor therapy. We currently recommend bilateral inguinal ultrasound and percutaneous biopsy of any suspicious lymph nodes prior to surgical planning to detect metastases that may have escaped inguinal palpation.

Special Considerations

Enlarged inguinal or pelvic lymphadenopathy, neoadjuvant chemotherapy or regional radiation should be considered relative contraindications as RAIL has not been validated as yet among such cohorts. We do not recommend RAIL in such patients outside of a clinical trial setting.

Preoperative Preparation

Informed Consent

Patients should be counseled on the general risks of lymphadenectomy such as cellulitis, abscess, seroma formation, prolonged drainage from

Electronic supplementary material: The online version of this chapter (doi:10.1007/978-3-319-45060-5_23) contains supplementary material, which is available to authorized users.

I.S. Jayaratnam, M.D. • S.F. Matin, M.D., F.A.C.S. (✉)
C.A. Pettaway, M.D.
Department of Urology, UT MD Anderson Cancer Center, 1515 Holcombe Blvd. Unit 1373, Houston, TX 77030, USA
e-mail: surmatin@mdanderson.org

drain sites, transient or permanent lymphedema of the extremities, or scrotum. The patient should also understand the risk of venous thromboembolism and the preventive measures taken to avoid thrombi, as well as other pulmonary and cardiovascular complications. We also make the patient aware that conversion to an open procedure could occur if there are concerns about ability to adequately view the relevant anatomy, failure to progress, or unintended vascular injuries that would optimally require an open approach for repair.

Documenting the preoperative mid-tibial calf circumference of both lower extremities can be helpful to measure the degree of lymphedema that develops postoperatively. Making patients aware that postoperative consultation with a lymphedema specialist (i.e., such as a physical therapist) can be useful for counseling on lymphedema prevention. Such measures include fitting them for graduated compression garments and extremity massage techniques.

Operative Setup

We currently use the da Vinci® Si HD Surgical System (Intuitive Surgical, Inc., Sunnyvale, CA). A four-trocar technique that includes one 12 mm camera port, two 8 mm robotic ports, and a 12 mm assistant port is used. The latter port is for the bedside assistant to retract tissue place surgical clips, suction, and remove tissue specimens. The base of the robot is positioned over the contralateral shoulder with the arms extending toward the groin. The assistant is seated lateral to the thigh, with the scrub technician positioned nearby with a table with robotic and laparoscopic instruments. The robotic tower is placed lateral to the contralateral lower extremity. Video screens should be present on both sides of the patient for easy viewing.

Having a standard setup will facilitate the transition to the other side for a bilateral procedure.

Patient Positioning

The patient is placed in the supine position on a table with stirrup leg supports (Fig. 23.1). Both hips externally rotated and separated to open up the groin for exposure. The lower extremity should be adequately supported and all pressure points should be padded, including the lateral malleolus of the foot, the lateral knee, and the greater trochanter of the femur. The feet are secured in the stirrup boot to prevent the patient from losing his position. Bilateral arms are to be tucked to the patient's side to allow proper robot positioning, with padding and wrist support to prevent nerve injury. The patient is draped with attention paid toward keeping the umbilicus and ASIS in view, as anatomic landmarks.

Trocar Placement

As seen in Fig. 23.2, the camera port is about three fingerbreadths inferior to the apex of the femoral triangle. The trocars for the right and left hand should have approximately one handbreadth separation from the camera port to avoid clashes between the camera and instrument arms. The assistant port is inserted between the camera and lateral trocar, slightly inferior to have enough working space below the robotic arms.

Instrumentation and Equipment List

Surgeon Equipment

da Vinci® Si HD Surgical System (Intuitive Surgical, Inc., Sunnyvale, CA)

Endowrist® Maryland bipolar forceps or PK dissector (Intuitive Surgical, Inc., Sunnyvale, CA)

Endowrist® curved monopolar scissors (Intuitive Surgical, Inc., Sunnyvale, CA)

Endowrist ® vessel sealer (Intuitive Surgical Corp, Sunnyvale, CA)

InSite® Vision System with 0° and 30° lens (Intuitive Surgical, Inc., Sunnyvale, CA)

Fig. 23.1 Patient positioning. Hips are externally rotated and relevant landmarks are kept in view

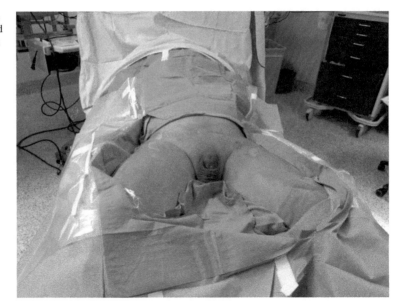

Fig. 23.2 Anatomy and port placement: anatomical landmarks and boundaries of dissection are illustrated here

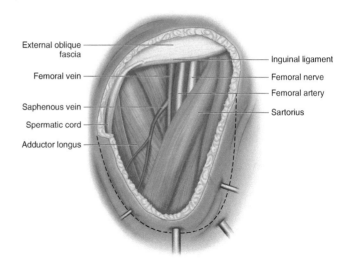

External oblique fascia
Femoral vein
Saphenous vein
Spermatic cord
Adductor longus
Inguinal ligament
Femoral nerve
Femoral artery
Sartorius

Trocars
12 mm balloon trocar (1)
8 mm robotic trocars (2)
12 mm trocar (1)

Recommended Sutures
Vascular Repair Rescue Stitch—4-0 Prolene on a RB needle cut to 6 in.

Assistant Equipment
Suction irrigator device

- Hem-o-lok® clip applier (Teleflex Medical, Research Triangle Park, NC)
- Small and Medium-Large Hem-o-lok® clips (Teleflex Medical, Research Triangle Park, NC)

10 mm specimen entrapment bag
Jackson Pratt/Blake closed suction Drain (2)

Step-by-Step Technique (Video 23.1)

Establishing Groin Access/ Insufflation and Trochar Placement

Access is obtained through a 2 cm skin incision, three fingerbreadths below the apex of the femoral triangle, dissecting through dermis and subcutaneous tissue to just above Scarpa's fascia. Using finger dissection in the cephalad direction, as well radially with a hemostat (Fig. 23.3) a working space is created that is large enough to accommodate a balloon dissector. This is then advanced as far cephalad as the inguinal crease and dilation proceeds from cephalad backward toward the camera port incision (Fig. 23.4). After this is completed, the dissector is deflated and the balloon port is placed and insufflation is started. Subsequently, the medial and lateral robotic trocars are placed under direct vision one handbreadth away from the camera port. The assistant port is then placed under direct vision between the lateral robotic port and the camera port (Fig. 23.5). After the robotic trocars and the assistant port are placed, the robot can be docked (Fig. 23.6).

Defining the Limits of Dissection

"The Roof"
Once the inguinal working space is created, the roof of the dissection is established by detaching any nodal or other tissue from below Scarpa's fascia (Fig. 23.7). Such tissue is cleaned off of the undersurface of Scarpa's fascia from the apex, all the way cephalad to the external oblique fascia and the spermatic cord.

The superior limit of dissection is the external oblique fascia, with the spermatic cord defining the superomedial limit. All lymphatic tissue is mobilized from this superior border inferiorly over the inguinal ligament inferiorly. These nodes are then removed with either the medial or lateral dissection packets depending on their relationship to the femoral artery. The midpoint of the adductor longus and Sartorius fascia define the medial and lateral limits, respectively, and their intersection at the apex of the femoral triangle is the inferior limit of the packet. The saphenous vein splits the packet in half and leads superiorly to the fossa navicularis where the femoral vein and artery are identified.

Medial Dissection
This portion of the dissection removes all lymphatic tissue from the midpoint of the adductor longus fascia medially to the lateral edge of the femoral vein and between the external oblique fascia superiorly and the apex of the femoral triangle inferiorly. At the inferior portion of the medial dissection, care is taken to proactively identify the saphenous vein to avoid inadvertent injury. At this apical level all nodal tissue is divided between large hemolock clips to try and avoid a prolonged postoperative lymph leak.

Fig. 23.3 Obtaining access: after incising the skin, hemostats are used to bluntly dissect down to Scarpa's fascia where the roof of the dissection will begin

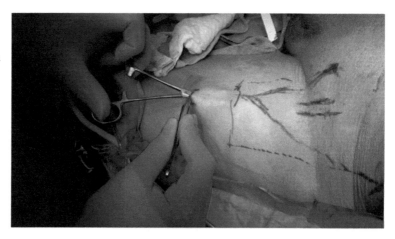

Fig. 23.4 Creating working space. Using the laparoscopic space maker through the access point, we create space starting at the most cephalad portion of dissection, down to the inferior limit

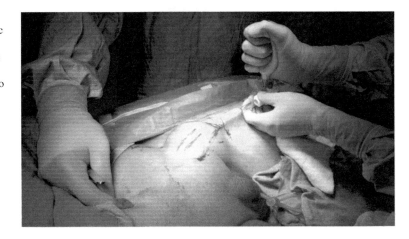

Fig. 23.5 Port placement. Ports are in place with insufflation activated. Notice adequate separation of the robotic ports to allow maximum mobility

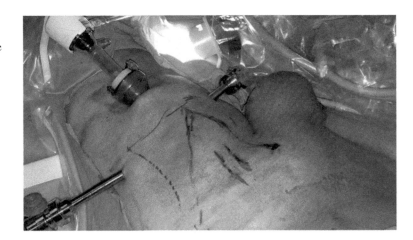

Fig. 23.6 Robot docking. Robotic arms are docked, taking care to angle the arms outward

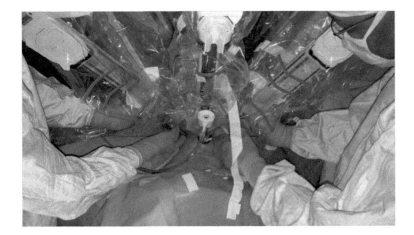

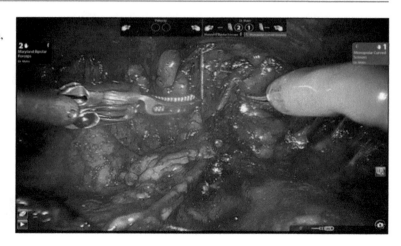

Fig. 23.7 "The Roof," all nodal tissue is dissected down, leaving Scarpa's fascia clean at the top of the screen

The specimen is then mobilized upwards toward the fossa ovalis using the saphenous vein below the fossa as the dividing line between the medial and lateral packets.

Lateral Dissection

The lateral dissection begins by mobilizing the nodal tissue from the lateral to medial direction, either over or underneath the fascia lata of the thigh (surgeons' preference), from the inguinal ligament superiorly to the apex of the femoral triangle inferiorly. Inferiorly at the lateral edge of the saphenous vein, the apical nodal tissue is divided between large hemolock clips, similar to the medial packet dissection. This packet is also rotated upward toward the fossa ovalis.

Dividing the Nodal Packet at the Level of the Fossa Ovalis

Using the previously identified saphenous vein, the lymphatic packet is divided in two from the saphenofemoral junction up to the inguinal ligament. The femoral vein is identified and the tissue is divided over the top of the vessel until the inguinal ligament is reached, and the packet is then rolled medially. Finally, starting inferiorly the packet is elevated and retracted cephalad and attachments are divided. The superior aspect is released at the femoral canal below the inguinal ligament and then amputated after placing a final clip.

We then direct our attention to the lateral packet, starting from the saphenous vein and dissecting the tissue away. This brings us down to the femoral artery, which is again meticulously dissected from caudal to cephalad until reaching the inguinal ligament. The free lateral edge of the packet is retracted medially and the remaining attachments are divided until the packet is free.

Femoral Artery Dissection

Care is taken during this step to not dissect lateral and below the artery in order to avoid injury to the femoral nerve.

Extraction and Drain Placement

The final two packets are placed in a laparoscopic specimen bag, and two Blake drains are placed after complete hemostasis is obtained. Alternatively, in order to facilitate more working space the complete medial dissection can be performed and the medial node packet removed. Subsequently, the lateral dissection can be completed and the packet removed. This two-step procedure is facilitated by using the 12 mm balloon port that allows one to extend the camera port incision to easily extract the specimen bag between the medial and lateral portions of the dissection.

Postoperative Management

Patients remain at bed rest for 48 h to decrease lymphatic flow usually associated with ambulation. Our goal is to facilitate collapsing the inguinal working space by allowing the inguinal roof to adhere to the inguinal floor. Our hypothesis is that this will allow earlier drain removal. On average, this leads to an in-hospital length of stay of approximately 4 days. Drains are kept until they have <30 mL of output per day for two consecutive days. Patches impregnated with chlorhexidine are used to cover the drain entry site in order to prevent drain tract infections [1]. Drains are removed one at a time once they achieve these criteria. Oral antibiotics are prescribed as long as the drains are in place.

Steps to Avoid Complications

- Use finger dissection initially to develop the working space prior to balloon dilation to develop the correct plane prior to balloon dilation
- Defining the boundaries of dissection is important to guarantee oncologic completeness in addition to proceeding safely with dissection.
- Meticulous attention to lymphatic sealing, with either clips (especially at the apex of the dissection) or a vessel sealing device (in other areas) is critical to preventing postoperative prolonged lymphatic leakage. The latter can lead to drain tract infections with prolonged drains in place or lymphocele formation if drains are removed earlier.
- Careful dissection around the femoral vessels is critical.
  - Avoid dissection lateral to and below the plane of the artery to avoid injuring the femoral artery
  - Utilize clips and careful cautery in order to keep the surgical field dry to preserve vision and prevent an inadvertent injury to the femoral artery or vein.

Reference

1. Chambers S, et al. Reduction of exit-site infections of tunnelled intravascular catheters among neutropenic patients by sustained-release chlorhexidine dressings: results from a prospective randomized controlled trial. J Hosp Infect. 2005;61(1):53–61.

Robotic Rectovesical Fistula Repair

Lawrence L. Yeung, James Mason, and Justin Dersch

Standardized Terminology

1. da Vinci® Surgical System (Intuitive Surgical, Inc., Sunnyvale, CA) as first citation then da Vinci® thereafter. The use of the da Vinci Si HD (versus standard, S or Xi) robot is assumed in each of the chapters unless specifically required or dictated by the procedure. As the Si HD is currently the most commonly used system, it is preferable to avoid describing procedures performed with standard or Xi systems as these are less relevant to the audience.
2. Trocar (not port)
3. Urethral catheter (not Foley catheter)
4. Electrocautery (not cautery)
5. Polyglactin (not Vicryl)
6. Hasson trocar (not Hassan)
7. Hem-o-lok (not Hemolok)

Electronic supplementary material: The online version of this chapter (doi:10.1007/978-3-319-45060-5_24) contains supplementary material, which is available to authorized users.

L.L. Yeung, M.D. (✉) • J. Dersch, M.D.
Department of Urology, University of Florida College of Medicine, 1600 SW Archer Rd, Box 100247, Gainesville, FL 32610, USA
e-mail: Lawrence.yeung@urology.ufl.edu

J. Mason, M.D.
Department of Urology, University of Iowa Healthcare, 200 Hawkins Drive, Iowa City, Iowa 52242, USA

Patient Selection

The indications for robotic rectovesical fistula (RVF) repair and open rectovesical fistula repair are identical. They include symptoms of RVF, which can include pneumaturia, fecaluria, and/or leakage of urine per rectum. The presence of rectovesical fistula can be confirmed with radiographic or endoscopic evidence (cystoscopy or colonoscopy) of a communication between the rectum and the bladder. Radiological studies that are useful include computed tomography with bladder or rectal contrast. Absolute contraindications to repair by the robotic approach include uncorrectable bleeding diatheses or the inability to medically tolerate general anesthesia. A transabdominal robotic-assisted laparoscopic technique also should not be used in patients with a more distal rectourethral fistula as the approach will likely give inadequate exposure for a successful repair.

Since rectovesical fistulas are generally iatrogenic in nature, the effects of prior abdominal and pelvic surgery are often encountered. Morbidly obese patients pose the additional challenges of respiratory compromise while in the steep Trendelenburg position, more limited working space, and instrument length limitations. Repeat RVF repairs are found to be even more complex and these scenarios should be avoided in a surgeon's early experience with robotic RVF fistula repair. Patients with prior surgical removal of the omentum or prior use of omental flaps may pose a greater technical challenge when attempting to interpose a vascularized flap, but this is not an absolute contraindication depending on the skill and experience of the surgeon as alternative vascularized flaps may be used.

Preoperative Preparation

Preoperative testing for surgical clearance is typically obtained within 30 days of surgery. This includes a complete blood count, basic metabolic panel, coagulation profile, EKG, chest x-ray, and urinalysis with culture as indicated. For more medically complex patients it is important to address their medical conditions prior to surgery, therefore general medicine or other medical subspecialties may need to be consulted for comprehensive preoperative medical optimization. Anticoagulants are held at least 7–10 days prior to surgery.

Imaging

A cystogram and retrograde urethrogram should be obtained to ascertain the location of the fistula between the rectum and urinary tract. A computer-assisted tomography (CT) cystogram is also useful in preoperative planning and provides more anatomic detail than a plain film cystogram. If the fistula is suspected and cannot be demonstrated by CT cystogram, a CT of the pelvis with rectal contrast can be performed in an attempt to identify the fistula.

Bowel Preparation

Starting the day before surgery patients are directed to take only clear liquids along with one bottle of citrate of magnesium. A Fleet Enema (C.B. Fleet Company, Inc., Lynchburg, VA) is administered the morning of surgery to ensure the rectal vault is clear of stool.

Informed Consent

Patients should be counseled on the known risks of surgery such as bleeding, infection, postoperative pain, incisional hernia, and the need of transfusion. They should also be aware of the potential for conversion to open surgery. A thorough discussion about the risk specific to robotic rectovesical fistula repair should also be had. This includes the risk of damage to adjacent intra-abdominal organs, recurrent fistula, urinary leak, bowel leak, new or worsened impotence, and new urinary or bowel symptoms.

Operative Setup

Operating room setup (see Fig. 18.1) for transabdominal robotic rectovesical fistula repair.

Operating room setup for robotic rectovesical fistula repair is similar to other robotic pelvic cases with the addition of equipment needed for the cystoscopy portion to start the case. Fluoroscopy is needed for the initial cystoscopic portion, and once this is completed the room can be adjusted for robotic use. Figure 18.1 illustrates the typical room layout for the robotic portion of the case. The surgeon console is in the corner of the room. The surgical assistant is at the patient's right with the surgical technician at the patient's left. The back table is typically placed to the left of the patient near the surgical technician with an additional table to the patient's right near the assistant with instruments available for quick access such as surgical clips.

Patient Positioning

Patient in split leg position on operative table (See Fig. 18.2). Note proper padding to protect all sites susceptible to pressure injury. The patient undergoes induction of general anesthesia and then positioning begins. First, the patient is placed in the dorsal lithotomy position using stirrups for the cystoscopic portion of the procedure as described later.

Next, the patient is placed in the supine split leg position as illustrated in Fig. 18.2. Foam padding is placed under each knee to prevent the legs from lying flat on the table and they are secured with tape. The legs are then split approximately 45° to allow for docking of the robot base near the foot of the bed. The left leg is lowered approximately 20°–30° so the fourth arm will not be in contact with the patient's left foot. After the lower body is positioned, foam padding is placed under the elbows and each arm is tucked along the patient's side. The patient's hands are covered with foam padding for protection during the case. The patient's upper body is secured to the table with foam padding and heavy tap across the upper chest.

Once the patient is fully secured we perform a test Trendelenburg position to ensure the patient does not slide. Next, the patient is prepped and draped and a 16 Fr urethral catheter is placed on the field. An oral gastric tube is placed by the anesthesia team and removed at the end of the procedure prior to extubation.

Trocar Configuration

Trocar configurations (See Fig. 18.3) for robotic RVF repair. Once pneumoperitoneum is established, the working trocars are placed. As shown in Fig. 18.3, a total of six trocars, including the camera port, are used: one 12 mm trocar for the camera, three intuitive 8 mm metal robotic trocars for the robotic arms, and a 5 and 12 mm trocar on the patient's right side for the assistant ports.

As is commonly recommended for transperitoneal robotic prostatectomy, we measure the distance between each trocar, ensuring there is at least 8 cm from the camera port to the first and third robotic arm ports and 8 cm between the third and fourth robotic arm ports. The assistant ports are offset from the first robotic arm port to the patient's right with the 12 mm trocar about 8 cm lateral to the first arm port and the 5 mm port about 8–10 cm cephalad and triangulated between the first robotic arm, the 12 mm assistant port, and the base of the penis.

Instrumentation and Equipment List

Equipment

- da Vinci Si Surgical System (Intuitive Surgical, Inc., Sunnyvale, CA)
- EndoWrist curved monopolar scissors (Intuitive Surgical, Inc., Sunnyvale, CA)
- EndoWrist ProGrasp forceps (Intuitive Surgical, Inc., Sunnyvale, CA)
- EndoWrist bipolar Maryland forceps (Intuitive Surgical, Inc., Sunnyvale, CA)
- EndoWrist needle driver (Intuitive Surgical, Inc., Sunnyvale, CA)
- EndoWrist mega suture cut needle driver (Intuitive Surgical, Inc., Sunnyvale, CA)
- InSite Vision System with 0° and 30° lens (Intuitive Surgical, Inc., Sunnyvale, CA)

Trocars

- 8-mm robotic trocar (3 if using a four-armed technique)
- 12-mm trocar (2)
- 5-mm trocar (1)

Recommended Sutures

- Rectal fistula closure: 2-0 polyglactin on UR-6 needle cut to 6 in.
- Bladder fistula closure: 2-0 polyglactin on UR-6 needle cut to 6 in.
- Bladder closure: 2-0 polyglactin × 2
- Suturing of omental flap: 2-0 polyglactin × 3
- Drain stitch: 2-0 nylon
- Skin Closure: 4-0 Monocryl

Instruments Used by the Surgical Assistant

- Laparoscopic needle driver
- Laparoscopic Scissors
- Blunt tip grasper
- Suction irrigator device

- Small, Large, and Extra Large Hem-o-lok clip appliers
- SURGICEL hemostatic gauze (Ethicon, Inc., Cincinnati, OH)
- 18 French urethral catheter
- Jackson-Pratt closed suction drain
- 10 mL syringe
- 60 mL catheter tip syringe
- 6 French JJ ureteral stent (length determined by measurement) (2)

Additional Equipment

- Rigid cystoscope, 22 French sheath and 30° lens for placement of nonconductive wire through the fistula and bilateral ureteral stent placement
- Open-End Flexi-Tip Ureteral Catheter, 5 Fr. (Cook Medical, Bloomington, IN) (1)
- Bentson Cerebral Guidewire (Cook Medical, Bloomington, IN) (1)
- Hydrophilic Guidewire (1)
- 16 French urethral catheter
- 10 mL syringe
- Fluoroscopy for ureteral catheter placement

Step-by-Step Technique (Figs. 24.1, 24.2, 24.3, 24.4, 24.5, 24.6, and 24.7)

Step 1: Cystoscopy, Bilateral Ureteral Stent Placement, and Fistula Canalization

For robotic laparoscopic rectovesical fistula repair with a combined retrovesical and transvesical approach, the patient is initially positioned in dorsal lithotomy position for cystoscopy and passage of a nonconductive wire (or ureteral catheter) through the fistula into the rectum to help later identify the fistula tract intraoperatively.

The bladder is entered transurethrally with a 22 F ridged cystoscope and 30° lens. Both ureteral orifices are identified as well as the fistula tract. A 6 F double J ureteral stent is placed into each ureter over a guidewire. Care is taken to place an appropriately sized stent to prevent the coil from obscuring the fistula site. This measurement is performed by using an end hole catheter to determine the distance from the ureteral orifice to the ureteropelvic junction. Two centimeters are subtracted from this measurement to choose the appropriate stent length. The

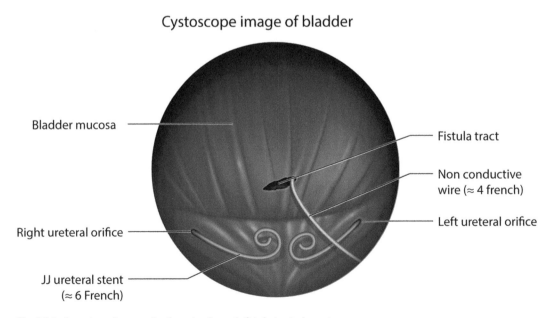

Fig. 24.1 Insertion of nonconductive wire through fistula tract via cystoscopy

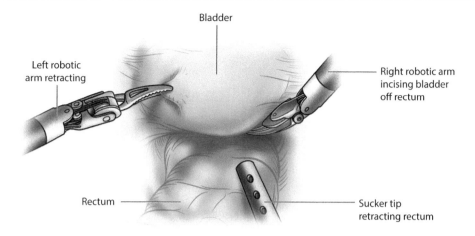

Fig. 24.2 Mobilization of bladder off rectum

Fig. 24.3 Identification of nonconductive wire through fistula

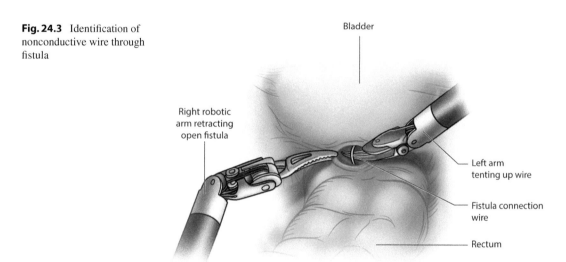

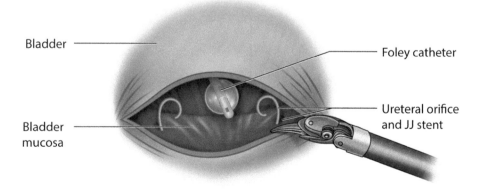

Fig. 24.4 Transverse cystotomy

placement of open-ended ureteral catheters is not optimal as they would obscure visualization of the fistula.

A nonconductive hydrophilic wire is then passed through the fistula tract cystoscopically. The surgeon's finger is placed into the rectum to pull the wire out and clamp it to the urethral end of the wire to achieve through-and-through access across the fistula tract. The external portion of the nonconductive wire is wrapped in a sterile towel, as this will be within the field during the robotic portion of the procedure. The patient is then undraped and repositioned as seen in Fig. 18.2 in the supine split leg position.

Refer to the section on patient positioning for specific directions on safely positioning the patient. An 18 F urethral catheter is placed transurethrally into the bladder on the sterile field.

Step 2: Trocar Placement and Robot Docking

Pneumoperitoneum is generally established with the Veress needle or alternatively the Hassan technique if there is concern for abdominal wall adhesions from prior surgery. The Veress needle is placed in the midline just below the umbilicus. Once sufficient insufflation to 15 mmHg is obtained, a 12-mm camera port is placed with a visual obturator and 0° camera lens just superior to the umbilicus, taking care to stay within 17 cm above the pubis as the robotic instruments are limited to a working length of 25 cm. Once inside the abdomen, the Veress needle is identified and removed. Inspection of the surroundings for injury secondary to Veress needle placement or bowel adhesions is quickly performed. The remaining trocars are placed under laparoscopic vision.

As shown in Fig. 18.3, a total of six trocars, including the camera port, are used: one 12 mm trocar for the camera, three 8 mm metal robotic

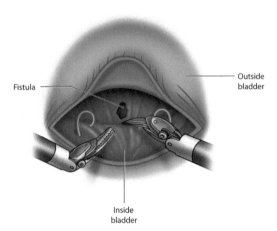

Fig. 24.5 Intravesical fistula dissection

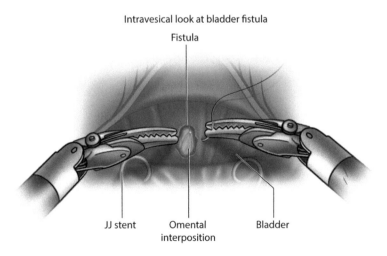

Fig. 24.6 Closure of intravesical fistula after omental flap interposition

trocars for the robotic arms, and a 5 and 12 mm trocar on the patient's right side for the assistant ports. Refer to the section on trocar configuration for specifics regarding trocar location.

Prior to making incisions for the robotic and assistant trocars, insufflation to 15 mmHg is established, 0.25% Marcaine is injected at each site, and the trocars are placed. Care is taken to adjust the assistant trocars based on the patient's body habitus to give the assistant a straight access to the pelvis. If the 12 mm assistant trocar is placed too laterally, there will be difficulty working along the ipsilateral side of the patient within the pelvis. Also, the 5 mm assistant trocar must be placed cephalad enough to allow the assistant to use both the 12 and 5 mm ports simultaneously without clashing with the external robotic arms. In many patients, the 5 mm assistant trocar will be within a several centimeters of the costal margin.

Once the trocars are placed, the patient is placed in a steep Trendelenburg position. The robot is moved into position between the patient's legs taking care to bring the base of the robot in close enough so that the camera port is within the working limits. Next, the robotic arms and instruments are inserted as well as a 30° lens in a downward configuration. The monopolar scissors are placed in the first robotic arm while the

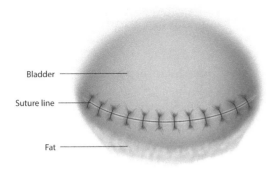

Bladder

Suture line

Fat

Fig. 24.7 Cystotomy closure

bipolar forceps are inserted into the left robotic arm. Both monopolar and bipolar electrocautery are set at 45 W throughout the procedure.

Step 3: Mobilization of Omentum (Table 24.1)

The initial step, after abdominal access, is mobilization of the omentum. Any adhesions between the omentum and the anterior abdominal wall or small bowel segments are lysed. Care must be taken to preserve the distal omentum and its blood supply for later use as a vascularized flap for interposition. A long tag suture may be placed in a dependent portion of the omentum to assist in bringing the omentum down to the pelvis when needed for interposition between the bladder and rectum.

Step 4: Separation of Bladder and Rectum

Next, attention is turned to the pelvis and the fourth arm is used to retract any redundant colon or small bowel that is lying in the pelvis. Adequate lysis of any adhesions may be necessary at this point to allow good mobility of bowel structures out of the pelvis.

The assistant can apply intermittent traction to the urethral catheter to assist the surgeon in identification of the plane between the bladder and rectum. This plane is carefully developed caudally with a combination of monopolar electrocautery via the scissors and sharp dissection. The assistant uses the suction irrigator device to maintain visibility by clearing the field of electrocautery smoke and blood. As the surgical plane is developed, the Maryland forceps are used to retract the bladder anteriorly while the assistant uses the suction irrigator device to provide countertraction posteriorly on the rectum.

Table 24.1 Mobilization of omentum: surgeon and assistant instrumentation

Surgeon instrumentation			Assistant instrumentation
Right arm	**Left arm**	**Fourth arm**	• Suction irrigator
• Monopolar scissors	• Maryland forceps	• ProGrasp forceps	• Hem-o-lock clip applier and clips
Endoscope lens: 30° down			

Step 5: Identification and Mobilization of Fistula

The dissection of the bladder–rectal plane is continued caudally until the fistula tract is encountered. Care must be taken during transection of the fistula tract to preserve the nonconductive wire in place that serves to localize the fistula. The dissection should be carried out past the fistula tract caudally and laterally to allow for adequate mobilization of the rectum for closure.

Step 6: Cystotomy

Once the plane between the bladder and rectum is adequately dissected, the next step is opening the bladder to provide better access and dissection of the most distal part of the fistula tract, which is typically difficult to expose via the retrovesical approach. A transverse cystotomy is created at the dome that is wide enough to allow movement of the camera and the two robotic working arms into the bladder.

Step 7: Intravesical Fistula Dissection (Table 24.2)

Once the cystotomy has been completed, the surgeon identifies stents in the ureteral orifices and notes their location so as to preserve them and avoid accidental injury. Next, the balloon of the urethral catheter is deflated followed by removal of the catheter. This permits visualization of the nonconductive wire as it emerges from the bladder neck and continues through the rectovesical fistula posteriorly.

The surgeon now sharply incises the bladder mucosa circumferentially around the intravesical portion of the fistula without the use of cautery.

The surgical assistant should provide optimal visualization by using the suction irrigation device to retract the bladder when necessary and clear the field of urine and blood. The bladder wall is undermined circumferentially to a distance of 1–2 cm around the fistula to allow for a tension-free closure of the bladder and rectal walls. This distance can be estimated with the knowledge that the scissor tips are approximately 1 cm in length. Care must be taken to avoid ureteral injury while undermining the bladder wall during this step.

Step 8: Rectal Defect Closure (Tables 24.3 and 24.4)

Next, attention is turned to closure of the rectal defect via the retrovesical plane. The edges of rectal mucosa are trimmed back to healthy tissue. The fistula must be adequately mobilized circumferentially to allow for a tension-free, watertight closure with apposition of healthy rectal mucosa.

A 2-0 polyglactin suture on a UR-6 needle cut to 6 in. is used to close the rectal defect in an interrupted fashion. The side of the fistula closest to the bladder neck can be difficult to access via the retrovesical approach, and it may be easier to close this location transvesically. Watertight closure of the rectal defect can be confirmed by filling the pelvis with water from the suction irrigator and then insufflating air into the rectum.

Step 9: Omental Interposition

After the rectal defect is closed, a vascularized omental interposition flap is interposed to decrease the chance of recurrence by eliminating overlapping suture lines. This is accomplished by identifying the previously mobilized omentum and

Table 24.2 Intravesical fistula dissection: surgeon and assistant instrumentation

Surgeon instrumentation			Assistant instrumentation
Right arm	**Left arm**	**Fourth arm**	• Suction irrigator
• Monopolar scissors	• Maryland forceps	• ProGrasp forceps	• 10 cm³ syringe
Endoscope lens: 30° down			

Table 24.3 Rectal defect mobilization: surgeon and assistant intrumentation

Surgeon instrumentation			Assistant instrumentation
Right arm	**Left arm**	**Fourth arm**	• Suction irrigator
• Monopolar scissors	• Maryland forceps	• ProGrasp forceps	• 10 cm^3 syringe
Endoscope lens: 30° down			
• Mega suture cut needle driver	• Needle driver	• ProGrasp forceps	• Laparoscopic needle driver
Endoscope lens: 30° down			• 2-0 Polyglactin suture

Table 24.4 Rectal defect closure: surgeon and assistant instrumentation

Surgeon instrumentation			Assistant instrumentation
Right arm	**Left arm**	**Fourth arm**	• Suction irrigator
• Mega suture cut needle driver	• Needle driver	• ProGrasp forceps	• Laparoscopic needle driver
Endoscope lens: 30° down			• 2-0 Polyglactin suture

bringing it to the pelvis. Four to five 2-0 polyglactin sutures are passed through the rectal wall superficially in a location distal to the closed rectal defect, and then the sutures are passed through the distal end of the omental flap and tied down. It is important to ensure complete interposition of the flap between the rectal and bladder repairs.

Step 10: Intravesical Fistula Neck Closure

After the omental flap has been interposed, the bladder side of the fistula is closed via the transvesical approach. This is performed with interrupted 2-0 polyglactin sutures on a UR-6 needle cut to 6 in.

Step 11: Bladder Closure

The next step of the procedure is cystotomy closure. This is done with a two-layer running closure using 2-0 polyglactin suture. First, an 18 French urethral catheter is placed through the urethra until the tip and balloon portion are within the bladder. The balloon is not inflated at this point to prevent the risk of puncturing it while closing the cystotomy. The first layer of the closure is performed by reapproximating the mucosal layer in a running fashion. For the second layer, the muscularis and serosa are run closed in an imbricated fashion. Once the cystotomy closure is complete, the integrity of the bladder closure is tested by injecting 150–200 mL of normal saline through the urethral catheter using a 60 cm^3 catheter tip syringe. Any leaks noted in the suture line are over sewn with 2–0 polyglactin suture in a figure of eight fashion. The urethral catheter balloon is then inflated with 10 mL of sterile water.

Step 12: Surgical Drain Placement and Exiting the Abdomen

The final step is placement of a surgical drain and exiting the abdomen. Surgical drain placement is important to monitor the bladder repair for a urine leak and to evacuate any fluid and blood in the pelvis. The surgical assistant passes a 10 French Jackson Pratt drain through the 12 mm assistant port. The surgeon grasps the end of the drain and places it within the pelvis but away from the cystotomy closure or fistula repair so as to prevent direct suction on these areas which could lead to fistulization. The drain is secured to the skin with a 2-0 nylon suture, and the robotic instruments and camera are removed and the robot is undocked. The 8 and 5 mm trocars generally do not require fascial closure, and the skin incisions are closed subcutaneously with a 4-0 monofilament absorbable suture. The fascia of the 12 mm camera trocar also generally does not require formal closure if a nonbladed, self-dilating trocar is used.

Postoperative Management

Postoperative pain control is titrated to provide the patient with enough comfort for good mobility, taking care not to cause excessive drowsiness or delayed return of bowel function. Intravenous narcotics are used as the mainstay for pain control with the addition of intravenous nonnarcotics such as ketorolac (as bleeding risk and renal function permit) or acetaminophen (as liver function permits) to minimize the narcotic need. The patient is transitioned to oral narcotics once return of bowel function is demonstrated. A clear liquid diet is given on postoperative day 1 and is advanced to a regular diet as tolerated. Stool softeners are given postoperatively and continued until postoperative day 14 to prevent constipation, which could cause failure of the rectal repair.

The pelvic drain is removed prior to discharge if the output is low, and there is no concern for a urinary leak. If the drain output is high, the fluid should be sent for creatinine. If the fluid is consistent with urine, the drain should be taken off of bulb suction and placed to gravity drain to prevent further siphoning of urine out of the bladder. The patient is discharged home with the urethral catheter in place to gravity drain for a duration of 14 days. A cystogram is performed on postoperative day 14 to ensure a successful repair. If a persistent urine leak is noted, the cystogram is repeated weekly until healing is demonstrated prior to urethral catheter removal.

Special Considerations

The surgeon attempting to perform robotic rectovesical fistula repair may encounter complex situations that they should be prepared to manage. For example, patients who have had prior bowel surgery may present with absent or shortened omentum that may not reach the deep pelvis. In this case, reasonable alternatives for tissue interposition include a peritoneal flap or epiploic appendage. Successful use of peritoneal flaps has been described for vesicovaginal fistula repairs. Fistula location must be considered as peritoneal flaps generally work best when fistula location is high enough for a well vascularized peritoneal flap to reach without requiring overly extensive dissection. An alternative option is a lengthy epiploic appendage found on a mobile cecum or caudally draping transverse colon.

Large fistula tracts can be more challenging to manage with a possible increased risk of failure. In cases of fistulas greater than 2 cm or in tenuous repairs, fecal diversion along with suprapubic catheter placement should be considered. Our preference for fecal diversion is with a laparoscopic diverting loop ileostomy performed by our colorectal surgeons. The ileostomy can be reversed 3–4 months after successful healing of the fistula. Placement of a suprapubic catheter allows for extended bladder drainage if needed, while avoiding additional irritation to the vesical fistula closure site from the urethral catheter balloon as it enters the bladder neck. These additional steps may lead to improved repair success and avoidance of the need for further repair attempts in an increasingly hostile abdomen from multiple surgeries.

Potential Complications and Steps to Avoid Them

There are several potential complications to avoid during robotic rectovesical fistula repair. This section aims to address situations that, if avoided, can improve the success and durability of fistula repair.

1. Omental devascularization—Knowledge of omental vascular anatomy can prevent damaging a good omental interposition flap while

obtaining pedicle length. If there is difficulty with obtaining sufficient omental length to reach the pelvic repair for interposition, the pedicle can be lengthened. Division of one of the gastroepiploic arteries and gastric attachments often allows for adequate pedicle length. Generally the right gastroepiploic artery is more robust. Therefore, division of the left gastroepiploic artery and short gastric arteries can be performed to lengthen the flap. Care must be taken to avoid gastric injury or ligation of the contralateral gastroepiploic artery.

2. Additional rectal injuries—This can occur during development of the plane between the bladder and rectum. It is critical to perform this step carefully as additional rectal injuries increase the size of defect needing closure, which can lead to increased risk for failure of the repair.

3. Ureteral injury—This can occur during separation of the bladder and rectum or during undermining of the bladder tissue during the transvesical approach. Placement of ureteral stents at the beginning of the case can aid in ureteral identification and help prevent these injuries.

4. Inadequate fistula closure—In a patient with a rectovesical fistula, further surgery becomes increasingly difficult. Therefore, the best chance for a durable repair is with the first attempt. The principles of fistula closure should be applied during a robotic rectovesical fistula closure to maximize chances of success. Those principles include a tension-free anastomosis, water or airtight closure, adequate mucosa to mucosa apposition, and nonoverlapping suture lines.

Reference

1. Modh R, Corbyons K, Tan S, Su L, Yeung L. Robotic repair of rectovesical fistula: combined anterior and posterior approach with omental flap interposition. Videourology. 2015;29(3). doi: 10.1089/vid.2014.0048.

Robotic Sacrocolpopexy

Mary E. Westerman, Daniel S. Elliott,
Mark S. Shimko, and George K. Chow

Abbreviations

ASC   Abdominal sacrocolpopexy
RALS   Robot-assisted laparoscopic surgery

Patient Selection

Pelvic organ prolapse negatively affects the quality of life of up to 40% of all women [1]. Abdominal sacrocolpopexy (ASC), first described in 1957, is considered the most durable repair for vaginal vault prolapse and can be done via an open abdominal, pure laparoscopic, or robot-assisted laparoscopic approach [2]. Given the potential morbidity associated with an open approach, the minimally invasive approach has become increasingly popular. However, the surgeon must take into account multiple factors when choosing the approach, as the success of the sacrocolpo-

pexy is largely dependent on appropriate patient selection [3]. Candidates for robot-assisted laparoscopic sacrocolpopexy (RALS) are those with recurrent prolapse following primary vaginal repair, high-grade apical prolapse (Baden-Walker 3 or 4) that may include a concomitant posterior or anterior vaginal vault defect (Fig. 25.1), and/or women who desire continued sexual function [4].

Preoperative Preparation

A thorough history and physical exam is conducted to evaluate for concomitant cystocele, rectocele, enterocele. In patients who have not had a hysterectomy, an evaluation for postmenopausal/abnormal uterine bleeding is carried out with a transvaginal ultrasound if indicated and documentation of pap smear history is verified [4].

During the preoperative visit, particular attention is paid to counseling and informed consent, as this has been shown to improve postoperative patient satisfaction [5]. Risks of the procedure including infection, bleeding, postoperative ileus, and/or possible injury to the bowel, bladder, ureters, and vagina should be discussed. Currently, we quote the likelihood of these complications at less than 1%. The risk of postoperative voiding dysfunction, dyspareunia, and mesh-related complications including erosion or extrusion are also discussed. Finally, the possibility of conversion is particularly emphasized

Electronic supplementary material: The online version of this chapter (doi:10.1007/978-3-319-45060-5_25) contains supplementary material, which is available to authorized users.

M.E. Westerman, M.D. • D.S. Elliott, M.D.
M.S. Shimko, M.D. • G.K. Chow, M.D. (✉)
Department of Urology, Mayo Clinic,
200 First Street SW, Rochester, MN 55905, USA
e-mail: chow.george@mayo.edu

Fig. 25.1 Sagittal section of female pelvis demonstrating apical vaginal vault prolapse; anatomical variation with posterior bladder wall draping over apex of vagina (*lower-left inset*); anatomical variation with posterior bladder wall recessed distally away from vaginal apex (*lower-right inset*)

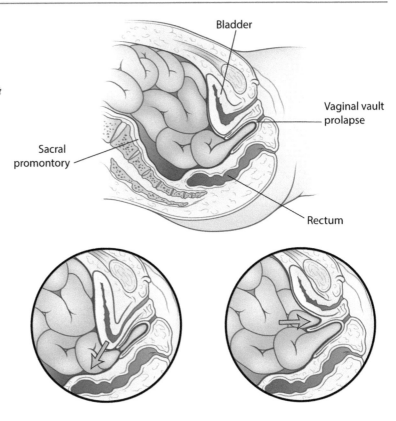

Operative Setup

The robotic system and operative suite is setup similar to the robot-assisted laparoscopic prostatectomy (Fig. 25.2). The surgeon console is in the corner of the room toward the foot of the operating table. The patient cart, when rolled in, should have its center column between the legs of the patient, with the base of the patient cart straddling the base of the operating table. The surgical assistant stands on the right side of the patient which allows access to the perineum during the procedure. The scrub nurse stands across from the assistant on the patient's left side.

in patients with a body mass index (BMI) greater than 30 kg/m^2 [6]. Preoperative anesthetic clearance is obtained when indicated. A type and screen is not needed, and we no longer give a laxative the night before surgery.

Patient Positioning and Preparation

The patient's legs are placed in cushioned, full supporting Allen stirrups. This keeps the patient in dorsal lithotomy throughout the procedure and allows access to the vagina before and after the patient cart is rolled in (Fig. 25.3). The lower extremity pressure points are padded, with specific attention given to the region behind the knees. To minimize the risk of plexus injuries, ensure that the stirrups do not place the lower extremities at excessive angles. A strap is secured across the chest below the breasts and the patient is then placed in Trendelenburg (between 15° and 20°). After padding the arm's pressure points, the arms are tucked beside the torso on arm boards. The abdomen below the level of the breasts, pelvis, vagina, and perineum is prepped for surgery. The vagina is left exposed during draping to allow for intraoperative placement of the handheld vaginal retractor (explained later in the

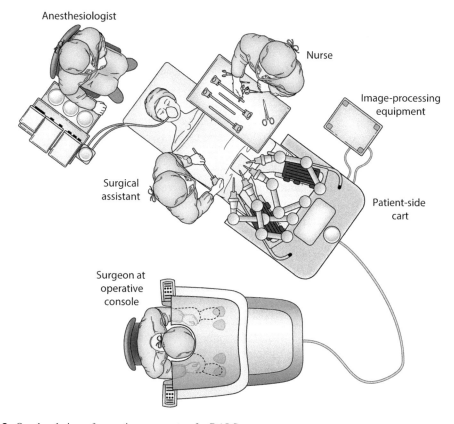

Fig. 25.2 Overhead view of operating room setup for RALS

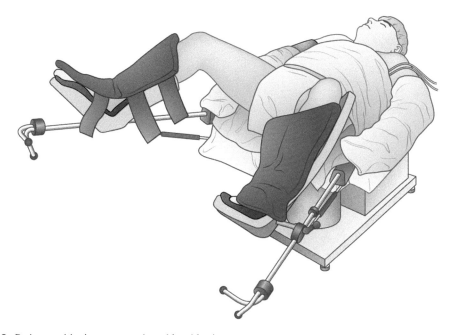

Fig. 25.3 Patient positioning on operative table with stirrups

description of RALS). A nasogastric tube, urethral catheter, and sequential compression devices
are placed prior to the start of the case. All patients
receive 24 h of perioperative antibiotics.

Trocar Configuration

RALS is performed using the da Vinci® Surgical
System (Intuitive Surgical, Inc., Sunnyvale, CA).
The initial placement of the central camera trocar
is based on the patient's pubic symphysis and
umbilicus (Fig. 25.4). Generally the initial central camera trocar is placed 12–15 cm above the
pubic symphysis but below the umbilicus. All
measurements are generalized and can change
based on a patient's body habitus. The placement
of trocars is started by placing the 12 mm disposable camera trocar (red trocar in Fig. 25.4). This
is placed 12–15 cm above the pubic symphysis
but staying below the umbilicus. The right and
left da Vinci® arm reusable 8 mm trocars (blue
trocars) are placed 10–12 mm from the central
camera trocar below the level of the camera trocar, lateral to the rectus muscles, and two finger-
breadths superior to the level of the anterior
superior iliac spine. The assistant 12 mm trocar
(lavender trocar) is placed two finger-breadths
below the subcostal margin and lateral to the rectus muscle, one hand-breadth (8–10 cm) away
from the right robotic 8 mm instrument trocar.

This trocar is approximately 10–12 cm from the
central camera trocar. An optional assistant 5 mm
trocar or possible third robotic arm (purple trocar) can be placed one hand-breadth (8–10 cm)
inferior-laterally from the assistant 12 mm trocar
at approximately the level of the umbilicus. This
trocar is approximately 10–12 cm from the central camera trocar. A bowel retraction suture may
be placed in the appendix epiploica of the sigmoid colon to retract it out of the way.
Alternatively, this site may be used to employ an
additonal robotic trocar for bowel retraction (X).

Instrumentation and Equipment List

Initially, standard laparoscopic instruments were
utilized in performing the RALS to assist in taking down adhesions and dissecting the vagina
from the posterior wall of the bladder. Now all of
the procedure, including the dissection of the
vagina is done with the da Vinci® robotic instrumentation. Regardless of the method used, the
sacrocolpopexy depends on the correct identification of the vaginal apex and ability to retract
the vagina inferiorly during dissection of the
anterior vaginal plane. We utilize a specialized
instrument engineered at our institution designated the hand-held vaginal retractor to visualize
the plane between the vagina and bladder

Fig. 25.4 Trocar
configuration for RALS

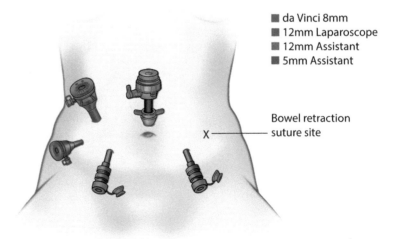

■ da Vinci 8mm
■ 12mm Laparoscope
■ 12mm Assistant
■ 5mm Assistant

Bowel retraction
X—————— suture site

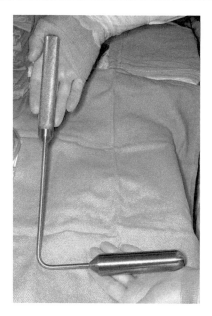

Fig. 25.5 Hand-held vaginal retractor

(Fig. 25.5). The laparoscopic and robotic instruments are listed as follows.

Equipment

- da Vinci® S Surgical System (Intuitive Surgical, Inc., Sunnyvale, CA)
- EndoWrist® curved monopolar scissors (Intuitive Surgical, Inc., Sunnyvale, CA)
- EndoWrist® ProGrasp™ forceps (Intuitive Surgical, Inc., Sunnyvale, CA)
- EndoWrist® needle drivers (2) (Intuitive Surgical, Inc., Sunnyvale, CA)
- InSite® Vision System with 0° and 30° lens (Intuitive Surgical, Inc., Sunnyvale, CA)

Trocars

- 12 mm trocars (2)
- 8 mm robotic trocars (2(2–3))
- 5 mm trocar (1)

Mesh Y-graft (polypropylene) (Fig. 25.6)

Recommended Sutures

- Retraction stitch for sigmoid colon: 2-0 Prolene suture full length on a Keith needle
- Fixation suture for polypropylene Y-graft: 2-0 GoreTex™ on CV-2 needle cut to 7 cm
- Y-graft mesh preparation: 2-0 monocryl
- Mesh retroperitonealization: 2-0 polyglactin on CT-1 cut to 7 cm

Instruments Used by the Surgical Assistant

- Laparoscopic needle driver
- Laparoscopic scissors
- Maryland grasper
- Suction irrigator device
- 16 Fr silicone urethral catheter
- Polypropylene Y-graft (AMS, Minnetonka, MN) (see Fig. 25.6)

Step-by-Step Technique (Videos 25.1, 25.2, 25.3, 25.4, 25.5 and 25.6)

RALS is performed using the da Vinci-S®, which allows three-dimensional visualization and six degrees of freedom of instrument movement to the surgeon through the modulated remote control. Docking the da Vinci® includes connecting the camera arm to the laparoscopic 12 mm trocar (red circle, Fig. 25.4), and connecting the instrument arms to the laparoscopic 8 mm trocars (blue circles, Fig. 25.4). During the entire procedure, a 30° lens in the downward view is placed via the camera trocar. We have started each description of our steps with an instrument index table which names the instrument used, the trocar used, and the handedness.

Step 1: Abdominal Access and Trocar Placement

Prior to placement of the laparoscopic trocars, a 16 Fr urethral catheter is placed for the entire procedure. As noted earlier, the initial placement

Fig. 25.6 Mesh Y-graft
(polypropylene)

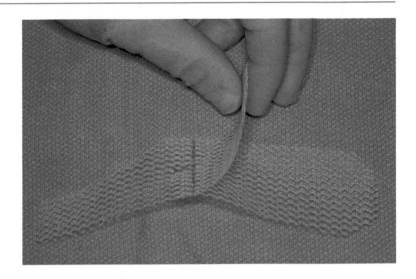

of the central camera trocar is based on the patient's pubic symphysis and umbilicus (Fig. 25.4). After abdominal insufflation using a Veress needle, we place a periumbilical Visiport optical trocar (Autosuture, Norwalk, CT) through a disposable 12 mm trocar under direct vision to avoid visceral or vascular injury. Generally, this initial trocar (camera) is placed 12–15 cm above the pubic symphysis but below the umbilicus. The assistant and robotic arm trocars are then placed under direct vision in the locations described earlier in section entitled "Trocar configuration" (Fig. 25.4).

Step 2: Vaginal Retractor Placement and Retraction of Sigmoid Colon (Table 25.1)

Initially all adhesions are taken down in the abdomen and pelvis with a ProGrasp™ in the left hand and monopolar curved scissors in the right hand. Adhesion takedown should allow exposure of the vagina and sigmoid colon. To avoid tissue damage along the planes between bladder and vagina, electrocautery is used judiciously at a setting of 30–40 W. To assist in dissection, the hand-held vaginal retractor is then placed in the previously prepped vaginal canal by the assistant to expose the vaginal apex (Fig. 25.7). Prior to vaginal dissection, the sig-

Table 25.1 Vaginal retractor placement and retraction of sigmoid colon: surgeon and assistant instrumentation

Robotic instruments	
Right arm	Left arm
• Curved monopolar scissors	• ProGrasp™ dissector
• Large needle driver	• Large needle driver
Assistant instruments	
Right hand	Left arm
• Hand-held vaginal retractor	

moid colon is reflected superior-laterally to the patient's left with a retracting suture. The site of the retraction suture is typically 8–10 cm lateral to the camera trocar at the level of the umbilicus (orange circle—Fig. 25.4). Retraction of the sigmoid is done with a 2-0 Prolene suture on a Keith needle which is introduced through the anterior abdominal wall 8–10 cm lateral to the camera trocar at the level of the umbilicus (orange circle—Fig. 25.4). Utilizing a needle driver in the right hand and a ProGrasp™ in the left hand, the Prolene suture is grasped from the anterior abdominal wall and placed through the tenia of the sigmoid colon. The suture is then brought out of the abdominal wall near its entrance site. The two ends of the suture are gently retracted together with a curved mosquito outside the body to expose the sacral promontory (Fig. 25.8).

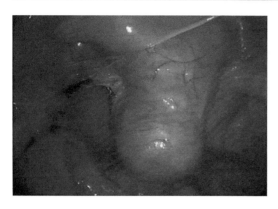

Fig. 25.7 Intraoperative view demonstrating insertion of hand-held vaginal retractor to delineate the vaginal apex

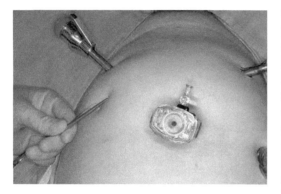

Fig. 25.8 Mosquito clamp holding retraction suture approximately one hand breadth lateral to camera trocar

Step 3: Vaginal Dissection (Table 25.2)

Utilizing monopolar curved scissors with electrocautery in the right hand and ProGrasp™ in the left hand, the plane between the anterior vagina and posterior bladder wall is dissected beginning with electrocautery to gently score the surface of the vagina. Thereafter, no electrocautery is used to dissuade devascularization of the vaginal wall. The hand-held vaginal retractor is used to deflect the vaginal apex inferiorly to allow better visualization of the plane between the vagina and bladder. It is important to note that anatomical variation exists between the anterior vaginal wall and posterior bladder wall that can make finding the correct plane difficult (please refer to the "Steps to Avoid Complications" section for further discussion).

Table 25.2 Vaginal dissection: surgeon and assistant instrumentation

Robotic instruments	
Right arm	Left arm
• Curved monopolar scissors	• ProGrasp™ dissector
Assistant instruments	
Right hand (assistant 5 mm—black circle)	Left hand (assistant 12 mm—green circle)
• Suction-irrigator • Hand-held vaginal retractor	• Maryland grasper

Utilizing scissors with electrocautery in the right hand and ProGrasp™ in the left hand, the plane between the anterior vagina and bladder is dissected with a spread and cut technique in combination with blunt dissection. The left hand instrument should be grasping the tissue anterior to the vagina and retracting superior to allow visualization of the apex of the vagina (Fig. 25.9a–d). If the surgeon is in the right plane, this dissection is generally bloodless. This plane between the anterior vagina and bladder wall is continued distally, as close as possible to the introitus, to maximize the support given by the Y-mesh graft. The plane between the rectum and posterior vagina generally requires less dissection and in some patients may be exposed to the level of the introitus. If dissection is needed in this plane, the same instruments and technique can be utilized as earlier for the anterior dissection.

Step 4: Exposing the Sacral Promontory and Placement of Gore-Tex Sutures (Table 25.3)

Window created in posterior peritoneum exposing the sacral promontory (Fig. 25.10a) and placement of GoreTex™ sutures into sacral promontory for later mesh fixation (Fig. 25.10b).

Utilizing curved monopolar scissors in the right hand and ProGrasp™ in the left hand, the peritoneal reflection above the proximal sacrum is gently scored with electrocautery to begin the dissection. Continue the dissection through the

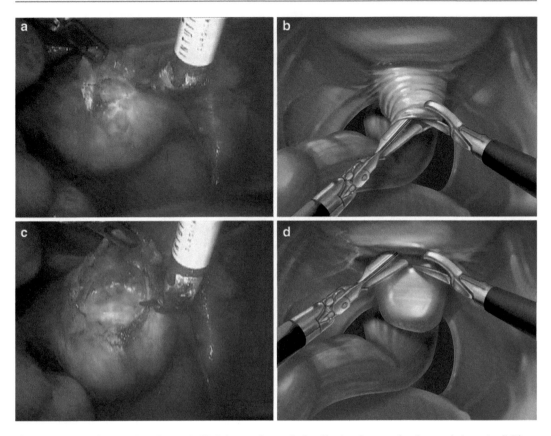

Fig. 25.9 (**a**, **b**) Bladder being dissected off of the anterior vaginal wall using the spread and cut technique. (**c**, **d**) Plane developed between bladder and anterior vagina

Table 25.3 Exposing the sacral promontory and placement of Gore-Tex sutures: surgeon and assistant instrumentation

Robotic instruments	
Right arm	Left arm
• Curved monopolar scissors	• ProGrasp™ dissector
• Needle driver	• Needle driver
Assistant instruments	
Right hand (assistant 5 mm—black circle)	Left hand (assistant 12 mm—green circle)
• Suction-irrigator	• Maryland grasper

tissues underlying the peritoneal reflection to visualize the sacral promontory (Fig. 25.10). It is important to note that severe bleeding is described by authors who have dissected and sutured mesh below the S-2 level in the transabdominal sacro-

colpopexy [7]. Because of this, our technique stays proximal on the sacrum during dissection and suture placement for mesh fixation (please refer to the "Steps to Avoid Complications" section for further discussion).

Utilizing needle drivers in both hands, individual 2-0 GoreTex™ sutures on a CV-2 needle approximately 7 cm in length are placed horizontally into the sacrum above the level of S2 (Fig. 25.10). The suture should be placed deep enough into the sacral promontory to sufficiently withstand moderate traction with the needle drivers. A total of three to four sutures with the needles left attached remain in the abdomen for mesh fixation. The surgical assistant typically uses a suction irrigator in the right hand (5 mm assistant trocar) and a Maryland grasper in the left hand (12 mm assistant trocar) for assistance and bowel retraction through this step.

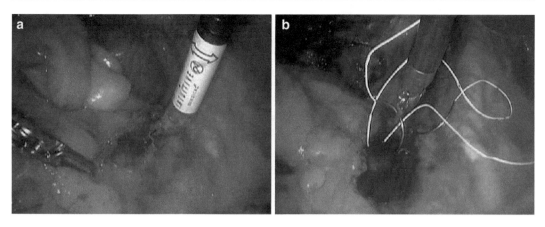

Fig. 25.10 (**a**) Window created in posterior peritoneum exposing the sacral promontory; (**b**) Placement of Gore-Tex sutures into sacral promontory for later mesh fixation

Table 25.4 Suturing mesh to vagina: surgeon and assistant instrumentation

Robotic instruments	
Right arm	Left arm
• Needle driver	• Needle driver
Assistant instruments	
Right hand (assistant 5 mm—black circle)	Left hand (assistant 12 mm—green circle)
• Suction-irrigator	
• Hand-held vaginal retractor	

Step 5: Suturing Mesh to Vagina (Table 25.4)

At this point in the procedure, the mesh Y-graft (polypropylene Y-graft; AMS, Minnetonka, MN) is prepared to introduce into the abdominal cavity. The anterior flap of the Y-graft is temporarily sutured back onto the tail of the Y-graft with 2-0 Monocryl suture outside the body (Fig. 25.11a). This maneuver keeps the flap from obscuring the surgeon's view and allows easier suturing of the posterior flap to the posterior vaginal canal. The mesh Y-graft is then introduced via the 12 mm assistant trocar with the posterior flap orientated along the posterior vaginal canal. The surgical assistant replaces the hand-held vaginal retractor into the vaginal canal and deflects it superiorly to reorientate the surgeon prior to placing sutures.

The surgeon then places the distal end of the posterior flap of the Y-mesh graft as close to the introitus as possible. The distal end of the Y-mesh graft's posterior flap is then sutured as close to the introitus as possible with individual 2-0 Gore-Tex sutures on a CV-2 needle approximately 7 cm in length. To obtain the best support of the apex, and posterior vagina, four to six total GoreTex™ sutures are used on the posterior flap of the Y-mesh graft. Figure 25.11b shows the suture configuration for mesh fixation to the vagina. The temporary Monocryl suture is then cut allowing the anterior flap to be manipulated to the anterior vagina. Due to fixating the posterior flap of the Y-mesh graft first, upward traction on the anterior flap allows easier and more precise mesh fixation and better visualization. The surgeon then places the distal end of the anterior flap of the Y-mesh graft as close to the introitus as possible.

Utilizing the needle drivers on both the right and left robotic arms, the distal end of the Y-mesh graft's anterior flap is sutured as close to the introitus as possible with individual 2-0 GorTex sutures on a CV-2 needle approximately 7 cm in length (Fig. 25.12a, b). To obtain the best support of the apex, and anterior vagina, four to six total Gore-Tex sutures are used on the anterior flap of the Y-mesh graft. Please see Fig. 25.11b which shows the suture configuration for mesh fixation to the vagina. All needles from the Gore-Tex suture are removed by the assistant.

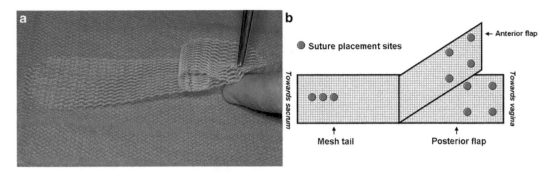

Fig. 25.11 (**a**) Mesh Y-graft's anterior flap sutured back onto tail in preparation for posterior flap suturing intracorporeally. (**b**) Suture configuration on mesh Y-graft

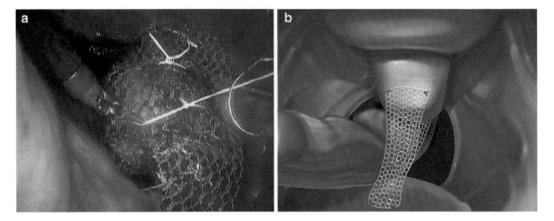

Fig. 25.12 (**a**) Mesh fixation to anterior vagina. (**b**) Schematic demonstrating completed fixation of the mesh to the anterior and posterior vagina

Table 25.5 Suturing mesh to sacrum: surgeon and assistant instrumentation

Robotic instruments	
Right arm	Left arm
• Needle driver	• Needle driver
Assistant instruments	
Right hand (assistant 5 mm—black circle)	Left hand (assistant 12 mm—green circle)
• Suction-irrigator	• Maryland grasper

Step 6: Suturing Mesh to Sacrum (Table 25.5)

Utilizing needle drivers in the right and left hands of the robot, the previously placed sacral sutures are used to tie the tail of the Y-mesh graft to the sacrum (Fig. 25.13a). Figure 25.11b shows the suture configuration on the tail of the Y-mesh graft.

The mesh should not be under tension but should approximate the apex of the vagina into a more normal anatomical position. By using the hand-held vaginal retractor, the assistant directs the vaginal apex into the normal anatomical configuration which allows the surgeon to tie the sutures without tension. The excess stem of the Y-mesh graft is excised and removed through the assistant trocar along with the GoreTex™ needles.

Step 7: Retroperitonealizing the Mesh and Exiting the Abdomen (Table 25.6)

Next, with the needle drivers on the robotic arms, a running 2-0 polyglactin suture on a CT-1 needle (7 cm in length) is used to reapproximate the

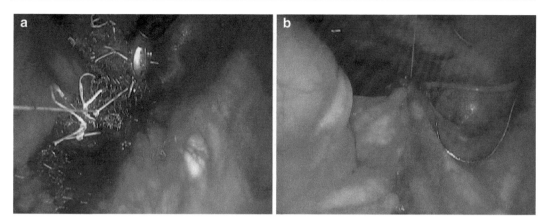

Fig. 25.13 (**a**) Mesh fixation to sacrum. (**b**) Retroperitonealization of mesh

Table 25.6 Retroperitonealizing the mesh and exiting the abdomen: surgeon and assistant instrumentation

Robotic instruments	
Right arm	Left arm
• Needle driver	• Needle driver
Assistant instruments	
Right hand (assistant 5 mm—black circle)	Left hand (assistant 12 mm—green circle)
• Suction-irrigator	• Maryland grasper

peritoneal reflection over the Y-mesh graft which is now tied to the sacrum (Fig. 25.13b). Figure 25.14 demonstrates what the final repair should resemble anatomically. The Y-mesh graft should approximate the vagina in a more normal anatomical position, but also support the anterior and posterior walls of the vaginal canal. After confirming hemostasis, trocar-site closure is done in the usual manner, using a trocar site closure device to close all wounds greater than 5 mm in diameter.

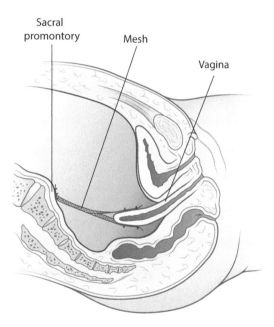

Fig. 25.14 Schematic diagram of sagittal section of female pelvis showing completed prolapse repair

Postoperative Management

At the end of the case, the nasogastric tube is removed and a vaginal pack is placed. RALS patients are managed with similar postoperative pathway as our robotic prostatectomy patients. The patient's diet is advanced to a regular diet by the morning of postoperative day #1. The vaginal pack and urethral catheter is removed on postop-erative day #1 and we ensure the patient is able to void spontaneously prior to discharge. For pain, we schedule Toradol and Tylenol and have oral narcotic pain medication available on an as-needed basis.

As the majority of the dissection is carried out between the bladder and vagina, we carefully observe vaginal drainage and urine color for any indication of bleeding as well as overall urine volume.

Special Considerations

Increased Body Mass Index

Obesity is a risk factor for the development of pelvic organ prolapse. While obesity has previously been reported to have no effect on durability after RALS [8], in our recent series of 83 patients we found that BMI was the only significant factor contributing to conversion from robotic to open surgery [6]. 34.7% (8/23) of patients with a $BMI \geq 30$ kg/m^2 underwent conversion to an open procedure [6]. Approximately $^1/_3$ of these conversions were related to difficulty with the presacral dissection due to increased retroperitoneal adiposity [6]. However, there was no significant difference in blood loss or operative time with increasing BMI [6]. Therefore while necessary to counsel patients with higher BMIs appropriately about their greater likelihood of conversion, BMI alone is not an absolute contraindication to a robotic approach.

Mesh Material

Synthetic meshes are used in the majority of patients undergoing a sacrocolpopexy as described in the literature [2]. A recent RCT found that at 5 years anatomical success rates for cadaveric fascia vs polypropylene mesh were 62% vs. 93% ($p=0.02$) [9]. Our preference is to use synthetic mesh (polypropylene) because of its initial pliability and long-term durability. A recent systematic review of the literature reported mesh erosion rates between 0 and 12% for sacrocolpopexy [10] while a 2004 review of ASC Nygaard et al. reported mesh erosion rates of 3.4% [2]. Currently in our series of RALS we report an erosion rate of 2.7% [11].

Concomitant Surgical Procedures

Eighty percent of our patients undergo an additional procedure at the time of RALS [6]. At our institution, the majority of RALS as well as those reported in the literature are performed in conjunction with an incontinence procedure [12]. It is the surgeon's preference to place an autologous transobturator urethral sling [13] at the time of sacrocolpopexy due to the ease of access and the potential unmasking of stress urinary incontinence following ASC if it is not already present. Halban culdoplasty is performed prior to retroperitonealizing the mesh on a case-by-case basis, determined by the depth of the cul-de-sac at the time of surgery.

Steps to Avoid Complications

Vaginal/Bladder Dissection and Anatomical Variations

In our experience, some patients with apical vaginal prolapse have a more difficult vaginal dissection due to the location of the bladder. A posterior bladder wall draping over the vaginal apex (Fig. 25.1; lower-left inset) or recessed along the anterior vaginal wall (Fig. 25.1; lower-right inset) may inhibit the surgeon from easily finding the bloodless plane between the bladder and vagina. In these situations, additional time and effort, as well as use of hand-held vaginal retractor is necessary to find the correct plane and avoid inadvertent perforation of the bladder, vagina, or rectum. Cases of inadvertent bladder or vaginal perforation during RALS at our institution were all due to the anatomical variations described in Fig. 25.1 (lower-left inset). In these two cases, the perforation was repaired and the sacrocolpopexy finished.

Intraoperative Hemorrhage

In order to minimize hemorrhage from unrecognized presacral blood vessels, mesh fixation at the sacral promontory is performed above S3 at our institution as opposed to S3 or S4 as traditionally reported [7]. Because of this, our dissection and suture placement is carried out proximally on the sacrum.

Acknowledgments The authors would like to thank our surgical assistants, especially Ms. Nancy Mork, for their contributions in the operative suite.

We would also like to thank the Medical Illustration and Audiovisual Departments at Mayo Clinic for their contributions.

References

1. Nygaard I, Barber MD, Burgio KL, Kenton K, Meikle S, Schaffer J, et al. Prevalence of symptomatic pelvic floor disorders in US women. JAMA. 2008;300(11): 1311–6.
2. Nygaard IE, McCreery R, Brubaker L, Connolly A, Cundiff G, Weber AM, et al. Abdominal sacrocolpopexy: a comprehensive review. Obstet Gynecol. 2004;104(4):805–23.
3. Elliott DS, Krambeck AE, Chow GK. Long-term results of robotic assisted laparoscopic sacrocolpopexy for the treatment of high grade vaginal vault prolapse. J Urol. 2006;176(2):655–9.
4. White WM, Pickens RB, Elder RF, Firoozi F. Robotic-assisted sacrocolpopexy for pelvic organ prolapse. Urol Clin North Am. 2014;41(4):549–57.
5. Kenton K, Pham T, Mueller E, Brubaker L. Patient preparedness: an important predictor of surgical outcome. Am J Obstet Gynecol. 2007;197(6):654.e1–6.
6. Linder BJ, Chow GK, Hertzig LL, Clifton M, Elliott DS. Factors associated with intraoperative conversion during robotic sacrocolpopexy. Int Braz J Urol. 2015;41(2):319–24.
7. Sutton GP, Addison WA, Livengood III CH, Hammond CB. Life-threatening hemorrhage complicating sacral colpopexy. Am J Obstet Gynecol. 1981;140(7):836–7.
8. Priyanka GSS, Lohse CM, McGee SM, Chow GK, Elliot DS. Impact of obesity of surgical outcomes after robotic-assisted laparoscopic sacrocolpopexy. World Congr Endourol. 2008.
9. Tate SB, Blackwell L, Lorenz DJ, Steptoe MM, Culligan PJ. Randomized trial of fascia lata and polypropylene mesh for abdominal sacrocolpopexy: 5-year follow-up. Int Urogynecol J. 2011;22(2):137–43.
10. Jia X, Glazener C, Mowatt G, Jenkinson D, Fraser C, Bain C, et al. Systematic review of the efficacy and safety of using mesh in surgery for uterine or vaginal vault prolapse. Int Urogynecol J. 2010;21(11):1413–31.
11. Linder BJ, Chow GK, Elliot DS. Long-term quality of life outcomes and retreatment rates after robotic sacrocolpopexy. Int J Urol. 2015;22(12):1155–8.
12. Elliott DS, Siddiqui SA, Chow GK. Assessment of the durability of robot-assisted laparoscopic sacrocolpopexy for treatment of vaginal vault prolapse. J Robot Surg. 2007;1(2):163–8.
13. Linder BJ, Elliott DS. Autologous transobturator urethral sling placement for female stress urinary incontinence. J Urol. 2015;193(3):991–6.

Robotic Vesicovaginal Fistula Repair

26

Eric A. Schommer, Steven P. Petrou, and David D. Thiel

Operative Setup

Briefing of the entire operative team including the surgeon, assistant, circulating nurse, scrub nurse, and anesthesiologist/nurse anesthetist is crucial to ensure case efficiency and proper operative setup. Concerns and questions may be addressed at this briefing to fill in any unknowns prior to the patient presenting to the operative suite.

Robotic vesicovaginal fistula (VVF) repair should be feasible with any of the commercially available da Vinci® robotic systems through Intuitive Surgical Corporation (Sunnyvale, CA, USA). Currently, our institution utilizes the da Vinci® Si HD Surgical System. We currently perform the procedure with three of the four arms available but the fourth arm may prove beneficial in certain cases and is available based on surgeon preference. This operation requires one bed-side surgical assistant and one scrub nurse. Figure 26.1 demonstrates the typical operating room setup. The assistant sits on the patients' right-hand side which gives sufficient access to the assistant 12 and 5 mm ports. A Mayo stand between the assistant and foot of the bed is readily accessible for common

instrumentation. The robot computer console and monitor are placed on the patients' right-hand side just outside of the Mayo stand. The suction as well as electrocautery is placed beside the robotic computer console. The scrub table as well as the scrub nurse is positioned on the patients' left-hand side. Once ports have been placed, the patient side robotic surgical cart is positioned between the patients' legs. Having a large operating room is a must to accommodate the large amount of equipment necessary for robotic surgery.

Patient Positioning

Patient positioning and anesthetic considerations are similar to robotic-assisted laparoscopic prostatectomy (See Chap. 21). Patients are placed in dorsal lithotomy position utilizing Allen stirrups with both arms tucked to the patient's side. The vagina, urethra, and abdomen should be prepared in the sterile operative field. Positioning should insure full intraoperative access to the vagina.

The patient is moved to the operative table in supine position with the buttock just superior to the removable foot portion of the table. Induction of general endotracheal anesthesia is performed by the anesthesiologist. Once anesthesia has released the patient for positioning by the operating room staff, the hands and elbows are padded bilaterally with egg-crate foam, ensuring that the intravenous access is still functioning accordingly. There are two draw sheets, one of which

E.A. Schommer, M.D. • S.P. Petrou, M.D.
D.D. Thiel, M.D. (✉)
Department of Urology, Mayo Clinic Florida,
4500 San Pablo Road South, Jacksonville,
FL 32224, USA
e-mail: Thiel.david@mayo.edu

Fig. 26.1 Operative room schematic

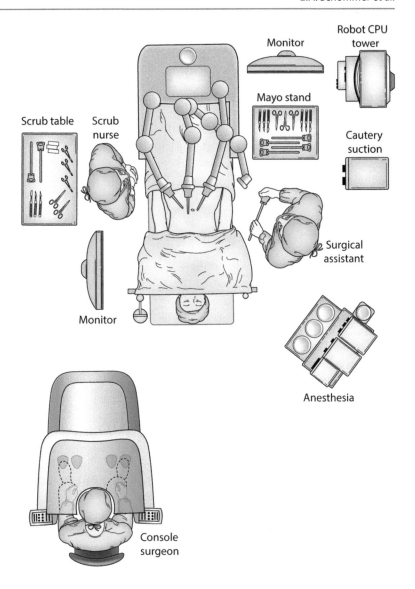

will remain on the table and one that will be used to tuck the arms. The patient is rolled by one operating room staff while another brings the upper draw sheet over the arm wrapping underneath the arm and tucked between the patient and bed. This is then repeated for the opposite arm. Care must be taken to ensure that the fingers are appropriately protected and the hands are in the thumb up position at their side. Thigh length sequential compression devices (SCDs) are then placed on the patient. Allen stirrups are then secured to the operative table. A pillow case or sheet is placed in each Allen stirrup. Simultaneously, each leg is placed in its respective Allen stirrup ensuring that the heels are

appropriately seated. Egg-crate foam is placed laterally just below the knee to protect the fibular nerve from any pressure. Egg-crate foam is also placed over the foot prior to securing the straps on the Allen stirrups. The SCDs are then attached to the pump. The foot end of the operative table is then removed. The stirrups are then manipulated to ensure a >90° angle about the knee, with the knees in line with the opposite shoulder. Stirrups are dropped to the low lithotomy split leg position as well as the high lithotomy position to ensure appropriate range of motion and positioning. They are then left in the low lithotomy position. Egg-crate foam is then placed across the patients' chest superior to the xiphoid. Two strips of heavy silk tape are then brought across the patients' chest over the foam and secured to the table. This should be snug but not too tight. Check with anesthesia to ensure the tidal volumes are still appropriate. A warming device or blanket may then be placed superior to the xiphoid per anesthesia preference. The patient is prepped from the xiphoid to below the perineum. The prep should be carried out laterally to the table and inferiorly to the mid-thigh bilaterally. The patient is then placed in 20° Trendelenburg for the initial portion of the case. A universal protocol time out is performed with all in attendance confirming correct patient, correct procedure, correct side (not applicable in this case), correct equipment, and any special considerations. All in attendance must verbally agree prior to the procedure start.

Trocar Configuration

A total of five trocars are utilized for the robotic portion of the case (Fig. 26.2). A 12 mm camera port is placed in the supra-umbilical midline. The left-sided 8 mm robotic trocar is placed 15 cm from the mid portion of the pubic bone and 8 cm from the midline. The right-sided 8 mm robotic trocar is placed 15 cm from the mid portion of the pubic bone and 8 cm from the midline. A 12 mm assistant trocar is placed 7 cm superolateral to the right-sided 8 mm robotic trocar. A 5 mm assistant trocar is placed 7 cm superolateral to the camera trocar on the patients' right-hand side. If a fourth arm is desired for the robot, a third 8 mm robotic trocar can be placed 10 cm lateral to the left 8 mm robotic trocar.

Instrumentation and Equipment List

Surgical instrumentation is similar to robotic-assisted laparoscopic radical prostatectomy and is listed in Table 26.1.

Additional Equipment for Robotic Portion

- da Vinci® Si HD Surgical System (Intuitive Surgical, Inc., Sunnyvale, CA)
- 10Fr round Jackson-Pratt closed suction pelvic drain
- 16Fr Urethral catheter
- Veress needle
- 12 mm trocar (2)
- 8 mm robotic trocar (2–3)

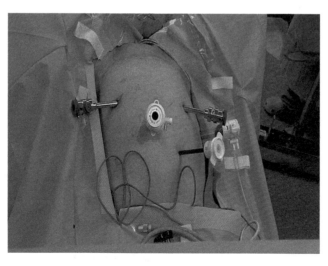

Fig. 26.2 Port placement. A 12 mm camera port is placed in the supraumbilical midline. 8 mm robotic ports are placed 15 cm from the pubic bone and 8 cm from the midline bilaterally. A 12 mm assistant port is placed 7 cm superolateral to the right side 8 mm robotic port. A 5 mm assistant port is placed 7 cm superolateral to the 12 mm camera port. Reprinted with permission. Rogers AE, Thiel DD, Brisson TE, Petrou SP. Robotic assisted laparoscopic repair of vesicovaginal fistula: The extravesicle approach. Can J Urol 2012; 19(5): 6474–6476

Table 26.1 Surgeon and assistant instrumentation

Surgeon instrumentation		Assistant instrumentation
Arm 1 (Right)	**Arm 2 (Left)**	• Suction irrigator
• EndoWrist® curved monopolar scissors (Intuitive Surgical, Inc., Sunnyvale, CA)	• EndoWrist® Maryland bipolar forceps (Intuitive Surgical, Inc., Sunnyvale, CA)	• Laparoscopic scissors
• EndoWrist® needle driver (Intuitive Surgical, Inc., Sunnyvale, CA)	• EndoWrist® needle driver (Intuitive Surgical, Inc., Sunnyvale, CA)	• Blunt tip grasper • Metal vaginal probe

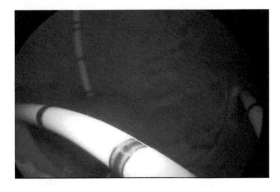

Fig. 26.3 Placement of ureteral catheters and fistula access cystoscopically. Bilateral ureteral catheters are placed to aid in intraoperative ureter identification. The supratrigonal fistula is cannulated with a yellow 5 French open-ended catheter. Reprinted with permission. Rogers AE, Thiel DD, Brisson TE, Petrou SP. Robotic assisted laparoscopic repair of vesicovaginal fistula: The extravesicle approach. Can J Urol 2012; 19(5): 6474–6476

- 5 mm trocar (1)
- 5 mm direct visualizing obturator trocar
- Laparoscopic camera
- 0° and 30° 5 mm laparoscopic lens
- Carter-Thomason® laparoscopic port closure system (Cooper Surgical, Inc. Trumbull, CT)
- Histoacryl® Topical Skin Adhesive (Tissue Seal, LLC, Ann Arbor, MI)

Equipment for Cystoscopy

- 22 French cystoscope sheath with 30° lens
- Laparoscopic camera with video monitor
- Straight Bard NiCore® Nitinol Guidewire (C. R. Bard, Inc., Covington, GA)
- Cook 5.0Fr/70 cm Open-End Ureteral Catheter—Yellow (Cook Incorporated, Bloomington, IN)
- (×2) Cook 6.0Fr/70 cm Open-End Ureteral Catheter—Green (Cook Incorporated, Bloomington, IN)

Suture

- (4) 8″ 2-0 Monocryl (Ethicon, Inc., Somerville, NJ) on SH needle
- 8″ 2-0 polyglactin on a CT2 needle

- 27″ 4-0 Monocryl (Ethicon, Inc., Somerville, NJ) on PS2 needle
- 0 Silk on CT1 needle
- (2) 0 polyglactin free tie

Step-by-Step Technique

Step 1: Cystoscopy and Placement of Catheters in Fistula and Ureters

Prior to achieving abdominal access, cystoscopy is performed to place localization catheters in the ureters as well as the VVF if possible (Fig. 26.3). These intraoperatively placed catheters aid in dissection of the VVF and intraoperative identification of the ureters. A 22Fr cystoscope sheath with obturator is thoroughly lubricated and introduced into the urethra. A 30° lens with video augmentation is used to identify the VVF and cannulate it with a Straight Bard NiCore® Nitinol Guidewire (C. R. Bard, Inc., Covington, GA). The wire is advanced until it loops back out of the vagina. A Cook 5.0Fr/70 cm Open-End Ureteral Catheter (Cook Incorporated, Bloomington, IN) is advanced over the Nitinol guidewire until it is visible looping back through the vagina. Vaginoscopy may be used to augment cannulation of the VVF (Fig. 26.4). This 5.0Fr catheter is yellow in color

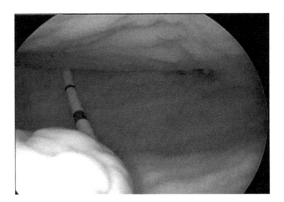

Fig. 26.4 5 French open-ended catheter cannulating VVF as seen on vaginoscopy

to differentiate it from the ureteral catheters that will be placed (green). Cannulation of the VVF preoperatively may not be possible and all cases.

The cystoscope is then removed leaving the yellow catheter in place. The cystoscope is then reintroduced into the bladder and both ureteral orifices are cannulated with the guidewire and a Cook 6.0Fr/70 cm Open-End Ureteral Catheter (Cook Incorporated, Bloomington, IN) is advanced up both ureters approximately 20 cm over the wire. The guidewire and cystoscope are removed and a urethral catheter placed. Vaginoscopy is completed. A 16Fr urethral catheter is then placed in the standard fashion and connected to bag drainage.

Step 2: Abdominal Access and Trocar Placement

Abdominal access and trocar placement are similar to that of robotic-assisted laparoscopic prostatectomy (See Chap. 21). Our technique for abdominal access and port placement is summarized later.

A 13 mm supra-umbilical midline incision is made and carried down to the fascia using electrocautery. The external rectus fascia is snared on each side of the midline with a nerve hook with the help of the surgical assistant. The fascia is lifted up away from the abdomen. A Veress needle is then introduced into the abdomen in standard fashion. Insufflation is then initiated to 20 mmHg for port placement. A 0° laparoscope with video augmentation and 5 mm direct visualizing trocar are then obtained. The Veress needed is withdrawn and the abdomen is entered with the 5 mm direct visualizing trocar and laparoscope. Port placement is noted in Fig. 26.2 and described earlier in the port placement section. An 8 mm robotic trocar is then placed 15 cm from the mid portion of the pubic bone and 8 cm from the midline on the left under direct visualization. A second 8 mm robotic trocar is then placed 15 cm from the mid portion of the pubic bone and 8 cm from the midline on the right under direct visualization. A 12 mm assistant trocar is then placed 7 cm superolateral to the right 8 mm robotic trocar. The laparoscope is then introduced into the right side assistant trocar. The supraumbilical trocar is removed under direct visualization and the 12 mm camera trocar is introduced through the same defect. Lastly, a 5 mm assistant trocar is introduced 7 cm superolateral the camera trocar on the right. At this point the pneumoperitoneum can be placed at 15 mmHg.

With the patient in maximum Trendelenburg position, the da Vinci® robot is then positioned between the patients' legs and the three robotic arms are docked to their respective trocars. Side docking of the robot has recently aided our ability to access the urethra cystoscopically during robotic reconstruction of the urinary tract if needed (VVF, bladder diverticulum, ureteral strictures) [5, 6]. We have not noted side docking to interfere with our ability to dissect structures in the pelvis. Side docking has also been well described by others performing urinary tract reconstruction and robotic prostatectomy in order to allow ureteroscopic/cystoscopic access to urologic organs intraoperatively [6, 7].

Robotic dissection of the fistula is completed with the da Vinci® 0° lens although a 30° lens may be used if needed. Dissection is completed with the EndoWrist® curved monopolar scissors (right hand) and the EndoWrist® Maryland bipolar forceps (left hand).

Fig. 26.5 Harvest of omental flap, ensuring enough length to reach the VVF

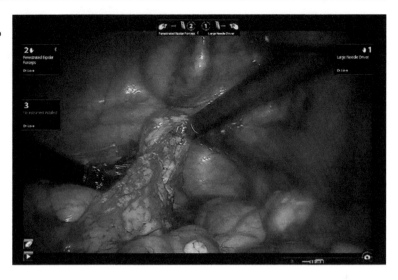

Step 3: Takedown of Abdominal Adhesions and Creation of Omental Flap

The right and left arm instrumentation remain the same as the prior step. Upon initial entry into the abdomen a survey is performed to look for relevant landmarks including the bladder, urachus, medial umbilical ligaments, urethral catheter balloon, and possible vaginal stump. An impression of the 5Fr ureteral catheter cannulating the VVF may be visible. Adhesions are frequently encountered around the VVF secondary to inflammation. Any adhesions present are taken down by applying downward traction with the left arm and sharply dissecting adhesions with the right arm. A metal dilator can be placed in the vagina by the surgical assistant to aid in visualization of the vagina during dissection. Once adhesions have been sharply dissected, adequate hemostasis is achieved with electrocautery.

Next an omental flap is obtained (Fig. 26.5). Omental interposition is essential to an adequate repair. If an omental flap is not freely available, a peritoneal flap or free bladder mucosal graft may be used. The most dependent portion of the omentum is localized and isolated. An adequate portion of omentum is mobilized by applying tension with the left hand and dissecting with monopolar scissors and electrocautery until there is sufficient length to reach the area of the VVF. The assistant may aid in this portion of the operation with suction irrigation and grasper counter-traction.

Step 4: Incision of the Peritoneum and Isolation of the VVF

The peritoneum over the area of the VVF is incised sharply with monopolar scissors (Fig. 26.6). The urethral catheter balloon and vaginal dilator may be manipulated by the surgical assistant to help in visualization of the VVF containing the yellow 5Fr ureteral catheter (Fig. 26.7). Proper exposure of the fistula allows adequate dissection, which in turn allows for a more adequate closure. Sufficient exposure of the VVF is required to permit room for a two-layer closure as well as the omental flap. The surgical assistant may provide retraction with a blunt tip grasper as well as exposure with a suction irrigator. Devascularized tissue should be removed to allow healthy tissue approximation at closure.

If the VVF cannot be localized extravesically, a formal midline cystotomy must be performed and the fistula located inside the bladder. Once the fistula is identified intravesically, it can be dissected free of the vagina. The vaginal mobilizer will aid in this dissection. Clamping the urethral catheter may aid in preventing loss of pneumoperitoneum if a large cystotomy is required [8].

Fig. 26.6 Incision of the peritoneum over the area of the VVF is incised sharply with the right hand using cold monopolar scissors. Reprinted with permission. Rogers AE, Thiel DD, Brisson TE, Petrou SP. Robotic assisted laparoscopic repair of vesicovaginal fistula: The extravesicle approach. Can J Urol 2012; 19(5): 6474–6476

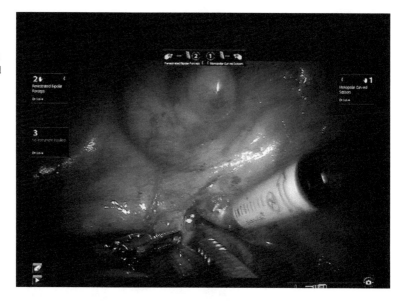

Fig. 26.7 Manipulation of metal vaginal dilator and yellow 5 French open-ended catheter to aid in dissection of VVF

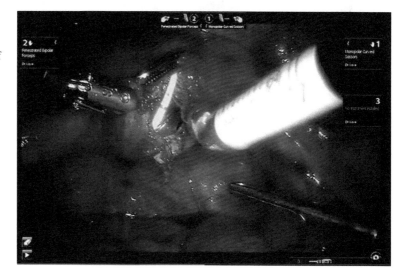

Step 5: Closure of the Vaginal Cuff

Once the VVF has been adequately dissected free and transected from the bladder, closure may begin. Adequate dissection of surrounding tissues is required to maintain a tension-free repair. Reconstruction is completed with EndoWrist® needle drivers (Intuitive Surgical, Inc., Sunnyvale, CA) in the right and left robotic arms. Closure is performed horizontally in two distinct layers with the second layer burying the first suture line. The vaginal cuff is closed with interrupted 2-0 monocryl on an SH needle (Fig. 26.8). Care should be taken that all needles are passed by the assistant through the 12 mm assistant trocar with a blunt tip grasper. The 5 mm assistant port is utilized solely for suction irrigation. The yellow ureteral catheter is left in the vaginal cuff until the last stitch needs to be thrown. A second running layer of 2-0 monocryl is then performed burying the previous suture line.

Step 6: Anchoring the Omental Flap

The previously mobilized omental flap is grasped with the left robotic arm and a stitch is thrown through the distal aspect of the flap (2-0 polyglactin

Fig. 26.8 The vaginal cuff is closed in two separate layers with interrupted 2-0 Monocryl on an SH needle

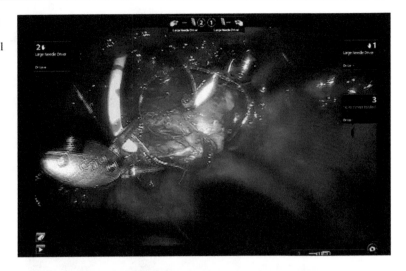

Fig. 26.9 Anchoring of the omental flap over the vaginal cuff closure

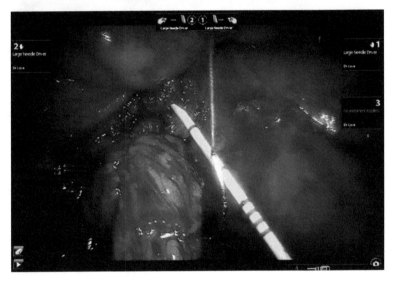

suture), ensuring a good purchase. Using the left hand for retraction/exposure at the site of vaginal cuff repair, the needle is then passed anterior and caudal to the vaginal cuff, between the bladder and vagina. This anchors the omental flap to the two-layer vaginal cuff repair (Fig. 26.9). A second or third stitch may be placed to ensure a good hold of the flap.

Step 7: Closure of the Bladder

Once the omental flap anchored in place, attention is turned to closure of the bladder. As in the closure of the vaginal cuff, this should be done in two layers with the second layer burying the first layer. This should also be a tension-free closure. While the vaginal cuff was closed horizontally, the bladder should be closed vertically to avoid overlapping suture lines. The assistant can help with retraction utilizing the suction irrigator or blunt tip grasper. The bladder is closed with a 2-0 monocryl on an SH needle in a running fashion (Fig. 26.10). When the initial layer is almost complete, the yellow ureteral catheter can be removed from the urethra and the first layer of closure completed. A second layer is also run burying the first suture line. If a large cystotomy

Fig. 26.10 Closure of cystotomy with running 2-0 Monocryl suture

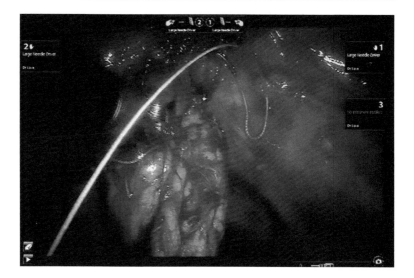

was required to isolate the VVF intravesically, the cystotomy will obviously require a larger closure and possibly more suture.

Step 8: Placement of Drain and Closure

The surgical site is irrigated appropriately and hemostasis ensured. A 10Fr round Jackson-Pratt closed suction pelvic drain is fed through the 5 mm assistant trocar in the RUQ. The surgeon grasps the drain with the right or left robotic arm and places it in the dependent pelvis. While the surgeon still has a hold of the drain, the 5 mm trocar is removed. The drain is sutured to the skin with a 0 Silk suture. The instruments are removed from the right and left robotic arms. The robotic camera is removed. A Carter-Thomason® laparoscopic port closure system (Cooper Surgical, Inc. Trumbull, CT) is used to close the lateral 12 mm assistant trocar site and the supraumbilical 12 mm camera trocar site. Pneumoperitoneum is discontinued and trocar caps removed to expel gas out of abdomen. Remaining laparoscopic trocars are then removed. Trocar skin sites are closed with running 4-0 monocryl on a PS2 needle. The patients' abdomen and genitals are washed and dried. Histoacryl® Topical Skin Adhesive (Tissue Seal, LLC, Ann Arbor, MI) is placed on all trocar sites. The green 6Fr ureteral

catheters can be removed at this time. The urethral catheter remains in place.

Postoperative Management

Oral and intravenous narcotic pain medications are provided on an as-needed basis. A clear liquid diet is started the evening of surgery. Diet is advanced on postoperative day 1. The Jackson-Pratt drain can be removed on postoperative day 1 assuming output is low. The patient can be discharged home on postoperative day 1 or 2 depending on hospital recovery and convalescence. A cystogram is performed postoperatively between days 7 and 14 to evaluate for water tight bladder closure. Urethral catheter can be removed after cystogram.

Steps to Avoid Common Complications

When performing repair of VVF, irrespective of approach, one must always ensure adequate exposure of the fistula, resect devascularized tissue, have tension-free closure on vagina and bladder sides, perform omental or tissue interposition, and have appropriate drainage while the repair heals. As with any operation, the more frequently the procedure is performed, the greater the consistency and quality of care provided. Having a dedicated team that works together frequently reduces errors and improves efficiency.

Ureteral catheters are placed at the beginning of the case to help with ureteral identification should the fistula be low on the posterior wall next to the intramural ureters. Should the ureter by injured or devascularized, a formal ureteral reimplant should be performed. This can be performed robotically and should be completed with the aid of a ureteral stent (See Chap. 31). With robotic surgery, care must always be taken to ensure that all working robotic arms are within the surgeons view. Good tissue interposition is crucial to minimize risk of VVF recurrence. One should always pay very close attention when passing sutures in and out of the abdomen, as a misplaced needle can be catastrophic in a patient positioned in steep Trendelenburg. The surgical assistant should always be careful and deliberate in passing instruments in and out of the abdomen, as the Iliac artery or vein can be damaged.

References

1. Leng WW, Amundsen CL, McQuire EJ. Management of female genitourinary fistulae: transvesical or transvaginal approach. Urology. 1998;160(6 pt 1):1995–9.
2. Rogers AE, Thiel DD, Brisson TE, Petrou SP. Robotic assisted laparoscopic repair of vesico-vaginal fistula: the extravesicle approach. Can J Urol. 2012;19(5): 6474–6.
3. Sundaram BM, Kalidasan G, Hemal AK. Robotic repair of vesicovaginal fistula: case series of five patients. Urology. 2006;67(5):970–3.
4. Hemal AK, Kolla SB, Wadhwa P. Robotic reconstruction for recurrent supratrigonal vesicovaginal fistulas. J Urol. 2008;180(3):981–5.
5. Daviduik AJ, Meschia C, Young PR, Thiel DD. Robotic-assisted bladder diverticulectomy: assessment of outcomes and modifications of technique. Urology. 2015;85(60):1347–51.
6. Chan ES, Yee CH, Lo KL, Chan CK, Hou SM. Side-docking technique for robot-assisted urologic pelvic surgery. Urology. 2013;82:1300–3.
7. Uffort EE, Jensen JC. Side docking the robot for robotic laparoscopic radical prostatectomy. JSLS. 2011;5:200–2.
8. Gupta NP, Mishra S, Hemal AK, et al. Comparative analysis of outcome between open and robotic surgical repair of recurrent supra-trigonal vesico-vaginal fistula. J Endourol. 2010;24(11):1779–82.

Sijo J. Parekattil and Jamin V. Brahmbhatt

Patient Selection

Selection for the various male infertility procedures is identical to the microsurgical arena. These patients tend to be fairly healthy, younger patients and all the procedures are performed in an outpatient setting. The robotic platform is used as an adjunct only for the microsurgical portion of the procedures once the skin incisions have been made and the tissues are exposed. Thus, body habitus and body mass index considerations are not as important as, for example, in intra-abdominal robotic applications (Video 27.1).

Preoperative Preparation

All patients are given an antibacterial soap to bathe in the night before and the morning of the surgery. Patients are asked to shave their scrotal and pubic areas the night before the surgery. Use of any blood thinners, aspirin, or vitamin E is avoided for 5 days before surgery. A broad-

Electronic supplementary material: The online version of this chapter (doi:10.1007/978-3-319-45060-5_27) contains supplementary material, which is available to authorized users.

S.J. Parekattil, M.D. (✉) • J.V. Brahmbhatt, M.D.
Department of Urology, The PUR Clinic, South Lake Hospital, Orlando Health, 1900 Don Wickham Drive, Clermont, FL 34711, USA
e-mail: sijo@orlandohealth.com

spectrum antibiotic such as cefazolin is administered intravenously 30 min before surgery.

Potential complications such as bleeding and infection are discussed with the patient. Most of the microsurgical procedures require that the patient is absolutely still for a prolonged period of time. The risks of general anesthesia are reviewed with the patient, since this is a comfortable and safe option for most patients. Intravenous sedation may be used in some cases as an alternative.

Operative Setup

At our institution we use the da Vinci® Si-HD system (Intuitive Surgical, Inc., Sunnyvale, CA) with a four-armed technique. Figure 27.1 illustrates the operative setup. The large high definition monitor at the foot of the patient allows the surgical assistant and the surgical nursing team to easily visualize the operative field and prepare instruments and suture for each step of the procedure. The robot is docked perpendicular to the operating table at the patient's side (Fig. 27.1).

Patient Positioning and Preparation

Figure 27.2 illustrates patient positioning for robotic male infertility procedures. The patient is placed in the supine position. The table is placed level (there is no Trendelenberg). The robot is brought in from the

Fig. 27.1 Operative setup for
male infertility robotic
procedures

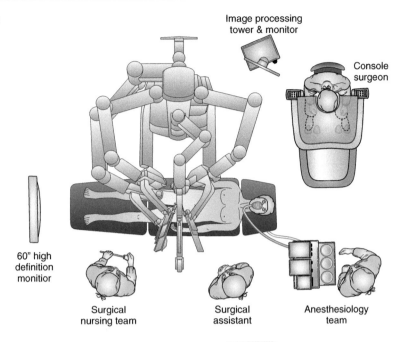

Fig. 27.2 Patient positioning
for robotic male infertility
procedures

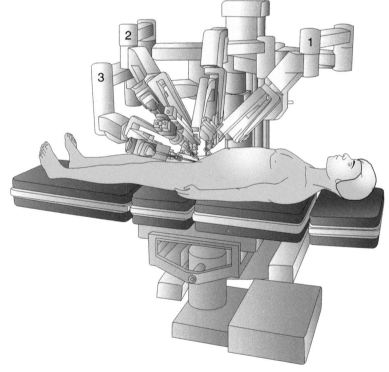

right side of the patient after skin incisions are made
and the operative tissues exposed. The arms of the
patient may be placed alongside (gently wrapped in
the draw sheets) or apart on arm boards with adequate padding to prevent any nerve compression
injuries. Sequential compression devices are placed
on the lower extremities to reduce the risk of deep
venous thrombus formation. A urethral catheter is
generally not utilized, however, if the procedure lasts
more than 2 h, the patient is usually straight catheter-
ized at the end of the procedure to drain the bladder
(before recovering the patient from anesthesia).

Trocar Configuration

The robot is positioned after skin incisions are made and operative tissues are exposed. The robot is used to perform the microsurgical components of the procedure. Since this is an open case, the trocars are loaded only to allow the instruments to function and to stabilize their movements outside the patient's body. Figures 27.2 and 27.3 illustrate the trocar placement and robotic arm placement. It is important to advance the instruments at least 4–5 cm beyond the tip of the trocar when positioning the robotic arms to optimize range of motion. The fourth robotic arm may be placed lateral to the left robotic arm to minimize instrument clashes. The 0° camera lens is used to optimize the visual field during procedures.

Instrumentation and Equipment List

Equipment

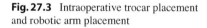

- da Vinci® Si Surgical System (four arm system; Intuitive Surgical, Inc., Sunnyvale, CA)

- EndoWrist® Black Diamond micro needle driver (Intuitive Surgical, Inc., Sunnyvale, CA)
- EndoWrist® Micro Potts Scissors (Intuitive Surgical, Inc., Sunnyvale, CA)
- EndoWrist® Micro bipolar forceps (Intuitive Surgical, Inc., Sunnyvale, CA)
- EndoWrist® curved monopolar scissors (Intuitive Surgical, Inc., Sunnyvale, CA)
- EndoWrist® Black Diamond micro needle driver (Intuitive Surgical, Inc., Sunnyvale, CA)
- InSite® Vision System with 0° lens (Intuitive Surgical, Inc., Sunnyvale, CA)

Trocars

- 12 mm trocar (2)
- 8 mm robotic trocars (3)

Recommended Sutures

- 10-0 nylon suture on double-armed fish-hook needles for vasal mucosal lumen anastomosis
- 9-0 nylon suture on micro needles for vasal muscularis and adventitial lumen anastomosis
- 6-0 prolene suture on micro needle for vasal

Fig. 27.3 Intraoperative trocar placement and robotic arm placement

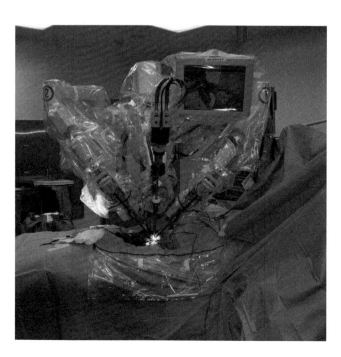

adventitial anastomosis and testicular tunical closure in microscopic TESE
- 3-0 silk suture ties (1.5 in. long) for vein ligation in varicocelectomy

Distal vas deferens is grasped (Fig. 27.4)

- 3-0 chromic suture for dartos layer and subcutaneous skin closure
- 4-0 chromic suture for scrotal skin closure
- 4-0 monocryl suture for subinguinal skin closure

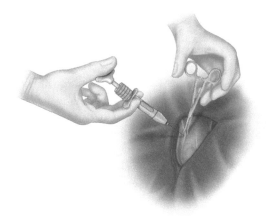

Fig. 27.4 Distal vas deferens is grasped

Instruments Used by the Surgical Assistant

- Micro Doppler Probe (Vascular Technology, Nashua, NH)
- 18-guage angiocatheter on a 10 cm^3 syringe for saline irrigation
- Weck micro sponge sticks
- Colored vessel loops for vessel identification during varicocelectomy
- Titanium or Metal small clips via automatic stapler to hold vessel loops during varicocelectomy

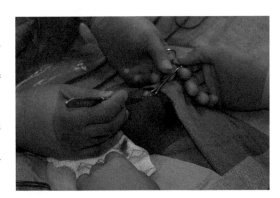

Fig. 27.5 Scrotal incision made over vas deferens

Step-by-Step Technique (Video 27.1)

Robot-Assisted Microsurgical Vasovasostomy

Step 1: Identifying the Distal Vas Deferens

The proximal (testicular side) and distal (beyond vasectomy site) vas deferens around the previous vasectomy site is palpated through the scrotal skin. The distal vas just above the vasectomy site is fixed with a towel clip through the scrotal skin (Fig. 27.4).

Step 2: Incising the Scrotum Over the Vas Deferens

A 1–2 cm vertical incision is made with a #15 blade scalpel inferiorly from the towel clip over the vas (Fig. 27.5).

Step 3: Dissection of the Vas Deferens

The distal and proximal vas ends are dissected free using fine electrocautery and sharp dissection (Fig. 27.6).

Step 4: Transection of the Proximal Vas and Examining Fluid Efflux

The proximal vas is carefully transected with an 11 blade scalpel and the fluid effluxing from the lumen is collected on a glass slide and examined under phase contrast microscopy to assess for the presence of any sperm (Fig. 27.7). If there is sperm found or the efflux is copious and clear or milky, then a vasovasostomy is performed on this side. If the efflux has no sperm and is thick and pasty, then a vasoepididymostomy is performed (described in the next section).

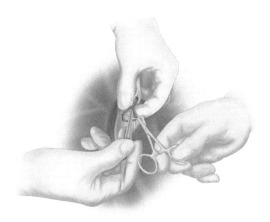

Fig. 27.6 Dissection of the vas deferens

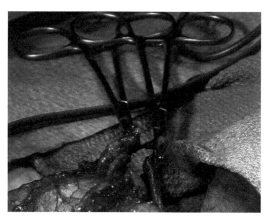

Fig. 27.8 Both ends of the vas brought up to prevent any tension

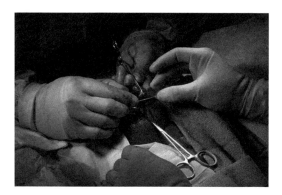

Fig. 27.7 Proximal vas is carefully transected and fluid examined

Step 5: Preparing the Ends of the Vasa for Vasovasostomy

The distal end of the vas is also transected and the two clean ends of the vas are now approximated to each other to allow a tension-free anastomosis. Small hemostats are placed on the adventitia next to each end of the vas to avoid any direct manipulation of the vas (Fig. 27.8). The same procedure is performed on the contralateral scrotal side through the same skin incision. The robot is now positioned to perform the microsurgical vasovasostomy as described in the patient and trocar positioning sections above.

Step 6: Robot-Assisted Microsurgical Vasovasostomy and Vasal Dilation (Table 27.1)

The left side vasovasostomy is performed first. The black diamond micro forceps are loaded on the right and left surgical robot arms. The 0° camera lens is loaded onto the robot camera arm. The micro Potts scissors are loaded onto the fourth robot arm. The two vas ends are placed over a 1/4″ Penrose drain. The assistant now irrigates the field with saline using a 10 cm³ syringe with an 18-gauge angiocatheter tip. Weck sponge sticks are used to dry the field. Each of the lumen of the vas is dilated with the black diamond forceps (Fig. 27.9).

Step 7: Passing the Suture to the Surgeon

The assistant now passes the 9-0 nylon suture in its inner packaging to the surgical field to allow the robot console surgeon to grasp the suture (using the black diamond right hand grasper) and cut it at about 2 in. length using the micro Potts scissors (left hand fourth arm) (Fig. 27.10).

Step 8: Posterior Vasal Muscularis Anastomosis

The 9-0 nylon suture is used to approximate the posterior muscularis layer of the two ends of the vas. The surgeon uses the black diamond forceps in both left and right arms as needle drivers. The fourth arm is used by toggling the surgeons left

Table 27.1 Robot-assisted microsurgical vasovasostomy and vasal dilation: surgeon and assistant instrumentation

Surgeon instrumentation			Assistant instrumentation
Right arm	**Left arm**	**Fourth arm**	• Irrigation syringe
• Black diamond micro needle driver	• Black diamond micro needle driver	Micro potts scissors	• Weck sponge sticks
Endoscope lens: 0°			

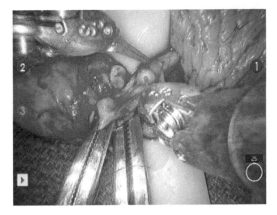

Fig. 27.9 Vas lumen dilated

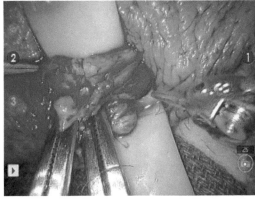

Fig. 27.11 Posterior 9-0 nylon muscularis suture placed

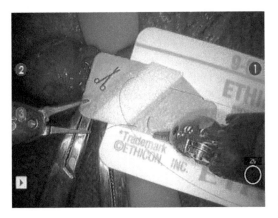

Fig. 27.10 Suture delivered to surgeon

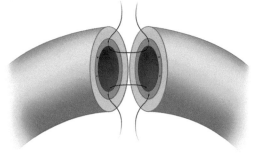

Fig. 27.12 Illustration of placement of the posterior 10-0 nylon sutures in the mucosal layer

arm to use the micro Potts scissors whenever suture needs to be cut (Fig. 27.11).

Step 9: Posterior Vasal Mucosal Lumen Anastomosis

Two or three double-armed 10-0 nylon sutures are now placed to re-anastomose the posterior mucosal lumen of the vas. The sutures are placed inside out to ensure good mucosal approximation. All sutures are placed before they are tied (Figs. 27.12 and 27.13).

Step 10: Anterior Vasal Mucosal Lumen Anastomosis

Three double-armed 10-0 nylon sutures are used to close the anterior mucosal lumen of the vas (Fig. 27.14).

Step 11: Anterior Vasal Muscularis Anastomosis

Five to six 9-0 nylon sutures are used to approximate the muscularis layer of the vasa (Figs. 27.15 and 27.16).

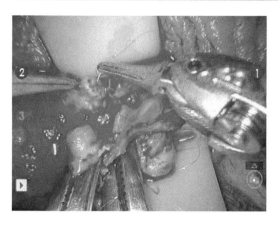

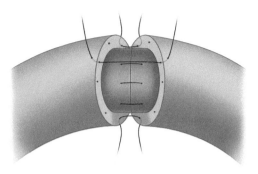

Fig. 27.15 Illustration of placement of anterior 9-0 nylon sutures in the muscularis layer

Fig. 27.13 Intraoperative image of placement of the posterior 10-0 nylon sutures in the mucosal layer

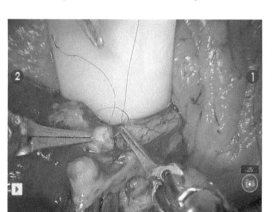

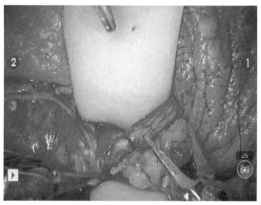

Fig. 27.14 Anterior 10-0 nylon sutures placed in mucosal lumen

Fig. 27.16 Intraoperative image of placement of anterior 9-0 nylon sutures in the muscularis layer

Step 12: Removal of Bridging Scar from the Vasal Ends

The surgical assistant excises the bridging scar tissue between the vasal ends using fine electrocautery (Fig. 27.17).

Step 13: Adventitial Anastomosis

The adventitia is approximated using a 6-0 prolene suture to relieve any tension in the anastomosis and to wrap the repair site (Fig. 27.18).

Step 14: Removal of Penrose Drain Scaffold

The Penrose drain is gently removed from under the repair. The vas is then replaced in the scrotal cavity (Fig. 27.19).

Step 15: Contralateral Vasovasostomy

The same procedure is now performed on the contralateral right side by repositioning the robot away from the patient to the right scrotum. The robotic vasovasostomy is performed on the right side as previously described.

Step 16: Skin Closure

The dartos layer is closed using a running 3-0 chromic suture for the scrotal skin incision. The skin is closed using a 4-0 chromic running suture. Bacitracin ointment is applied to the incision and fluff dressings with an athletic support are applied. An ice pack is carefully applied to the scrotum in the recovery room.

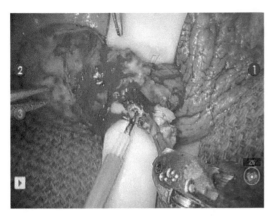

Fig. 27.17 Removal of bridging scar from the vasal ends

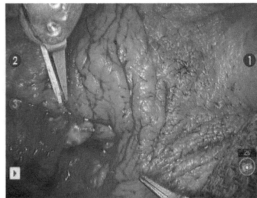

Fig. 27.19 Removal of the Penrose drain from behind the anastomosis

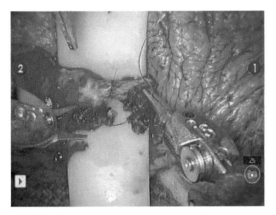

Fig. 27.18 Approximating the adventitia with a 6-0 prolene suture to relieve any tension across the anastomosis and to wrap the anastomosis

Robot-Assisted Microsurgical Vasoepididymostomy

Step 1: Preparing the Epididymis and Docking of the Robot (Table 27.2)

The first four steps of the robot-assisted microsurgical vasovasostomy procedure (listed above) describe the preparation of the vas for vasoepididymostomy. The robotic vasoepididymostomy procedure starts from step 4 above if there is no sperm in the fluid from the proximal vas and the fluid is thick and pasty. The scrotal incision is enlarged by another 1–2 cm inferiorly, the testicle is delivered and the tunica is incised to expose the epididymis. The adventitial layer of the epididymis is incised above the level of epididymal obstruction (blue/grey zone with dilated epididy-

mal tubules above this area). The black diamond micro forceps are used in the left and right robotic arms. An ophthalmologic micro blade is held in the fourth arm with black diamond micro forceps. The 0° camera lens is used. Two 10-0 nylon double-armed suture needles are placed longitudinally through a single epididymal tubule to expose the tubule. This tubule is then incised longitudinally using the micro blade between the two suture needles to create a lumen in the tubule (Fig. 27.20).

Step 2: Vasal Adventitial to Epididymal Tunica Anastomosis

A 6-0 prolene suture is utilized to approximate the adventitia of the epididymis to the muscularis of the vas. This prevents tension in the vas mucosa to epididymal lumen anastomosis (Fig. 27.21).

Step 3: Involution Vasoepididymostomy

The two double-armed 10-0 nylon needles in the epididymal tubule are advanced through and then all four of the needle ends are brought inside out on the vas mucosal lumen to involute the epididymal tubule lumen into the vas lumen (Figs. 27.22, 27.23 and 27.24).

Step 4: Vasal Muscularis to Epididymal Tunica Anastomosis

Five to six 9-0 nylon sutures are placed circumferentially to approximate the muscularis of the

Table 27.2 Preparing the epididymis and docking of the robot: surgeon and assistant instrumentation

Surgeon instrumentation			Assistant instrumentation
Right arm	**Left arm**	**Fourth arm**	• Irrigation syringe
• Black diamond micro needle driver	• Black diamond micro needle driver	Black diamond micro needle driver	• Weck sponge sticks
Endoscope lens: 0°			

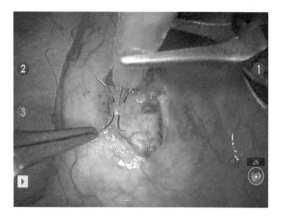

Fig. 27.20 Incision of epididymal tubule

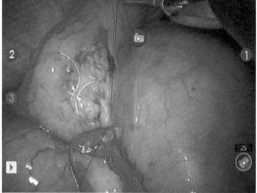

Fig. 27.21 Placement of 6-0 prolene anchor suture

Fig. 27.22 Illustration of the placement of 10-0 double-armed nylon sutures to involute epididymal tubule into the vas mucosal lumen

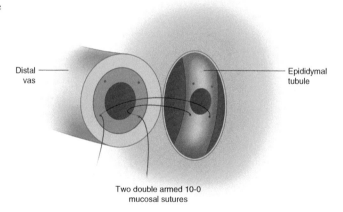

vas to the adventitia of the epididymal tubule (Figs. 27.25, 27.26 and 27.27).

Step 5: Testicular Repositioning and Skin Closure

The testicle and anastomosis are carefully delivered back into the scrotum. The dartos layer is closed using a running 3-0 chromic suture. The skin is closed using a 4-0 chromic running suture. Bacitracin ointment is applied to the incision and fluff dressings with an athletic support are applied. An ice pack is carefully applied to the scrotum in the recovery room.

Robot-Assisted Microsurgical Varicocelectomy

Step 1: Subinguinal Skin Incision

A 2–3 cm subinguinal incision is made over the location of the external inguinal ring (Fig. 27.28).

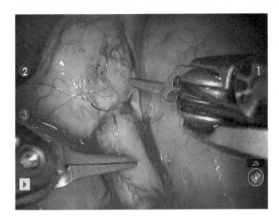

Fig. 27.23 Placement of the 10-0 nylon sutures

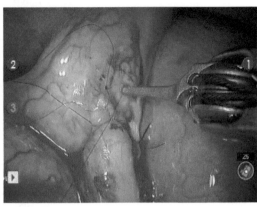

Fig. 27.24 Completion of the 10-0 nylon anastomosis

Fig. 27.25 Illustration of the circumferential placement of the 9-0 nylon vas muscularis to epididymal adventitia sutures

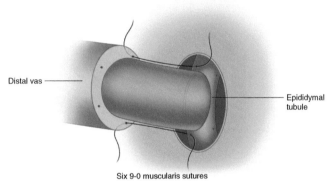

Distal vas

Epididymal tubule

Six 9-0 muscularis sutures

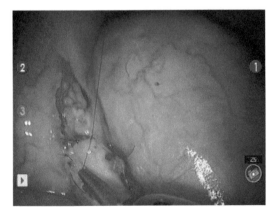

Fig. 27.26 Placement of the 9-0 nylon sutures

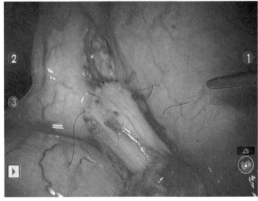

Fig. 27.27 Completion of the 9-0 nylon anastomosis

Step 2: Spermatic Cord Preparation, Robot Docking, and Dissection of Cremasteric Muscles (Table 27.3)

The spermatic cord is carefully dissected and then raised through the skin incision. A ½″ inch Penrose drain is placed under the cord to keep it elevated. A sterile tongue blade is placed through the Penrose drain under the cord to further elevate and spread the cord. The robot is positioned from the patient's right side as described in the beginning of this section. The black diamond micro forceps are used in the right robotic arm, the micro bipolar forceps in the left arm, and the curved monopolar scissors in the fourth arm. For left-sided cases, a 0° camera lens is utilized; for right-sided cases, a 30° (down) lens is utilized. The cremasteric sheath of the spermatic cord in now incised to separate the cord structures (Fig. 27.29).

Step 3: Identification of Testicular Artery with Intraoperative Doppler Ultrasound

Real-time intraoperative Doppler ultrasound is utilized to localize the testicular artery and ensure that no injury occurs to this vessel (Fig. 27.30).

Step 4: Dissection and Ligation of Testicular Veins

Enlarged veins are carefully dissected and then ligated using 3-0 silk suture ties. Doppler ultrasound verification of each vessel before it is ligated is performed to ensure that no arteries are ligated. The curved monopolar scissors or Potts scissors in the fourth arm is used to cut the vessels after being tied (Fig. 27.31).

Step 5: Optional Closure of Spermatic Cord Sheath

After all the veins are ligated, the spermatic cord sheath is now closed using a 6-0 prolene running suture. This step is optional (Fig. 27.32).

Step 6: Release of Spermatic Cord

The tongue blade is removed from within the Penrose. The Penrose is now carefully removed and the spermatic cord is released. The testicle is gently pulled down to retract the spermatic cord completely into the incision (Fig. 27.33).

Step 7: Skin Closure

The skin incision is closed at the subcutaneous layer using a 3-0 polyglactin suture. The skin is closed using a running subcuticular 4-0 monocryl suture and skin glue.

Robot-Assisted Microsurgical Testicular Sperm Extraction (TESE)

Step 1: Scrotal Skin Incision and Robot Docking (Table 27.4)

A vertical 4–5 cm incision is made in the scrotal skin along the median raphe (Fig. 27.34). The

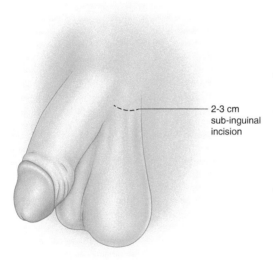

2-3 cm sub-inguinal incision

Fig. 27.28 Subinguinal skin incision

Table 27.3 Spermatic cord preparation, robot docking, and dissection of cremasteric muscles: surgeon and assistant instrumentation

Surgeon instrumentation			Assistant instrumentation
Right arm	**Left arm**	**Fourth arm**	• Irrigation syringe
• Black diamond micro needle driver	• Micro bipolar forceps	• Curved monopolar scissors or micro potts scissors	• Weck sponge sticks
Endoscopelens: 0°			• Micro Doppler probe
			• Colored vessel loops
			• Small metal clip applier

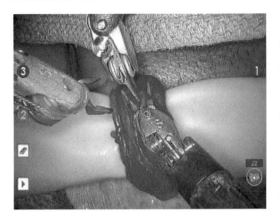

Fig. 27.29 Incision of the cremasteric sheath of the spermatic cord

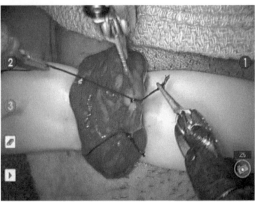

Fig. 27.31 Ligation of enlarged vein in the spermatic cord

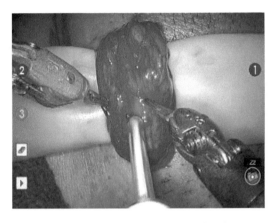

Fig. 27.30 Real-time intraoperative Doppler ultrasound of the testicular artery

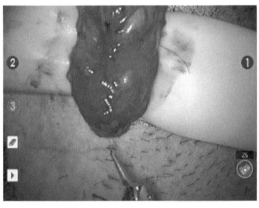

Fig. 27.32 Closure of the spermatic cord sheath

incision is carried down to the tunica vaginalis of the scrotum and then this is incised as well to deliver the testicle. The robot is now positioned from the patient's right side as described in the beginning of this section. The black diamond micro forceps are placed in the left robotic arm. The curved monopolar scissors are placed in the right robotic arm. Another black diamond micro forceps is placed in the fourth arm of the robot.

Step 2: Tunical Incision

Once the testicle is exposed, a 2–3 cm transverse incision in made in the tunica of the testicle to expose the seminiferous tubules (Figs. 27.35 and 27.36).

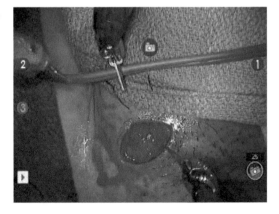

Fig. 27.33 Retraction of the spermatic cord into the incision

Table 27.4 Scrotal skin incision and robot docking: surgeon and assistant instrumentation

Surgeon instrumentation			Assistant instrumentation
Right arm	**Left arm**	**Fourth arm**	• Irrigation syringe
• Black diamond micro needle driver	• Curved monopolar scissors	• Black diamond micro needle driver	• Weck sponge sticks
Endoscope lens: 0°			

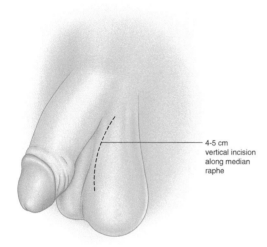

4-5 cm vertical incision along median raphe

Fig. 27.34 Robotic TESE scrotal skin incision

Step 3: Testicular Exploration

The testicular lobules are carefully dissected through to find areas that appear to have larger seminiferous tubules (Fig. 27.37).

Step 4: Testicular Sperm Extraction

These areas are sampled and the specimens are examined immediately with phase contrast microscopy. The assistance of trained embryologists in the operating room optimizes the identification and retrieval of sperm (Fig. 27.38). Sampling is performed till abundant sperm sufficient for multiple assisted reproductive technique cycles are collected. These sperm are either cryopreserved or used for fresh transfer techniques.

Step 5: Deep Dissection

In cases where no sperm are readily found, the testicle is thoroughly evaluated. Dissection through the deeper lobules of the testicle is per-formed and sampling of any enlarged tubules is performed (Fig. 27.39). The additional black diamond micro forceps in the fourth robotic arm can be very helpful in deep dissection to help retract the superficial lobules out of the way as the surgeon is evaluating the deeper lobules.

Step 6: Polar Dissection of the Testicle

In men who have enlarged testicles, or if the upper or lower poles of the testicle cannot be reached through the mid-transverse testicular incision, an additional 1–2 cm transverse incision is made in the upper or lower pole to assess these areas (Fig. 27.40).

Step 7: Tunical and Skin Closure

Once adequate sperm has been retrieved or adequate sampling has been performed, the tunical incisions in the testicle are closed with 6-0 prolene running suture. The testicle in placed back into the tunica vaginalis cavity within the scrotum and this layer is closed with running 3-0 chromic suture. The dartos muscle layer of the scrotum is closed using 3-0 chromic running suture and then the scrotal skin is finally closed with 4-0 chromic running suture. Bacitracin ointment is applied to the incision and fluff dressings with an athletic support are applied. An ice pack is carefully applied to the scrotum in the recovery room.

Postoperative Management

Robotic surgical procedures for male infertility are generally performed as outpatient procedures. A scrotal support is placed prior to awaking the patient. The patient is asked to use this support for 2–3 weeks after surgery. The patient is instructed to have limited activity and have bed rest for

Fig. 27.35 Incisions in the testicle

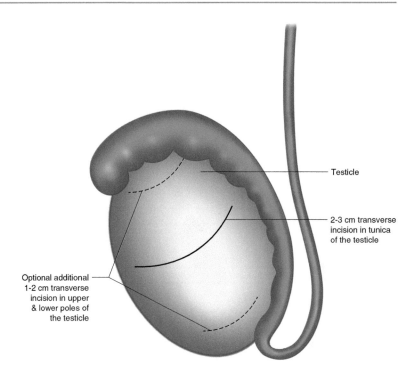

Testicle

2-3 cm transverse incision in tunica of the testicle

Optional additional 1-2 cm transverse incision in upper & lower poles of the testicle

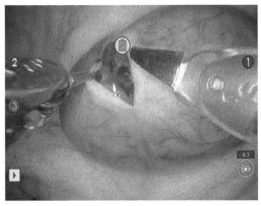
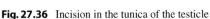

Fig. 27.36 Incision in the tunica of the testicle

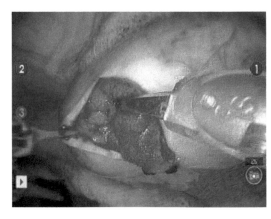

Fig. 27.37 Dissecting through the testicular lobules to identify enlarged seminiferous tubules

about 1 week after surgery. No strenuous activity or heavy lifting is allowed for 4 weeks postoperatively. All patients are provided prescriptions for narcotics for a brief period and antibiotics (keflex) for a few days. Ketorolac is usually avoided to minimize the risk of scrotal hematoma develop-

ment. Patients are instructed to utilize ice packs (30 min on and off) for the first week postoperatively to minimize the use of narcotics. In the case of vasectomy reversal, patients are instructed to refrain from masturbation or ejaculation for at least 6 weeks postoperatively.

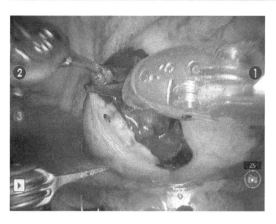

Fig. 27.38 Sampling seminiferous tubules that appear to be enlarged

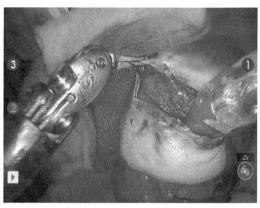

Fig. 27.40 Upper pole testicular dissection and sampling

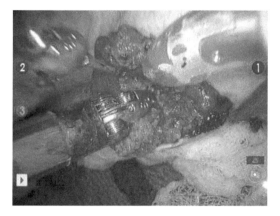

Fig. 27.39 Deeper sampling within the testicle

tissues and thermal injury to the patient. The surgical assistant must pass the sutures to the surgical field with the sutures still in the original inner packing. This allows the surgeon to remove the suture from the pack under magnified vision and reduces that risk of misplacing fine suture and needles.

Cocuzza et al. [1] have recently shown that the systematic use of intraoperative Doppler during microsurgical varicocelectomy can significantly decrease the risk of inadvertent testicular artery injury. Thus, we routinely utilize this modality during varicocelectomy to optimize patient safety.

Steps to Avoid Complications

During robot docking, care must be taken to ensure that the tip of the endoscope lens is at least 5–10 cm away from the operative field as the heat that emanates from the light within the endoscope may potentially cause desiccation of the

Reference

1. Cocuzza M, Pagani R, Coelho R, Srougi M, Hallak J. The systematic use of intraoperative vascular Doppler ultrasound during microsurgical subinguinal varicocelectomy improves precise identification and preservation of testicular blood supply. Fertil Steril. 2010;93(7):2396–9.

Complications and Management of Robotic Lower Urinary Tract Procedures

28

Weil R. Lai and Raju Thomas

Introduction

Robotic-assisted radical prostatectomy (RARP) is the most common robotic pelvic procedure performed in urology. Despite the learning curve associated with laparoscopy and robotic surgery, one has to be cognizant about the potentials of complications at every step. One has to start with careful positioning of patients for robotic surgery because positioning-related complications can be a major post-operative management issue. Intra-operative complications can occur because every prostatectomy or cystectomy (RARC) presents with its own anatomy and challenges, and therefore, vigilance has to be exercised. Post-operative complication rates for RARP have been well documented. In a large series evaluating the complications associated with RARP in 3337 consecutive patients between January 2005 and December 2009 at a tertiary referral center, Agarwal et al. reported an overall complication rate of 9.8%, with 81.3% of the complications occurring within the first 30 days after surgery [1].

W.R. Lai, M.D.
R. Thomas, M.D., F.A.C.S., M.H.A. (✉)
Department of Urology, Tulane University School of Medicine, 1430 Tulane Avenue, SL-42, New Orleans, LA 70112-2632, USA
e-mail: rthomas@tulane.edu

The most common complications during the operative and immediate post-operative periods included anemia requiring blood transfusions (2.2%), urine leak, and ileus. An extensive meta-analysis of peri-operative outcomes and complications after RARP found similar overall complication (9%) and transfusion rates (2%) [2]. The meta-analysis also reported mean rates of lymphocele/lymphorrhea (3.1%), urine leak (1.8%), and reoperation (1.6%). As much of the robotic lower urinary tract surgery done worldwide is RARP, other procedures such as RARC are also gaining momentum. Thus, we will discuss complications associated with these robotic pelvic surgical procedures in this chapter.

The complications encountered with robotic pelvic surgery have been divided into three categories:

1. Positioning-related complications
2. Intra-operative complications
3. Post-operative complications

Positioning-Related Complications

Positioning-related complications are divided into two major categories:

1. Musculoskeletal-related adverse events
2. Non-musculoskeletal-related adverse events

© Springer International Publishing Switzerland 2017
L.-M. Su (ed.), *Atlas of Robotic Urologic Surgery*, DOI 10.1007/978-3-319-45060-5_28

Musculoskeletal-Related Adverse Events

Proper positioning of the patient is crucial in minimizing positioning-related complications. Robotic lower urinary tract surgery is typically performed in concurrent lithotomy and steep Trendelenburg positions to improve lower abdominal exposure and to facilitate gravitational retraction of the bowels. These patients have to be secured to the operating table in such a way as to prevent cephalad sliding of the patient as well as to alleviate against any pressure points on the joints, vasculature, and peripheral nerves. Thus, if the patient is not properly secured to the operating room table, he is at risk of sliding in the Trendelenburg position. Patient slippage with the robot docked can lead to incisional tearing which can potentially risk incisional hernia and increased post-operative abdominal pain [3]. Additionally, if the patient is in stirrups, it can lead to increased pressure at the flexed knee, and one has to be aware of pressure on the common peroneal nerve and additionally the increase in the risk of compartment syndrome of the calves (Fig. 28.1). To reduce these risks secondary to slippage, experts have advised the use of memory foam, gel mattress, or bean bag to secure

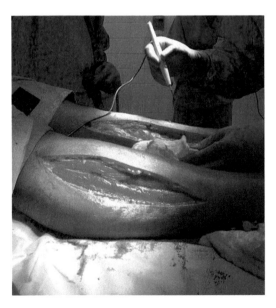

Fig. 28.1 Fasciotomies of both calves to successfully manage compartment syndrome after RARP

the patient to the operating room table. Recently, the marketplace has seen several new kits available which reduce the risk of these complications, albeit at a small price. Examples include the Pink Pad (Xodus Medical Inc., New Kensington, PA), Trendelenburg Stabilizer (Alimed, Dedham, MA), Devon SLT Kit (Covidien, Mansfield, MA), Trendelenburg Positioning Kit (Soule Medical, Lutz, FL), VacuPad (Vmed Technology, Mill Creek, WA), and Badillo/Trendelenburg restraint (Medos Healthcare Solutions, Chelsea, AL). In an observational study of 22 women undergoing robotic-assisted gynecologic procedures in Trendelenburg position (i.e., in a similar position as RARP or RARC), egg-crate pink foam was shown to minimize patient shifting, with a median shift distance of 1.3 cm [4]. These cases were done without shoulder braces or straps, as the use of shoulder braces have been shown to be associated with brachial plexus injuries [5]. We do not recommend shoulder braces or straps.

The two common positions for the lower extremities during RARP include dorsal lithotomy position using stirrups and the split-leg position. The stirrups used in these patients should be multi-positional and adequately padded. While positioning the patients in these stirrups, the use of additional foam material is recommended to prevent any unexpected pressure on the nerves or joints. We recommend taking the additional minute or two to ensure all pressure points are adequately padded. The arms are usually tucked alongside the torso with the hand positioned in a closed fist action holding a roll of foam. This is the least traumatic positioning of the arms, considering that these cases can exceed 2–3 h of operative time. Periodic evaluation of the patient's positioning to ensure lack of slippage and warmth of the extremities is highly encouraged. Positioning is done in conjunction with the anesthesia personnel so as to ensure adequate access to anesthesia-required parenteral lines and monitoring equipment.

In a cohort of 179 patients who underwent RARP or RARC in lithotomy position, 6 (1.68%) developed post-operative lower extremity neuropathy [6]. At 9 months of follow-up, only one of those six patients had neuropathic symptoms limiting daily activities. In comparison, in a retrospective study of 377 patients who underwent RARP in split-leg position, 5 (1.3%) developed lower extremity neuropathy [7]. Three of those patients had femoral mononeuropathy. Those authors noted that they often hyperextended the hips by 20°–25° to allow docking of the da Vinci® S and Si Surgical Systems (Intuitive Surgical, Inc., Sunnyvale, CA). While age, height, weight, and body mass index were not significantly associated with lower extremity neuropathy, the authors noted that the five patients with lower extremity neuropathy had significantly higher mean operative time (496.2 min) compared to the entire cohort (377.9 min).

Extra caution must be exercised with morbidly obese patients. Increased pressure on the brachial plexus must be alleviated with additional padding, and one should not subject the arms to be tightly secured close to the abdomen. Doing so produces additional pressure on the brachial plexus because of subaxillary fat pad in these patients. These patients may not be able to grip objects with their hands for 24–72 h. Such obese patients have impaired arterial oxygenation and have higher risk for hypercapnia [8]. In rare instances, one may be faced with a diagnosis and management dilemma of rhabdomyolysis. In an epidemiologic study of major urologic procedures from the National Inpatient Sample from 2003 to 2011, 870 (0.1%) of 1,016,074 patients developed rhabdomyolysis [9]. Independent risk factors included younger age, male sex, diabetes, chronic kidney disease, obesity, and perioperative bleeding (which were noted to serve as a surrogate for prolonged operating room time).

At our institution, we secure the patient on the operating room table, which is lined with egg-crate foam. The foam is taped to the table to prevent slippage of egg-crate foam. To minimize the risk of brachial plexus injury, we immobilize the patient's upper extremities to his side with a draw sheet that is sandwiched in place between the egg-crate foam and the operating room table. Chest straps are not routinely used or recommended. The elbows and wrists are supported in neutral position to reduce the risk of ulnar and radial nerve injuries, respectively. With the da Vinci® Si robot, the patient's lower extremities

are placed in low lithotomy position with Yellofin® stirrups (Allen Medical, Acton, MA) to allow robot docking between the patient's lower extremities. With the da Vinci® Xi robot, we use the split-leg position in those cases without hyperextending the hips, as the robot docks to the patient from the side without the risk of collision between the split-leg positioners and the robot arms. These split-leg positioning attachments are standard with most operating room tables but must be special ordered. Details regarding appropriate positioning are described in the chapter on patient positioning in this book.

Non-musculoskeletal Adverse Events

Even though the majority of adverse events are related to the musculoskeletal system, one must be cognizant of other potential complications associated with positioning. In cases of prolonged Trendelenburg position, robotic pelvic surgery has also been associated with laryngeal edema, posterior ischemic optic neuropathy, and sanguinous otorrhea [10–12]. Cardiac-related complications have been a concern in these patients not only from the positioning but also age and pre-operative cardiac status concerns.

Patients who are morbidly obese or those with COPD may have pulmonary-related complications because of prolonged Trendelenburg position [13].

Intra-operative Complications

A variety of intra-operative complications can be encountered. This is not only during one's robotic learning curve but also in the very experienced robotic surgeon as well [14]. This is thought to be because the experienced robotic surgeon is willing to tackle the more complex and complicated cases, and these patients are prone to their own share of complications. The intra-operative complications can be broadly categorized as follows:

1. Vascular complications
2. Non-vascular complications

Vascular Complications

Amongst the most acute of intra-operative complications are those associated with vascular injuries and subsequent hemorrhage. Injuries to the vasculature may present themselves during key components of robotic lower urinary tract surgery. Vascular injury can be initiated as early as initiating pneumoperitoneum because of the Veress needle and trocars, which can cause both vascular and non-vascular complications. We highly recommend following all recommended practice guidelines for creation of safe pneumoperitoneum. Safe use of Veress needle technique or the Hassan technique are recommended for initiating pneumoperitoneum. Following this, we recommend that the trocars be placed as much as possible under direct laparoscopic guidance.

The most common vascular injury associated with robotic pelvic surgery is laceration of the inferior epigastric vessels during trocar placement [15]. This type of injury is often recognized intra-operatively and is usually caused during insertion of the pararectus trocars [16]. If the bleeding is persistent despite judicious use of electrocautery and/or clipping, Stolzenburg et al. recommend placing a suture through the abdominal wall (with a straight needle or with the Carter-Thomason device) to encircle the bleeding vessel and tying down the suture extracorporeally for hemostasis [16]. The suture can then be removed from the skin on post-operative day 2 unless it is a self-absorbing suture. Even without bleeding during initial placement of the trocars, the authors have also advised laparoscopic inspection of all trocar sites for active bleeding after trocar removal, at the end of the procedure, and at lower pneumoperitoneum pressures, as unrecognized small bleeders can lead to large abdominal and/or secondary scrotal hematomas.

The incidence of major vascular injuries from Veress needle and initial trocar placement is approximately 0.1% [17]. The common iliac vessels and the aorta are the most common major vessels associated with Veress needle placement [18, 19]. To decrease the risk of overshooting the needle and puncturing those blood vessels, Sotelo et al. recommended advancing the Veress needle into the patient at a 45° angle to avoid advancing the needle too far into the abdomen [17]. For obese patients, they recommend using a 90° angle placement to traverse the more considerable skin to fascia distance.

Another source of vascular injury during robotic pelvic procedures is during standard and extended pelvic lymphadenectomy. This can be secondary to avulsion, laceration, or electrocautery injury. In rare cases, failure of laparoscopic insulation can lead to arcing of the electrocautery current directly into the vessel and lead to a thermal injury [20]. Venous injuries, such as laceration of the external iliac vein, can be controlled with the combination of temporary increase in pneumoperitoneum (to 20–25 mmHg), moderate compression of the vein, judicious compression and suctioning of the operative field by the bedside assistant, and precise suturing. A mini-laparotomy pad may be used to not only mop up excess blood in the operative field but also tamponade the operative site, while limiting the loss of pneumoperitoneum from the bedside assistant's suction irrigator. Suturing can be accomplished with the use of a non-absorbable monofilament suture (e.g., 4-0 polypropylene) tagged with Lapra-Ty (Ethicon, Somerville, NJ) (a.k.a., "rescue stitch") to minimize the need to physically tie down the suture. This maneuver saves precious time in the face of ongoing active bleeding. Other groups, such as Sotelo et al., advocated the use of a multifilament suture (e.g., 4-0 polyglactin on a RB-1 needle) with Hem-o-lok clip (Teleflex, Morrisville, NC) attached to the end, as such sutures have minimal memory and may be easier to throw in a continuous fashion [17]. Such simple technical modifications can save significant time in controlling bleeding. In the cases of bleeding that could not be controlled laparoscopically, the surgeon should be prepared to convert to an open procedure.

While significant bleeding from the dorsal venous complex (DVC) is less commonly encountered in RARP and RARC compared to open surgical techniques, the excess blood can stain the tissue planes as visualized with the robot and prolong the operative time by making other parts of the operation more visually difficult to complete, especially during the suturing of the vesico-urethral anastomosis or intracorporeal urinary diversion. As the bleeding is venous, it can be decreased and/or tamponaded with a temporary increase in pneumoperitoneal pressure. This is followed by oversewing the cut end of the DVC with a 2-0 polyglactin suture in a continuous running fashion. For persistent bleeding, an alternative is to apply pressure against the DVC such as with an inflated urethral catheter balloon (placed on stretch extracorporeally) for a few minutes to initiate hemostasis and to allow time for the appropriate sutures and hemostatic agents to be prepared, such as SURGICEL (Ethicon, Somerville, NJ) on the back table.

Of course, in patients where bleeding is anticipated, one need not to be reminded that adequate type and cross-matched blood products should be available, and appropriate informed consent should be obtained beforehand. Moreover, post-operative management will have to include close post-operative monitoring, including possible intensive unit care.

Non-vascular Complications

These complications can also start with the initiation of pneumoperitoneum and up until the end of the robotic surgical procedure. Once again, vigilance and early recognition are the keys to successful outcomes of unexpected complications.

Bowel Injury

Patients who have had prior abdominal surgery are at higher risk for intestinal adhesions and thereby should be managed accordingly. These patients need to be consented for the risk of enterotomies and the need for consultation with other surgical services as needed.

In patients who have had prior abdominal surgery, we recommend using an off-site trocar placement under direct laparoscopic visual guidance. Using the visual obturator is highly recommended. Once the peritoneum has been entered, then the abdomen is inspected for adhesions, and these are then released using instruments through the off-site trocar and additional trocars (which can be placed under direct visualization). If intestinal adhesions are excessive and overly time-consuming, the robotic surgeon may need to resort to other non-robotic techniques to complete the procedure. If lysis of intestinal adhesions is successfully completed, then the procedure is continued after appropriate placement of the robotic trocars and subsequent docking of the robot.

In order of gravity, the duodenum, colon, and the rest of the small bowel are to be respected for the most severe of complications, during trocar placement. Therefore, prompt diagnosis is crucial, and furthermore obtaining prompt general surgery consultation in managing these bowel injuries is highly recommended. More often than not, these bowel complications may present themselves post-operatively, and at this point general surgery consultation is considered mandatory.

As we focus on robotic pelvic surgery, the most common complications are injuries to the rectum. Patients who have undergone prior radiation treatment, obesity, and locally extensive cancers make rectal entry a risky possibility. During RARC, there is an additional risk of entry into the cecum and colon, especially during the extended pelvic lymph node dissection. Diagnosing rectal entry intra-operatively and making appropriate management decisions will decrease any post-operative complications such as vesico-rectal fistula, ensuing sepsis from fecal spillage, and so forth.

In a comprehensive review of records from six institutions (representing 6650 patients who underwent transperitoneal RARP), 11 patients sustained rectal injury (0.17%) [21]. Eight of those cases were recognized intra-operatively, with five being noted during dissection of the posterior prostate plane, one during seminal vesicle dissection, and two during apical dissection. In those recognized cases, they were full-thickness lacerations, with seven done with sharp scissors and one done by stapler inclusion. All eight underwent primary repair, with one patient additionally also received diverting colostomy per general surgery recommendations. The majority of the repairs were performed with at least a 2-layer closure with 3-0 polyglactin suture, thorough pelvic irrigation, and testing of the repair with air insufflation. Of the seven managed with primary repair alone intra-operatively, one did require a subsequent colostomy and suprapubic catheter to allow spontaneous closure of the recto-urethral fistula. None of the recognized cases developed pelvic abscess.

In contrast, the three patients whose rectal injuries were not recognized at the time of RARP all presented with signs and symptoms of recto-urethral fistula [21]. The fistulae were confirmed with Gastrografin enemas, were managed with diverting ileostomy or colostomy, and later repaired in delayed fashion with rectal advancement flap 16–24 weeks later. Interestingly, the authors report no long-term adverse effect on urinary and bowel function.

Of note, we use the rectal air insufflation technique to diagnose or rule out rectal injury intra-operatively. For this test, we recommend using a 20 French red rubber catheter into the rectum via the anus. The bedside assistant fills the pelvis with irrigation fluid. Air is then instilled through the red rubber tubing into the rectum. If air bubbles are seen in the irrigation fluid in the pelvis, then rectal injury is suspected, which is then located and treated with the suturing technique described above.

In the series from Henry Ford reported by Kheterpal et al., 10 of 4400 patients (0.2%) who underwent RARP sustained rectal injury [22]. All ten injuries were recognized intra-operatively and repaired primarily without tissue interposition. The one patient who subsequently developed recto-urethral fistula underwent a diverting colostomy, followed by delayed repair of the fistula. The same patient also had gross fecal spillage at the time of the rectal injury. Potential risk factors identified in these patients included six who underwent wide excision at the time of surgery because of concern for rectal wall involvement and one who previously had undergone saturation biopsies with 85 cores.

In the non-robotic literature, the incidence of rectal injury in open and laparoscopic radical prostatectomy is similarly low. In the series of 11,452 patients who underwent radical prostatectomy (10,183 radical retropubic, 1269 laparoscopic) at Johns Hopkins from 1997 to 2007,

rectal injuries were present in 12 (0.12%) and 6 (0.47%) of the open and laparoscopic cases, respectively [23]. Sixteen of the injuries were identified intra-operatively and repaired primarily in multiple layers without fecal diversion. Omental interposition was used in four cases. Of the cases without omental interposition, two developed recto-urethral fistula and were either managed with prolonged urethral catheterization (9 weeks) or diverting colostomy with delayed fistula repair. For the two injuries not identified intra-operatively, they presented as recto-urethral fistula within 4 days in the post-operative period. Those cases were initially managed with prolonged urethral catheterization and fecal diversion with colostomy. Because of persistence of the fistula, both underwent rectal advancement flap to repair the fistula.

In a Japanese radical prostatectomy database of 35,099 patients who underwent either open or laparoscopic radical prostatectomy, 151 (0.43%) were identified with rectal injury [24]. The authors studied whether mechanical bowel preparation provided benefit in reducing perioperative morbidity associated with rectal injury. Based on multivariate analyses (on infectious complications, requirement of delayed colostomy formation, length of stay, and cost), they found no difference between groups of patients who used mechanical bowel preparation and those who did a non-mechanical bowel preparation.

Though we do not routinely recommend preoperatively bowel preparation in our institution, we do recommend patients at risk for rectal injury to undergo bowel preparation.

Obturator Nerve Injury

The rate of obturator nerve injury cited in literature ranges from 0.2 to 5.7% [25]. Sequelae of the obturator nerve injury include adductor weakness, thigh paresthesia, leg pain, and abnormal leg movements and gait. In a retrospective case series of 3558 prostatectomies from a high-volume institution (of which 2531 and 1027 represent extraperitoneal laparoscopic radical prostatectomy and RARP, respectively), Gozen et al. identified five cases of obturator nerve injury [25]. In all cases, the injuries occurred during pelvic lymphadenectomy and were recognized intra-operatively. In three patients who underwent laparoscopic radical prostatectomy, surgical clips were inadvertently placed on the proximal aspect of the obturator nerve. Those clips were removed once the injury was recognized. (We recommend caution during removal of the clips, as exertion of too much force might lead to avulsion of the nerve.) In two patients who underwent RARP, the nerve was transected proximally. The nerve edges were re-approximated with 6-0 polypropylene monofilament suture in a tension-free manner. Additional treatments, if needed, included physiotherapy and neurotropic medication (in the form of Vitamin B6) in four and three of the patients, respectively. Per the authors, these patients did recover with no permanent defects in obturator nerve function, but they did not define the duration of their follow-up period.

Based on the literature review carried out by the same authors, they proposed a risk map for obturator injury during pelvic lymphadenectomy, with 7 and 2 cases from other groups representing injuries to the proximal and distal parts of the obturator nerve, respectively [25]. The proximal aspect of the obturator nerve was defined as the location where the nerve passes close to the external iliac vein and the internal iliac artery. Their recommendation was to retract the peritoneum more medially to increase visualization of this space. Sotelo et al. recommended medial retraction of the nodal packet and visualization of the nerve prior to placement of clips on the nodal packet [3]. The clips should be placed in parallel to the nerve to decrease the risk of clipping the nerve.

Ureteral Injury

Ureteral injuries may occur during posterior bladder neck dissection, extended pelvic lymphadenectomy, dissection of the seminal vesicles, and isolation of the vas deferens. Caution should be exercised when performing RARP in patients with large prostates and those with large median lobe. The J-hooking or displacement of the lower ureter by the intravesical median lobe or large posterior lobes can make the lower ureters vulnerable to injury during dissection. Mechanisms of injury have included transection, ligation, and edema of the ureteral orifice. In an updated series of 6442 patients who underwent RARP at Henry Ford, three patients sustained ureteral injuries that were not recognized intra-operatively [26]. One patient had presented with persistent high fluid output from a trocar site, with subsequent CT scan demonstrating a right distal ureteral injury with associated urinoma. The injury was initially managed with percutaneous drainage of the urinoma, percutaneous nephrostomy tube, and ureteral stent placement. After removal of the stent, the ureter re-obstructed, and he underwent robot-assisted ureteral reimplant approximately 1 year after RARP. The second patient sustained left ureteral transection during salvage prostatectomy and later underwent an open transureteroureterostomy. The third patient developed anuria secondary to transection of the transplant kidney's ureter. This was repaired with robotic ureteroureterostomy during the same hospital admission.

In comparison, in a large laparoscopic radical prostatectomy series of 2164 patients from Heilbronn, three patients sustained ureteral injuries [27]. These injuries were all recognized intra-operatively, with two complete and one partial transections. The two complete transection injuries likely occurred at the time of bladder neck dissection, with one patient having prior episodes of prostatitis (making identification of vas deferens difficult) and the other patient with a large prostate with associated intravesical median lobe. The partial transection occurred during extended pelvic lymphadenectomy. The complete transections were managed with Lich-Gregoir extravesical ureteral reimplant. The partial transection was managed with primary repair. Using the posterior approach for RARP can place the lower ureters at risk for injury, and caution is advised.

In conclusion, maintaining a high index of suspicion in certain patients such as the big median lobe of the prostate can minimize any possible trauma of the lower ureter. Unusual and persistent output from the drainage tube post-RARP should raise an alarm about possible ureteral or vesico-urethral etiologies. As mentioned above, prompt diagnosis is important, and if detected intra-operatively, can be corrected with known options such as end-to-end ureteroureterostomy, ureteral reimplantation, and so forth. If the diagnosis is delayed exceeding 7 days, then one has to decide on the most appropriate treatment algorithm. This is when proximal drainage with nephrostomy tube and drainage of any urinoma precedes any definitive subsequent surgical management.

Post-operative Complications

Post-operative complications may present themselves in short order or in a delayed fashion. These delayed complications may be for bleeding, bowel related, lymphoceles, or urinary tract related.

Bleeding

Robot pelvic surgeries rarely present with post-operative and post-discharge bleeding episodes. However, slow hemorrhage can be encountered in the face of mild to moderate oozing in the pelvis or from active small bleeding points. With the widely popular nerve-sparing radical prostatectomy and nerve-sparing radical cystectomy, the use of thermal energy is discouraged. This can lead to some bleeding points which may accelerate in the post-operative period and can present with abdominal pain and ileus accompanied by anemia, hypotension, weakness, etc. Diagnosis is made with serial hematocrits and imaging with CT scans. Management decisions such as further observation, percutaneous drain versus open incisional evacuation of hematoma and placement of drains will have to be decided on an individual to individual patient basis. With the increasing use of anti-coagulants for cardiac-related diagnoses, a slow oozing hematoma can become symptomatic in short order and complicate management decisions. Prompt diagnosis and management strategy will need to be individualized.

Additionally, one must not ignore other sources of bleeding such as trocar sites, injury to the inferior epigastric vessels, and during the pelvic lymphadenectomy procedure. Appropriate imaging will diagnose these sites.

Vesico-urethral Anastomotic Leak

One of the remarkable accomplishments of RARP has been the dramatic decrease in the incidence of bladder neck contractures and disruption of the vesico-urethral anastomosis [28, 29]. This decreased incidence is attributed to the superior 3-D visualization and precise vesico-urethral anastomosis. Despite this, the incidence of vesico-urethral anastomotic leak ranges from 3.5 to 13.6% [29]. The precise incidence of persistent anastomotic leak remains unknown as it is rare. The most common area of the leak is at the posterior aspect of the anastomosis. Risk factors include an incompletely reapproximated mucosa-to-mucosa anastomosis, pelvic hematoma (which distracts the anastomosis), and migration of surgical clip. Prolonged leak has been associated with scar formation and development of bladder neck contracture. The leak classically presents with increased surgical drain output and with elevated drain fluid creatinine. Urine leak may also present as contrast extravasation on fluoroscopic cystogram done as part of the surgeon's post-prostatectomy protocol to identify patients at risk of developing the urinary leak (e.g., extensive bladder neck reconstruction of a wide bladder neck, large median lobes, etc.). Figure 28.2a, b show an example of a leak involving the posterior aspect of the vesico-urethral anastomosis.

The initial management of the vesico-urethral anastomotic leak is prolonged urethral catheter drainage. If the gap, between the urethra and the bladder, associated with the leak is large, there may be concern for the morbidity of prolonged catheter drainage and the increased risk of the development of significant bladder neck contracture. In those cases, one may consider early laparoscopic or robotic repair of the vesico-urethral anastomosis. In a series of 391 laparoscopic radical prostatectomy patients [30], 14 patients

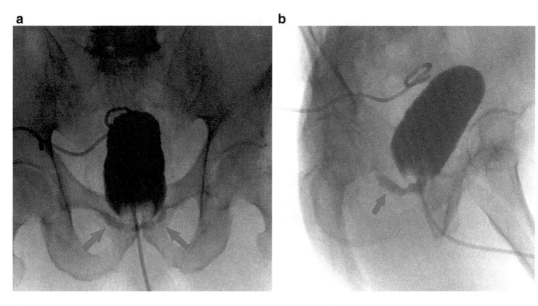

Fig. 28.2 Post-RARP cystogram in (**a**) anterior–posterior and (**b**) oblique view shows persistent contrast leak (as denoted by *red arrows*), even after percutaneous drainage of urinoma

had persistent anastomotic leak. While ten did heal with "conservative measures", the remaining four underwent laparoscopic repair of the vesico-urethral anastomosis. Those four patients had at least one-third dehiscence of the anastomosis noted at the time of the repair. Two of the patients had their entire anastomosis redone.

Alternatively, other authors have reported their experience with endoscopic management of such persistent leaks. Lim et al. reported their technique of cystoscopic injections of *N*-butyl-2-cyanoacrylate, followed by fibrin glue injection into the gaps contributing to the anastomotic leaks [29]. Out of 1828 patients in their series, they performed the injections in ten patients (0.5%) because of persistent or large anastomotic leaks. The urethral catheters remained in place for an additional average of 7.7 days. At a follow-up of approximately 2 years, all ten patients remained fully continent.

Bladder Neck Contracture

Though RARP has markedly decreased the incidence of bladder neck contracture (BNC), it still ranges from 0 to 2% for RARP [28], with risk factors including post-operative gross hematuria, vesico-urethral anastomotic leak, and urinary retention. Treatment options include urethral dilation and transurethral incision of BNC. Some groups, including Vanni et al., have demonstrated efficacy with intralesional injection of mitomycin C after performing transurethral cold knife incision of BNC [31]. In their series, the 18 patients had at least one failed prior transurethral incision procedure. At a median follow-up of 1 year after the procedure with intralesional mitomycin C injection, a patent bladder neck was noted in 13 patients (72%) after 1 procedure, 3 patients after 2 procedures (17%), and 1 after 4 procedures.

In comparison, Eltahawy et al. performed intralesional triamcinolone injection into BNC after incising the BNC with a Holmium laser at 3 and 9 o'clock positions [32]. In the 24 patients represented in the series, most had prior attempts to treat the BNC, including dilation, internal urethrotomy, transurethral resection, and open surgery. Their technique was performed once in 17 patients and twice in 7 patients. At a mean follow-up of 2 years, 19 (83%) had patent bladder neck. These management strategies are at risk of causing urinary incontinence, and thus, 11 of those patients in this series ultimately underwent artificial urinary sphincter placement for urinary incontinence.

Symptomatic Lymphoceles

Lymphoceles can present in patients who undergo pelvic lymphadenectomy during RARP or RARC. They can be asymptomatic or present with a multitude of symptoms, including fevers, leukocytosis, acute onset urinary incontinence (from extrinsic compression on the bladder), venous thrombolic events, lower extremity edema, pelvic pain, and superficial phlebitis. In a series of 521 patients who had undergone extended pelvic lymphadenectomy as part of RARP, 46 (9%) were diagnosed with lymphoceles on screening pelvic ultrasound 1 month after surgery [33]. The lymphoceles remained persistent on screening ultrasound in 11 patients at both 3 and 6 months after surgery. Of the 46 patients, 13 had symptoms associated with the lymphoceles. In that group, the most common sign and symptoms were fevers and leukocytosis suggestive of infection. Seven patients underwent percutaneous drain placement with Interventional Radiology, with the drains left indwelling until the drain output was ≤ 10 mL/ day. None of those patients required repeat treatment. Based on these results, the authors recommended a screening pelvic ultrasound at 3 months after surgery (as a majority of the lymphoceles resolved between 1 and 3 months), and that if lymphoceles are detected, they recommended percutaneous drainage because of the higher risk of developing infected lymphoceles.

One recently published technique to pre-emptively reduce the risk of lymphocele formation comes from a group from Lahey clinic [34]. They proposed the creation of a peritoneal interposition flap to the bladder to reduce the risk of lymphocele formation. In their prospective series of 155 patients undergoing RARP with pelvic lymphadenectomy, 78 patients underwent the additional interposition flap procedure. Lymphocele formation was noted in 11.6% in the standard group (with mean detection time of lymphocele approximately 30 days) and 0% in the flap group.

Surgical Clip Migration

Migration of surgical clip into the bladder and/ or the vesico-urethral anastomosis is rare but has been reported in case reports [35–40] and noted in personal operative experience. When the clip gets in contact with urine, it can serve as a nidus for stone formation and urinary tract infections [37]. Symptoms of surgical clip migration into the urinary tract may include gross hematuria, intractable lower urinary tract symptoms, and persistent urinary tract infections. In a retrospective review of records for the etiology of BNC in 524 RARP patients [36], the authors found that two BNC cases were associated with Hem-o-lok clip migration into the vesico-urethral anastomosis, one BNC case associated with Hem-o-lok clip migration into the bladder, and one non-BNC case (i.e., anastomotic leak) with Hem-o-lok clip migration into the bladder neck. These clips were removed endoscopically.

In more unusual scenarios, there have been case reports of repeat Hem-o-lok migration into the bladder on a single patient [40], metal clip migration into the bladder [39], and Hem-o-lok migration into the rectum [38]. For the case of the clip in the rectum, the clip was incidentally found as a rectal mass on colonoscopy done for evaluation of colonic diverticulosis.

We highly recommend prompt removal of each surgical clip when it could not be deployed, and therefore all the loose clips in the abdomen should be removed to prevent any migration.

Discussion

The key to minimizing complications during pelvic robotic surgery is to anticipate them before they occur. Some patients, especially those undergoing salvage prostatectomy, are at higher risk of complications. Even before making the first incision, it is important to properly position the patient on the operating room table to minimize the risk of positioning-related injuries. For surgical teams new to robotics, commercial products exist to simplify patient positioning for procedures requiring steep Trendelenburg position, which is often done for robotic lower urinary tract procedures. For readers interested in additional information on positioning-related injuries in robotic urologic procedures, comprehensive literature reviews may be found in Sukhu and Krupski [41] and Akhavan et al. [5].

In our opinion, many of the intra-operative complications can be avoided with attention to detail on surgical anatomy. Because there is no haptic feedback with the robot, it is important to be vigilant of the intracorporeal locations of the robotic instruments, the bedside assistant's instruments, and suture needles, as such sharp objects can easily lacerate or avulse pelvic structures when they are passed in and out of the body. When using electrocautery, it is important to make sure that the insulation is intact and also important to keep the conductive parts of the instruments away from major vessels, bowel, ureter, and nerve. When such structures are injured (especially the rectum), repair of such organs should be performed at the time of surgery to minimize post-operative sequelae.

Like open and laparoscopic surgery, robotic surgery has its share of post-operative complications in RARP and RARC cases. In the case of large vesico-urethral anastomotic leaks with concern for anastomotic disruption, re-exploration with robotics or laparoscopy in the early post-operative period may be done safely to repair or redo the anastomosis. The rate of BNC has decreased with robotic surgery. However, the quality of the literature in the management of post-prostatectomy BNC has been limited to small case series, and the treatment of BNC raises the risk for the development of persistent urinary incontinence. For pelvic lymphoceles after pelvic lymphadenectomy, the majority will resorb within 3 months after surgery. The ones that persist have a higher risk of infection and should be drained. Presence of gross hematuria, worsening lower urinary tract symptoms, and/or prolonged vesico-urethral anastomotic leaks should raise suspicion for migration of surgical clip into the lower urinary tract.

Conclusion

Overall complications from robotic lower urinary tract surgery remain low. As the most common robotic pelvic procedures performed in urology, RARP and RARC have been well studied and documented in its positioning-related, intra-operative, and post-operative complications. Many of these complications can also be found in other lower urinary tract procedures (e.g., cystectomy, ureteroneocystostomy, nephroureterectomy with bladder cuff excision, simple prostatectomy). In addition to having a skilled surgeon with expert knowledge of pelvic anatomy, a surgical team dedicated to robotic surgery helps to minimize these complications and manage them in a safe manner when they occur.

References

1. Agarwal PK, Sammon J, Bhandari A, Dabaja A, Diaz M, Dusik-Fenton S, et al. Safety profile of robot-assisted radical prostatectomy: a standardized report of complications in 3317 patients. Eur Urol. 2011;59(5):684–98.
2. Novara G, Ficarra V, Rosen RC, Artibani W, Costello A, Eastham JA, et al. Systematic review and meta-analysis of perioperative outcomes and complications after robot-assisted radical prostatectomy. Eur Urol. 2012;62(3):431–52.
3. Sotelo RJ, Haese A, Machuca V, Medina L, Nunez L, Santinelli F, et al. Safer surgery by learning from complications: a focus on robotic prostate surgery. Eur Urol. 2016;69(2):334–44.
4. Klauschie J, Wechter ME, Jacob K, Zanagnolo V, Montero R, Magrina J, et al. Use of anti-skid material and patient-positioning to prevent patient shifting during robotic-assisted gynecologic procedures. J Minim Invasive Gynecol. 2010;17(4):504–7.
5. Akhavan A, Gainsburg DM, Stock JA. Complications associated with patient positioning in urologic surgery. Urology. 2010;76(6):1309–16.
6. Manny TB, Gorbachinsky I, Hemal AK. Lower extremity neuropathy after robot assisted laparoscopic radical prostatectomy and radical cystectomy. Can J Urol. 2010;17(5):5390–3.
7. Koc G, Tazeh NN, Joudi FN, Winfield HN, Tracy CR, Brown JA. Lower extremity neuropathies after robot-assisted laparoscopic prostatectomy on a split-leg table. J Endourol. 2012;26(8):1026–9.
8. Nishio I, Noguchi J, Konishi M, Ochiai R, Takeda J, Fukushima K. The effects of anesthetic techniques

and insufflating gases on ventilation during laparoscopy. Masui. 1993;42(6):862–6.

9. Pariser JJ, Pearce SM, Patel SG, Anderson BB, Packiam VT, Shalhav AL, et al. Rhabdomyolysis after major urologic surgery: epidemiology, risk factors, and outcomes. Urology. 2015;85(6):1328–32.

10. Phong SV, Koh LK. Anaesthesia for robotic-assisted radical prostatectomy: considerations for laparoscopy in the Trendelenburg position. Anaesth Intensive Care. 2007;35(2):281–5.

11. Weber ED, Colyer MH, Lesser RL, Subramanian PS. Posterior ischemic optic neuropathy after minimally invasive prostatectomy. J Neuroophthalmol. 2007;27(4):285–7.

12. Cohen A, Ledezma-Rojas R, Mhoon E, Zagaja G. Bloody otorrhea after robotically assisted laparoscopic prostatectomy. Can J Urol. 2015;23(3):7834–5.

13. Kilic OF, Borgers A, Kohne W, Musch M, Kropfl D, Groeben H. Effects of steep Trendelenburg position for robotic-assisted prostatectomies on intra- and extrathoracic airways in patients with or without chronic obstructive pulmonary disease. Br J Anaesth. 2015;114(1):70–6.

14. Ellison JS, Montgomery JS, Wolf Jr JS, Hafez KS, Miller DC, Weizer AZ. A matched comparison of perioperative outcomes of a single laparoscopic surgeon versus a multisurgeon robot-assisted cohort for partial nephrectomy. J Urol. 2012;188(1):45–50.

15. Stolzenburg JU, Truss MC. Technique of laparoscopic (endoscopic) radical prostatectomy. BJU Int. 2003; 91(8):749–57.

16. Stolzenburg JU, Rabenalt R, Do M, Lee B, Truss MC, McNeill A, et al. Complications of endoscopic extraperitoneal radical prostatectomy (EERPE): prevention and management. World J Urol. 2006;24(6):668–75.

17. Sotelo R, Nunez Bragayrac LA, Machuca V, Garza Cortes R, Azhar RA. Avoiding and managing vascular injury during robotic-assisted radical prostatectomy. Ther Adv Urol. 2015;7(1):41–8.

18. Catarci M, Carlini M, Gentileschi P, Santoro E. Major and minor injuries during the creation of pneumoperitoneum. A multicenter study on 12,919 cases. Surg Endosc. 2001;15(6):566–9.

19. Schafer M, Lauper M, Krahenbuhl L. Trocar and Veress needle injuries during laparoscopy. Surg Endosc. 2001;15(3):275–80.

20. Lorenzo EI, Jeong W, Park S, Kim WT, Hong SJ, Rha KH. Iliac vein injury due to a damaged Hot Shears tip cover during robot assisted radical prostatectomy. Yonsei Med J. 2011;52(2):365–8.

21. Wedmid A, Mendoza P, Sharma S, Hastings RL, Monahan KP, Walicki M, et al. Rectal injury during robot-assisted radical prostatectomy: incidence and management. J Urol. 2011;186(5):1928–33.

22. Kheterpal E, Bhandari A, Siddiqui S, Pokala N, Peabody J, Menon M. Management of rectal injury during robotic radical prostatectomy. Urology. 2011;77(4):976–9.

23. Roberts WB, Tseng K, Walsh PC, Han M. Critical appraisal of management of rectal injury during radical prostatectomy. Urology. 2010;76(5):1088–91.

24. Sugihara T, Yasunaga H, Horiguchi H, Matsuda S, Fushimi K, Kattan MW, et al. Does mechanical bowel preparation ameliorate damage from rectal injury in radical prostatectomy? Analysis of 151 rectal injury cases. Int J Urol. 2014;21(6):566–70.

25. Gozen AS, Aktoz T, Akin Y, Klein J, Rieker P, Rassweiler J. Is it possible to draw a risk map for obturator nerve injury during pelvic lymph node dissection? The Heilbronn experience and a review of the literature. J Laparoendosc Adv Surg Tech A. 2015;25(10):826–32.

26. Jhaveri JK, Penna FJ, Diaz-Insua M, Jeong W, Menon M, Peabody JO. Ureteral injuries sustained during robot-assisted radical prostatectomy. J Endourol. 2014;28(3):318–24.

27. Teber D, Gozen AS, Cresswell J, Canda AE, Yencilek F, Rassweiler J. Prevention and management of ureteral injuries occurring during laparoscopic radical prostatectomy: the Heilbronn experience and a review of the literature. World J Urol. 2009;27(5):613–8.

28. Wang R, Wood Jr DP, Hollenbeck BK, Li AY, He C, Montie JE, et al. Risk factors and quality of life for post-prostatectomy vesicourethral anastomotic stenoses. Urology. 2012;79(2):449–57.

29. Lim JH, You D, Jeong IG, Park HK, Ahn H, Kim CS. Cystoscopic injection of N-butyl-2-cyanoacrylate followed by fibrin glue for the treatment of persistent or massive vesicourethral anastomotic urine leak after radical prostatectomy. Int J Urol. 2013;20(10):980–5.

30. Castillo OA, Alston C, Sanchez-Salas R. Persistent vesicourethral anastomotic leak after laparoscopic radical prostatectomy: laparoscopic solution. Urology. 2009;73(1):124–6.

31. Vanni AJ, Zinman LN, Buckley JC. Radial urethrotomy and intralesional mitomycin C for the management of recurrent bladder neck contractures. J Urol. 2011;186(1):156–60.

32. Eltahawy E, Gur U, Virasoro R, Schlossberg SM, Jordan GH. Management of recurrent anastomotic stenosis following radical prostatectomy using holmium laser and steroid injection. BJU Int. 2008;102(7):796–8.

33. Keskin MS, Argun OB, Obek C, Tufek I, Tuna MB, Mourmouris P, et al. The incidence and sequela of lymphocele formation after robot-assisted extended pelvic lymph node dissection. BJU Int. 2016;118(1):127–31.

34. Lebeis C, Canes D, Sorcini A, Moinzadeh A. Novel technique prevents lymphoceles after transperitoneal robotic-assisted pelvic lymph node dissection: peritoneal flap interposition. Urology. 2015;85(6):1505–9.

35. Banks EB, Ramani A, Monga M. Intravesical Weck clip migration after laparoscopic radical prostatectomy. Urology. 2008;71(2):351.e3–4.

36. Blumenthal KB, Sutherland DE, Wagner KR, Frazier HA, Engel JD. Bladder neck contractures related to the use of Hem-o-lok clips in robot-assisted laparoscopic radical prostatectomy. Urology. 2008;72(1):158–61.

37. Tugcu V, Polat H, Ozbay B, Eren GA, Tasci AI. Stone formation from intravesical Hem-o-lok clip migration

after laparoscopic radical prostatectomy. J Endourol. 2009;23(7):1111–3.

38. Wu SD, Rios RR, Meeks JJ, Nadler RB. Rectal Hem-o-lok clip migration after robot-assisted laparoscopic radical prostatectomy. Can J Urol. 2009;16(6):4939–40.

39. Kadekawa K, Hossain RZ, Nishijima S, Miyazato M, Hokama S, Oshiro Y, et al. Migration of a metal clip into the urinary bladder. Urol Res. 2009;37(2):117–9.

40. Tunnard GJ, Biyani CS. An unusual complication of a Hem-o-lok clip following laparoscopic radical prostatectomy. J Laparoendosc Adv Surg Tech A. 2009;19(5):649–51.

41. Sukhu T, Krupski TL. Patient positioning and prevention of injuries in patients undergoing laparoscopic and robot-assisted urologic procedures. Curr Urol Rep. 2014;15(4):398. doi:10.1007/s11934-014-0398-1.

Part IV

Robotic Pediatric Surgery

Pediatric Robotic Pyeloplasty

29

Bruce J. Schlomer and Craig A. Peters

Patient Selection

With the increased use of prenatal ultrasound, most ureteropelvic junction obstructions (UPJO) are found prior to birth. Initial workup usually includes a renal ultrasound and voiding cystourethrogram (VCUG) as well as nuclear renal scan, especially when significant UPJO is suspected. Prophylactic antibiotics are controversial but are usually recommended at least until the above-mentioned studies are done. If at any point the child develops urinary tract infections or nausea/vomiting/flank pain suspected to be related to the UPJO, then robotic pyeloplasty is offered to the parents and patient as an interventional option. Also, if on initial nuclear renal scan, the differential kidney function is <40% or there has been a change of >10% differential, then intervention with robotic pyeloplasty is discussed. Non-resolving high-grade hydronephrosis becomes a relative indication based on parental and physician preferences.

Electronic supplementary material: The online version of this chapter (doi:10.1007/978-3-319-45060-5_29) contains supplementary material, which is available to authorized users.

B.J. Schlomer, M.D. • C.A. Peters, M.D. (✉)
Pediatric Urology, Children's Medical Center,
University of Texas Southwestern,
1935 Medical District Dr., Mail Stop F4.04, Dallas,
TX 75235, USA
e-mail: craig.peters@childrens.com

Preoperative Preparation

Bowel Preparation

All patients are asked to have a clear liquid (apple juice, Jell-o, ginger ale, water, broth) diet for 24 h before surgery to reduce the bulk of stool in the colon. They are also given one Dulcolax® suppository (Boehringer Ingelheim Pharmaceuticals, Inc., Ridgefield, CT) for the night before.

All patients and family should understand that the procedure will be performed by the surgeon, not the "robot." Some families are concerned about this issue due to misinformation or misperceptions. The family and patient should always be made aware of the possibility of conversion to open surgery. This is emphasized to be used in cases where the ability to complete the procedure or safety are of concern. If a family is hesitant or unwilling to consent to this uncertainty, open surgery should be recommended so they know what to expect. The risks of general anesthesia must also be presented to the patient. Other risks that need to be relayed during informed consent include the realization that renal function could remain the same or even worsen after surgery. Continued flank pain, nausea, vomiting, recurrent urinary tract infections, urine leak, injury to abdominal structures, and the possibility of reoperation for recurrent obstruction also need to be discussed.

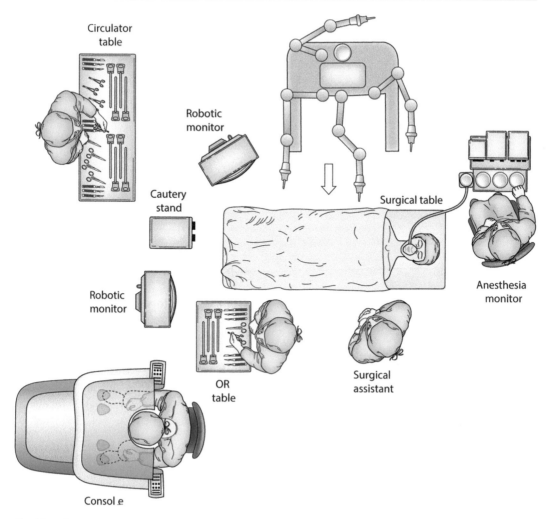

Fig. 29.1 Operating room setup for right robotic pyeloplasty demonstrating standard configuration of operating room personnel and equipment

Operative Setup

At our institution we use the da Vinci® with a three-armed technique. An assistant and the scrub technician are positioned on the side of the patient opposite the robot. Video monitors are placed for easy viewing by all team members. Overhead views of the room setup for right and left pyeloplasties are shown, respectively, in Figs. 29.1 and 29.2. We recommend having a dedicated operating room and operating room team for the da Vinci® to decrease room turnover delays and possible equipment damage due to transporting the robot from one room to another.

Patient Positioning and Preparation

Initially, place the patient in lithotomy or froglegged position for retrograde ureteral stent (if planned) and urethral catheter placement. Next, place the patient in modified flank with a 30° wedge under the ipsilateral side where the pyeloplasty will be performed with padding and tape across chest and thighs. Folded towels and tape are placed over the patient's arms but under the abdomen (Fig. 29.3). If an antegrade stent placement is planned, we will prep in the penis in males and prep in a pre-placed council catheter in females. Flexible cystoscopy with a pediatric flexible cystoscope or ureteroscope can then

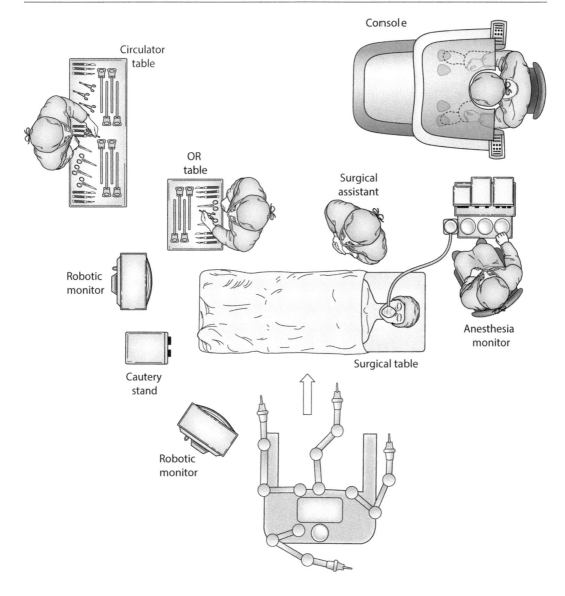

Fig. 29.2 Operating room setup for left robotic pyeloplasty demonstrating standard configuration of operating room personnel and equipment

be performed to confirm stent position, in females using a wire to gain access to bladder can make the process faster. Rotate the table so that the patient's abdomen is flat while obtaining trocar access, then rotate to 60° (30° wedge plus 30° table rotation) just prior to docking the robot. The anesthesia team should place an NG or OG tube before access.

Trocar Configuration

The trocar configuration for a left versus right pyeloplasty is basically a mirror image of itself (Figs. 29.4 and 29.5). One notable difference is the possibility of needing an extra trocar for liver retraction during a right pyeloplasty, although the renal pelvis can be accessed adequately in most

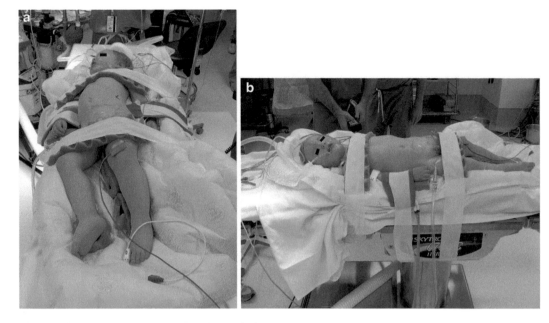

Fig. 29.3 Patient positioning shown for a left pyeloplasty. (**a**) Inferior view. (**b**) Side view

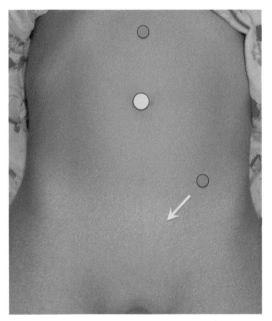

Fig. 29.4 Trocar configuration for left robotic pyeloplasty. *Yellow port* is for the camera and the *orange ports* are for the working instruments. In smaller children, very large renal pelvis or a lower renal pelvis, the inferior working port should be moved inferior and medial as indicated by the *yellow arrow*

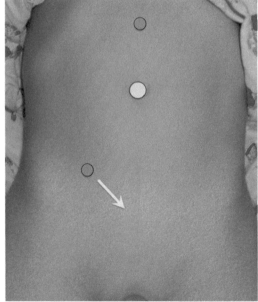

Fig. 29.5 Trocar configuration for right robotic pyeloplasty. *Yellow port* is for the camera and the *orange ports* are for the working instruments. In smaller children, very large renal pelvis or a lower renal pelvis, the inferior working port should be moved inferior and medial as indicated by the *yellow arrow*

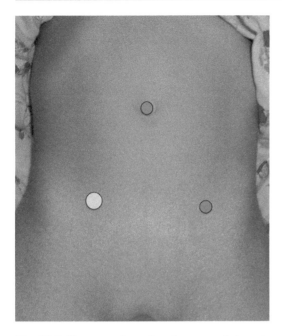

Fig. 29.6 Trocar configuration for concealed ports (HIDES) technique. *Yellow port* is for the camera and the *orange ports* are for the working instruments

cases without this extra trocar. We typically use the 5 mm trocars for robotic arm access when the patient is younger than 8–10 years, otherwise the 8 mm trocars are used.

Alternatively, the trocar configuration can be shifted caudally so that the camera port is a couple finger breadths above the pubic bone and the working ports placed at umbilicus and in ipsilateral lower quadrant. This would eliminate the scar in the midline of upper abdomen in place of a scar in low midline presumably under the underwear line (Fig. 29.6) [1].

We have found that an assistant port is not needed in most cases. If an assistant port is needed, we typically place this lateral to the contralateral rectus muscle between the upper working port and camera port.

Instrumentation and Equipment List

Equipment

- da Vinci® Surgical System (3-arm system; Intuitive Surgical, Inc., Sunnyvale, CA)

- EndoWrist® Monopolar Hook, 5 or 8 mm (Intuitive Surgical, Inc., Sunnyvale, CA)
- EndoWrist® Maryland Dissector, 5 or 8 mm (Intuitive Surgical, Inc., Sunnyvale, CA)
- EndoWrist® DeBakey Forceps, 5 or 8 mm (Intuitive Surgical, Inc., Sunnyvale, CA)
- EndoWrist® Curved Monopolar Scissors, 8 mm (Intuitive Surgical, Inc., Sunnyvale, CA)
- EndoWrist® Round Tip Scissors, 5 or 8 mm (Intuitive Surgical, Inc., Sunnyvale, CA)
- EndoWrist® Needle Driver, 5 or 8 mm (Intuitive Surgical, Inc., Sunnyvale, CA)
- InSite® Vision System with 30° lens (Intuitive Surgical, Inc., Sunnyvale, CA)

Trocars

- 10 mm trocar
- 8 mm robotic trocars (2, if child is older than 6 years)
- 5 mm robotic trocar (option for smaller patients, although the 5 mm instruments are not as precise or dexterous as the 8 mm instrument) (usually 2; if you need liver retraction during a right pyeloplasty then you will need 3, or a 3.5 mm cannula)
- Recommended sutures:
- Preplaced fascial box stitch: 2-0 or 3-0 polyglactin suture
- Hitch stitch: 2-0 or 3-0 PDS on SH needle
- Pyeloplasty anastomosis: Monocryl or polyglactin suture, size depending upon age (we use: neonate to 6 months 6–0, 6 months to teen years 5–0; Length of suture approximately 12–14 cm).
- Skin Closure: 4-0 or 5-0 monocryl suture

Recommended Ureteral Stent

- Ages 0–6 years: 3.7 Fr double J and 0.028 in. wire; length: age plus 10 cm
- Ages over 6: 4.8 Fr double J and 0.035 in. wire
- Alternatively can use 4.8 Fr double J stent in all ureters that accommodate this size and only use smaller size stent in ureters that will not.

Instruments Used by the Surgical Assistant

- Maryland grasper
- Suction irrigator device
- Cold scissors for cutting sutures

Step-by-Step Technique (Video 29.1)

Step 1: Ureteral Stent Placement

With the patient in lithotomy or frog-legged position, perform a retrograde pyelogram and place ureteral stent on the affected side up to the area of obstruction. Leave a string attached to the ureteral stent and tape string to inside of leg. This permits removal in clinic at a later date without cystoscopy.

Alternatively, ureteral stent placement can be done antegrade later in the operation (see below). This allows possible improved ease of dissection of renal pelvis and UPJ with pelvis still full and not drained by ureteral stent.

We do not perform a retrograde pyelogram for typical cases of UPJ obstruction with classic imaging findings in which an antegrade stent is planned. However, we have a low threshold to obtain a retrograde pyelogram and will always obtain one if history is unusual or if anatomy is atypical (fusion or malrotation, concern for ureteral polyp, etc.).

Step 2: Abdominal Access and Trocar Placement

For a left UPJO, reposition the patient in a left modified flank position as noted above; then, for trocar placement, rotate the table so the patient's abdomen is 0°. The 10 mm camera trocar is placed in the area of the umbilicus, using the Hasson open technique with 2-0 polyglactin suture on a UR-6 needle or a 3-0 polyglactin suture on a CT-2 needle bent accordingly. These are pre-placed fascial box stitches (used later for closure). Working trocars are then placed sharply under direct vision after pre-placing the fascial box stitches. Rotate the patient to approximately 60° (30° from table rotation and 30° from the wedge placed earlier) and dock the robot.

Step 3: Access to Ureteropelvic Junction (Table 29.1)

Displace small bowel away from the surgical field and toward the midline. At this point, if the UPJO is obvious through the mesentery, then a transmesenteric approach may be followed to gain access to the ureteropelvic junction (UPJ) (Fig. 29.7). Otherwise, continue as below. Retract the colon medially and identify the white line of Toldt. Pick up the parietal peritoneum and make an incision extending from above the likely area of the renal pedicle to the aortic bifurcation using the hook electrocautery (5 mm or 8 mm) or hot scissors (8 mm) (Fig. 29.8). Expose the ureter distal to the UPJ being careful not to jeopardize the segmental blood supply in the area. Also, be aware of the gonadal vessels running parallel to the ureter in this area. Dissect proximally along the ureter. As the kidney is approached, look for lower pole vessels that are common with this anomaly (Fig. 29.9). Isolate and dissect around these vessels. Do not ligate them as this could lead to segmental renal ischemia. Before excessive mobilization, determine whether the vessels appear to be contributing to the obstruction if possible. This will determine

Table 29.1 Access to ureteropelvic junction: surgeon and assistant instrumentation

Surgeon instrumentation		Assistant instrumentation
Right arm	**Left arm**	• Suction-irrigator
• Monopolar hook tip cautery (5 or 8 mm)	• Maryland dissector (5 mm cold; 8 mm bipolar)	
• Monopolar scissors (8 mm)		
Endoscope lens: 30° down		

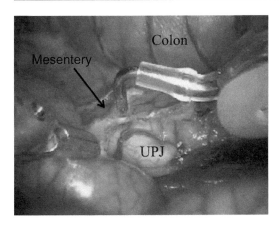

Fig. 29.7 Transmesenteric approach. In children, as opposed to adults, a transmesenteric approach to the kidney is reasonable and usually preferred. The thin colonic mesentery is seen here just above the ureteropelvic junction (UPJ)

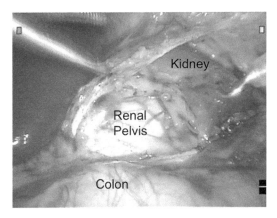

Fig. 29.8 Retraction of the colon. The colon is retracted medially and dissection is made along the *white line* of Toldt exposing the underlying kidney and renal pelvis

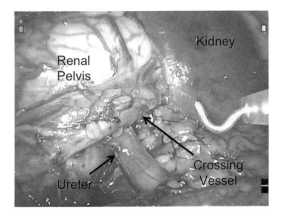

Fig. 29.9 Crossing vessels are often encountered, as shown here

whether ureteral transposition anterior (usually) to the vessels is needed.

Step 4: Placement of Hitch Stitch (Table 29.2)

Once adequate access to the renal pelvis, UPJ, and proximal ureter is achieved (Fig. 29.10), switch the monopolar electrocautery out for a needle driver. Pass a 2-0 or 3-0 PDS stitch on an SH needle that has been partially straightened through the abdominal wall lateral to the kidney and just at the costal margin. Place this stitch through the medial aspect of the renal pelvis, back out the abdominal wall and then hold in place with a hemostat. This is used as a "hitch-stitch" to elevate the renal pelvis, providing stability and lifting the operative field out of any collection of urine or blood (Fig. 29.11). Tension is adjustable.

Table 29.2 Placement of hitch stitch: surgeon and assistant instrumentation

Surgeon instrumentation		Assistant instrumentation
Right arm	**Left arm**	• Suction-irrigator
• Needle driver	• Maryland dissector	
Endoscope lens: 30° down		

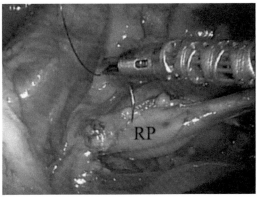

Fig. 29.10 Exposure of the renal pelvis (RP), UPJ, and proximal ureter. Obtaining excellent mobilization of the UPJ at this point in the surgery helps later on during the anastomosis

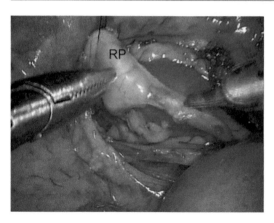

Fig. 29.11 Hitch stitch. The hitch stitch should easily lift the renal pelvis and proximal ureter. *RP* renal pelvis

Table 29.3 Pyelotomy and ureteral spatulation: surgeon and assistant instrumentation

Surgeon instrumentation		Assistant instrumentation
Right arm	**Left arm**	• Suction-irrigator
• Round tip scissors (5 mm) or hot shears (8 mm)	• Maryland dissector	
Endoscope lens: 30° down		

Step 5: Pyelotomy and Ureteral Spatulation (Table 29.3)

Place the scissors in the right hand. Pyelotomy is performed with a diamond-shaped incision into the renal pelvis superomedial to inferolateral below the UPJ (Fig. 29.12). Use the remaining renal pelvis on the ureter as a handle for manipulation. Perform a lateral spatulating incision of the ureter through the UPJ and distally to where the ureter appears normal in diameter (Fig. 29.13).

Step 6: Anastomosis of Renal Pelvis to the Ureter (Table 29.4)

With a needle driver in the right hand, begin anastomosis of the renal pelvis to the ureter using a running Monocryl or polyglactin suture (6-0 for infants to age 6 months, 5-0 to teens; 12–14 cm in

length) passed through one of the working trocars. The first stitch is placed in the vertex of the ureteral spatulation and the posterior side of the collecting system is usually sewn first (Figs. 29.14 and 29.15). This depends upon the orientation of the pelvis and the relative angle of the instruments. After completion of the first side, the ureteral stent can be positioned into the pelvis. If a stent has not been pre-placed, a stent is fed over a wire passed through the abdominal wall through a 14 or 16 G angiocatheter and down the ureter (Fig. 29.16). Length should be generous to ensure bladder positioning. We like to tie the second side anastomotic suture at vertex of ureteral spatulation and pelvis prior to placing antegrade stent. Cystoscopy can then be performed by the assistant to confirm distal coil of stent is in good position in bladder while the second side anastomosis is started. The redundant renal pelvis tissue is removed (Fig. 29.17). The second side is anastomosed from the vertex of the ureteral spatulation upward and any extra opening of the pelvis is closed with this suture as well. The distal part of the ureter used as a handle can be excised at this time. A third suture may be needed if the pyelotomy is large (Figs. 29.18 and 29.19). All sutures are cut by temporarily replacing the needle driver with the round tip scissors or conventional laparoscopic scissors. Needles and suture are brought in and removed through the right 5 or 8 mm robotic trocar by the assistant with the laparoscopic needle driver.

Postoperative Management

Postoperatively, the patient is placed on 1.5× maintenance fluids, usually D5 ½ NS. He or she is started on a clear liquid diet with orders to advance as tolerated. Perioperative antibiotics (usually cefazolin 50–100 mg total over 24 h divided in three doses) are continued for 24 h. Pain control includes morphine (0.1 mg/kg IV) every 3–4 h p.r.n. pain as well as Tylenol® with codeine elixir (0.5–1 mg/kg po) every 4 h p.r.n. pain, or an equivalent. At our institution, we usually also place orders for oxybutynin (0.1 mg/kg po initially post-op) every 8 h p.r.n. bladder

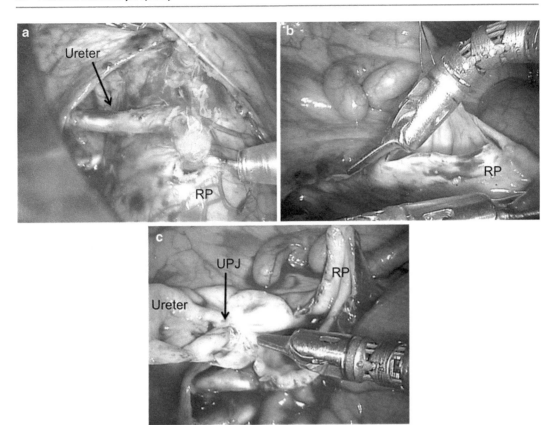

Fig. 29.12 Pyelotomy (right kidney shown). (**a**) The pyelotomy is begun by making a sharp incision superomedial on the renal pelvis just below the hitch stitch. *RP* renal pelvis. (**b**) The incision is continued inferolaterally. (**c**) A tight UPJ was noted in this patient as seen here

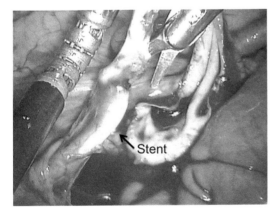

Fig. 29.13 Lateral spatulating incision of the ureter. Notice the preplaced stent seen through the wall of the ureter

Table 29.4 Anastomosis of renal pelvis to the ureter: surgeon and assistant instrumentation

Surgeon instrumentation		Assistant instrumentation
Right arm	**Left arm**	• Suction-irrigator
• Needle driver	• Maryland dissector	• Laparoscopic needle driver
• Round tip scissors (5 mm) or hot shears (8 mm)		
Endoscope lens: 30° down		

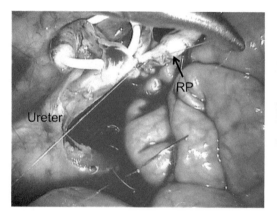

Fig. 29.14 A vertex stitch is placed to start the anastomosis. *RP* renal pelvis

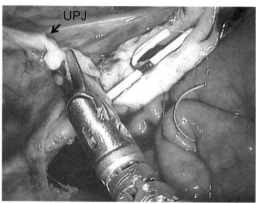

Fig. 29.17 Removal of UPJ. The UPJ is removed and sent for pathology

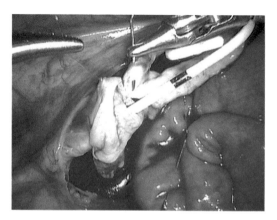

Fig. 29.15 Posterior running stitch. The first running stitch demonstrated here is usually placed posteriorly as it eases anterior running stitch placement later

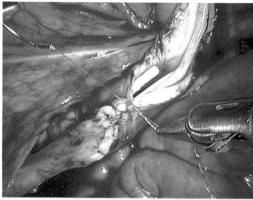

Fig. 29.18 Completion of anterior anastomosis. The anterior anastomosis is now completed. In case of a large pyelotomy, once this anastomosis is complete, the running stitch or additional sutures may be used to close the pyelotomy

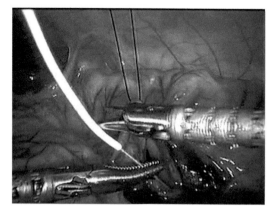

Fig. 29.16 Antegrade stent placement. After the first running stitch is completed, antegrade stent placement can be performed if a stent was not placed initially. An angiocatheter (14 G) is passed through the abdominal wall and the needle removed. A.035 guide wire loaded with a 4.7 Fr. Double J stent is passed through the angiocatheter and guided into the ureter. The stent and wire are guided inferiorly under direct vision using the robotic instruments

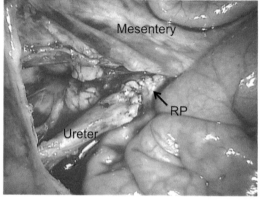

Fig. 29.19 Depiction of completed pyeloplasty. *RP* renal pelvis

spasms as well as ondansetron (0.1 mg/kg) every 8 h p.r.n. nausea. We also have used ketorolac (0.5 mg/kg IV, maximum 15 mg IV) every 6 h × 6 doses routinely without any issues in cases with a normal contralateral kidney. On the morning of postoperative day 1, the oxybutynin is held and the patient's urethral catheter is removed. If a string is attached to the stent, the urethral catheter should be gently twisted to avoid dislodging the stent. Most patients are ready for discharge by the afternoon on postoperative day 1.

Special Considerations

Patient selection is always a critical factor in any surgical procedure and the issue of patient age and size is often raised with respect to robotic procedures. With increasing experience, the authors have not limited use of robotic pyeloplasty to any specific age group. While it may be argued that infants may not benefit as much as older children and adolescents, it is unclear where to draw a line. Our experience and others have confirmed that robotic pyeloplasty may be safely and efficiently performed in children of all ages [2–6].

Use of the vascular hitch procedure is often considered and has been reported to some degree [7], yet it seems to be more of a compromise surgery than the best means to correct a clinical problem with a high degree of certainty. It is not recommended in any way due to the unpredictability of its outcome [8].

In most children, transmesenteric access to the UPJ is readily accomplished, particularly with the aid of the "hitch-stitch" [5, 9]. If the mesentery is thick with fat and the ureter is not easily visualized, the left colon should be reflected. For right-sided pyeloplasty, the hepatic flexure is reflected medially to expose the pelvis. In most cases, the pelvis may be exposed without using a liver retraction trocar.

Retroperitoneal robotic pyeloplasty in children can be successfully performed, even in smaller children [10] with the theoretical advantage of not violating the peritoneal space. The positioning can be challenging but this should be equally effective.

Some authors have performed a stent-less pyeloplasty with reported satisfactory results [11, 12]. We have used this in highly selected cases without problems, but it remains our preference to use a double J stent, which eliminates the need for a wound drain and limits the risk of extravasation or temporary clinically significant obstruction.

Reoperative pyeloplasty follows the same steps, but may require more aggressive exposure to permit safe mobilization of the renal pelvis [13].

Steps to Avoid Complications

The major concerns specific to pyeloplasty include searching for a crossing vessel, both to avoid injury as well as recognizing its presence and determining if the ureter needs to be transposed. Patients with an intrarenal pelvis require care during mobilization of the pelvis to avoid injury to the hilar vessels. Avoid excessive mobilization of the ureter to limit devascularization and limit direct grasping of the ureter to the excess pelvis used as a handle.

References

1. Gargollo PC. Hidden incision endoscopic surgery: description of technique, parental satisfaction and applications. J Urol. 2011;185(4):1425–31.
2. Autorino R, Eden C, El-Ghoneimi A, Guazzoni G, Buffi N, Peters CA, et al. Robot-assisted and laparoscopic repair of ureteropelvic junction obstruction: a systematic review and meta-analysis. Eur Urol. 2014;65(2):430–52.
3. Avery DI, Herbst KW, Lendvay TS, Noh PH, Dangle P, Gundeti MS, et al. Robot-assisted laparoscopic pyeloplasty: multi-institutional experience in infants. J Pediatr Urol. 2015;11(3):139.e1–5.
4. Kutikov A, Nguyen M, Guzzo T, Canter D, Casale P. Robot assisted pyeloplasty in the infant-lessons learned. J Urol. 2006;176(5):2237–9; discussion 9–40.
5. Lee RS, Retik AB, Borer JG, Peters CA. Pediatric robot assisted laparoscopic dismembered pyeloplasty: comparison with a cohort of open surgery. J Urol. 2006;175(2):683–7; discussion 7.
6. Minnillo BJ, Cruz JA, Sayao RH, Passerotti CC, Houck CS, Meier PM, et al. Long-term experience and outcomes of robotic assisted laparoscopic pyeloplasty in children and young adults. J Urol. 2011;185(4):1455–60.

7. Gundeti MS, Reynolds WS, Duffy PG, Mushtaq I. Further experience with the vascular hitch (laparoscopic transposition of lower pole crossing vessels): an alternate treatment for pediatric ureterovascular ureteropelvic junction obstruction. J Urol. 2008;180(4 Suppl):1832–6; discussion 6.

8. Menon P, Rao KL, Sodhi KS, Bhattacharya A, Saxena AK, Mittal BR. Hydronephrosis: comparison of extrinsic vessel versus intrinsic ureteropelvic junction obstruction groups and a plea against the vascular hitch procedure. J Pediatr Urol. 2015;11(2):80.e1–6.

9. Passerotti C, Peters CA. Pediatric robotic-assisted laparoscopy: a description of the principle procedures. ScientificWorldJournal. 2006;6:2581–8.

10. Olsen LH, Jorgensen TM. Computer assisted pyeloplasty in children: the retroperitoneal approach. J Urol. 2004;171(6 Pt 2):2629–31.

11. Rodriguez AR, Rich MA, Swana HS. Stentless pediatric robotic pyeloplasty. Ther Adv Urol. 2012;4(2):57–60.

12. Silva MV, Levy AC, Finkelstein JB, Van Batavia JP, Casale P. Is peri-operative urethral catheter drainage enough? The case for stentless pediatric robotic pyeloplasty. J Pediatr Urol. 2015;11(4):175.e1–5.

13. Passerotti CC, Nguyen HT, Eisner BH, Lee RS, Peters CA. Laparoscopic reoperative pediatric pyeloplasty with robotic assistance. J Endourol. 2007;21(10):1137–40.

Robotic Partial Nephrectomy

30

Craig A. Peters

Patient Selection

Robotic-assisted laparoscopic partial nephrectomy in children most commonly involves patients who have a nonfunctioning moiety in a duplex renal system. Specific indications that would lead to discussion with the patient and parents of intervention include recurrent urinary tract infections, flank pain, or nausea/vomiting suspected to be related to the nonfunctioning moiety. Asymptomatic patients raise the concern about the long-term risks of developing symptoms, generally related to infection.

When a duplicated renal moiety shows some level of function on a renal scan, a drainage procedure may be considered. This can be a proximal or distal ureteroureterostomy, or less often a ureteral reimplantation. Even in some nonfunctioning segments, a drainage procedure may be the most efficient with less risk of injury to the remnant moiety. The advantage of a partial nephrectomy includes avoiding prolonged follow-up, which is often appropriate for reconstructive procedures. In general, however, partial nephrectomy is somewhat more complex, includes the risk of a residual urinoma, and poses a small risk of devascularization of the remnant pole. Both upper and lower partial nephrectomies can be performed with equal success. Upper pole procedures are usually performed for ectopic ureters or ureteroceles with duplication, while lower ole procedures are for lower pole reflux or ureteropelvic junction obstruction associated with nonfunction. The author's practice has been to perform salvage procedures when there is function or when there is limited function but the upper pole is not markedly dilated. In the older child, often with marked dilation of the upper pole, a partial nephrectomy is preferred. Lower pole preservation is only offered when there is demonstrable function in the affected segment, although there are no guidelines as to the appropriate amount of function [1].

Preoperative Preparation

Bowel Preparation

All patients are asked to have a clear liquid (apple juice, Jell-O, ginger ale, water, broth) diet for 24 h before surgery to reduce the bulk of stool in the colon. They are also given one Dulcolax® suppository for the night before. They are then NPO for at least 3 h prior to the case. Specific to

Electronic supplementary material: The online version of this chapter (doi:10.1007/978-3-319-45060-5_30) contains supplementary material, which is available to authorized users.

C.A. Peters, M.D. (✉)
Pediatric Urology, Children's Medical
Center, University of Texas Southwestern,
1935 Medical District Dr., Mail Stop F4.04,
Dallas, TX 75235, USA
e-mail: craig.peters@childrens.com

infants or young children is the use of milk of magnesia (cherry flavor, refrigerated) one to two teaspoons, daily for 2 days before surgery. For 3 days prior to surgery, older children are asked to use senna liquid, one to two teaspoons up to twice daily for 3 days before surgery or ex-lax® squares (chocolate covered senna): ½ to 1 square, repeating twice daily until cleaned out. Teenagers may use Dulcolax® tabs: 20 mg BID the day prior to surgery.

Informed Consent

All patients and family should understand that the surgeon, NOT the "robot", will perform the procedure. The da Vinci® is actually a "master–slave" micromanipulator where the operator is in total control. The robot is not in any way autonomous. Some families are concerned about this issue due to misinformation or misperceptions. The family and patient should always be made aware of the possibility of conversion to open surgery. This is emphasized to be used in cases where the ability to complete the procedure or safety are of concern. If a family is hesitant or unwilling to consent to this uncertainty, open surgery should be recommended so they know what to expect. The risks of general anesthesia must also be presented to the patient. Other risks that need to be relayed during informed consent include the possibility of continued flank pain, nausea, vomiting, recurrent urinary tracts infections, and reoperation.

Operative Setup

At our institution we use the da Vinci® Si with a three-armed technique. An assistant and the scrub technician are positioned on the side of the patient opposite the robot. Video monitors are placed for easy viewing by all team members. An overhead view of the room setup for right and left partial nephrectomies are shown, respectively, in Figs. 30.1 and 30.2.

Patient Positioning and Preparation

Place the patient in modified flank position with a 30° wedge under the ipsilateral side where the partial nephrectomy will be performed with padding and tape across chest and thighs. Also, place folded towels and tape over the patient's arms but under abdomen (Fig. 30.3). Rotate the table so that the patient's abdomen is flat while obtaining trocar access, then rotate to 60° (30° wedge plus 30° table rotation) just prior to docking the robot. The anesthesia team should place an NG or OG tube prior to access.

Trocar Configuration

Trocar configurations for left and right partial nephrectomies are shown in Figs. 30.4 and 30.5. One notable difference is the possibility of needing an extra trocar for liver retraction during a right partial nephrectomy. Again, we typically use the 5 mm trocars when the patient is younger than 8–10; otherwise, the 8 mm trocars are used.

Instrumentation and Equipment List

Equipment
- Da Vinci® Surgical System (3-arm system; Intuitive Surgical, Inc., Sunnyvale, CA)
- EndoWrist® Monopolar Hook Electrocautery, 5 or 8 mm (Intuitive Surgical, Inc., Sunnyvale, CA)
- EndoWrist® Maryland Dissector, 5 mm or Bipolar Maryland Dissector, 8 mm (Intuitive Surgical, Inc., Sunnyvale, CA)
- EndoWrist® Curved Monopolar Scissors, 8 mm (Intuitive Surgical, Inc., Sunnyvale, CA)
- EndoWrist® Round Tip Scissors, 5 mm (Intuitive Surgical, Inc., Sunnyvale, CA)
- EndoWrist® Needle Driver, 5 or 8 mm (Intuitive Surgical, Inc., Sunnyvale, CA)
- Articulated Suction device, 8 mm (Intuitive Surgical, Inc., Sunnyvale, CA)
- InSite® Vision System with 30° lens (Intuitive Surgical, Inc., Sunnyvale, CA)

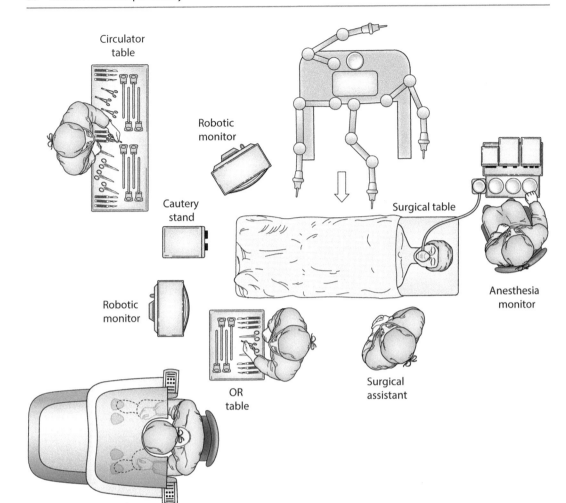

Fig. 30.1 Operating room setup for right partial nephrectomy demonstrating standard configuration of operating room personnel and equipment

Trocars

- 10 mm trocar—camera port
- 8 mm robotic trocars (2, if child is older than 8 years)
- 5 mm trocar (usually 2, if you need liver retraction during a right partial nephrectomy then you will need a 3 mm or 5 mm port for a lifting/retraction device)

Recommended Sutures

- Preplaced fascial box stitch: 2-0 or 3-0 poly- glactin suture

- Vessel ligation and closure of renal defect: 3-0 and/or 4-0 polyglactin suture, length 12–14 cm by age
- Skin Closure: 4-0 or 5-0 monocryl suture

Instruments Used by the Surgical Assistant

- Laparoscopic needle driver
- Maryland grasper
- Suction irrigator device
- Laparoscopic Kittner
- 5 mm titanium clip applier, medium (two are always kept in room)

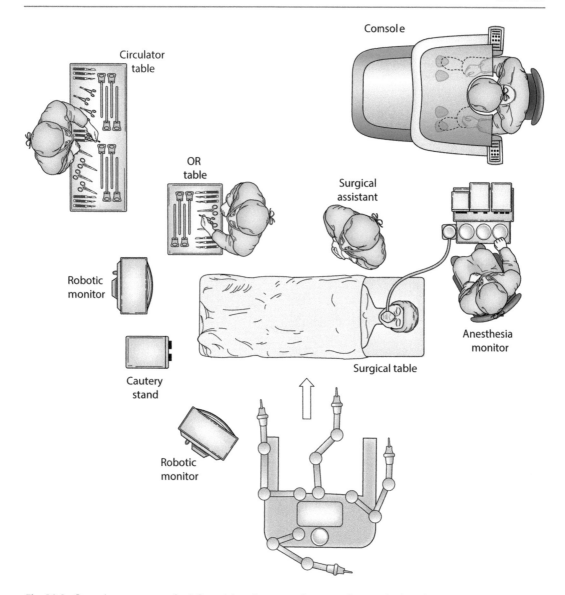

Fig. 30.2 Operating room setup for left partial nephrectomy demonstrating standard configuration of operating room personnel and equipment

Step-by-Step Technique (Video 30.1)

Step 1: Abdominal Access and Trocar Placement

For a right partial nephrectomy, reposition the patient in a right modified flank position as noted above then, for trocar placement, rotate the table

so the patient's abdomen is 0°. The 12 mm camera trocar is placed in the area of the umbilicus, using the Hasson open technique with 2-0 polyglactin suture on a UR-6 needle or a 3-0 polyglactin suture on a CT-2 needle bent accordingly. These are pre-placed fascial box stitches (used later for closure). Working trocars are then placed sharply under direct vision after pre-placing the fascial box stitches. For right-sided operation, a fourth trocar is placed for liver retraction. This trocar is

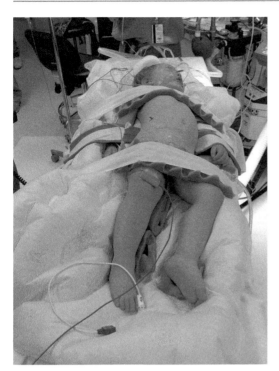

Fig. 30.3 Patient positioning shown for a left partial nephrectomy

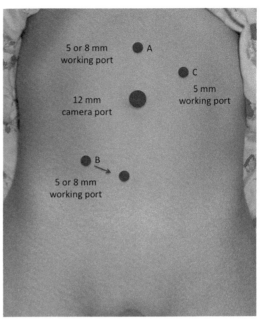

Fig. 30.4 Trocar configuration for right partial nephrectomy. (*A*) Working port is roughly half the distance between the umbilicus and the xiphoid. (*B*) Working port is roughly 2/3 the distance between the umbilicus and the anterior superior iliac spine (ASIS), but if the area of interest is in the lower retroperitoneum or the child is small, may be adjusted medially and inferiorly. (*C*) Working port is for retraction of the liver

placed in the left upper quadrant to permit passing between the camera and upper working trocar without interference and to lift the liver for exposure. Either a blunt Kittner dissector or a grasping tool is passed under the liver edge, lifted and pushed against the opposite abdominal sidewall to stabilize the instrument and liver. Rotate the patient to approximately 60° (30° from table rotation and 30° from the wedge placed earlier) and dock the robot.

Step 2: Accessing the Nonfunctioning Moiety (Table 30.1)

Reflect the colon away from the renal hilum and upper pole to permit full exposure of the upper aspect of the kidney (for upper pole partial) A hitch stitch can be placed through the abdominal wall to the upper pole for better exposure and retraction (Fig. 30.6). Expose the affected ureter at the lower pole of the kidney and separate it from the lower pole ureter carefully (Fig. 30.7).

The dilated upper pole ureter is then dissected upward and under the hilar vessels with care. It must be sufficiently mobilized to permit being passed under the vessels.

Step 3: Transection of Ureter and Vessels to Nonfunctioning Pole (Table 30.2)

Once mobilized, the ureter is ligated with polyglactin suture unless markedly dilated. If maintained somewhat distended, future dissection will be easier. The affected ureter is then transected between sutures and mobilized under the vessels and used to expose the upper pole. This permits better identification of the upper pole vessels and subsequent control. Vessels supplying the upper pole may be clipped or ligated with silk suture (Fig. 30.8). It is important to assess the effect of vessel ligation each time and make sure there are no lower pole

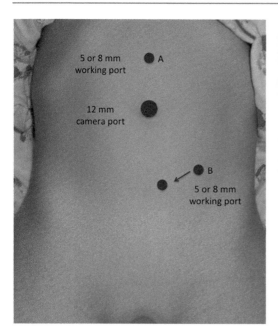

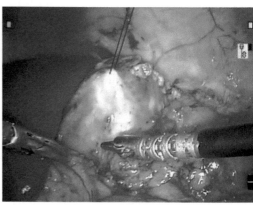

Fig. 30.6 Exposure of the upper pole collecting system using a hitch stitch to lift and stabilize the upper pole

Fig. 30.5 Trocar configuration for left partial nephrectomy. (*A*) Working port is roughly half the distance between the umbilicus and the xiphoid. (*B*) Working port is roughly 2/3 the distance between the umbilicus and the anterior superior iliac spine (ASIS), but if the area of interest is in the lower retroperitoneum or the child is small, may be adjusted medially and inferiorly

Table 30.1 Accessing the nonfunctioning moiety: surgeon and assistant instrumentation

Surgeon instrumentation		Assistant instrumentation
Right arm	Left arm	• Suction-irrigator
• Monopolar hook electrocautery	• Maryland dissector	• Laparoscopic Kittner
Endoscope lens: 30° down		

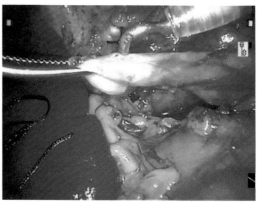

Fig. 30.7 Dissection of upper pole (UP) ureter at the level of the lower pole and moving superiorly to the hilum and under the renal vessels

collaterals being clipped. If multiple vessels are encountered, individual suture ligation may be preferable to avoid dislodging clips.

Step 4: Dissection of Nonfunctioning Moiety (Table 30.3)

Once the vessels and ureter are controlled, the affected upper pole is dissected free by establishing the plane between the upper pole collecting system and the lower pole parenchyma. This usually leaves a rim of tissue that is easily transected with electrocautery (Fig. 30.9). The collecting system should be removed as completely as possible to avoid a post-operative urinoma (Fig. 30.10).

Step 5: Closure of Defect (Table 30.4)

Once the affected pole is removed, the defect is closed using 2–3 polyglactin mattress sutures over a bolster of local fat (Figs. 30.11 and 30.12). If the lower pole collecting system is violated, it

Table 30.2 Transection of ureter and vessels to nonfunctioning pole: surgeon and assistant instrumentation

Surgeon instrumentation		Assistant instrumentation
Right arm	Left arm	• Suction-irrigator
• Needle driver	• Maryland dissector	• Laparoscopic Kittner
• Round tip scissors		• Laparoscopic needle driver
Endoscope lens: 30° down		

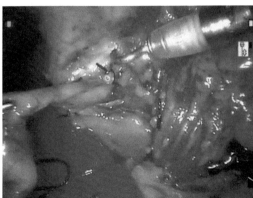

Fig. 30.9 Dissection of upper pole collecting system. The hook cautery or hot shears can be used to incise the rim of renal parenchyma of the upper pole

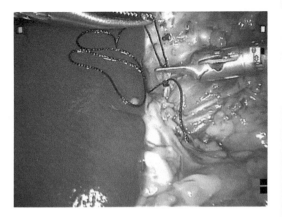

Fig. 30.8 Ligation of the upper pole vessels. Silk sutures are being used with these multiple small vessels to avoid dislodging vascular clips

Table 30.3 Dissection of nonfunctioning moiety: surgeon and assistant instrumentation

Surgeon instrumentation		Assistant instrumentation
Right arm	Left arm	• Suction-irrigator
• Monopolar hook electrocautery	• Maryland dissector	• Laparoscopic Kittner
Endoscope lens: 30° down		

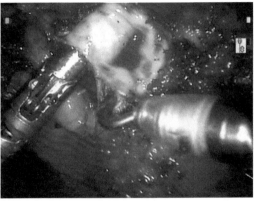

Fig. 30.10 Removal of the upper pole collecting system sitting on top of the lower pole

is closed and a drain is left in place; otherwise, there is no drain used. While it may be acceptable to leave the defect open, there seems to be a relationship with developing post-operative urinomas when the defect has not been closed. These may not cause clinical problems, but are always of concern to families. Whenever possible, the defect is closed in a manner similar to what was performed with open procedures.

Table 30.4 Closure of defect: surgeon and assistant instrumentation

Surgeon instrumentation		Assistant instrumentation
Right arm	Left arm	• Suction-irrigator
• Needle driver	• Maryland dissector	• Laparoscopic Kittner
• Round tip scissors		• Laparoscopic needle driver
Endoscope lens: 30° down		

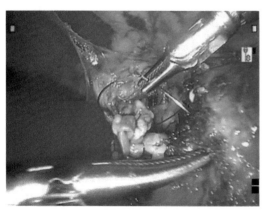

Fig. 30.11 Closure of renal defect by suturing a bolster of retroperitoneal fat into the defect and secured using mattress sutures of PDS

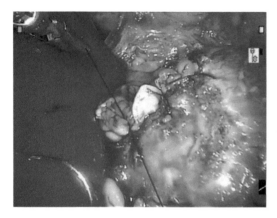

Fig. 30.12 Appearance of the closed defect on the upper aspect of the lower pole of the kidney

Table 30.5 Further dissection and removal of affected ureter: surgeon and assistant instrumentation

Surgeon instrumentation		Assistant instrumentation
Right arm	Left arm	• Suction-irrigator
• Monopolar hook electrocautery	• Maryland dissector	• Laparoscopic Kittner
• Needle driver		• Laparoscopic needle driver
• Round tip scissors		
Endoscope lens: 30° down		

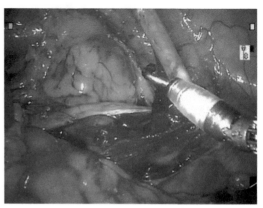

Fig. 30.13 Resection of affected ureter. Resection is performed by lifting ureter as shown here, and progressively releasing attachments with hook electrocautery. The ureter can usually be taken to just below the iliac vessels without difficulty

Step 7: Exiting the Abdomen

The operative area is irrigated, cleared, and inspected. The robot is undocked. Trocars are removed under direct vision. The two specimens (nonfunctioning moiety and ureter) are removed through the umbilical trocar. Preplaced fascial box stitches are tied, and a subcuticular Monocryl suture is used for skin closure.

Post-operative Management

Post-operatively, the patient is placed on 1.5× maintenance fluids, usually D5 ½ NS. A clear liquid diet is started on the operative day with

Step 6: Further Dissection and Removal of Affected Ureter (Table 30.5)

The affected ureter is resected as low as convenient, which is usually to the iliac vessels. It is tied off with polyglactin suture if refluxing (clips are not secure), or left open if obstructed without reflux (Fig. 30.13). If refluxing and obstructed, it should be ligated as close to the bladder neck as possible. This may require re-positioning the robot.

orders to advance as tolerated. Perioperative antibiotic (usually cefazolin) is continued for 24 h. Pain control includes morphine (0.1 mg/kg IV) every 3–4 h p.r.n. pain as well as Tylenol® with codeine elixir (0.5–1 mg/kg po) every 4 h p.r.n. pain. The urethral catheter is removed prior to leaving the operating room. If a drain is placed, it is monitored to ensure low output and is then usually removed on the morning of post-op day 1. Most patients are ready for discharge by midday on post-op day 1.

Special Considerations

Lower pole partial nephrectomy is performed in a similar manner, usually for lower pole reflux with nonfunction. The ureter is more easily controlled, but similar care must be taken to avoid upper pole vessel injury. Some authors use a ureteral catheter in the remnant pole to inject blue dye to identify collecting system leaks, but we have not found this to be necessary. The ability to efficiently close the polar defect has eliminated the occurrence of urinomas that have been reported in laparoscopic partial nephrectomy when the polar defect is not closed [2].

Handling of the distal ureter is based on practicality in terms of the extent of resection. Some authors claim it is important to remove as much as possible, but there are few reports to indicate a real risk of complications with the exception of a refluxing and obstructed segment. If it is felt that entire removal of the ureter is needed, or if it is necessary to perform a contralateral anti-reflux operation, the robotic system is re-docked in the lower position for bladder access and the dissection performed.

Post-operative follow-up involves a renal ultrasound at 4–6 weeks to ensure that the remnant pole is not obstructed in any way and that there is no urinoma. The vascular integrity of the lower pole can be assessed using Doppler flow and there is no need for a renal scan unless there is specific concern for injury. In the few reports where remnant pole injury has been demonstrated, patients presented with clear clinical symptoms of pain or fever.

The presence of a urinoma is best managed with reassurance and monitoring [3]. There is little chance it will become symptomatic. In one instance, a post-operative urinoma was aspirated to calm the family but it rapidly recurred, only to eventually resolve spontaneously.

Steps to Avoid Complications

The most significant complication for partial nephrectomy in children with duplication anomalies is injury to the lower pole, usually through vascular injury or spasm [4]. Great care must be taken to minimize manipulation of the hilar vessels and to carefully identify the vessels associated with the affected pole. They may be small and branched or a single vessel. Observation of the color of the remnant pole is useful to avoid inadvertent clamping of the remnant vessels. Vessels can be tied or clipped. Papaverine solution can be instilled through a long laparoscopic needle if spasm is evident.

References

1. Peters CA, Mendelsohn K. Ectopic ureter and uretero-cele. In: Wein A, Kavoussi L, Partin A, Peters C, editors. Campbell-Walsh urology, vol. 4. 11th ed. Philadelphia: Elsevier; 2016.
2. Mason MD, Anthony Herndon CD, Smith-Harrison LI, Peters CA, Corbett ST. Robotic-assisted partial nephrectomy in duplicated collecting systems in the pediatric population: techniques and outcomes. J Pediatr Urol. 2014;10(2):374–9.
3. Lee RS, Sethi AS, Passerotti CC, Retik AB, Borer JG, Nguyen HT, et al. Robot assisted laparoscopic partial nephrectomy: a viable and safe option in children. J Urol. 2009;181(2):823–8; discussion 8–9.
4. Wallis MC, Khoury AE, Lorenzo AJ, Pippi-Salle JL, Bagli DJ, Farhat WA. Outcome analysis of retroperitoneal laparoscopic heminephrectomy in children. J Urol. 2006;175(6):2277–80; discussion 80–2.

Micah Jacobs and Craig A. Peters

Patient Selection

Patients with vesicoureteral reflux (VUR) initially come to our attention because of either a prenatal finding of hydronephrosis or a febrile urinary tract infection in the first few years of life. If not already done, initial workup includes a renal ultrasound and possibly a VCUG. Prophylactic antibiotics are often recommended at least until the above-mentioned studies are done. Once the diagnosis of reflux is established, treatment options include surveillance, surveillance with prophylactic antibiotics, and anti-reflux surgery. In general, conservative measures are initially employed and if those fail (e.g., breakthrough febrile urinary tract infections on prophylactic antibiotics), anti-reflux surgery is discussed. At all interactions during the course of patient care, the patient and parents are educated on the nature of reflux and treatment options so they may make educated decisions. At our institution, robotic anti-reflux surgery is most often approached by an extravesical ureteral reimplant. Although intravesical approaches have also been described, this chapter is limited to the extravesical technique.

Preoperative Preparation

Bowel Preparation

In order to reduce the bulk of stool in the colon, patients are asked to have a clear liquid (apple juice, Jell-o, ginger ale, water, broth) diet for 24 h before surgery. They are also given one Dulcolax® suppository the night before.

Informed Consent

All patients and family should understand that the procedure will be performed by the surgeon, NOT the "robot." Some families are concerned about this issue due to misinformation or misperceptions. The family and patient should always be made aware of the possibility of conversion to open surgery. It is emphasized that this would only occur in cases where the ability to complete the procedure or safety are of concern. If a family is hesitant or unwilling to consent to this uncertainty, open surgery should be recom-

Electronic supplementary material: The online version of this chapter (doi:10.1007/978-3-319-45060-5_31) contains supplementary material, which is available to authorized users.

M. Jacobs, M.D., M.P.H.
Department of Urology, Children's Medical Center, University of Texas Southwestern, Dallas, TX, USA

C.A. Peters, M.D. (✉)
Pediatric Urology, Children's Medical Center, University of Texas Southwestern, 1935 Medical District Dr., Mail Stop F4.04, Dallas, TX 75235, USA
e-mail: craig.peters@childrens.com

mended so they know what to expect. The risks of general anesthesia are also presented to the patient. Other risks that need to be relayed during informed consent include the realization that renal function could remain the same or even worsen after surgery. Continued flank pain, nausea, vomiting, recurrent urinary tract infections, and the possibility of reoperation also need to be discussed.

Operative Setup

At our institution we use the da Vinci® Si with a three-armed technique. An assistant and the scrub technician are positioned on opposite sides of the table and the robot is brought in from the direction of the patient's feet. Video monitors are placed for easy viewing by all team members. An overhead view of the room setup for ureteral reimplant is shown in Fig. 31.1. We recommend

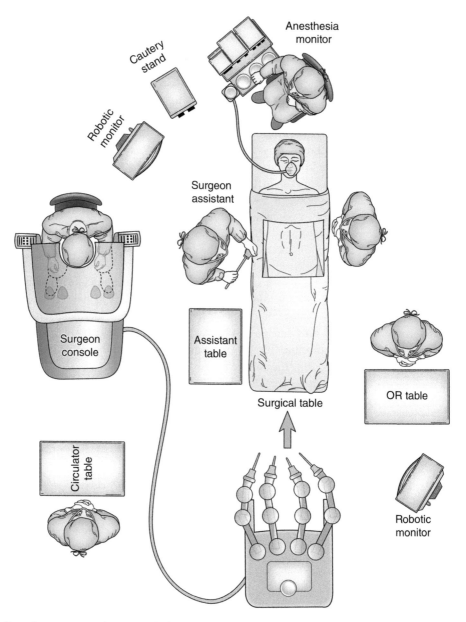

Fig. 31.1 Operating room setup for extravesical ureteral reimplant demonstrating standard configuration of operating room personnel and equipment

having a dedicated operating room for the da Vinci® to decrease room turnover delays and possible equipment damage due to transporting the robot from one room to another.

Place padding and tape across chest and lower thighs and place a folded towel and tape over arms but under abdomen. The anesthesia team should place an NG or OG tube prior to access.

Patient Positioning and Preparation

Initially, frog leg the patient (Fig. 31.2) to prep and place urethral catheter in the sterile field. Placement of a rectal tube for decompression may also be helpful. Then adjust legs to have patient in supine position for obtaining access (Fig. 31.3).

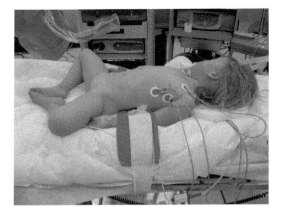

Fig. 31.2 Initial positioning for reimplant. "Frog leg" positioning helps with initial placement of urethral catheter on the sterile field in female patients

Trocar Configuration

Trocar configuration for an extravesical ureteral reimplant is shown in Fig. 31.4. The 5 mm trocars can be used when the patient is younger than 8–10 years, otherwise the 8 mm trocars are used. Adjust the patient to moderate Trendelenburg position prior to docking robot.

Instrumentation and Equipment List

Equipment

- da Vinci® Si Surgical System (Intuitive Surgical, Inc., Sunnyvale, CA)
- EndoWrist® Monopolar Hook Electrocautery, 5 or 8 mm (Intuitive Surgical, Inc., Sunnyvale, CA)
- EndoWrist® Maryland Dissector, 5 or 8 mm (Intuitive Surgical, Inc., Sunnyvale, CA)

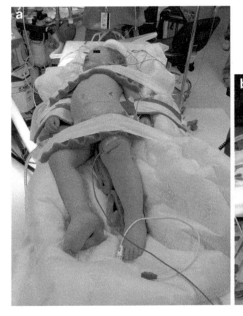

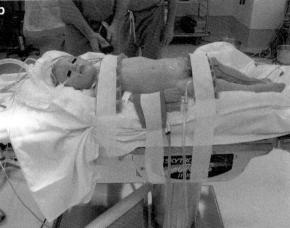

Fig. 31.3 Final positioning for reimplant. After catheter is placed, the patient is readjusted to the supine position

Fig. 31.4 Trocar configuration for extravesical ureteral reimplant

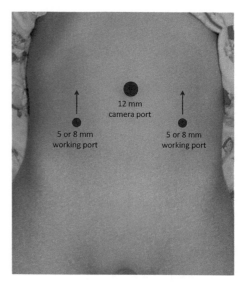

Working Ports are roughly 2/3 the distance between the umbilicus and the anterior superior iliac spine (ASIS). In small infants, the working ports should be moved more superiorly to prevent restrictive proximity to bladder and ureters.

- EndoWrist® DeBakey Forceps, 5 or 8 mm (Intuitive Surgical, Inc., Sunnyvale, CA)
- EndoWrist® Curved Monopolar Scissors, 8 mm (Intuitive Surgical, Inc., Sunnyvale, CA)
- EndoWrist® Round Tip Scissors, 5 or 8 mm (Intuitive Surgical, Inc., Sunnyvale, CA)
- EndoWrist® Needle Driver, 5 or 8 mm (Intuitive Surgical, Inc., Sunnyvale, CA)
- Articulated irrigation device, 8 mm (Intuitive Surgical, Inc., Sunnyvale, CA)
- InSite® Vision System with 30° lens (Intuitive Surgical, Inc., Sunnyvale, CA)

Trocars

- 8.5/10 mm Camera trocar
- 8 mm Robotic trocars (2, only if child is older than 8–10)
- 5 mm Trocar (2)

Recommended Sutures

- Preplaced fascial box stitch: 2-0 or 3-0 polyglactin suture
- Hitch stitch: 3-0 or 4-0 polyglactin
- Bladder mucosal tears: 6–0 chromic, 14 cm length
- Detrusor tunnel: 4-0 polyglactin, 14 cm length
- Skin closure: 4-0 or 5-0 monocryl suture

Instruments Used by the Surgical Assistant

- Maryland grasper
- Suction irrigator device

Step-by-Step Technique (Video 31.1)

Step 1: Abdominal Access and Trocar Placement

As noted above, the urethral catheter may be easily placed on the sterile field prior to adjusting the patient from frog-legged to supine position. The 12 or 8.5 mm camera trocar is placed in the area of the umbilicus, using the Hasson open technique with 2-0 polyglactin suture on a UR-6 needle or a 3-0 polyglactin suture on a CT-2 needle bent accord-

Table 31.1 Ureteral mobilization: surgeon and assistant instrumentation

Surgeon instrumentation		Assistant instrumentation
Right arm	Left arm	• Suction-irrigator
• Monopolar hook electrocautery (or monopolar scissors)	• Maryland dissector	
Endoscope lens: 30° down		

ingly. These are pre-placed fascial box stitches (used later for closure). Working trocars are then placed sharply under direct vision after pre-placing the fascial box stitches. Dock the robot.

Step 2: Ureteral Mobilization (Table 31.1)

Access is transperitoneal to the posterior aspect of the bladder. The ureter is identified through the peritoneum, exposed by incising the peritoneum transversely lateral to the midline, posterior to bladder and anterior to uterus in girls (Fig. 31.5). The ureter is mobilized for about 5–6 cm proximal to UVJ (Fig. 31.6a, b), staying close to the ureter

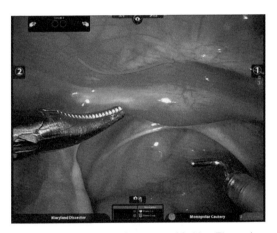

Fig. 31.5 Transperitoneal access to bladder. The peritoneum is incised just over the ureter of interest (*red line*), along the vesico-uterine fold of the peritoneum

without disrupting its adventitia. A combination of blunt and electrocautery dissection is used. If there is difficulty in identifying the ureter anterior to the uterus, this can be accomplished more proximally and dissected down toward the bladder.

Step 3: Placement of Hitch Stitch (Table 31.2)

Often visualization of the posterior bladder and distal ureter is adequate once the bladder has been completely emptied, but if necessary a hitch stitch can be placed. In order to do this the bladder wall is exposed and hitched upward by passing a 3-0 polyglactin suture on an SH needle through the abdominal wall, then through the bladder lateral to the anticipated upper point of the tunnel, looping around itself once, then taking another bite of the bladder on the opposite side of the tunnel with another loop, then back through the abdominal wall on the opposite side and securing it in place with a hemostat. The two-point fixation of the

Table 31.2 Placement of hitch stitch: surgeon and assistant instrumentation

Surgeon instrumentation		Assistant instrumentation
Right arm	Left arm	• Suction-irrigator
• Needle driver	• Maryland dissector	
Endoscope lens: 30° down		

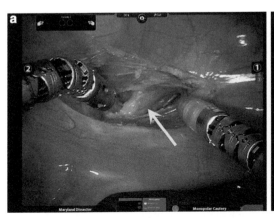
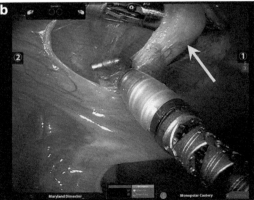

Fig. 31.6 Mobilization of ureter (**a**) Exposure of the ureter (*yellow arrow*). (**b**) With the ureter elevated, lateral attachments may be cauterized away from the ureter (*yellow arrow*), taking care to stay close to the ureter without injuring the vascularity

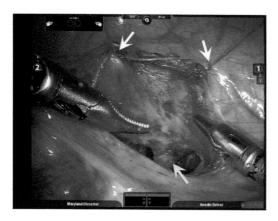

Fig. 31.7 Bladder hitch stitch. For unilateral or bilateral procedures, a two-point hitch is used with vicryl suture passed through the abdominal wall jus above the pubis and being passed through the bladder wall in two places (*white arrows*) to lift and stretch the posterior bladder wall and expose the ureter (*yellow arrow*)

for the complete dissection. The bladder is partially filled with saline to provide wall tension and visualization of the mucosa, which facilitates dissection; this can be varied through the procedure depending upon the exposure (Fig. 31.8a–c). Any puncture of the mucosa is closed with 6-0 chromic figure-of-eight stitch. Detrusor muscle flaps are elevated on each side of the incision, wide enough to wrap around the ureter. Two approaches are used to manage the hiatus. The hiatus can be completely dissected circumferentially around the ureter and an advancement stitch as originally described by Zaontz et al. placed. Alternatively an inverted Y incision of the detrusor around the hiatus is made and no advancement stitch is placed. The relative utility of these options has not been defined.

Table 31.3 Creation of detrusor tunnel: surgeon and assistant instrumentation

Surgeon instrumentation		Assistant instrumentation
Right arm	Left arm	• Suction-irrigator
• Monopolar hook electrocautery (or monopolar scissors)	• Maryland dissector	
Endoscope lens: 30° down		

bladder lifts it upward and spreads the wall to provide tension on the detrusor, facilitating tunnel creation. Another option in patients with a very thick abdominal wall is to tie this suture to the posterior abdominal wall (Fig. 31.7).

Step 4: Creation of Detrusor Tunnel (Table 31.3)

The ureteral hiatus is exposed enough to permit creation of the detrusor tunnel, but no more, to avoid unnecessary injury to perivesical nerves. A detrusor incision is made to the level of the mucosa to create a tunnel for the ureter. It is most efficient to begin at the top of the tunnel, farthest from the hiatus to permit identification of the depth of the mucosal layer and use this as a guide

Step 5: Placement of Ureter into Tunnel (Table 31.4)

An interrupted closure of the tunnel over the ureter using 4-0 polyglactin suture (length 14 cm—three knots can be tied) is performed in one of two approaches:

(a) Distal to proximal: this necessitates passing the needle under the ureter with each stitch, but the ureter is not in the way of suturing and the detrusor trough is visible for each stitch.
(b) Proximal to distal: this starts with the initial stitch that brings the ureter into the tunnel. Subsequent stitches are more easily placed, but there is limited visibility of the intramural ureter with each stitch. The first stitch is slightly difficult to tie as the ureter is under some tension. This is best done with the ipsilateral instrument under the ureter as the knot is tied, lifting the ureter into the tunnel (Fig. 31.9a, b).

Usually four to six stitches are placed, creating a tunnel of 2.5–3.5 cm. The robotic needle holder may be used to estimate tunnel length and its patency. Note that the ureter may appear to be under tension when tented by the pneumoperitoneum, particularly with a hitch stitch in place, but should not be as the abdomen is desufflated (Fig. 31.10).

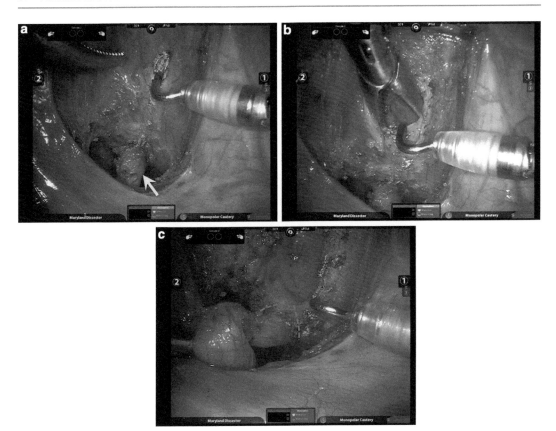

Fig. 31.8 Creation of detrusor tunnel. (**a**) With the bladder partially filled, an outline of the tunnel is scored. From what will be the proximal aspect of the tunnel to the ureteral hiatus (*yellow arrow*). (**b**) The Maryland dissector is used to help manipulate the detrusor flaps as dissection is continued. Notice the bluish hue of the mucosa. The Maryland dissector can be gently placed between the mucosa and detrusor muscle to further flap creation. (**c**) The detrusor muscle fibers adjacent to the ureteral hiatus are cut (*dashed red line*) to permit complete wrapping of the muscle over the ureter. A full circumferential incision is performed by some

Table 31.4 Placement of ureter into tunnel: surgeon and assistant instrumentation

Surgeon instrumentation		Assistant instrumentation
Right arm	Left arm	• Suction-irrigator
• Needle driver	• Maryland dissector (or needle driver)	• Laparoscopic needle driver
• Round tip scissors		
Endoscope lens: 30° down		

Step 6: Reapproximation of the Peritoneum

The hitch stitch may now be removed. The peritoneum can be closed with a running 4-0 polyglactin suture (Fig. 31.11).

Step 7: Exiting the Abdomen

The operative area is irrigated, cleared, and inspected. The robot is undocked. Trocars are removed under direct vision, the preplaced fascial box stitches are tied, and a subcuticular Monocryl suture is used for skin closure.

Postoperative Management

For uncomplicated unilateral procedures, a bladder catheter is not essential, but for bilateral cases, this is left in place at least overnight. Postoperatively, the patient is placed on 1.5× maintenance fluids, usually D5 ½NS. He or she is started on a clear liquid diet with

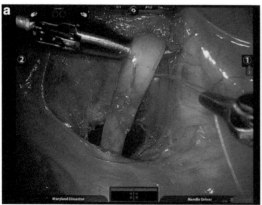
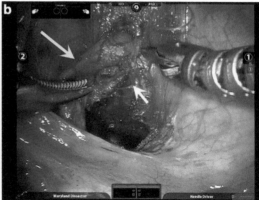

Fig. 31.9 Initiation of proximal to distal closure of tunnel. (**a**) Beginning of a proximal to distal closure, the stitch has been placed under the ureter and through the lateral detrusor flap. The ureter is elevated while tying this stitch by placing the left robotic arm under the ureter. (**b**) Placing subsequent stitches is facilitated by the ureter (*yellow arrow*) being elevated and the detrusor trough being exposed. The needle (*white arrow*) is seen passing through the right-sided detrusor flap

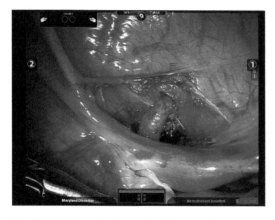

Fig. 31.10 Completed tunnel with ureter in position. With the hitch stitch removed the ureter should have a straight course superiorly

orders to advance as tolerated. Perioperative antibiotics (usually cefazolin 50–100 mg total over 24 h divided in three doses) are continued for 24 h then prophylactic antibiotics are continued until at least the first follow-up clinic visit. Pain control includes morphine (0.1 mg/kg IV) every 3–4 h p.r.n. pain as well as Tylenol® with codeine elixir (0.5–1 mg/kg po) every 4 h p.r.n. pain. At our institution, we usually also place orders for ondansetron (0.1 mg/kg) every 8 h p.r.n. nausea. Most patients are ready for discharge by midday on postoperative day 1.

Special Considerations

This method can be used for duplex ureters as long as a slightly wider dissection of the detrusor flaps is performed. This method has also been used for dilated ureters with both plication and excisional tapering, with resection of the obstructive distal segment.

Intravesical transtrigonal ureteral reimplantation has been performed as well as the extravesical technique, although it is more challenging and results have not been as robust [1].

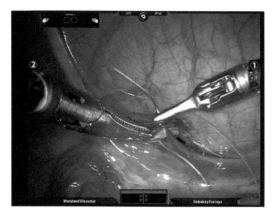

Fig. 31.11 Peritoneal closure using 4-0 vicryl

Steps to Avoid Complications

Protection of the vas deferens in boys is important. The peritoneum is incised beyond the vas and the vas is retracted by sweeping the peritoneum, rather than the vas itself. Continue to monitor the location of the vas throughout the procedure, particularly at the hiatal dissection where the vas is looping around the ureter medially [2].

No stents are left in place in most cases, but a double-J stent would be placed for a solitary kidney.

Due to the risk of postoperative urinary retention following bilateral extravesical anti-reflux surgery, attempts have been made to perform a nerve-sparing procedure [3]. While the presumed cause of retention is neural injury, this has not been proven and the local nerves are not macroscopically visible, nor associated with a marker structure as in the periprostatic nerves. The most efficient approach is to stay as close to the ureters as possible with limited extra dissection. Even so the risk is present. Our experience has been to leave the bladder catheter in overnight, and if the first voiding trial fails, to discharge the child home with a catheter to be removed in 3–5 days [4]. The incidence of retention is lower than for open surgery, but not likely to be absent.

Recently reported results have not shown the same level of success in correcting reflux as initial reports [5, 6], although the specific reasons are unclear. The impact of patient selection, tunnel length, dissection of the hiatus, and other technical aspects may be relevant.

References

1. Peters CA, Woo R. Intravesical robotically assisted bilateral ureteral reimplantation. J Endourol. 2005;19:618–21; discussion 21–2.
2. Passerotti C, Peters CA. Pediatric robotic-assisted laparoscopy: a description of the principle procedures. Sci World J. 2006;6:2581–8.
3. Casale P, Patel RP, Kolon TF. Nerve sparing robotic extravesical ureteral reimplantation. J Urol. 2008;179:1987–9; discussion 90.
4. Smith RP, Oliver JL, Peters CA. Pediatric robotic extravesical ureteral reimplantation: comparison with open surgery. J Urol. 2011;185(5):1876–81.
5. Akhavan A, Avery D, Lendvay TS. Robot-assisted extravesical ureteral reimplantation: outcomes and conclusions from 78 ureters. J Pediatr Urol. 2014;10(5):864–8.
6. Grimsby GM, Dwyer ME, Jacobs MA, Ost MC, Schneck FX, Cannon GM, Gargollo PC. Multi-institutional review of outcomes of robot-assisted laparoscopic extravesical ureteral reimplantation. J Urol. 2015;193(5 Suppl):1791–5.

Complications in Pediatric Robotic Surgery

32

Craig A. Peters

Introduction

While the benefits of robotic surgery in pediatric urologic practice have become progressively evident, concern remains as to the potential risk for complications, particularly in small children. There are three key elements to limit the potential impact of complications in robotic and laparoscopic surgery children. These are prevention, recognition, and management. These three will be discussed in some detail and they are all interdependent with each other during any particular surgery.

Prevention

Of course prevention of a complication should be the highest priority and involves several important elements. One should always be aware of the possible risks for particular surgery in a particular patient. One should anticipate the possibility of complications both in the procedure as a whole, as well as in particular parts of the procedure that may be more prone to problems. A key

C.A. Peters, M.D. (✉)
Pediatric Urology, Children's Medical
Center, University of Texas Southwestern, 1935
Medical District Dr., Mail Stop F4.04, Dallas, TX
75235, USA
e-mail: craig.peters@childrens.com

element of this is to recognize the complication prone situation. This can occur during access where there are any difficulties in initially obtaining what should be routine access or in the child with prior abdominal surgery where there may be adhesions. Situations in which there is limited vision either due to the anatomy, proximity or due to fogging, also increase the potential for inadvertent injuries. Any case in which there is prior surgical or inflammatory scarring also increases the potential for inadvertent injury, particularly vascular injury. In children, unusual anatomy is typically the basis for surgery and one should always be anticipating and alert for variations in normal structure. This can be particularly the case in duplication anomalies where identification and localization of the various components, both ureteral and renal, are very important. Renal ectopia, particularly pelvic kidney with malrotation, poses challenges as well, and one should always be cognizant of the potential for complex vascular anomalies in these children. This is also the situation with horseshoe kidneys.

In all steps of any procedure, safe technique should be followed. This is certainly very important with access, using either the Veress needle, although no technique is truly risk-free [1, 2]. During dissection, the practice of touching a cold instrument with an electrified instrument to provide for tissue cautery is risky, particularly if one cannot see all of the electrified elements of the cold instrument. Inadvertent burn injuries to

© Springer International Publishing Switzerland 2017
L.-M. Su (ed.), *Atlas of Robotic Urologic Surgery*, DOI 10.1007/978-3-319-45060-5_32

bowel or vascular structures then become more possible.

Just as with open surgery, the surgeon must always be aware of their surroundings from an anatomic perspective. A three-dimensional mental image of the surroundings of the operative field should always be maintained in the surgeon's mind. If there is uncertainty as to the orientation or proximity, a brief pause to reassess location and context is useful. In dissecting the right renal pelvis, for example, the close proximity of the duodenum and IVC should always be in mind.

In pediatric practice of both laparoscopy and robotics, the largest fraction of complications occur during access. This occurs in both open and Veress needle techniques. During open technique one should never attempt cannula insertion until the open space of the peritoneum has been visualized. If pre-placed fascial sutures are to be used, they should not be passed until after the peritoneum is opened and the cavity visualized. Pre-placed fascial sutures have a significant advantage particularly in children, because they provide for counter-traction as the cannula is being placed through the abdominal wall. The natural resistance of the child's abdominal wall is limited and without counter-traction it is possible, even with a blunt cannula, to injure peritoneal or retroperitoneal structures.

If the Veress needle technique is being used, strict adherence to safe steps and practices is important. The author still strongly recommends the saline test with aspiration to ensure that the bowel or a vascular structure has not been inadvertently entered. The drop test confirming intraperitoneal placement, while not definitive, is certainly reassuring. If there is any uncertainty as to the placement of the needle, insufflation should not be started. With the initial passage of the needle it is important to avoid vigorous pressure and potential past pointing, with the risk for inadvertent puncture of an intra-abdominal structure.

During the actual operative procedure, safe technique includes continual awareness of the visible and hidden anatomy. As noted above, maintenance of a three-dimensional anatomic image in the surgeon's mind is particularly useful.

Keeping surgical instruments within the visual field, particularly in small children, reduces the potential for inadvertent injury by working instruments. Accidental thermal injury due to cautery is probably the most common procedural complication, and carries the potential for profound and highly morbid sequelae.

As noted above, it is advisable not to use indirect cautery through a cold instrument. One should also be particularly cautious when using the 8 mm instruments, that the operator is certain about which instrument is being electrified during coagulation.

Tissue control during any procedure is important to provide adequate exposure and surgical precision. Excessive manipulation and handling, however, particularly in small children, can produce potentially significant tissue damage and failure of healing. Controlling the tissue and fully visualizing before either cautery or suture manipulation will also prevent potential problems. One should always visualize the tissue to be cut with cold or cautery technique. When applying vascular clips, complete visualization is also strongly recommended, including the distal tip of the clip to ensure that it has both surrounded the tissue of interest as well as come together appropriately without scissoring.

Recognition

While prevention of complications is the foundation of safe surgery, recognition of an evolving complication is equally important. Recognition can occur during access, intraoperatively, as well as postoperatively.

During access, using Veress technique, aspiration will reveal the potential for needle entry into the bowel or into a vascular structure. If insufflation is undertaken before this is recognized, a minor complication becomes a major one. With initial insufflation, intraperitoneal pressure should be monitored and the ideal is that the pressures remain relatively low during initial insufflation and only rise as the capacity of the peritoneum is reached. Awareness of the patient's hemodynamics, particularly during initial insufflation is important and is a shared responsibility between the anesthesia and the surgical team. Sudden desaturation or loss of perfusion indicates either respiratory compromise or CO_2 embolus. Watching for signs of bleeding that may not be obvious during initial visualization of the peritoneal space can reveal possible injury to the inferior epigastric vessels, for example. A pool of blood in the small bowel area or in one of the gutters can indicate a vascular injury that has not yet been recognized. As always, early recognition can limit the potential impact of any complication.

During the operative procedure ongoing bleeding can be recognized with a slow diminution of illumination. Even though the puddle of blood may not be directly visible, the absorption of reflected light by the blood can reduce the overall field illumination significantly. Similarly, the loss of the space of the operative field, which can be gradual, signifies loss of the pneumoperitoneum and may reflect a significant leak or dislodgment of one of the cannulas. The compromised operative field can limit one's ability to respond to a problem, increase the potential risk of inadvertent injury, and dislodgment of one of the ports obviously would limit one's ability to respond to that problem.

Postoperative recognition of ongoing complications can occur in several ways. If there is persistent leakage from one of the port sites, the possibility of a urinary leak should be considered, although some ports will normally show oozing of blood for 1 or 2 days. The classic signs of a possible bowel injury include fever and leukocytosis, however these are not always definitively present. It has sometimes been reported that these patients can show a reduction in their peripheral white blood cell count. The addition of port site pain is also seen as an indication of intra-abdominal problems, particularly a bowel injury. Port site pain can also reflect a incisional port site hernia. Local tenderness and distention will be present but it may not be possible to definitively identify a defect, particularly in small children. Imaging studies maybe useful. A particularly problematic postoperative issue is persistent ileus. While this can simply reflect the response to manipulation as well as analgesics, an ileus can also signal an ongoing intra-abdominal process such as obstruction, intestinal injury or urinary leak.

Some specific complications can occur with particular surgical procedures. Placement of double-J ureteral stents intraoperatively can be a source of problems. This can cause ureteral perforation or elevation of a mucosal flap. Intraoperative confirmation of safe placement of a stent using ultrasound, plain x-ray, or cystoscopy are good options to limit the potential impact of a misplaced stent by early recognition.

Management

Effective management of any intraoperative complication is enhanced by early recognition, but one must be prepared to rapidly manage potentially catastrophic complications as well. These really are limited to major vascular injuries, carbon dioxide embolus, or surgical hemorrhage. The major vascular injuries during pediatric laparoscopy have largely been due to access injuries and lack of recognition. Once recognized, rapid control through pressure is the first step. Exposure and access is the second critical element concurrent with initiating stabilization measures. Careful and precise communication within the team is essential [3]. The determination of the need for conversion to open access must be made rapidly and communicated effectively.

It is important to maintain a focus on dealing with an evolving problem, particularly bleeding, in such a way that will not escalate the problem from being manageable robotically to necessitating conversion. Minor bleeding can become a major problem with rapid careless attempts to control it. The temptation to drop a tissue that starts bleeding should be avoided, as lifting will often compress and slow bleeding. If it is clearly a larger vessel, simple compression can temporize until the necessary tools are brought into play, including suction and irrigation to permit visualization and control, and suture for ligature control. If only two ports are being used, a third working port may be placed to permit suction and still maintain two instruments for control. For most renal cases in children, this would optimally be in the upper quadrant, just off the midline contralaterally. Alternatively, it can be more lateral on the same side as the affected kidney.

Evidence of retroperitoneal bleeding, such as an obvious hematoma, should be observed for progression. If expanding, it should be explored, cleared, and any bleeding controlled. Intra-abdominal pressure should be lowered for several minutes to ensure that the hematoma will not expand without a pneumoperitoneum.

Bowel injury that is recognized intra-operatively should be managed depending upon the extent of the injury. A small isolated burn can be over-sewn with a figure of eight suture, as would a small enterotomy. The surrounding tissues should be carefully inspected for thermal injury and if in doubt, resected. While most pediatric urologists are completely comfortable with bowel surgery, it is recommended to obtain a general surgical opinion if in doubt.

Concern for a ureteral injury may arise during any ureteral surgery, particularly ureteral reimplantation. If the ureter is overtly damaged or appears pale, retrograde placement of a ureteral stent is probably the best initial step to permit healing without leakage. Direct repair of a small ureterotomy is appropriate, unless there is concern for a more extensive thermal injury. In such cases, either a stent or wound drain is the most conservative measure as well.

Conclusion

Pediatric urological robotic surgery has shown a very safe track record, but it is likely that with increased use, complications will occur [4, 5]. As this technology becomes more widely used, it will be difficult to maintain appropriate vigilance due to the infrequency of these complications and a sense of complacency may become equally widespread. This must be avoided. We must maintain a constant mind-set of prevention, recognition and always have a plan for management of those complications.

References

1. Passerotti CC, Nguyen HT, Retik AB, Peters CA. Patterns and predictors of laparoscopic complications in pediatric urology: the role of ongoing surgical volume and access techniques. J Urol. 2008;180(2):681–5.
2. Jansen FW, Kolkman W, Bakkum EA, de Kroon CD, Trimbos-Kemper TC, Trimbos JB. Complications of laparoscopy: an inquiry about closed- versus open-entry technique. Am J Obstet Gynecol. 2004;190(3):634–8.
3. Acero NM, Motuk G, Luba J, Murphy M, McKelvey S, Kolb G, et al. Managing a surgical exsanguination emergency in the operating room through simulation: an interdisciplinary approach. J Surg Educ. 2012;69(6):759–65.
4. Dangle PP, Akhavan A, Odeleye M, Avery D, Lendvay T, Koh CJ, et al. Ninety-day perioperative complications of pediatric robotic urological surgery: a multi-institutional study. J Pediatr Urol. 2016;12(2):102 e1–6.
5. Bansal D, Defoor Jr WR, Reddy PP, Minevich EA, Noh PH. Complications of robotic surgery in pediatric urology: a single institution experience. Urology. 2013;82(4):917–20.

Part V

Single Port Robotic Surgery: Current Status and Future Considerations

Single-Port Robotic Surgery: Current Status and Future Considerations

33

Pascal Mouracade, Daniel Ramirez, and Jihad H. Kaouk

Introduction

The application of robotics in urologic surgery has been widely adopted secondary to the advantages it provides over standard laparoscopy. These advantages include three-dimensional vision, improved ergonomics, and enhanced precision and dexterity offered by Endowrist technology. The improvements offered by robotic technology ultimately resulted in robotics being adopted in laparoendoscopic single-site surgery (LESS) in order to overcome the challenges associated with suturing, intra-abdominal triangulation, and instrument clashing.

Our center reported the first series of robotic laparoendoscopic single-site surgery (RLESS) in 2008 and found that intracorporeal dissection and suturing were easier when compared to traditional LESS techniques [1]. Since that time, our center has published several studies describing RLESS, improvements in techniques, and its application to several different urologic surgeries [2–4]. Several studies have gone on to compare outcomes between RLESS and other laparoscopic approaches, including standard robotic, laparoscopic, or LESS surgery [2, 5, 6]. Though

P. Mouracade, MD, PhD • D. Ramirez, M.D.
J.H. Kaouk, M.D. (✉)
Glickman Institute of Urology and Nephrology,
Cleveland Clinic, 9500 Euclid Ave, Q10-1,
Cleveland, OH 44195, USA
e-mail: kaoukj@ccf.org

these series have been limited by their small sample sizes and retrospective designs, they still demonstrate similar outcomes with the potential for improved cosmesis associated with RLESS. Despite the benefits offered by robotic technology, there still exist limitations which are inherent to a single-site approach. These limitations include instrument clashing secondary to a bulky external mechanics, limited space for the bedside assistant, failure to integrate the fourth robotic arm and challenges with re-creating intracorporeal triangulation. While several improvements in technique has been offered to address these challenges [7, 8], RLESS continues to be an evolving approach and has not yet been widely adopted [9].

The RLESS approach has many similar properties when compared to traditional robotic surgery, including the arrangement of the operative theater, instrumentation, suture, and draping. Docking the robotic console is also comparable, though the angle of the ports will influence the angle at which the robotic arms are docked, and this may be performed differently in RLESS to reduce instrument clashing. Surgical steps of each distinct procedure are also the same, though several improvisations are executed during RLESS to work around the limited available space. Other tactics can be employed to limit robotic arm and instrument clashing, for example concomitant movement of the camera and robotic arms. This chapter reviews the necessary tools and techniques for various different

© Springer International Publishing Switzerland 2017
L.-M. Su (ed.), *Atlas of Robotic Urologic Surgery*, DOI 10.1007/978-3-319-45060-5_33

urologic procedures that are specific to RLESS and focuses on their differences from traditional robotic surgery.

Single-Site vs. Single-Port Surgery

When describing access for an RLESS approach, a critical distinction must be made between single-site access and single-port access. The chief difference between the two is how many fascia incisions are made and utilized for port placement. Single-site access uses a single skin incision through which multiple fascial incisions are made for placement of multiple ports (Fig. 33.1). Single-port access also utilizes a single skin incision, but for this access, a single fascial incision is made in order to introduce an access platform that allows multiple channels to be used (Fig. 33.2). The site of entry may be at the umbilicus or elsewhere, depending on the surgery being performed. Umbilical entry has been the most commonly described technique for RLESS as it allows access for various areas of the body and provides improved cosmesis as the scar may be easily hidden [10].

Single-site access involves the use of a single skin incision with multiple fascial incisions to gain access into the abdominal cavity. The typical access site for single-site access is the umbilicus. A 3–4.5 cm incision is made intraumbilically and the umbilicus is dissected free from the rectus fascia to create a potential space between the fascia and skin. Once this is done, a 2 cm incision is created traversing the linea alba through which a multichannel port can be introduced. The robotic ports are placed through the same skin incisions but separate stab incisions are made through the fascia at the desired location, depending on the operation being performed. The ports are tunneled to their desired location to achieve triangulation around the specific area of interest.

Single-port access involves the use of a single skin and fascial incision for access to the abdominal cavity with a multiport access device. Various different devices exist of single-port access, including the GelPort (Applied Medical, Rancho Santa Margarita, CA) and the TriPort (Advanced Surgical Concepts, Bray, Ireland). Access is typically gained via a 2–5 cm periumbilical incision, which can be made in a semicircular fashion to hide the incision within the fold of the umbilicus. The umbilicus is released from the fascia. A 3–4 cm incision is made in a vertical fashion through the linea alba in order to obtain access into the peritoneum and allow placement of the single-port device. Care must be taken not to make the fascial incision too large as this may result in a gas leak during insufflation. If this

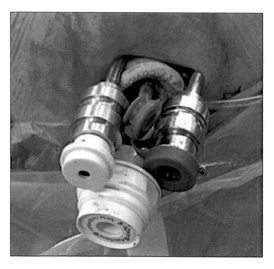

Fig. 33.1 Single-site access using SILS Port (Covidien, Minneapolis, MN)

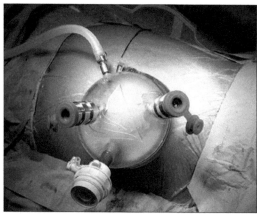

Fig. 33.2 Single-port access with GelPort (Applied Medical, Rancho Santa Margarita, CA)

does occur, it may be remedied by placement of a fascial holding suture or petroleum gauze at the area of the leak.

Multichannel Port Selection

Various multichannel ports exist for performing RLESS (Table 33.1). No studies exist to directly compare outcomes between each device, though many studies have described their individual use, noting their advantages and disadvantages. In the initial RLESS series, Kaouk et al. employed the R-Port device (Advanced Surgical Concepts, Bray, Ireland) [1]. This device is comprised of an insufflation cannula, two 5 mm ports, and one 12 mm channel to accommodate a laparoscopic lens. This port accommodates a 12–25 mm fascial incision and is placed using the open Hasson technique. It is designed to expand both radially and length wise in order to adjust to a larger abdominal wall thickness of up to 10 cm and to decrease the risk of gas leakage during insufflation. Stein et al described the use of the GelPort for four cases of RLESS upper tract procedures and reported flexibility with port placement, an easy access for the bedside assistant and facilitation with specimen removal, especially in cases of RLESS nephrectomy [2]. White et al. reported a series of 50 cases using the SILS port (Covidien, Minneapolis, MN), R-Port, and GelPoint devices [11]. They reported a preference for the SILS port due to the ability to freely exchange the cannulas allowing placement of various sized cannulas.

trocars, ease of passage for clips, suture and stapling devices by the assistant and finally, for its durability. The authors also noted that gas leakage was experienced with use of all the devices, usually secondary to fascial incisions that were made to large during initial placement of the multichannel device. Lee et al. have published the largest series of RLESS procedures using a homemade multichannel device fashioned from an Alexis retractor (Applied Medical) and a sterile surgical glove, size 7 [12]. The wound retractor is placed and the sterile glove is stretched over the opening. Up to four trocars may be placed through the glove fingers. The main advantage for this homemade multichannel port is decreased cost and availability of components, but it is limited in the fact that the surgical glove is easily torn, especially with high insufflation pressures.

Robotic Docking

Subtle differences exist when comparing traditional robotic docking with docking used for RLESS procedures. In regards to the robotic platform, the da Vinci Si or Xi models are preferred over the S model secondary to enhanced visualization, improved ergonomic control at the surgeon console, and, most importantly, a more-compact, sleeker bedside profile which assists with minimizing external clashing of the robotic arms [11, 13]. For RLESS procedures, typically only two robotic instrument arms are used due to limited working space.

Table 33.1 Advantages and disadvantages of available multichannel access ports

Multichannel port	Manufacturer	Advantages	Disadvantages
GelPOINT/GelPORT	Applied Medical	Flexible placement of trocars	Requires larger incision
		Larger working space to decrease clashing	Gas leak with long procedures
		Easier extraction of specimen	
SILS port	Covidien	Flexible placement	Difficult insertion through thick abdominal wall
		Accommodates three ports	
R-Port/TriPort	Advanced Surgical Concepts	Compact	Difficult insertion
		Expands to decrease leakage of gas	Inability to change cannula
Homemade using Alexis retractor	Applied Medical	Low cost	Easily tears
		Flexible placement widely available	Balloon of glove at high insufflation pressures

Other tactics have been described in order to minimize external clashing of robotic arms. The "chopstick" technique popularized by Joseph et al. minimizes external instrument clashing by crossing the instruments at the level of the fascia in order to create more space between the robotic arms outside of the body [7, 14]. This technique was previously employed during single-site laparoscopic surgery but proves to be very challenging secondary to the crossing of instruments resulting in "reverse handedness." This benefit of using the robotic platform is that the robotic instruments are controlled electronically, allowing the left- and right-hand joystick hand effectors to be interchanged, thus removing this challenge. The main drawback of this method is intra-abdominal arm clashing. The surgeon must always remain cognizant as to the position of each instrument to avoid clashing and counter-springing.

RLESS Instrumentation

The standard selection of robotic instruments has been the most commonly utilized tool for performing RLESS procedures, as only a limited quantity of RLESS-specific appliances have been developed [4, 11, 12]. The benefit for using the existing 8 mm da Vinci robotic instruments is familiarity and employment of EndoWrist technology. Five millimeter instruments can also be deployed, but it is important to note that 5 mm instruments deflect rather than articulate, which maintains their range of motion.

Intuitive surgical has developed various tools specific for RLESS, including a multichannel platform specialized for their robotic platform (Fig. 33.3), which includes two curved cannulas, two straight cannulas, and a valve to allow insufflation. The curve of the lateral cannulas allows for institution of intracorporeal triangulation. Similar to the "chopstick" technique, the instruments are crossed at the level of the fascia, necessitating electronic reversal of the effector controls between the surgeon console and patient-side cart. This platform was utilized by Cestari et al. in performing RLESS pyeloplasty in nine patients [15]. All nine cases were performed with a mean

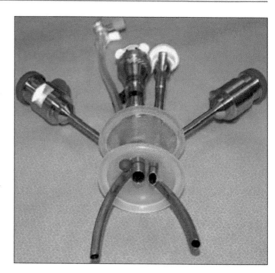

Fig. 33.3 Da Vinci curved cannula system for RLESS

OR time of 166 min, no need for additional ports or need for operative conversion.

Various lens arrangements have been described for RLESS procedures. In their series of RLESS prostatectomy, White et al. primary employed the use of a 0° scope but found that the utilization of a 30° has the advantage of positioning the camera out of the path of the robotic instruments potentially decreasing the degree of instrument clashing [4]. Various arrangements have been used for upper tract RLESS procedures. When considering which lens to use during RLESS, the surgeon must take into account port placement and potential for clashing. Having both 30° and 0° lenses available during an early experience may be beneficial in assessing which configuration is preferred for a specific procedure.

Pelvic Surgery

Radical Prostatectomy

Our institution described our initial experience with single-site laparoscopic radical prostatectomy in 2007 and found that the procedure is technically feasible but difficult to perform [16]. The robotic platform serves as an invaluable adjunct for performing single-site prostatectomy, ultimately reducing the learning curve and improving technical challenges encountered with the LESS approach, namely intracorporeal suturing of the anastomosis. Docking and patient positioning are identical to standard robotic-assisted prostatectomy with the patient in steep Trendelenburg lithotomy position and the patient-side cart positioned between the patient's legs.

We prefer a single-site access with use of a multichannel port. The robotic instrument ports are placed through the same skin incision but introduced intra-abdominal via separate fascial sites. Initially, a 3–5 cm intraumbilically incision is made on the inferior aspect of the umbilicus in a semilunar fashion as to hide the incision at the end of the case. The umbilicus is completely freed from its fascial attachments and a 2 cm incision is made through the linea alba for placement of a single-site access port. We prefer the SILS Port (Covidien) for this endeavor as it accommodates three variable-sized ports and expands to prevent leakage of insufflation. Once the multichannel port is placed through our incision in the linea alba, the 8 mm robotic instrument ports are placed. These ports are placed at the inferior lateral edge of our skin incision and tunneled as far laterally as possible to emulate their position during a standard robotic prostatectomy. The fourth robotic arm is not utilized for our RLESS approach. A 12 mm trocar is placed via the SILS port for placement of the robotic camera. The instruments are not crossed in a "chopstick" fashion for RLESS prostatectomy. Having both a 30° and 0° lens available is beneficial.

Bladder mobilization is performed with 8 mm curve monopolar scissors in the right robotic arm and a 5 mm Schertel grasper or 8 mm ProGrasp forceps in the left robotic port. A 30° upward lens may be of benefit during this dissection if the urachus is not in view. The urachus is transected with cautery and the peritoneum is opened laterally to either side of the medial umbilical ligaments and the bladder is dropped from its position on the anterior abdominal wall, as is done during the standard approach. The anterior surface of the prostate is cleared of fatty tissue and the endopelvic fascia is incised on either side to expose the levator ani muscles bilaterally. The muscle fibers are detached from the prostate, typically with blunt dissection. At times, accessory pudendal arteries or peri-prostatic veins are encountered during this dissection and may need to be ligated with suture or clips. Once this dissection has been performed, the prostatic apex is defined by incising the puboprostatic ligaments in order to identify the dorsal venous complex (DVC). Ligation of the DVC is performed with a 2-0 braided polyglactin suture placed in a figure-of-eight fashion using an 8 mm robotic needle driver.

Once this is performed, the anterior bladder neck is identified superior to the prostatic base. This area can be better defined by manipulating the catheter and by identifying the base of the prostate at the opening of the endopelvic fascia. It is beneficial to have the catheter balloon deflated prior to this time, as the balloon may distort the bladder neck, making its identification more difficult. Once the anterior bladder neck is open and the catheter is seen, the catheter is pulled into the field secured to the anterior abdominal wall with the use of a 2-0 suture in a "marionette" fashion, as described in our initial RLESS series [1]. Since the third robotic instrument is not available during RLESS, this move allows anterior retraction of the prostate which facilitates dissection of the posterior bladder neck and initial dissection of plan posterior the prostate. The posterior bladder neck is opened and gradually separated from the prostatic base. Care is taken to identify and avoid the ureteral orifices. Once the bladder is completely separated from the prostate, the anterior layer of Denovilliers fascia is opened in order to expose bilateral vas deferens and seminal vesicles. In cases where nerve-sparing is not performed, a 5 mm harmonic scalpel may be used. In cases where nerve-sparing is being performed, Hem-o-lok clips are used to maintain an athermal technique, maintaining an interfascial approach for neurovascular bundle release.

Once the posterior plane is complete, our attention is taken to the apex of the prostate. The DVC is transected using cautery from the 8 mm monopolar scissors and the anterior urethra is transected sharply. We typically preserve the longest urethral length possible, taking into account any cancer that is present at the prostatic apex to ensure a negative margin, as the apex is the most common site of a positive margin during robotic prostatectomy. Once the anterior urethra is incised and the catheter is identified, the catheter is retracted into the anterior urethra to expose the posterior urethral edge, which is then divided sharply. The prostate is then completely freed and placed outside of the pelvis. We routinely perform pelvic lymph node dissection in patients with intermediate and high-risk disease. Bilateral pelvic lymph node dissection is performed identically to standard robotic prostatectomy technique. Lymphatic tissue from the external iliac chain and obturator foramen are removed.

Vesicourethral anastomosis is completed with an 8 mm robotic needle driver in the left and right robotic ports to facilitate intracorporeal suturing and is completed with a 2-0 poliglecaprone 25 (Monocryl) suture on an RB-1 needle. The anastomosis is performed in a running fashion from the 6 o'clock to the 12 o'clock position. We typically use a dyed and undyed suture, with the dyed suture on the right-hand side to facilitate identification of the suture. Both ends are tied together once the anastomosis is complete. A 10 mm Jackson Pratt drain is routinely left in place via a separate stab incision made through the fascia, but the drain is brought out through the skin via the same initial incision used for the multichannel port. All specimens are placed in a laparoscopic specimen bag and removed via the gel port site.

Robotic Single-Port Transvesicle Enucleation of the Prostate

Our experience with robotic-assisted single-port transvesicle enucleation of the prostate (R-STEP) was published in 2010 [17]. This procedure involves the use of the Applied Medical GelPort through a suprapubic incision that allows port placement directly into the bladder for transvesicle enucleation.

Patients are placed in low lithotomy position and cystoscopy is performed prior to obtain transvesicle access in order to define the apical limits of the prostate with a Collins knife incision. The bladder is filled with irrigation and the skin incision is marked from the level of the dome of the bladder downward toward the pubis. Identification of the cranial-most extent of the incision is facilitated with the use of a spinal needle placed under cystoscopic vision directly into the bladder. Once this limit is defined, a 3 cm skin incision is made through the fascia, and the perivesicle fat is dissected to expose the underlying detrusor. Two-stay sutures are placed along both side of the detrusor opening at this point. The bladder is opened transversely between the stay sutures. A 16 Fr catheter is placed into the bladder and its balloon is inflated with 5 cm^3 of sterile water. The GelPort is then placed through the wound in order to allow access into the bladder. We use a 12 mm port at the 6 o'clock position for the robotic camera and insufflation, two 5 mm ports on the right and an 8 mm robotic instrument port on the left. The GelPort gel pad comes with a pre-made hole in the center to assist with trocar placement. The hole is closed prior to placement of the gel pad over the wound retractor as it is not used in this technique. Once all the ports are placed, insufflation of the bladder is obtained and set to 20 mmHg. An upward facing 30° scope is used during this procedure to improve with visualization and limit instrument clashing. The 5 mm harmonic scalpel is used in the right arm and a 5 mm deflecting Schertel grasper is placed in the left. A circular incision is made around the prostatic adenoma between the prostate and bladder neck. Care is taken to identify and avoid bilateral ureteral orifices during this initial dissection. The avascular plane is developed between the prostatic adenoma and prostate capsule and enucleation is carried from the prostatic base to the apex. The incision made at the apical prostate at the beginning of the case assists with identification of the apex during this dissection. Once this is complete and bleeding is controlled, a 24 Fr 3 way hematuria catheter is placed into the bladder with 30 cm^3 of sterile water in the balloon. The specimen is removed from the bladder via the GelPort site and the bladder is closed in a running fashion with 2-0 absorbable suture. The rest of the wound is closed in the standard fashion, using 0-0 PDS for fascial closure.

Perineal Robotic Radical Prostatectomy

Our institution has been evaluating the use of a completely novel approach for robotic radical prostatectomy from a perineal approach [18]. This technique may be advantageous in patients who have had prior extensive abdominal surgery, radiation, or in patients with urinary or gastrointestinal diversions. In addition, this approach offers the same advantages of a posterior, space of Retzuis-sparing technique by preserving endopelvic fascia, DVC, and the pelvic floor diaphragm [19–21].

Initially, we make a midline, transverse, semilunar incision in the perineum between the ischial tuberosities, similar to the incision made for open perineal radical prostatectomy, but we only utilize an incision about two-thirds the size of the open technique. Once this incision is made, the central tendon is divided and a GelPOINT multichannel access port (Applied Medical, Rancho Santa Margarita, CA) is placed into the wound after the potential space is created and the apex of the prostate is identified. We utilize a 12 mm camera port, two 8 mm robotic ports, and a second 12 mm port for the bedside assistant.

Thus far we have reserved a robotic perineal approach for patients in whom a retropubic or transperitoneal approach is deemed challenging, such as those patient with prior extensive rectal and/or colonic resection and other history of prior pelvic surgery. Thus far we have performed this procedure on two patients with promising results [22], though currently our unpublished series consists of five patients. This approach is feasible and thus far we have not had to convert to standard open, robotic or laparoscopic techniques using a single-site perineal approach. This novel technique is still in its infancy and our future experience with this approach is forthcoming.

Upper Tract and Renal Surgery

Radical Nephrectomy

Patient positioning and robotic docking for RLESS radical nephrectomy (RLESS-RN) is the same as the conventional approach for traditional robot-assisted nephrectomy, with the patient in a modified flank position and the robot docked over the ipsilateral shoulder and flank. Only three arms for the robot platform are utilized as there is limited room for the fourth arm in docking through a single port. A variety of multichannel access ports have been described for use during RLESS radical nephrectomy. Stein et al. described RLESS nephrectomy with use of the GelPort device as being greatly beneficial as the specimen is easily extracted through the port itself [2]. Once the multichannel port is selected, placed and robot docked, the steps of dissection for RLESS-RN is the same as for conventional laparoscopic or robotic nephrectomy. Standard 8 mm robotic instruments are typically utilized. Initially, the white line of Toldt is incised and the colon is mobilized medially. The ureter and gonadal vessels are identified and controlled. The hilum is found by following anatomical landmarks and the renal vessels are controlled and ligated by the use of a vascular cutting stapler passed through the assistant port. Small vessels, gonadal vessels, and ureter can be controlled by use of a Hem-o-lok clips either placed by the assistant or robotically using the robotic clip applier. At our institution, we reserve use of the robotic clip applier only for angles that are not accessible by the assistant in order to decrease disposable costs associated with robotic instrumentation. Once the hilum is ligated and other attachments to the kidney are released, it is placed into a laparoscopic specimen bag and extracted through the GelPort access site.

In regards to perioperative outcomes comparing conventional laparoscopic nephrectomy and RLES-RN, our institution performed a retrospective comparative matched analysis published in 2011 [3]. Patients were matched 1:1 based on ASA score, BMI, and tumor size. Both GelPort and SILS ports were used in the RLESS group. No difference was seen when comparing EBL, postoperative pain, OR time, or rate of complications. The study found a lower post-operative narcotic requirement (25.3 vs. 37.5 morphine equivalents; $p=0.05$) and a shorter length of stay (2.5 vs. 3.0 days; $p=0.03$) in the RLESS-RD group.

Partial Nephrectomy

Initial patient positioning and docking of the robot for RLESS partial nephrectomy (RLESS-PN) is identical to RLESS-RN, with the patient in a modified flank position with 60° of flexion, using three robotic arms, as there is little available room for the fourth. Eight-millimeter conventional robotic instruments are used. The dissection and exposure is also the same for standard robotic partial nephrectomy (RPN). Once the hilum is identified, the tumor is exposed and delineated with a laparoscopic ultrasound device that is introduced through the assistant port. At our institution, we prefer the ProART™ Robotic Ultrasound Transducer made by BK Medical as it allows the robotic surgeon to directly control the ultrasound probe with the use of robotic ProGrasp forceps. Use of the ultrasound probe will delineate the margins of the tumor and guide initial resection. The decision for type of hilar clamping is left to the surgeon's discretion and is typically decided on once the tumor has been exposed and analyzed with the ultrasound probe. Resection and renorrhaphy are performed in the standard fashion, similar to conventional RPN techniques.

Lee et al. published the largest series of RLESS-PN in 2011 [12]. This series of 68 RLESS cases utilized a homemade access port as previously described, and included 51 consecutive patients who underwent RLESS-PN. Average tumor size and EBL were 3.0 cm and 322 cm^3, respectively with a transfusion rate of 14%. This high rate of transfusion was attributed to renal bleeding during tumor resection and one incidence of renal vein injury. Two patients (3.9%) required conversion to open procedure for management of hilar bleeding in one, and for difficulty accessing the renal tumor in the other.

Arkoncel et al. performed a comparative analysis of 35 patients who underwent "two-port" RLESS-PN [5]. These patients were matched 1:1 based on tumor complexity with patients who underwent standard RPN. In these RLESS-PN cases a "two-port" technique was used. A homemade single-site access port was created with the use of an Alexis tissue retractor and a sterile surgical glove. The second port consisted of a 12 mm assistant port that was placed outside of the homemade port and a separate incision site. In regards to OR time, transfusion rate, EBL, complications, length of stay, and pain control, no difference was seen in either group. They study described increased difficulty with the RLESS approach for partial nephrectomy specifically commenting on the restrictive nature of the robotic arms and increased instrument clashing. Secondary to these technical challenges, RLESS-PN has not been widely adopted.

Dismembered Pyeloplasty

Our center initially described RLESS dismembered pyeloplasty in our initial RLESS series from 2008 [1]. Patient positioning and robotic docking is similar to partial nephrectomy. The patient is placed in modified flank position with 60° of table flexion. Our initial series described performing RLESS pyeloplasty with use of an R-Port, though use of other ports has been described, including the SILS and GelPoint multichannel access ports [2, 6, 14]. A ureteral stent is placed prior to robotic docking via cystoscopy and fluoroscopic guidance. Initial exposure is performed in the standard fashion. Attention is taken to the proximal ureter and renal pelvis. The stenotic ureteropelvic junction (UPJ) is excised and sent to pathology, the ureter spatulated laterally, and reconstructive tailoring of the renal pelvis is performed. Water-tight anastomosis is created with interrupted or running suture with the stent left in place with the proximal coil in the renal pelvis. Once the anastomosis is complete, a 10 mm Jackson–Pratt drain is left in place and brought out of the body via the incision at the umbilicus.

Patients with UPJ obstruction may be the best candidates for an RLESS approach as this population is typically younger and the surgery is performed for a benign indication. No large specimen is extracted from the body, thus the incision may remain small in size making it easier to hide the incision within the fold of the umbilicus. Single port pyeloplasty was initially performed via a LESS approach, but the adoption of the robotic platform has improved our ability to perform these cases. Olweny et al. publish a retrospective comparative analysis of LESS and RLESS pyeloplasty in 2012 with ten patients in each arm [6]. They found no significant difference between the group regarding pain control, EBL, complications, or length of stay. They did find however that the RLESS group had a significantly longer operative time (226 vs. 188 min; $p = 0.007$). Ultimately, the authors felt that the robotic platform improved the single-site procedure by employing improved optics with three-dimensional vision and intracorporeal wrist articulation.

The use of the curved cannula single-port access device developed for RLESS by Intuitive Surgical (Fig. 33.3) was assessed in nine patients undergoing RLESS pyeloplasty in a study by Cestari et al. [15]. This device employs the current Si da Vinci robotic system, and consists of curved robotic instruments and curved cannula that allow crossing of the instruments at the level of the fascia, similar to the previously described "chop-stick" technique. Crossing of the instruments minimizes instrument clashing while maintaining intracorporeal triangulation. No complications or conversion to open or traditional laparoscopic techniques were encountered in their series of nine patients, but they described a major limitation of the curved cannula system in the lack of instruments articulation that is offered by conventional robotic instrumentation.

Future of Single-Site Robotic Surgery

Since its inception, the notion of minimally invasive surgery has inspired urologists to push the limits of available technology and to improve on the current techniques in order to devise new methods and instrumentation. The concept of laparoendoscopic single-site surgery (LESS) was conceived with the main objective of easing patient recovery, improving cosmesis, and enhancing quality of life outcomes, but its widespread adoption has yet to materialize secondary to intrinsic challenges compared to standard laparoscopic or robotic techniques.

Combining LESS with the robotic platform has greatly enhanced our surgical capability by offering increased articulation and stability for precise suturing and dissection. Since the publication of our initial series, multiple institutions have adopted the technique and published series of their own. While the da Vinci robotic system has substantially improved our ability to perform single site surgery, it was not originally designed for this purpose. Because of this, an innovative device precisely designed for RLESS (da Vinci single-port, SP999) has been designed. In contrast to the original robotic design for single-site surgery that requires the use of multiple separate ports, the SP999 da Vinci© single-port system only uses a single port to introduce the instruments and camera (Fig. 33.4). This system uses the same base of the patient side cart as the Xi da Vinci robotic system and is adapted onto a single arm (Fig. 33.5).

Our institution was one of the first to utilize the new single-port robotic system in a clinical series [23]. We have performed single-site robotic surgery using this novel technology in 19 patients, 11 of which underwent single-site robotic prostatectomy. There were no conversions to

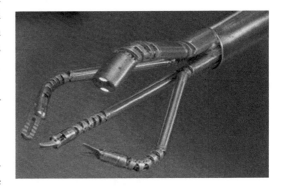

Fig. 33.4 SP999 single-port da Vinci platform

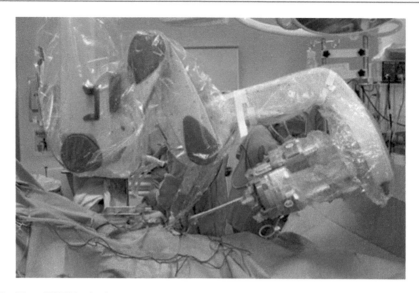

Fig. 33.5 Docking of SP999 robotic system

open, contemporary robotic or laparoscopic techniques and high-grade complications only occurred in two patients. Functional outcomes over a 3-year follow-up were comparable to standard techniques. This new single-port robotic technology represents a step forward in minimally invasive surgery. It is unique as it allows for intracorporeal triangulation while eliminating instrument clashing seen with other methods of performing single-site surgery. The new da Vinci SP surgical system (model SP1098; Intuitive Surgical, Sunnyvale, CA, USA) represents an evolution of the second-generation robotic system (SP999) with upgraded technology designed specifically for extraperitoneal single-site surgery. We used the SP1098 to perform retroperitoneal R-LESS radical nephrectomy (n=1) and bilateral partial nephrectomy (n=4) on the anterior and posterior surfaces of the kidney in a preclinical study [24]. Similar to the SP999, the SP1098 consists of three main components: a surgeon console, a patient side cart, and a vision cart. The designs of the articulating endoscopic camera and three double-jointed articulating endoscopic instruments (Fig. 33.6), which enter the patient through a multichannel robotic port, are unchanged. As before, four robotic manipulators, or instrument drives, that control the camera and instruments are mounted on an instrument

arm that is attached to the patient side cart. The surgeon console is identical to the second-generation robotic system (SP999) with a foot pedal that allows control of the instrument arm. Unique to this robotic system is the ability to clutch and pivot the instrument arm about its remote center without moving each individual instrument. In effect, an instrument can be stationed at one location in the surgical field (e.g., for retraction) while the instrument arm is clutched and reoriented to a separate site, where the remaining instruments can be deployed without disturbing the stationary instrument. This improvement overcomes the constraint of multiple instruments entering the body through a fixed point, effectively expanding the workspace and improving maneuverability (Fig. 33.7). The new vision cart is similar to the previous generation with upgraded resolution to accommodate the improved camera optics.

Conclusions

The adaptation of the robotic platform to the LESS technique has greatly improved the ability to perform single incision urologic procedure, mainly by instituting improved optics and articulating wrist technology as offered by robotic

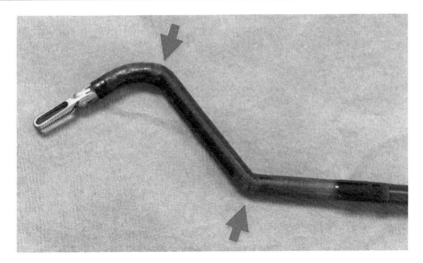

Fig. 33.6 EndoWrist forceps showing the double-jointed distal end with elbow and articulating wrist joints that facilitate triangulation at the surgical site

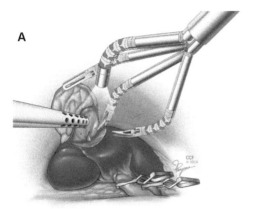
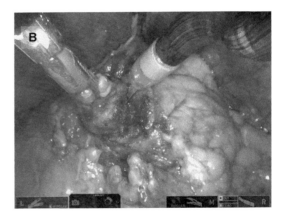

Fig. 33.7 Illustration showing parenchymal excision using the SP1098 (**A**) and intraoperative photograph of the same task (**B**)

instrumentation. While this approach has improved over time, there has still not been widespread adoption of RLESS secondary to innate challenges that still exist, including instrument clashing and limited bed-side access for the surgical assistant. A novel device specifically designed or single-port robotic surgery will be introduced in the near future and will improve our ability to perform these procedures. The field on minimally invasive surgery continues to expand its horizon with each new technique and device that comes to market. There is no doubt that these new approaches will continue to push the limits of minimally invasive urology.

References

1. Kaouk JH, Goel RK, Haber GP, Crouzet S, Stein RJ. Robotic single-port transumbilical surgery in humans: initial report. BJU Int. 2008;103:366–9.
2. Stein RJ, White WM, Geol RK, Irwin BH, Haber GP, Kaouk JH. Robotic laparoendoscopic single-site surgery using GelPort as the access platform. Eur Urol. 2010;57:132–7.
3. White MA, Autorino R, Spana G, et al. Robotic laparoendoscopic single-site radical nephrectomy: surgical techniques and comparative outcomes. Eur Urol. 2011;59:815–22.
4. White MA, Haber GP, Autorino R, et al. Robotic laparoendoscopic single-site radical prostatectomy: technique and early outcomes. Eur Urol. 2010;58:544–50.

5. Arkoncel FR, Lee JW, Rha KH, et al. Two-port robot-assisted vs standard robot-assisted laparoendoscopic single-site partial nephrectomy: a matched-pair comparison. Urology. 2011;78:581–5.

6. Olweny EO, Park SK, Tan YK, Gurbus C, Caddedu J, Best SL. Perioperative comparison of robotic assisted laparoendoscopic single-site (LESS) pyeloplasty versus conventional LESS pyeloplasty. Eur Urol. 2012;61:410–4.

7. Joseph RA, Goh AC, Cuevas SP, et al. Chostick surgery: a novel technique improves surgeon performance and eliminates arm collision in robotic single-incision laparoscopic surgery. Surg Endosc. 2010;24:1331–5.

8. Haber GP, White MA, Autorino R, et al. Novel robotic da Vinci instruments for laparoendoscopic single-site surgery. Urology. 2010;76:1279–82.

9. Janetschek G. Robotics: will they give a new kick to single-site surgery? Eur Urol. 2014;66:1044–5.

10. Kaouk JH, Autorino R, Kim FJ, et al. Laparoendoscopic single-site surgery in urology: worldwide multi-institutional analysis of 1076 cases. Eur Urol. 2011; 60:998–1005.

11. White MA, Autorino R, Spana G, Hillyer S, Stein RJ, Kaouk JH. Robotic laparoendoscopic single site urological surgery: analysis of 50 consecutive cases. J Urol. 2012;187:1696–701.

12. Lee JW, Arkoncel FRP, Rha KH, et al. Urologic robot-assisted laparoendoscopic single-site surgery using a homemade single-port device: a single-center experience of 68 cases. J Endourol. 2011;25:1481–5.

13. Seideman CA, Yung KT, Faddegon S, et al. Robot-assisted laparoendoscopic single-site pyeloplasty: technique using the da Vinci Si robotic platform. J Endourol. 2012;26:971–4.

14. Joseph RA, Salas NA, Johnson C, et al. Chopstick surgery: a novel technique enables use of the da Vinci robot to perform single-incision laparoscopic surgery [video]. Surg Endosc. 2010;24:3224.

15. Cestari A, Buffi NM, Lista G, et al. Feasibility and preliminary clinic outcomes of robotic laparoendo-scopic single-site (R-LESS) pyeloplasty using a new single-port platform. Eur Urol. 2012;62: 175–9.

16. Kaouk JH, Goel RK, Haber GP, et al. Single port laparoscopic radical prostatectomy. Urology. 2008;72: 1190–3.

17. Fareed K, Zaytoun OM, Autorino R, et al. Robotic single port suprapubic transvesicle enucleation of the prostate (R-STEP): initial experience. BJU Int. 2012; 110:732–7.

18. Laydner H, Akca O, Autorino R, Eyraud R, Zargar H, Brandao LF, Khalifeh A, Panumatrassamee K, Long JA, Isac W, Stein RJ, Kaouk JH. Perineal robot-assisted laparoscopic radical prostatectomy: feasibility study in the cadaver model. J Endourol. 2014;28(12):1479–86.

19. Avant OL, Jones JA, Beck H, et al. New method to improve treatment outcomes for radical prostatectomy. Urology. 2000;56(4):658–62.

20. Galfano A, Ascione A, Grimaldi S, et al. A new anatomic approach for robotic-assisted laparoscopic prostatectomy: a feasibility study for completely intrafascial surgery. Eur Urol. 2010;58(3):457–61.

21. Galfano A, Di Trapani D, Sozzi F, et al. Beyond the learning curve of the Retzius-sparing approach for robot-assisted laparoscopic radical prostatectomy: oncologic and function results of the first 200 patients with 1 year follow up. Eur Urol. 2013;64(6): 974–80.

22. Akca O, Zargar H, Kaouk JH. Robotic surgery revives radical perineal prostatectomy. Eur Urol. 2015;68(2): 340–1.

23. Kaouk JH, Haber GP, Autorino R, Crouzet S, Ouzzane A, Flamand V, Villers A. A novel robotic system for single-port urologic surgery: first clinical investigation. Eur Urol. 2014;66(6):1033–43.

24. Maurice MJ, Ramirez D, Kaouk JH. Robotic laparoendoscopic single-site retroperitioneal renal surgery: initial investigation of a purpose-built single-port surgical system. Eur Urol 2017;71(4):643–7.

Part VI

Robotic Platforms: Past, Present, Future Perspectives

Robotic Surgery: Past, Present, and Future

S. Duke Herrell

Background

Robots are able to perform varied precise and accurate tasks including existing in hazardous environments and handling hazardous materials with minimal risk to humans. They excel at performing highly repetitive tasks and have been widely adopted into industrial manufacturing due to many of these advantages. Overall, robots are often categorized by type of control mechanisms. Robotic control can be defined as active, where the robot is actually performing the action without human control usually under a programmed command structure; semi-active, where the robot is responsible for some of the control but is overseen during the task by a human who is able to add control; and, finally, passive (master–slave) system architecture where the system only performs movements that are input directly from the human controller. No autonomous movement is present in the commercial surgical robotic system created for abdominal and thoracic minimally invasive surgery, although this is an area of active research. The success of robotic industrial manufacturing has demonstrated that robots can be tireless, accurate, and capable of speed and precision that is far beyond that of a human. However, industrial robots are also dangerous as their speed, size, and movements can result in significant damage to surrounding structures or life forms if there are errors in command or control.

Pure laparoscopic surgery provides the gold standard benefits of minimally invasive surgery including decreased pain, improved cosmesis, reduced hospitalization, reduced recovery, and overall shorter convalescence. Negatives of minimally invasive surgery include the constraints of instrumentation and visualization. The human hand and wrist has a full 7° of freedom (DOF) of motion whereas a standard non-dexterous laparoscopic straight instrument contains only 4° of motion. The fulcrum effect of the trocar and instrument in combination limits access to some workspace areas and can result in potential transmission of tremor. The extended length of instrumentation can result in non-optimal angles and vectors of approach for tasks such as suturing and cutting. Multiple authors have noted significant learning curves with the performance of minimally invasive surgery via laparoscopic and endoscopic minimally invasive approaches. Complex tasks such as suturing require a significant learning curve.

History of Surgical Robotics

Industrial robotics preceded surgical robotics by many years. Adaptation of industrial robots to surgery was first performed in 1985 when the

S.D. Herrell, M.D. (✉)
Department of Urologic Surgery, Vanderbilt University Medical Center, A-1302, Medical Center North, Nashville, TN 37232-2765, USA
e-mail: duke.herrell@vanderbilt.edu

© Springer International Publishing Switzerland 2017
L.-M. Su (ed.), *Atlas of Robotic Urologic Surgery*, DOI 10.1007/978-3-319-45060-5_34

PUMA (Programmable Universal Machine for Assembly, or Programmable Universal Manipulation Arm) robot (Unimation Corp./ Westinghouse Corp.) was used to perform neurosurgical targeted biopsies using CT guidance [1]. The PUMA was used to enhance the precision of stereotactic brain biopsy techniques versus manual techniques. While the system proved accurate, it was not adopted for widespread use due to workflow and operative time requirements.

Urology had a key and early role in robotics with the development of a transurethral prostate resection robot by Davies et al. based on a PUMA 560 robot [2]. The system used intraoperative ultrasound imaging and was shown in the lab setting to be feasible. Despite showing the potential of robotics in urology, widespread use did not follow. The industrial robot manufacturer eventually limited access to continued development due to concerns about safety. Of note, the PUMA robot was designed for industrial use with a barrier area to prevent contact or collision with people and objects. Safety concerns continue to this day regarding the use of robots, especially autonomous control, in the surgical environment. The research team at the Imperial College of London went on to develop the PROBOT for resection of benign prostatic hypertrophy, which was not based on the 560 PUMA [3]. It utilized image-guided, model-based anatomy to perform a successful resection of the prostate and was, interestingly, an entirely automated system for transurethral resection. Interestingly, the system had multiple degrees of freedom (7 DOF) and was able to perform an automated transurethral resection by being coupled to a motorized component that maneuvered and operated the resectoscope. The desired volume of prostate resection and tissue removal was captured based on preoperative prostate volume and shape from data by transrectal ultrasound scan. It is indeed fascinating that some of the first clinical utilizations of robotics in surgery incorporated the concepts of image-guided surgery (IGS). A small cohort of patients underwent the PROBOT procedure; however, the need for subsequent surgeon-performed electrocautery hemostasis and concerns over accuracy of ultrasound in selection of planned resection volume resulted in abandonment of the developing

platform. Interestingly, there is now renewed interest in robotic systems for BPH management based on both new tissue removal techniques and ablative technologies. These robotic systems are programmed to limit their treatments to preoperatively and intraoperatively obtained tissue volumes based on imaging [4, 5].

Simultaneously, other specialties, such as orthopedics, were also exploring development of robotic surgical systems. ROBODOC, created by Integrated Surgical Systems, Inc. (ISS) (Sacramento, CA), developed a system to precisely mill the femur cavity for an artificial hip replacement [6]. The ROBODOC received 510(k) approval from the FDA and has found some commercial success. The system is comprised of a computer workstation, which allows three-dimensional preoperative surgical planning, and the ROBODOC surgical assistant, a computer-controlled robotic system for drilling and precision milling the appropriate areas of bone. Literature studies have shown that robotically milled bone defects provide improved contact with the prostheses [7]. A variety of other orthopedic systems have followed including the OrthoPilot (Aesculap AG, Tuttlingen, Germany), Acrobot (Acrobot Company Ltd, London, England), and MAKOplasty system (Stryker Corp. Kalamazoo, MI) [8].

Spurred by the exciting initial developments in robotic surgery of the late 1990s, several groups around the world developed other "robotic" surgical systems. A team headed by Dan Stoianovici PhD at Johns Hopkins University developed several novel robotic systems including systems for holding and maneuvering needles under image guidance. A variety of potential applications were explored with promising improvements in accuracy results including prostate radioactive seed placement, organ biopsy, and stereotactic injections [9–11].

Laparoscopy

Several research teams began in the 1980s and 1990s to work on improving the potential of robotics application to the burgeoning field of laparoscopic minimally invasive surgery. These research teams worked on a concept of improved end-effector manipulators, which were superior to standard "straight stick" laparoscopy with the addition of surgeon remote control of the device (telepresence). Computer Motion, Inc. (Santa Barbara, CA), a startup created by Yulun Wang, Ph.D. in 1989, had the first FDA-approved robotic system that consisted of a camera and lens holding robotic arm, which was under the control of the surgeon. The AESOP (Automated Endoscopic System for Optimal Positioning) consisted of a robot arm with motorized joints that controlled the position of the minimally invasive laparoscope and was typically under command of the surgeon via speech recognition. The AESOP was sold extensively in the United States and became part of many surgeons' preferences in the operating room. The early advantages of robotics such as surgeon control, tirelessness, and accuracy were apparent even on these early platforms. Computer Motion also developed separate patient-side manipulators, which were able to move and control surgical end-effector tools via a remote control console. These patient-side manipulators, surgical tools, and the endoscope manipulation system were combined together to form the Zeus surgical system. In this system, the surgeon sat in a telepresence console and was in control of multiple separate patient-side manipulator arms and end-effector instruments attached to the operating room table. The surgeon interacted with the machine/human interface controls on their console to control the position and actions of all of the robotic end-effectors.

Other robotic surgical systems were also under development via collaborations between academic researchers and federally funded government institutes. Some of these projects aimed at the ability to operate in space or remotely operate in a dangerous environment such as the frontlines of a battlefield and involved funding and support from NASA (National Aeronautics and Space Administration) and the DOD (Department of Defense). Early development of systems took place at the Stanford Research Institute (SRI). The initial SRI concept was developed by roboticist Phil Green, Ph.D. and had initially developed

a telemanipulation device to allow improvements in microsurgery for nerve and vascular surgery of the hand. SRI eventually developed a robotic platform for potential use inside of a military mobile surgical unit that would be present at the frontlines during battlefield situations. Medics and others would place the injured soldier into the operating pod while surgeons remotely performed stabilizing maneuvers from a safe and remote site. The "SRI Green Telepresence Surgery System" was designed for battlefield telemanipulative open surgery. The SRI-developed system was used for basic animal surgeries and also to manipulate an endoscope similar to the system under development by Computer Motion, Inc. As DOD funding and interest waned on this system, the private sector moved in and the commercial rights to the system were licensed to Frederic Moll, M.D. who saw the potential applications to minimally invasive surgery. Moll licensed the system in 1995 and created the startup company of Intuitive Surgical Systems (Sunnyvale, CA). The system used a master–slave telepresence computer-assisted surgical technology based on the initial SRI platform, which has come to be called a surgical "robot".

Computer Motion and Intuitive Surgical were both developing surgeon-controlled robotic platforms for advanced manipulation of tools in the field using wristed instruments, camera control, advanced visualization, etc. In 1999, Computer Motion introduced the Zeus system consisting of an AESOP camera control arm and three additional patient side-manipulator robotic arms. The system was advantageous in that it was directly mounted to the operating room table and therefore could move with movement of the patient to allow for repositioning during complicated procedures. In the Zeus system, the AESOP portion was controlled by the surgeon via voice commands, while the patient-side manipulators were under the telepresence control of the surgeon seated in a console. The operative field was visualized on a 2D monitor. Later in development, polarizing glasses were added to create a 3D viewing effect. The end-effectors on the Computer Motion system were limited to six degrees of freedom (6DOF). Zeus was introduced to the European market and was initially used for studies on early cardiac surgery procedures and nephrectomy. Meanwhile, Intuitive Surgical continued strategic development of the da Vinci system for advanced minimally invasive laparoscopic surgery. One of the major differences from Zeus being that the patient-side manipulators were all mounted on a mobile robotic stand, which was maneuvered into position next to the patient but did not move with the bed movements. Early da Vinci systems had three arms consisting of two end-effector patient-side tool manipulators and a patient-side manipulator to control the camera movements.

The machine/human interface of the da Vinci was designed into a separate but electronically linked self-contained "cockpit" type arrangement (console) where the surgeon put their head into a visualization hood, which displayed the images from the endoscope system. The da Vinci also added 3D visualization by using a camera with binocular lenses and the images were fused to create a three-dimensional visual field display in the hood. Perhaps the largest advantage of the da Vinci was the proprietary wrist design that allowed for seven degrees of freedom with the instrument tip under control of the surgeon. This EndoWrist™ provided surgeons a very "intuitive" interaction with the robotic instruments as an extension of the surgeon's hand and finger motions. The manipulators were grasped between the surgeon's fingers in a very similar way to standard surgical instrument hand and finger manipulation. This allowed the da Vinci to achieve a control hand/machine interface that was created with great enthusiasm by surgeons as compared to the Zeus system. Later systems incorporated a fourth arm to allow for surgeon control of retraction.

Early Use

Starting in March 1997, Cadiere and group in Belgium performed the first robotic-assisted laparoscopic surgeries using the da Vinci surgical system [12]. Development of the Zeus to market was in a similar timeframe. Initially, both companies entered the market with some early sales and success. However, both companies became embroiled in litigation against each other regarding various patents and developments. In March 2003, the two companies merged with Intuitive taking over the single company and the product line of Computer Motion and development of alternative systems was rapidly ended. The next decade saw the rise of a single commercially available robotic system in the form of the da Vinci created by Intuitive Surgical.

Da Vinci Robotic Platform Overview

Once the da Vinci platform became the only commercially available system for robotic minimally invasive surgery, sales and applications rapidly followed. The FDA had cleared the da Vinci as an endoscopic instrument control system for use in laparoscopic abdominal procedures in July 2000. The following March 2001, the FDA cleared the da Vinci for non-cardiac thoracoscopic surgical procedures such as surgery on the lung and esophagus. One of the early goals of the Intuitive Surgical development team was to use the machine for internal mammary artery harvest and combine this with robotic coronary bypass surgery. Interestingly, early adopters in Europe and the United States utilized the da Vinci to aid in the burgeoning interest in performing laparoscopic radical prostatectomy. The French team lead by Guillonneau and Vallancien had developed the pure laparoscopic procedure [13] but translation to acceptance amongst non-laparoscopic-trained surgeons, especially urologic oncologists, was challenging. Even skilled laparoscopic surgeons found the learning curve of laparoscopic radical prostatectomy including prostate dissection, nerve-sparing, and reconstruction of the urethrovesical anastomosis extremely demanding. The first robotic radical prostatectomies were performed in 2000 in Europe by a variety of groups and published [14–16]. After a frustrating attempt to learn laparoscopic radical prostatectomy from the French, early acquisition and adoption of the da Vinci for radical prostatectomy by Menon from Henry Ford Hospital in Detroit, Michigan lead the way for the development and popularization of robotic radical prostatectomy in the US [17, 18]. The EndoWrist® Intuitive Surgical allowed movements similar to the human wrist and markedly shortens the learning curve for complex laparoscopic tasks such as suturing. As of 2015, more than 2000 da Vinci surgical systems have been installed worldwide.

The initial da Vinci has been revised and improved with several new models since introduction. Starting with the S and Si systems, a fourth arm carrying a third surgeon-controlled instrument became available. The fourth arm could be used for a variety of tasks but was typically used for retraction. This allowed increased surgeon control of the surgical field and retraction was superior to depending on multiple bedside assistants. Additionally, the ability to switch between the various instrument arms allowed the surgeon set a retractor in place under their precise control. In this author's opinion, the ability to provide additional surgeon direct-controlled retraction in the field has been amongst the greatest advantages brought forward on the da Vinci system. Upgrades to the da Vinci S surgical system also allowed for improved visualization, rapid instrument exchange and docking, and increased work volume, which is referred to as "multiquadrant access" by the manufacturer. Along the way, additional improved interfaces have been developed including a touchscreen monitor to allow for interactive proctoring of the surgeon who is operating the console (telestration), and an input into the display (Tile Pro™) allowing additional view of patient information, stored preoperative imaging, or active intraoperative display of imaging such as ultrasound. The da Vinci Si was released in 2009 and continued upgrades including the potential for continued improvement in three-dimensional vision enhancement, upgraded user and OR software integration, as well as the potential of dual console capability to aid in support and training. The dual console system has multiple potential advantages including the ability for two surgeons to swap control back and forth allowing different types of surgeons to interact quickly within the surgical field. Perhaps the most interesting application potential of the dual console system is in the training for easier adaptation to new procedures and more complex procedures [19].

Intuitive has also recently come out with an immersive virtual environment training skills simulator [20]. The "backpack" attaches to a Si console and allows surgeons a platform to practice different surgical skills utilizing the simulator. This platform has built-in metrics to track progress. The software system allows additional practice modules to be incorporated. Most modules at this point focus on basics such as manipulation of the wrist, camera movement and clutching to allow for improved workflow during actual surgery, exercises regarding the system setup, and exercises regarding needle control and suturing. This is a very important skill as effective and efficient management of tool position and hand and instrument geometry is one of the keys to developing skills. Another skill category includes the use of different energy-based hemostatic instruments. During these modules, users are able to practice the use of both monopolar and bipolar energy on virtual blood vessels during dissection tasks. A variety of other commercial vendors have produced and commercialized virtual reality training systems for robotic surgery [21].

As previously mentioned, the design of the da Vinci platform is really a master–slave architecture telepresence robotic system and falls squarely into the arena of computer-assisted surgery (CAS). The da Vinci platform, which has gone through various iterations, consists of several basic parts. The surgical cart serves as a motorized stand on which multiple arms are mounted in tree architecture. Each arm has passively positioned hinged arms which allow the true "robot" portion which hangs from each hinged arm to be brought into alignment and triangulation similar to a laparoscopic surgical case. Older systems such as the da Vinci S and Si were limited in the camera only being placed in the central arm designed for camera control. The newer Xi version allows the camera to be switched to any of the various robotic arms allowing for improvements in angles of visualization and adjustment for more complex surgical interventions.

There are a variety of proprietary da Vinci tools that can be placed into the patient-side robots, called PSMs (patient-side manipulators). These instruments allow for seven degrees of freedom and are available in a variety of configurations that allow for cutting, suturing, stapling, clip application, various traumatic and atraumatic graspers, suction, and hemostatic energy in the form of bipolar and vessel sealing. There are also multiple control points on the surgeon console allowing for ergonomic positioning for surgeon comfort. Additional foot pedals and finger controls provide interactions that control electrocautery, bipolar, instrument manipulation, and camera focusing and movement. Newer systems also contain fluorescence vascular imaging capability and the ability to bring in images from other sources into the surgeon's visual field in the console using the TilePro device. The most common use of TilePro is to allow the surgeon to visualize real-time intraoperative ultrasound images that can be performed either by an assistant using a laparoscopic ultrasound or with a robotic-compatible drop-in ultrasound probes that are now available from several manufacturers. The Xi da Vinci platform system has a new and unique patient side cart that allows for additional freedom in positioning the robotic arms stand and provides improved ease of docking for the OR staff.

Design of the da Vinci places the surgeon's visual and hand control interface in a similar triangular approximation of both open and laparoscopic surgery. The hand/machine interface controls are extremely intuitive to use and allow even novices to quickly master complex manipulation such as knot tying. However, it must be remembered that although complex tasks such as suturing are eased by the design, the knowledge of how to approach the surgical field, provide appropriate retraction, and avoid complications and injury lies with the surgeon and is not part of a telepresence manipulator such as the current da Vinci robotic platform.

Future: Other Potential Manufacturers/Platforms

Note: The following is not an exhaustive list of the current manufacturer landscape in surgical robotics but simply represents a listing of several of the current companies and groups with interesting robotic platforms that may have future impact on urology.

SOFAR: This Italian company SOFAR (Milan, Italy) has developed the TELELAP Alf-X system in collaboration with the European Commission's Joint Research Center of the Institute For the Protection and Safety of the Citizen [22]. This is a remote telepresence operated robotic system that utilizes a system of remote arms that are brought in from individual stands around the patient bed. The surgeon uses a remote teleoperation console similar to the da Vinci console. Early versions of the system reported to feature haptic feedback, an eye tracking system for endoscope positioning, and reusable endoscopic instruments. The eye tracking system is designed to control not only the position of the endoscope and surgical view but also allows instrument control using screen icon activation via eye tracking. The manufacturer notes that up to four different manipulators may be placed into the patient. The company has targeted surgical specialties including gynecology, urology, general surgery, and thoracic surgery. A three-dimensional screen display is present on the surgeon console and the use of eye tracking technology is purported to reduce the need for the surgeon to disengage from manual control of the instruments. Their corporate website stresses the potential of reusable instrumentation to reduce cost although acquisition and maintenance costs are not readily available. The system has been approved in Europe and has regulatory clearance in the European Union (Europe CE Mark 2012). A phase 2 study was recently reported in Surgical Endoscopy and involved over 140 human surgeries [23]. At the time of the creation of this chapter, the SOFAR Company and Alf-X platform were involved in a potential acquisition deal by the North Carolina based company TransEnterix (Research Triangle Park, North Carolina). The system is not available in the US at present.

TransEnterix: Is based in North Carolina and was founded in 2006. The company initially developed the non-robotic SPIDER surgical system, a single port manually controlled instrument platform, consisting of flexible instruments along with a linked endoscope to allow for improved triangulation in a reduced work volume for laparoscopic single-site surgery. The company calls this improvement "flexible laparoscopy". They received European CE Mark regulatory approval and a variety of procedures were performed in both the US in Europe by various surgical disciplines although the majority were focused at general surgical applications. In urology, Leveillee et al. have utilized the system for successful procedures [24]. Over the past several years the company moved toward "roboticizing" this platform and created a platform targeted at single-site surgery called the SurgiBot. According to website and marketing materials this platform is aimed at outpatient single-site surgery procedures such as cholecystectomy. In this system, the surgeon is sterilely scrubbed at the patient side and controlling the end-effector instrumentation of the suspended "robotic" system. The design allows for triangulation and a small work volume and the flexible robotic controlled instrumentation allows achieving end-effector angulation despite the lack of a distal true wrist configuration. The end-effectors are capable of multiple degrees of freedom and come in a variety of standard instrumentation designs. The company has submitted 510 (K) application to the FDA for the system. As noted above, the company raised additional capital and is acquiring the Alf-X (SOFAR) robotic platform, which may allow them to move rapidly to compete for standard laparoscopic and robotic multiport procedures.

Titan Medical: Titan Medical is based into Toronto, Ontario, Canada and is a publicly traded company that has been in process of entering the robotic surgical market for several years with a variety of early platform prototypes. One early prototype concept, Amadeus, looked very similar to the da Vinci multi-armed system with a surgeon console and patient side robotic manipulators. More recently, the company is targeting the single port procedural interventions and has created the SPORT (Single Port Orifice Robotic Technology) system. This consists of a 25 mm single access port robot system containing articulating instruments and a three-dimensional visualization endoscope and camera system. The company is targeting gynecology, urology, and gastrointestinal surgery as markets for this potential system. Titan is targeting approval and potential commercial availability for both the European and US markets hopefully in 2016–2017. The surgeon sits at a workstation with a 3-D endoscopic display while a patient side cart holds the suspended robotic system in position over the patient. Once the robotic cannula is inserted into the patient's body cavity, it can deploy into a working configuration involving three-dimensional visualization and multiple articulating snake-like instruments. Prototypes are in development and lab trials according to the company website.

Raven Project: The Raven platform was initially developed at the University of Washington. It has now gone through multiple generations of development. The project has sought to develop an open source platform for research on telerobotic surgery. The system software control uses an open operating system called Robot Operating System, allowing individual labs that acquired the system to access and alter the programming for development. The robotic system research collaboration by several universities using Raven is aimed at supporting open source materials development and advancing new and important robotics research by eliminating the proprietary nature of system control software. Some of projects involving the Raven platform are targeted at cardiovascular and otolaryngology sinus surgery research. The platform is available as a research tool but is not targeted for clinical care at this point in time.

Medrobotics: Medrobotics Corporation was formed in 2005 and is based on technology from researchers at Carnegie Mellon University. Their Flex Robotic System is a unique articulating multifaceted linked endoscope designed for robotic steering along nonlinear paths that are not currently possible with straight endoscopes. The scope is composed of flexible and maneuverable controlled segments that are advanced and manipulated with computer control. Once advanced to the interventional workspace, the flexible system can be locked into stability due to its multiple mechanical linkages. It forms a rigid platform carrying illumination and visualization. The surgeon then passes flexible 3 mm instruments along parallel access ports to the workspace. The system contains two working channels and accommodates proprietary instrumentation, which have a "wristed" design as well as potentially third-party instruments. Movement and rotation of these instruments is based on manual control of the surgeon. The system received European CE Mark approval in 2014 and FDA clearance in July 2015 for transoral procedures in the mouth and throat area [25, 26].

Hansen Medical: Hansen Medical (Mountain View, CA), founded by Dr. Moll, has developed a robotically controlled catheter system called Sensei™. The physician provides telepresence manipulation of the catheters from a control console. A computer-controlled patient-side module uses robotic control to steer specialized flexible wire-controlled catheters. The system is approved in the US and Europe for manipulation, catheter control, and use in electrophysiology cardiac procedures. While the current system is targeted at cardiac ablation procedures, an early prototype system was used for a small series of flexible endoscopic urologic interventions at the Cleveland clinic [27]. The overall goal of the company is to develop technology for the accurate, efficient, and improved control of flexible catheter movement during therapeutic procedures for a variety of specialties.

Future Robotic Platforms in Urologic Surgery: Research at Vanderbilt University

Emerging robotic platforms are being developed at many institutions to improve performance of a wider variety of surgical interventions. At Vanderbilt, using a trans-institutional collaboration between surgeons and engineers, we are developing approaches beyond the standard minimally invasive robotic urologic surgeries conducted presently with the da Vinci platform. These newer platforms and instruments are designed to incorporate significant potential advantages of CAS, robotics, and other technologies to improve the safety and outcomes of transurethral bladder cancer surgery and surveillance, improve transurethral prostate surgery, and allow for previously impossible needle access and ablation delivery. The design and kinematic engineering of the da Vinci incorporates a wire and pulley driven end-effector with computer-control. This type of underlying mechanical structure and materials limits the size of the instrument diameter to 5 mm or greater. As previously discussed the da Vinci tower is not modular and, while highly adaptable, is constrained by the motion of the patient side manipulators (PSMs) and collision avoidance, although this has been improved on the recent da Vinci Xi. The da Vinci is a marvel of design and adaptability and has allowed many innovative clinicians to use the platform for a wide variety of surgical approaches in urologic, abdominal, thoracic, oral, and cardiac surgery. The next step for robotic surgical intervention may utilize development of alternative platforms, which allow for even more affordable, adaptable, less invasive, and purpose-specific surgical robotics.

This section reviews several robotic interventional platforms under development by the author and colleagues in collaboration with the School of Engineering at Vanderbilt University. All are applicable to urologic surgery as well as a variety of other surgical and interventional specialties.

Transurethral Bladder Tumor (TURBT): Potential for Robotics

Transurethral resection of bladder tumor (TURBT) is a gold standard surgical intervention for initial pathological staging and treatment of non-muscle invasive bladder cancer (NMIBC). Initial TURBT has been shown in multiple clinical series to often be inadequate for clinical staging, result in incomplete tumor removal, and potentially have a role in recurrence [28–30]. TURBT presents a number of technical challenges, which may be addressed by creation, and incorporation of new tools and imaging modalities. Indeed, the recent interest in photodynamic diagnostic imaging and improved optical imaging has shown the potential to improve detection. The geometric anatomic constraints of access to some regions of the bladder make it difficult to bring the bladder wall into the reachable workspace of the rigid resectoscope without external manipulation. The wall thickness and distension properties of the bladder layer can contribute to bladder perforations and incomplete resections. Current TURBT is carried out piece-meal for all but <1 cm tumors, possibly contributing to seeding and recurrence [31]. En-bloc TURBT has been demonstrated clinically, but the approach remains difficult with the limitations of current endoscopic technology [32–34]. Instrumentation limitations include lack of intravesical tooltip dexterity, a limited instrumentation repertoire, and lack of in-vivo feedback and precise depth control. Robotics hold promise to improve surgical outcomes by enhancing safety, dexterity and accuracy of resection, offering complete and potentially augmented visualization coverage for bladder surveillance, and facilitating en-bloc TURBT. Improving the initial technique of TURBT could potentially reduce the rate of re-resection, patient morbidity and discomfort, treatment costs, and ultimately improve prognosis.

Key improvements: (1) Improve surveillance and detection, (2) Improve resection accuracy, dexterity, and instrument reach to allow better staging, (3) Provide means for delivering future in-vivo imaging modalities, (4) Provide a means for monitoring resection depth and enforcing methods to minimize perforation risks while optimizing obtaining definitive pathology and wall layers for staging.

The tremor dampening stability and micro-movement control of a robotic platform would seem ideal to improve TURBT and would support intravesical augmented visualization and in-vivo sensory tool deployment, such as photodynamic diagnosis, OCT (optical coherence tomography), and US. Control algorithms can be developed to provide confirmation for full surveillance coverage and support improved telemanipulation control modes to increase dexterity of tools. Improvement of the instrumentation for transurethral endoscopic urologic procedures has been an area of active interest in clinical and engineering research groups [35, 36].

Working collaboratively with the lab of renowned robotics researcher Nabil Simaan PhD, we have developed a prototype concept robot shown in Fig. 34.1 [37]. This robot fits through a standard endoscope sheath with an inner bore larger than 5 mm. The robot has eight actuators and a two-segment snake-like device that allows each segment to bend on two Degrees of Freedom (DOF). The snake robot has three working channels that allow the deployment of a standard biopsy tool, a fiberscope, and integrated light source, and a third working channel that is used for delivering a resection device. The robot is axially actuated along the resectoscope sheath axis until deployed in the bladder where dexterous telemanipulation can begin (Fig. 34.2).

We recently published on our initial ex-vivo experiments in the bovine bladder [38]. The dexterity of the robot allows for pivoting about the contact point and performing potential en-bloc resection. Augmentation of control mechanisms such as depth of resection setting and augmented visualization modalities are planned for subsequent prototype generations.

HOLEP FOR BPH: Potential for Robotics

There has been recent renewed interest in developing robotic technology to assist with transurethral surgery. Some of the earliest research on surgical robotics focused on TURP, with the goal to improve safety and accuracy of prostate resection [39]. HOLEP has recently emerged with excellent outcomes for even huge glands and has shown clinical advantage in a variety of RCTs [40–44]. HOLEP with its clinical advantages, limited dissemination, and steep learning curve might be an ideal procedure for improvements through computer-assisted surgery (CAS) (robotic) technology [45–49]. Thus, we sought to conceptualize, design, and develop a CAS

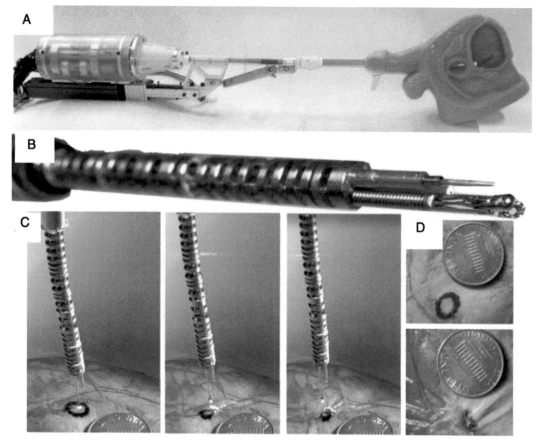

Fig. 34.1 (**a**) Prototype dexterous manipulator robot deployed through sheath into bladder model (**b**) dexterous segment and end-effectors including laser, grasper, and fiberscope camera deployed. (**c**) Laser ablation of target circle on tissue (**d**) before and after laser ablation of target

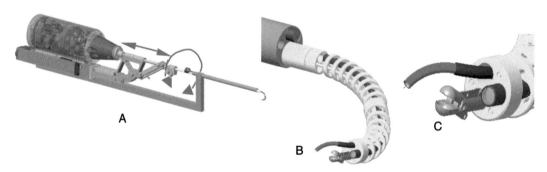

Fig. 34.2 Prototype. (**a**) Deployment through resectoscope type sheath (**b**) rigid scope (*green*) will carry rod lens for wide visual guidance with irrigation and outflow. (**c**) Dexterous snake robot (*yellow*) will carry additional optical fiberscope and end-effectors

system with the goal of increasing utilization of HOLEP [50].

The overall system design is based on the premise of concentric tubes, which utilize concentrically nested, precurved, elastic Nitinol tubes as the end-effectors. The basic robotic system consists of three main modules: the user interface, the transmission, and the endoscope

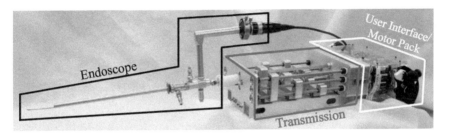

Fig. 34.3 The current configuration of the robotic platform consists of a user interface and transmission module which is passed through an offset rigid nephroscope

(Fig. 34.3). The user interface consists of two handles, each with an embedded joystick and trigger. The user interface controls motors responsible for driving the concentric manipulators. Maneuvering the trigger and joysticks produces corresponding fine motions of the concentric tube manipulators. Gross movement of the endoscope is accomplished by using coordinated motions of both hands to manually manipulate the entire unit keeping the surgeon at the field and in control of the system. The device is suspended on a counterbalanced arm to assist the surgeon in supporting the weight of the robot and allow for ease of scope motions while using end-effector controls.

The current endoscope utilized is a continuous flow rigid nephroscope (Storz, Inc.), which was chosen as the offset lens design allows passage of the cannula tools through the working channel. The endoscope contains integrated light sources and optics, a 5 mm working channel through which two concentric tube manipulators are introduced. We have shown that our novel concentric tube endoscopic system is capable of performing complex movements of the end-effectors within a small working space in both phantom and ex-vivo experiments (Mitchell et al. J Endourology, [51]). Our initial work has shown that this robot has the ability to effectively perform tasks that could potentially decrease the technical challenges encountered during laser enucleation of the prostate.

We believe that this type of technology will be valuable for performing and disseminating HOLEP and could have potential to create novel endoscopic instrumentation.

Concentric Tube Robots: Steerable Needles and Beyond

"Steerable" needles come in a variety of designs and configurations and have the potential to alter the "linear path only" approach of current needles [51]. Webster et al. have described a steerable needle configuration based on nested, precurved concentric Nitinol tubes (Fig. 34.4) [52, 53]. As the number of tubes and complexities of the curves and path route increases, the kinematics and control necessitate the use of motorized drive and computer-assisted control (robotics) [54]. Nitinol, the same material used in cardiac stents, provides memory, strength, and flexibility. The computer-controlled robotic system coordinates the linear and rotational motion of all of the tubes and is able to steer the curved needle along specified paths. These needles can be made in a large range of diameters and curvatures. Potential roles for steerable needles in Urologic Surgery include biopsy and ablation delivery to previously unreachable or inaccessible areas combined with precise control and nonlinear path control [55, 56]. The significant customizability of this device is one of its strengths. These robots can carry a wide variety of surgical instruments through their central working channel. Ablation technology or lasers can be delivered through them and forceps or other small tools can be mounted to their tips. Burgner et al. recently described the use of multiple of these concentric tubes as the arms of a miniature tentacle-like surgical robotic device [56].

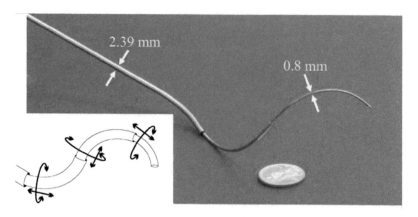

Fig. 34.4 Concentric tube steerable needle. Picture has three nested Nitinol precurved tubes. Diagram shows four nested segments [37] © Copyright 2016 IEEE

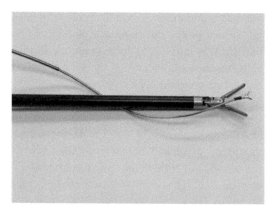

Fig. 34.5 Concentric tube robot with microlaparoscopic sized end-effector manipulator (grasper) compared to standard da Vinci instrument

In Urology and a variety of other surgical fields, these robots offer many potential advantages. Current da Vinci instruments are limited in their size by the underlying wire and pulley architecture (Fig. 34.5). Concentric tube robots have now reached an exciting stage and we are currently using them in laboratory studies in the contexts of biopsy, thermal ablation, as a micro-laparoscopic robotics platform, and to create new types of trans-endoscopic robotic instrumentation.

Conclusion

Robotic surgical platforms, as evidenced by the adoption of the da Vinci, have had a rapid and far-reaching impact on the performance of minimally invasive surgical procedures in urologic surgery as well as other disciplines. Further developments in robotics will continue and will likely impact many surgical fields. Additional new versions of da Vinci, new commercial manufacturers, and futuristic robotic platforms and tools will leverage the benefits of robotics in surgery in increasingly effective ways. Urologic surgery as a field has been an early adopter and research leader in robotic surgery developments and should be extremely proud of its role in innovation and adoption. Continued developments in the fields of robotics, computing, and imaging promise to continue this ongoing technologic revolution in the operating room.

References

1. Kwoh YS, Hou J, Jonckheere EA, Hayati S. A robot with improved absolute positioning accuracy for CT guided stereotactic brain surgery. IEEE Trans Biomed Eng. 1988;35(2):153–60.
2. Davies BL, Hibberd RD, Coptcoat MJ, Wickham JE. A surgeon robot prostatectomy—a laboratory evaluation. J Med Eng Technol. 1989;13(6):273–7.
3. Harris SJ, Arambula-Cosio F, Mei Q, Hibberd RD, Davies BL, Wickham JE, et al. The Probot—an active robot for prostate resection. Proc Inst Mech Eng H. 1997;211(4):317–25.
4. Russo S, Dario P, Menciassi A. A novel robotic platform for laser-assisted transurethral surgery of the prostate. IEEE Trans Biomed Eng. 2015;62(2):489–500.
5. Faber K, de Abreu ALC, Ramos P, Aljuri N, Mantri S, Gill I, et al. Image-guided robot-assisted prostate

ablation using water jet-hydrodissection: initial study of a novel technology for benign prostatic hyperplasia. J Endourol. 2015;29(1):63–9.

6. Taylor RH, Joskowicz L, Williamson B, Guéziec A, Kalvin A, Kazanzides P, et al. Computer-integrated revision total hip replacement surgery: concept and preliminary results. Med Image Anal. 1999;3(3):301–19.

7. Nishihara S, Sugano N, Nishii T, Miki H, Nakamura N, Yoshikawa H. Comparison between hand rasping and robotic milling for stem implantation in cementless total hip arthroplasty. J Arthroplasty. 2006;21(7):957–66.

8. Lang JE, Mannava S, Floyd AJ, Goddard MS, Smith BP, Mofidi A, et al. Robotic systems in orthopaedic surgery. J Bone Joint Surg Br. 2011;93(10):1296–9.

9. Cleary K, Melzer A, Watson V, Kronreif G, Stoianovici D. Interventional robotic systems: applications and technology state-of-the-art. Minim Invasive Ther Allied Technol. 2006;15(2):101–13.

10. Cleary K, Watson V, Lindisch D, Taylor RH, Fichtinger G, Xu S, et al. Precision placement of instruments for minimally invasive procedures using a "needle driver" robot. Int J Med Robot. 2005;1(2):40–7.

11. Allaf M, Patriciu A, Mazilu D, Kavoussi L, Stoianovici D. Overview and fundamentals of urologic robot-integrated systems. Urol Clin North Am. 2004;31(4):671–82. vii.

12. Cadière GB, Himpens J, Germay O, Izizaw R, Degueldre M, Vandromme J, et al. Feasibility of robotic laparoscopic surgery: 146 cases. World J Surg. 2001;25(11):1467–77.

13. Guillonneau B, Cathelineau X, Barret E, Rozet F, Vallancien G. Laparoscopic radical prostatectomy: technical and early oncological assessment of 40 operations. Eur Urol. 1999;36(1):14–20.

14. Binder J, Kramer W. Robotically-assisted laparoscopic radical prostatectomy. BJU Int. 2001;87(4):408–10.

15. Binder J, Jones J, Bentas W, Wolfram M, Bräutigam R, Probst M, et al. Robot-assisted laparoscopy in urology. Radical prostatectomy and reconstructive retroperitoneal interventions. Urologe A. 2002;41(2):144–9.

16. Abbou CC, Hoznek A, Salomon L, Lobontiu A, Saint F, Cicco A, et al. Remote laparoscopic radical prostatectomy carried out with a robot. Report of a case. Prog Urol. 2000;10(4):520–3.

17. Menon M, Tewari A, Baize B, Guillonneau B, Vallancien G. Prospective comparison of radical retropubic prostatectomy and robot-assisted anatomic prostatectomy: the Vattikuti Urology Institute experience. Urology. 2002;60(5):864–8.

18. Tewari A, Peabody J, Sarle R, Balakrishnan G, Hemal A, Shrivastava A, et al. Technique of da Vinci robot-assisted anatomic radical prostatectomy. Urology. 2002;60(4):569–72.

19. Smith AL, Scott EM, Krivak TC, Olawaiye AB, Chu T, Richard SD. Dual-console robotic surgery: a new teaching paradigm. J Robotic Surg. 2013;7(2):113–8.

20. Liu M, Curet M. A review of training research and virtual reality simulators for the da Vinci surgical system. Teach Learn Med. 2015;27(1):12–26.

21. Sethi AS, Peine WJ, Mohammadi Y, Sundaram CP. Validation of a novel virtual reality robotic simulator. J Endourol. 2009;23(3):503–8.

22. Gidaro S, Buscarini M, Ruiz E, Stark M, Labruzzo A. Telelap Alf-X: a novel telesurgical system for the 21st century. Surg Technol Int. 2012;22:20–5.

23. Fanfani F, Monterossi G, Fagotti A, Rossitto C, Alletti SG, Costantini B, et al. The new robotic TELELAP ALF-X in gynecological surgery: single-center experience. Surg Endosc. 2015;4.

24. Leveillee RJ, Castle SM, Gorin MA, Salas N, Gorbatiy V. Initial experience with laparoendoscopic single-site simple nephrectomy using the TransEnterix SPIDER surgical system: assessing feasibility and safety. J Endourol. 2011;25(6):923–5.

25. Johnson PJ, Rivera Serrano CM, Castro M, Kuenzler R, Choset H, Tully S, et al. Demonstration of transoral surgery in cadaveric specimens with the medrobotics flex system. Laryngoscope. 2013;123(5):1168–72.

26. Remacle M, Prasad VMN, Lawson G, Plisson L, Bachy V, Van der Vorst S. Transoral robotic surgery (TORS) with the Medrobotics Flex™ System: first surgical application on humans. Eur Arch Otorhinolaryngol. 2015;272(6):1451–5.

27. Desai MM, Grover R, Aron M, Ganpule A, Joshi SS, Desai MR, et al. Robotic flexible ureteroscopy for renal calculi: initial clinical experience. J Urol. 2011;186(2):563–8.

28. Maruniak NA, Takezawa K, Murphy WM. Accurate pathological staging of urothelial neoplasms requires better cystoscopic sampling. J Urol. 2002;167(6):2404–7.

29. Brausi M, Collette L, Kurth K, van der Meijden AP, Oosterlinck W, Witjes JA, et al. Variability in the recurrence rate at first follow-up cystoscopy after TUR in stage Ta T1 transitional cell carcinoma of the bladder: a combined analysis of seven EORTC studies. Eur Urol. 2002;41(5):523–31.

30. Herr HW, Donat SM. Quality control in transurethral resection of bladder tumours. BJU Int. 2008;102(9 Pt B):1242–6.

31. Ray ER, O'Brien TS. Should urologists be spending more time on the golf course? BJU Int. 2007;100(4):728–9.

32. Ukai R, Kawashita E, Ikeda H. A new technique for transurethral resection of superficial bladder tumor in 1 piece. J Urol. 2000;163(3):878–9.

33. Ukai R, Hashimoto K, Iwasa T, Nakayama H. Transurethral resection in one piece (TURBO) is an accurate tool for pathological staging of bladder tumor. Int J Urol. 2010;17(8):708–14.

34. Lodde M, Lusuardi L, Palermo S, Signorello D, Maier K, Hohenfellner R, et al. En bloc transurethral resection of bladder tumors: use and limits. Urology. 2003;62(6):1089–91.

35. Sánchez de Badajoz E, Jiménez Garrido A, García Vacas F, Muñoz Martínez VF, Gómez de Gabriel J, Fernández Lozano J, et al. New master arm for

transurethral resection with a robot. Arch Esp Urol. 2002;55(10):1247–50.

36. de Badajoz ES, Jiménez Garrido A, Muñoz-Martinez VF, Gómez-Degabriel J, García-Cerezo A. Transurethral resection by remote control. Arch Esp Urol. 1998;51(5):445–9.

37. Goldman RE, Bajo A, MacLachlan LS, Pickens R, Herrell SD, Simaan N. Design and performance evaluation of a minimally invasive telerobotic platform for transurethral surveillance and intervention. Trans Biomed Eng. 2013;60(4):918–25.

38. Pickens RB, Bajo A, Simaan N, Herrell D. A Pilot ex vivo evaluation of a telerobotic system for transurethral intervention and surveillance. J Endourol. 2015;29(2):231–4.

39. Davies BL, Hibberd RD, Ng WS, Timoney AG, Wickham JE. The development of a surgeon robot for prostatectomies. Proc Inst Mech Eng H. 1991 ;205(1):35–8.

40. Cornu J-N, Ahyai S, Bachmann A, la Rosette de J, Gilling P, Gratzke C, et al. A systematic review and meta-analysis of functional outcomes and complications following transurethral procedures for lower urinary tract symptoms resulting from benign prostatic obstruction: an update. Eur Urol. 2015; 67(6):1066–96.

41. Chen Y-B, Chen Q, Wang Z, Peng Y-B, Ma L-M, Zheng D-C, et al. A prospective, randomized clinical trial comparing plasmakinetic resection of the prostate with holmium laser enucleation of the prostate based on a 2-year followup. J Urol. 2013; 189(1):217–22.

42. Elshal AM, Elkoushy MA, El-Nahas AR, Shoma AM, Nabeeh A, Carrier S, et al. GreenLight™ laser (XPS) photoselective vapo-enucleation versus holmium laser enucleation of the prostate for the treatment of symptomatic benign prostatic hyperplasia: a randomized controlled study. J Urol. 2015;193(3):927–34.

43. Kuntz RM, Lehrich K, Ahyai S. Transurethral holmium laser enucleation of the prostate compared with transvesical open prostatectomy: 18-month follow-up of a randomized trial. J Endourol. 2004;18(2):189–91.

44. Naspro R, Suardi N, Salonia A, Scattoni V, Guazzoni G, Colombo R, et al. Holmium laser enucleation of the prostate versus open prostatectomy for prostates >70 g: 24-month follow-up. Eur Urol. 2006;50(3):563–8.

45. Bhojani N, Gandaglia G, Sood A, Rai A, Pucheril D, Chang SL, et al. Morbidity and mortality after benign prostatic hyperplasia surgery: data from the American College of Surgeons national surgical quality improvement program. J Endourol. 2014;28(7): 831–40.

46. El-Hakim A, Elhilali MM. Holmium laser enucleation of the prostate can be taught: the first learning experience. BJU Int. 2002;90(9):863–9.

47. Seki N, Mochida O, Kinukawa N, Sagiyama K, Naito S. Holmium laser enucleation for prostatic adenoma: analysis of learning curve over the course of 70 consecutive cases. J Urol. 2003;170(5):1847–50.

48. Placer J, Gelabert-Mas A, Vallmanya F, Manresa JM, Menéndez V, Cortadellas R, et al. Holmium laser enucleation of prostate: outcome and complications of self-taught learning curve. Urology. 2009;73(5): 1042–8.

49. Shah HN, Mahajan AP, Sodha HS, Hegde S, Mohile PD, Bansal MB. Prospective evaluation of the learning curve for holmium laser enucleation of the prostate. J Urol. 2007;177(4):1468–74.

50. Hendrick RJ, Herrell SD, Webster RJ. A multi-arm hand-held robotic system for transurethral laser prostate surgery. In: IEEE International Conference on Robotics and Automation (ICRA), p. 2850–5; 2014.

51. Mitchell CR, Hendrick RJ, Webster RJ, Herrell SD1. J Endouro. Toward Improving Transurethral Prostate Surgery: Development and Initial Experiments with a Prototype Concentric Tube Robotic Platform. J Endourol. 2016 Jun;30(6):692–6. doi: 10.1089/ end.2016.0155. Epub 2016 May 20.

52. Webster RJI, Okamura AM, Cowan NJ. Toward active cannulas: miniature snake-like surgical robots. In: 2006 IEEE/RSJ International Conference on Intelligent Robots and Systems. IEEE; 2006. 7p.

53. Webster RJ III, Romano JM, Cowan NJ. Design and mechanics of active cannulas. In: IEEE Transactions on Robotics; 2008.

54. Rucker DC, Jones BA, Webster RJ. A geometrically exact model for externally loaded concentric-tube continuum robots. IEEE Trans Robot. 2010; 26(5):769–80.

55. Burgner J, Swaney PJ, Lathrop RA, Weaver KD, Webster RJ. Debulking from within: a robotic steerable cannula for intracerebral hemorrhage evacuation. IEEE Trans Biomed Eng. 2013;60(9):2567–75.

56. Burgner J, Rucker DC, Gilbert HB, Swaney PJ, Russell PT, Weaver KD, et al. A telerobotic system for transnasal surgery. IEEE ASME Trans Mechatron. 2014;19(3):996–1006.

Index

© Springer International Publishing Switzerland 2017
L.-M. Su (ed.), *Atlas of Robotic Urologic Surgery*, DOI 10.1007/978-3-319-45060-5